SURGICAL TREATMENT OF TRAUMA

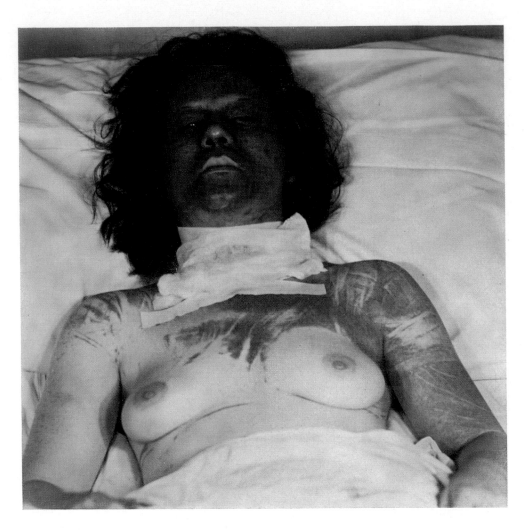

Traumatic Asphyxia

This characteristic discoloration results from sudden severe compression of the chest, and is due to multiple thromboses in the venules and capillaries. (*see* Chapter 27, p. 359).

Library of Congress Catalog Card No. 59-9126

Printed in Austria

SURGICAL TREATMENT
OF TRAUMA

Edited by

PRESTON A. WADE, M.D.

With 35 Contributors

GRUNE & STRATTON   New York and London 1960

CONTENTS

CONTRIBUTORS V
PREFACE XI
FOREWORD XII

I. TREATMENT – GENERAL PRINCIPLES

1. FUNDAMENTAL PRINCIPLES OF WOUND HEALING. *Frank Glenn* 3
2. BONE METABOLISM. *Melvin Horwith* 12
3. THE METABOLIC RESPONSE TO INJURY. *James A. Nicholas* 20
4. TRAUMATIC SHOCK. *John M. Beal* 26
5. THE PRINCIPLES OF FIRST AID TREATMENT. *Preston A. Wade* 31
6. ANESTHESIA FOR THE SURGERY OF TRAUMA. *Joseph F. Artusio, Jr.* 37
7. ANTIBIOTICS IN TRAUMA. *Peter Dineen* 42
8. THE CARE OF MULTIPLE INJURIES. *Preston A. Wade* 46
9. THE TREATMENT OF MASS CASUALTIES. *Paul W. Braunstein* 59
10. MANAGEMENT OF BURNS. *Herbert Conway* 67

II. FRACTURES – GENERAL CONSIDERATIONS

11. THE X-RAY IN FRACTURE TREATMENT. *Nathaniel Finby* 95
12. OPEN FRACTURES. *Robert Lee Patterson, Jr.* 109
13. OPERATIVE TREATMENT OF FRACTURES. *Preston A. Wade* 120
14. TREATMENT OF NONUNION. *Preston A. Wade* 158
15. EARLY MOBILIZATION OF JOINTS IN TREATMENT OF FRACTURES. *Preston A. Wade* 179
16. PATHOLOGIC FRACTURES. *Robert Lee Patterson, Jr., and Sidney N. Eichenholtz* .. 188
17. FRACTURES IN CHILDREN. *Preston A. Wade* 203

III. HEAD, NECK AND SPINE

18. MANAGEMENT OF HEAD INJURIES. *Bronson S. Ray* 235
19. EYE INJURIES. *John M. McLean* 245
20. FRACTURES OF THE MANDIBLE. *Stanley J. Behrman* 252
21. INJURIES OF SOFT TISSUES AND BONES OF THE FACE. *Herbert Conway* ... 278
22. TRACHEOTOMY. *James A. Moore* 301
23. FRACTURES AND DISLOCATIONS OF CERVICAL SPINE. *P. D. Wilson, Sr., and J. Paul Harvey, Jr.* 306
24. FRACTURES OF DORSAL AND LUMBAR SPINE. *H. Balensweig* 321
25. INJURIES TO THE SPINAL CORD. *Herbert Parsons* 333
26. ACUTE BACKACHE. *Peter-Cyrus Rizzo* 345

IV. CHEST AND ABDOMEN

27. INJURIES TO THE CHEST. *Cranston W. Holman* 353
28. INJURIES TO THE ABDOMEN. *S. W. Moore* 362
29. TRAUMA TO KIDNEY, URETERS AND BLADDER. *Victor F. Marshall* 372
30. INJURIES TO THE URETHRA AND GENITALIA. *John W. Draper* 382
31. FRACTURE OF THE PELVIS AND COMPLICATING INJURIES. *Paul W. Braunstein and John W. Draper* 388

V. THE EXTREMITIES

32. FRACTURE DISLOCATIONS OF THE SHOULDER GIRDLE. *Philip D. Wilson, Jr.* 405
33. FRACTURE OF THE HUMERUS. *William Cooper* 412

34. Injuries to the Elbow. *Preston A. Wade* 416
35. Fractures of the Forearm. *Paul W. Braunstein* 447
36. Colles' Fracture. *Rolla D. Campbell, Jr.* 460
37. Fractures and Dislocations of Carpal Bones. *Howard D. Balensweig and Irvin Balensweig* 495
38. Fractures in the Hand. *Lee Ramsay Straub* 506
39. Injuries to the Hand. *Lee Ramsay Straub* 521
40. Fractures of Acetabulum and Dislocation of Hip. *Preston A. Wade* 530
41. Intracapsular Fractures of Femoral Neck. *Preston A. Wade* 559
42. Intertrochanteric Fractures of the Femur. *Carleton M. Cornell and Rendel Levonian* 584
43. Fractures of the Femur. *Preston A. Wade* 596
44. Injuries to the Menisci and the Ligaments of the Knee Joint. *Frederick Lee Liebolt* 617
45. Fractures of the Knee. *Frederick Lee Liebolt* 626
46. Treatment of Tibial Shaft Fractures. *Rolla D. Campbell, Jr.* 635
47. Wounds of Extremities, Cross-leg Flaps and Other Reconstructive Procedures on the Soft Tissues. *Herbert Conway* 673
48. Injuries of the Ankle. *Robert L. Patterson, Jr. and Paul W. Braunstein* 701
49. Fractures and Dislocations of Foot and Tarsus. *Howard Balensweig* 722
50. Amputations. *T. Campbell Thompson* 734
51. Peripheral Nerve Injuries. *Howard S. Dunbar* 736
52. Acute Arterial Injuries. *Jere W. Lord, Jr.* 746
53. Ruptures of Tendons and Muscles. *J. Paul Harvey, Jr.* 752

Index 761

VI

THE AUTHORS

ARTUSIO, JOSEPH F., JR., B. S., M. D.
Professor of Anesthesiology in Surgery, Professor of Anesthesiology in Obstetrics and Gynecology, Cornell University Medical College; Anesthesiologist-in-Chief, New York Hospital, New York City.

BALENSWEIG, HOWARD, B. S., M. D., F. A. C. S. Instructor in Surgery, Cornell University Medical College; Assistant Attending Surgeon, New York Hospital, New York City.

BALENSWEIG, IRVIN, B. S., M. D., F. A. C. Assistent Professor of Clinical Surgery (Orthopedics), Cornell University Medical College; Attending Surgeon (Orthopedics), New York Hospital; Attending Orthopedic Surgeon, Hospital for Special Surgery, New York City.

BEAL, JOHN M., B. S., M. D.
Associate Professor of Clinical Surgery, Cornell University Medical College; Attending Surgeon, New York Hospital, New York City.

BEHRMAN, STANLEY J., B. S., D. D. S., F. A. C. D.
Assistant Professor of Clinical Surgery (Dental Surgery), Cornell University Medical College; Associate Attending Oral Surgeon, New York Hospital, New York City.

BRAUNSTEIN, PAUL W., B. S., M. D., F. A. C. S. Assistant Professor of Clinical Surgery, Cornell University Medical College; Assistant Attending Surgeon, New York Hospital, New York City.

CAMPBELL, ROLLA D., JR., A. B., M. D.
Assistant Professor of Clinical Surgery (Orthopedics), Cornell University Medical College; Assistant Attending Surgeon (Orthopedics), New York Hospital; Assistant Attending Orthopedic Surgeon, Hospital for Special Surgery; Assistant Attending in Surgery (Orthopedics) and Attending Orthopedic Surgeon to Out Patients, Roosevelt Hospital, New York City.

CONWAY, HERBERT, M. B., B. S., M. D., F. A. C. S., M. S.
Professor of Clinical Surgery (Plastic Surgery), Cornell University Medical College; Attending Surgeon-in-Charge of Plastic Surgery, New York Hospital; Consultant in Plastic Surgery, United States Veterans Hospital; Consultant in Plastic Surgery for Hospital for Special Surgery, New York City.

COOPER, WILLIAM, B. S., M. D., F. A. C. S.
Associate Professor of Clinical Surgery (Orthopedics), Cornell University Medical College; Associate Attending Surgeon (Orthopedics), New York Hospital; Attending Orthopedic Surgeon, Hospital for Special Surgery, New York City.

CORNELL, CARLETON M., M. D., F. A. C. S.
Instructor in Surgery, Cornell University Medical College; Assistant Attending Surgeon, Bellevue Hospital Second Surgical Division; Attending Surgeon, Manhattan Eye & Ear Hospital, New York City.

DINEEN, PETER, M. D.
Assistant Professor of Clinical Surgery, Cornell University Medical College; Assistant Attending Surgeon, New York Hospital, New York City.

DRAPER, JOHN W., A. B., M. D.
Associate Professor of Clinical Surgery (Urology), Cornell University Medical College; Associate Attending Surgeon (Urology), New York Hospital; Visiting Surgeon in Charge of Second Urological Service, Bellevue Hospital, New York City.

DUNBAR, HOWARD S., A. B., M. D.
Assistant Professor of Clinical Surgery (Neurosurgery), Cornell University Medical College; Assistant Attending Surgeon (Neurosurgery), New York Hospital; Associate Visiting Surgeon, Bellevue Hospital; Associate Attending Surgeon, Roosevelt Hospital, New York City.

EICHENHOLTZ, SIDNEY N., B. S., M. A., M. D., F. A. C. S.
Attending Orthopedic Surgeon, Yonkers General and St. Joseph's Hospital, Yonkers, N. Y.; Assistant Attending Orthopedic Surgeon, Hospital for Special Surgery; Instructor in Orthopedic Surgery, Cornell University Medical College, New York City.

FINBY, NATHANIEL, A. B., M. D.
Associate Professor of Radiology, Cornell University Medical College; Assistant

Attending Radiologist, New York Hospital, New York City.

GLENN, FRANK, M.D., F.A.C.S.
Lewis Atterbury Stimson Professor of Surgery, Cornell University Medical College; Surgeon-in-Chief, New York Hospital, New York City.

HARVEY, J. PAUL, JR., M.D.
Associate Attending Surgeon (Orthopedics), New York Hospital; Research Fellow, Hospital for Special Surgery; Instructor in Orthopedic Surgery, Cornell University Medical College, New York City.

HOLMAN, CRANSTON W., A.B., M.D., F.A.C.S.
Professor of Clinical Surgery, Cornell University Medical College; Attending Surgeon, New York Hospital; Director, Second Surgical Division, Bellevue Hospital, New York City.

HORWITH, MELVIN, B.S., M.D.
Assistant Professor of Medicine, Cornell University Medical College; Assistant Attending Physician, Acting Head, Division of Metabolism & Endocrinology, Department of Medicine, New York Hospital, New York City.

LEVONIAN, RENDEL, M.D.
Assistant Resident Second Surgical Cornell Division, Bellevue Hospital, New York City.

LIEBOLT, FREDERICK LEE, A.B., M.D., Sc.D., LL.D., F.A.C.S.
Associate Professor of Clinical Surgery (Orthopedics), Cornell University Medical College; Attending Surgeon (Orthopedics), New York Hospital; Attending Orthopedic Surgeon, Hospital for Special Surgery, New York City.

LORD, JERE W., JR., A.B., M.D., F.A.C.S.
Professor of Clinical Surgery, New York University Postgraduate Medical College; Visiting Surgeon, Fourth Division, Bellevue Hospital, New York City.

MARSHALL, VICTOR F., M.D., F.A.C.S.
Professor of Clinical Surgery (Urology), Cornell University Medical College; Attending Surgeon-in-Charge, Urology, James Buchanan Brady Foundation of the New York Hospital; Associate Attending Surgeon, Memorial Hospital, New York City.

McLEAN, JOHN M., M.D., M.E.
Professor of Clinical Surgery (Ophthalmology), Cornell University Medical College; Attending Surgeon-in-Charge of Ophthalmology, New York Hospital, New York City.

MOORE, JAMES A., B.S., M.D., F.A.C.S.
Associate Professor of Clinical Surgery (Otolaryngology), Cornell University Medical College; Attending Surgeon-in-Charge of Otolaryngology, New York Hospital, New York City.

MOORE, SAMUEL W., B.S., M.D., F.A.C.S.
Professor of Clinical Surgery, Cornell University Medical College; Attending Surgeon, New York Hospital; Consultant to Surgery Staff, Mount Vernon Hospital; Consultant to Surgery Staff, Hospital for Special Surgery, New York City.

NICHOLAS, JAMES A., A.B., M.D.
Assistant Professor of Clinical Surgery (Orthopedics), Cornell University Medical College; Assistant Attending Orthopedic Surgeon, Hospital for Special Surgery; Assistant Attending Surgeon (Orthopedics), New York Hospital; Adjunct Orthopedic Surgeon, Lenox Hill Hospital, New York City.

PARSONS, HERBERT, A.B., M.D.
Associate Professor of Clinical Surgery (Neurosurgery), Cornell University Medical College; Associate Attending Surgeon (Neurosurgery), New York Hospital; Associate Neurosurgeon, Memorial Hospital; Visiting Surgeon, Bellevue Hospital, New York City.

PATTERSON, ROBERT L., JR., A.B., M.D.
Associate Professor of Clinical Surgery (Orthopedics), Cornell University Medical College; Attending Surgeon (Orthopedics), New York Hospital; Attending Orthopedic Surgeon, Hospital for Special Surgery, New York City.

RAY, BRONSON S., B.S., M.D., F.A.C.S.
Professor of Clinical Surgery (Neurosurgery), Cornell University Medical College; Attending Surgeon-in-Charge of Neurosurgery, New York Hospital; Consulting Neurosurgeon, New York Hospital, Westchester Division; Neurosurgeon, Memorial Hospital; Visiting Surgeon-in-Charge of Neurosurgical Service, Bellevue Hospital, New York City.

RIZZO, PETER-CYRUS, M.D., F.A.C.S., D.O.S., A.A.O.S.
Assistant Professor of Clinical Surgery (Orthopedics), Cornell University Medical

College; Associate Attending Surgeon (Orthopedics), New York Hospital; Attending Orthopedic Surgeon, Hospital for Special Surgery, New York City; Consulant, New York Infirmary.

STRAUB, LEE RAMSAY, M. D., C. M.
Associate Professor of Clinical Surgery (Orthopedics), Cornell University Medical College; Attending Surgeon (Orthopedics), New York Hospital; Attending Orthopedic Surgeon, Hospital for Special Surgery, New York City.

THOMPSON, T. CAMPBELL, A. B., M. D., M. Sc. D., F. A. C. S.
Professor of Clinical Surgery (Orthopedics), Cornell University Medical College; Attending Surgeon-in-Charge (Orthopedics), New York Hospital; Surgeon-in-Chief (Orthopedics) and Director, Hospital for Special Surgery, New York City.

WADE, PRESTON A., A. B., M. D., F. A. C. S.
Professor of Clinical Surgery, Cornell University Medical College; Attending Surgeon, New York Hospital; Consulting Surgeon, Hospital for Special Surgery, New York City; Past-Chairman of Committee on Trauma, American College of Surgeons; Chief of Combined Fracture Service, New York Hospital-Hospital for Special Surgery.

WILSON, PHILIP D., B. A., M. D., F. A. C. S.
Professor of Clinical Surgery Emeritus (Orthopedics), Cornell University Medical College; Consultant in Orthopedics, New York Hospital; Surgeon-in-Chief Emeritus and Director of Research, Hospital for Special Surgery, New York City.

WILSON, PHILIP D., JR., M. D.
Assistant Professor of Clinical Surgery (Orthopedics), Cornell University Medical College; Associate Attending Surgeon (Orthopedics), New York Hospital; Associate Attending Orthopedic Surgeon, Hospital for Special Surgery, New York City.

PREFACE

In 1956 Cornell University Medical College presented the first of a series of annual postgraduate courses on "Fractures and Other Trauma." The full week's course was planned to cover the entire field of trauma, including the general principles of trauma and the injuries sustained in specific areas, involving many specialties. The organization of the course included fifty-five lecture periods from thirty minutes to one hour and a series of demonstrations of application of traction and plaster of Paris. Discussion periods followed each lecture. At the end of each day, a conference was held in which a varied group of cases were presented and discussed by the lecturers and the students. The lecturers were chosen from the faculty of Cornell University Medical College, all of whom are associated with The New York Hospital or its affiliated orthopedic hospital, The Hospital for Special Surgery.

The purpose of the course was to give to the practicing surgeon, general surgeon, orthopedic surgeon, general practitioner and resident, a very practical review of the current methods used in the treatment of each subject under consideration. No attempt was made to cover the history of the subject or to discuss old and obsolete methods except insofar as they applied to the present treatment. The course was planned to supply a need for practical instruction in the treatment of traumatic conditions which the practicing surgeon faces daily.

The courses have been enthusiastically received and well attended and are an established postgraduate effort of Cornell University Medical College. There have been many requests for a written review of the various lectures, and the preparation of this book is a response to these requests.

Since this book is a compilation of many lectures prepared by thirty-five different authors, no attempt has been made to standardize the form of presentation. Each lecturer has been asked to present the subject in the manner he considers most suitable to accomplish the major objective of good instruction. There is necessarily a repetition of discussion of several subjects, but since the material is presented by different authors, this is considered valuable in presenting various points of view in certain important areas. The student is reminded of the fact that there may be many equally proper methods of treatment for a single lesion, and each lecturer gives his point of view and advises what he considers to be the best form of treatment in his hands. This book, therefore, presents the combined experience of some thirty-five surgeons of the Cornell University — New York Hospital Medical Center actively engaged in the treatment of trauma.

In presenting this volume, Cornell University Medical College hopes to add to the knowledge and wisdom of the practicing surgeon and so improve the treatment given those individuals who are subject to the violence of modern living.

PRESTON A. WADE, M.D.

FOREWORD

The problems of the injured are as old as surgery itself. The control of hemorrhage, the fixing of fractured bones and the conservation of the soft tissues are part of the day's work of the surgeon, be it in the home, office or hospital. Many of the fundamental principles involved have had little added to them over the years. On the other hand, there have been advances superimposed on these principles which have made the correction and the treatment of such injuries much safer for the patient and have enabled them to be accomplished with less discomfort.

It is one of the avowed functions of a teaching medical center to be concerned with the problems of health in the present day environment. Each decade sees considerable change in the activities of the individuals of any community. Occupation, transportation and the mechanical accessories of a household are responsible for the type and extent of the wounds that are incurred. Therefore, it behooves the surgeon who is to care for these individuals not only to understand the hazards they are exposed to and which result in injuries, but also to be ever mindful of the demands that will be made on these individuals after they recover. Thus, it is important that treatment be directed not only at preservation of life and conservation of part but also at restoration of function compatible with what will be required of the individual to permit him to remain an independent person capable of caring for himself and earning a livelihood.

The matter of trauma as a medical problem has been given greater consideration in recent years in both graduate and undergraduate training programs. Great progress has been made in the handling of patients in the larger hospitals. It is hoped that the developments that accrue under the more favorable circumstances in the midst of adequate facilities and highly trained personnel will continue. Thus, such institutions should not only contribute to improvement in the care of the injured in our own community, but should make available to others their experience, including their mistakes, so that they may profit from them.

This book presents the clinical approaches with their underlying concepts of a group of surgeons at the New York Hospital-Cornell Medical Center. The successes as well as the failures are included in an effort to direct attention to the more common sequelae and complications that may occur when the injury is given more attention than the individual as a whole. Emphasis has been placed on the centering of the responsibility of the injured patient on one surgeon, leaving it to him to secure such assistance as he may deem necessary.

FRANK GLENN, M. D.

I. TREATMENT — GENERAL PRINCIPLES

FUNDAMENTAL PRINCIPLES OF WOUND HEALING

Frank Glenn, M.D.

This chapter on wound healing will be molded in the direction of clinical observations and the practice of surgery; nevertheless, it is based on well documented theoretic conceptions implemented by a consistent philosophy of approach. The dictionary defines surgery as follows: "Surgery is that branch of medical science, art and practice, which is concerned with the correction of deformities and defects, the repair of injuries, the diagnosis and care of diseases, the relief of suffering and the prolongation of life by manual and instrumental operation." Wound healing is common to all surgical problems. It is the fundamental process on which rests the many and diverse interests of the surgeon in attaining his objectives. All surgeons should possess the available knowledge concerning wound healing so that they may be able to facilitate the phenomenon when possible and so that they may avoid those actions and practices that may interfere with it.

Those wounds that the surgeon produces in the course of practicing the art and science of surgery can often be placed and fashioned so that there will be minimal interference with healing. In the course of an operation, actually the development of a wound, one should attempt to visualize the healing process that may be anticipated and seek to make every provision for this to take place as rapidly as possible with a minimal requirement of new tissue. The generalization that a long incision heals as quickly as a short one holds within reasonable bounds. Certainly the experienced surgeon assures himself of adequate exposure to facilitate his objective, but the trauma, the injury of tissues, should be minimal. The advantages of a sharp knife, a direct incision, and the preservation of an adequate circulation are well recognized. It is equally important that the incised tissues be further injured as little as possible by retraction, crushing and tearing by blunt dissection. Meticulous hemostases, the individual ligature of divided blood vessels rather than massive occlusion of adjacent tissues, will do much to allow the wound to begin the repair process without having first to remove the excess blood clot and/or necrotic tissue. [7] The wound that is carefully repaired by the meticulous reapproximation of divided or separated structures with suture material that evokes little foreign body reaction will more closely resemble the normal appearance of a part than that in which there has been inadequate hemostasis with excess clot formation within the wound, and which has been repaired with coarse and irritating suture material that approximates the opposing surfaces under tension. [2]

Careful surgeons pay great attention to the production and repair of their wounds. Gentle handling of tissues and accurate anatomic reconstruction do more than satisfy the eye. They pave the way for early and efficient wound healing and impose minimal discomfort on the patient. Protection against infection by aseptic technic supported with chemotherapy when indicated provides additional insurance that the healing process may continue uninterrupted until the repair is complete.

Contaminated wounds and those associated with considerable tissue destruction such as are often seen among automobile accident victims, confront the surgeon with problems that are different from those he may produce on an elective basis, but can in just as great a degree be benefited by careful and meticulous management.

Classification of Wounds

Clean Incised Wounds Closed Primarily: A simple incision by a scalpel produces a minimum of trauma. If infection is prevented, healing may take place by first intention. As soon as the incision is made, blood from the capillaries pours into the wound. Quite quickly, perhaps within five minutes, this blood clots. On the surface, a crust of clotted plasma fills the incision. This crust is rather impermeable and is distinctly bactericidal, protecting the depths of the wound. The fibrin forms a mesh in the plasma, fixing the blood cells. The circulation to the area increases, there is swelling grossly, and an exudate appears in the tissues adjacent to the wound. The exudate contains plasma, macrophages, polymorphonuclears, lymphocytes, endothelial cells and histiocytes.

A.   **B.**

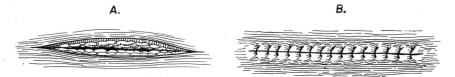

Fig. 1—Clean incised wound closed primarily.

The polymorphonuclears come from the blood stream, as do the macrophages and wandering cells. The endothelial cells arise from the cut ends of the capillaries, the histiocytes and fibroblasts from the tissue spaces. All of these cells are concerned with repair and with combating the invading organisms that are usually present in varying numbers. Clotting is the first phase of wound healing, and second is the removal of the debris, which is accomplished chiefly by the macrophages, reticuloendothelial cells and histiocytes. Third is the formation of capillary loops from the endothelial cells, and fourth is development of fibroblasts from fibrocytes and formation of collagen. Thus, as the break in the continuity of the tissue is bridged, fibroplasia takes place, with the cells increasing in size and adherence to give tensile strength to the wound. The process of wound healing begins as soon as the injury is incurred, and it progresses rapidly for almost fourteen days. Then it gradually terminates over the succeeding months until a thin scar remains as the only residue of repair.

These facts as stated are an oversimplification of what goes on in wound healing. Actually it is a very complex physiologic process. We can visualize new capillary formation into the clot, followed by phagocytosis and later fibroplastic proliferation and the appearance of intercellular material such as collagen and reticulum. Epithelization, of course, is readily observed. There is much that goes on in any healing wound that the eye cannot see. The complicated biochemical, physiochemical, and physiologic reactions are influenced by a myriad of factors. [1] Many of these we believe we recognize, and we attempt to control them in an effort to facilitate the healing process. We realize, of course, that there are others that we do not yet know about. Actually we seem to be more familiar with the factors that interfere with wound healing rather than those that accelerate it.

Contaminated Wounds Débrided and Closed Primarily: Many of the wounds in modern day life involve simple division of structures with minimal destruction of tissue. These are, of course, contaminated. The likelihood

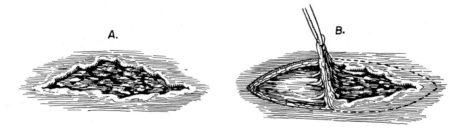

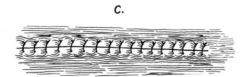

Fig. 2—Contaminated wound débrided and closed primarily.

of infection [4] in these wounds to the extent that the process of healing will be impaired varies greatly. In the past, time has served as a criterion for determining whether or not a primary closure should be done. Prior to the advent of chemotherapeutic agents, much was written about the "golden first six hours." With systemic antibiotics this period has been extended up to 24 hours if there is not too much tissue damage. Carefully performed débridements followed by meticulous reapproximation further enable us to accomplish healing by primary intention more frequently than heretofore. However, what is actually done in any one of the three types of wounds is dependent on many factors, local and systemic, that have a bearing on healing.

Contaminated Wounds, Débrided and Secondarily Closed by (A) Secondary Closure and (B) Granulation or Secondary Intention: The distinction between

this category and that just discussed is admittedly one of degree. For the
most part the wounds are of greater extent, i. e., often they involve a greater
variety of structures and tissues and not infrequently these are contaminated
from sources outside the body or from within, as in wounds involving the
gastrointestinal tract. These are in general the larger wounds and are sometimes
multiple. In approaching them, three objectives are to be kept in mind in the

A.

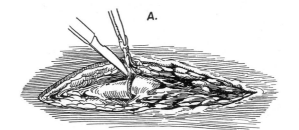

B.

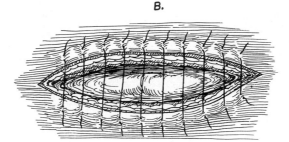

C.

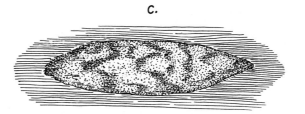

Fig. 3–Contaminated wound. (A) Débridement. (B) Closure by secondary suture.
(C) Closure by granulation.

following order: (1) saving life, (2) conservation of tissue and (3) restoration
of function. Systemic factors may dictate when and to what extent local
measures may be accomplished. Débridement, reduction of a fracture,
diversion of the fecal stream, for example, may better be delayed for hours

in a patient in shock. Extensive tissue injury or avulsion of a part may render wound closure untenable. In the past decade considerably more has been accomplished earlier because of improved methods for combating shock, covering exposed surfaces with skin grafts and providing greater protection against infection by chemotherapy.

Special Tissues

In the care and management of any of the three groups of wounds just described, consideration must include the nature of the tissues that are injured. Do they have the ability to regenerate? Are they repaired by inert scar tissue? Briefly we can list these tissues as follows:

Epithelium: One has the greatest opportunity to observe wound healing on the surfaces covered by skin or mucous membrane. It is a rapid process of regeneration that provides for the chief function of the skin as a protection but does not replace such functional tissues within the skin as sweat glands and hair follicles. On the other hand sensory nerves may grow into such skin and be of assistance in rendering it more nearly normal in over-all function.

Mesothelium: The serous membranes, such as the pleura and the peritoneum, are capable of early and rapid regeneration following injury. They have an additional characteristic. When surfaces of the peritoneum are brought together by suture, they readily adhere with a small amount of exudate that in time is replaced by a small amount of scar tissue which has considerable tensile strength. This is seen in the suturing of intestine to intestine by approximation of peritoneum to peritoneum. When the mucosal surfaces are approximated, they behave in a similar manner.

Bone: An injured or fractured bone heals by regeneration that appears to arise from the periosteum, the haversian canals, and the endosteum. Osteoblasts that extend into the granulation are the base for a strong callus that becomes firm with the deposition of calcium.

Tendons: Tendons may be said to make an attempt at regeneration. Tendons that are divided and approximated are held in continuity first by exudate and later by granulation tissue. Into the latter, cells from the tendon project for shorter distances as compared to the regenerated areas of the skin or peritoneum.

Cartilage: In articular cartilage there is no true regeneration, whereas injury to costal cartilage is seen to regenerate from intact perichondrium.

Muscle: Muscle lacks the ability to regenerate and heals by scar tissue laid down in the granulation.

Nerve Tissue: Nerve tissue may regenerate if the neurilemma sheath remains viable. If nerve cells are destroyed they do not regenerate. Thus, if a peripheral nerve is divided it may grow in the peripheral direction with restoration of function. Destroyed brain and spinal cord tissue heals by scar tissue, not by regeneration.

Local Factors in Wound Healing

The extent and site of a wound as well as the nature of the trauma may determine to some extent its healing course. Injuries from tearing, crushing, burning by friction and contusion are different in appearance from those resulting from a sharp knife. The zone of tissue injury is indistinct. Muscle, skin, bone and nerve tissue, for instance, vary in their local response to trauma. The relationship of the injured tissue to various regions of the anatomy also plays a role. Whether the wound is on the head, near a joint or within the abdomen may determine the anticipated course, which may vary greatly.

The blood supply to a wound may determine what may be anticipated in maintaining viability following repair. Certain areas, such as the face and head, have a luxuriant blood supply and an extensive collateral circulation, and necrosis from ischemia is rare. On the other hand, injuries to an extremity, such as a crushing injury with a fracture about the knee, may jeopardize the blood supply to the leg and foot. The occlusion of the venous blood return from an extremity, though less important than arterial occlusion because of the proportional collateral channels, may cause edema and impair the arterial circulation. Arterial ischemia, uncorrected, is incompatible with tissue survival. Necrotic tissue provides fertile soil for bacterial growth. If bone, tendon or any necrotic tissue is not removed by phagocytosis it may well become a nidus that requires surgical extirpation if infection is to be overcome. Site of injury, extent of vascular occlusion, position and systemic factors are some of the variables that determine the degree of impairment of the circulation in relation to a wound.

Radiation injuries, including burns from atomic explosions, are complicated by both local and systemic effects which may vary greatly. [6] The local effect may result in marked tissue injury with little systemic effect. On the other hand there may be little local trauma, but systemic damage that precludes healing of a part and may result in radiation sickness and death. Because the systemic reaction may not be predictable, patients with nuclear explosion injuries, no matter how apparently slight as evidenced by local reaction, should be most carefully observed. This is a new field and we should seek to keep informed on new advances in it.

Systemic Factors in Wound Healing

An immediate and profound disturbance of body metabolism follows trauma, [8] regardless of type, if it is of significant magnitude. The extent of the disturbance is influenced by age, health, and well-being of the individual. Likewise the duration, or the lag period before recovery begins and becomes established is dependent on the same factors. Specific observations support this. During the first few days following trauma, a negative nitrogen balance develops with a potassium loss and a retention and accumulation of sodium. These are well within tolerable ranges for the young and healthy, but in those without reserve, such as the elderly, those with systemic disease, and the malnourished, situations difficult to reverse may become established. Their correction requires precision management. For example, in the elderly anemic patient who becomes oliguric or anuric. haphazard administration of water and electrolytes, including chloride and potassium may be disastrous. When parenteral routes only are available for maintaining the patient, overloading of the circulation, as well as administration not only beyond metabolic requirements but in toxic amounts is not uncommon.

What goes on within the wound itself depends a good deal on the host as a whole. He must possess the materials needed to contribute to healing and must have an adequate circulatory system to deliver the materials to the wound as needed. The materials required include oxygen, water, electrolytes, protein, fat, carbohydrates, vitamins and hormones, to mention the obvious. The blood stream is affected by, and its elements vary with, the presence of many physiologic conditions, which may range from shock to occlusive arterial disease. If sufficient oxygen is not present, the vital metabolic processes are curtailed. The basic food materials of protein, fat and carbohydrates have long been recognized as necessary to healing, and this need is fairly well understood. Closely associated with the normal food requirements are the essential vitamins A, B and C and, to a lesser degree, D, K and T, which we do not understand nearly so well. Vitamin A deficiency, for example, delays the entire process of wound healing. A lack of vitamin B blocks certain metabolic processes. When vitamin C is absent, the collagen laid down is devoid of holding power. This intracellular cement is of great importance to the tensile strength of healing wounds. [3]

It is generally agreed that protein is of the greatest importance in wound healing. Actually, the materials that compose any new tissue are mostly protein. An excess of protein does not accelerate wound healing or result in greater tensile strength. A lack of proteins, a hypoproteinemia, on the other hand, does inhibit wound healing. There are many facets to the relation of protein to wound healing. It is essential to a normal colloid osmotic pressure of plasma and to cellular membrane function. In its absence or dearth, balance of water and electrolytes is impaired, and if these tend to accumulate outside blood vessels, edema results. Thus, usual orderly processes in wound healing may be slowed to a complete standstill where proteins are not available or are grossly inadequate. The same degree of impairment does not result from lack of any one of the other important materials needed for the healing process, including fat, carbohydrate, vitamins, etc.

In recent years, the relation of hormones to wound healing has been the subject of much study. Dr. Cannon long ago pointed out the role of epinephrine in initiating adrenocortical activity in response to trauma. In one of his observations, the protecting hemostasis that results during emergency is described. Closer study demonstrated that the water-retaining and sodium-retaining effects of adrenocortical discharge during the mobilization of cell water and protein combine effectively after injury to bolster extracellular water and plasma volume. The relations among sodium, potassium, and water and their associated interaction with nitrogen metabolism, need much more study. Good progress has been made, but we hope that these relations will be better understood in the future. Recent voluminous reports have given ACTH the spotlight at the present time. In my opinion, ACTH is only one of the substances produced by the neuroendocrine [5] axis that may be isolated. Its use, however, may serve as a model for future studies. We know that the endocrine response to injury, insofar as the adrenocortical hormone is concerned, is one that will influence the healing process. The logical step following isolation of a growth-stimulating hormone would be to increase its concentration in the postoperative patient in order to stimulate the wound healing process.

The effects of ACTH as thus far reported are not completely understood. The substance does seem to produce some alteration in the mesenchymal structures of the body. There is retarding of fibrous tissue growth and an apparent stimulating effect on epithelialization. There also appears to be a blunting of the hypersensitive responses in the chemical reactions associated with trauma, such as loss of potassium and retention of sodium. Howe makes the observation that "a hormone-like substance which can stop such defense mechanisms as the sprouting of new blood vessels and fibroplasia is not only significant in itself, but conversely the finding suggests that an offsetting mechanism must likewise exist whenever a wound heals." We could therefore concern ourselves with whether a number of clinical postoperative problems may not have their solution in what we may term a "hyponormal" hormone production response. Specifically, I refer to liver shutdown, kidney failure, thromboembolism, wound dehiscence and that salvage heap of "death postoperatively, cause undetermined."

Summary

Many factors, both local and systemic, are involved in the process of healing in even the most simple wound. As has been emphasized, there are additional factors in the more complex wounds. Taken together, these provide certain basic rules that should enable us to facilitate this important reparative process. Strict attention to these is essential if the optimum conditions for healing are to be established and maintained in the surgical management of any wound, whether it be elective or otherwise.

Preservation of life, conservation of the part, and restoration of function are the objectives in the surgery of wounds. They are always but a part of the patient and in a sense respond as an individual responds. Above all, wounds are not solely mechanical distortions of normal anatomic relationships to be corrected by machine controlled realignment. Rather, they require an approach that recognizes the myriad of cells with their variations that make up the part or region. Complex repair with minimal scarring is indicative of efficiency in wound healing.

References

[1] ALTEMEIER, W. A. and STEVENSON, JEAN M.: Physiology of wound healing. Christopher's Textbook of Surgery, ed. 6. Philadelphia, W. B. Saunders Co., 1956, chap. 2, p. 23.

[2] HALSTED, W. S.: Ligature and suture material: The employment of fine silk in preference to catgut and the advantages of transfixion of tissues and vessels in control of hemorrhage. J. A. M. A. *60:* 1119, 1913.

[3] LANMAN, T. H., and INGALLS, T. H.: Vitamin C deficiency and wound healing. Ann. Surg. *105*, 616, 1937.

[4] MELENEY, F. L.: Clinical Aspects and Treatment of Surgical Infections. Philadelphia, W. B. Saunders Co., 1949.

[5] MOORE, F. D., and BALL, M. R.: Metabolic Response to Surgery. Springfield, Ill. Charles C Thomas, 1952.

[6] MORTON, J. J., Jr.: Radiation burns due to atomic explosions. Ann. Surg. (in press).

[7] REID, M. R.: Some considerations of the problems of wound healing. New England J. Med. *215*: 753, 1936.

[8] SANDBLOOM, P.: Effect of injury on wound healing. Ann. Surg. *129*: 305, 1949.

CHAPTER 2

BONE METABOLISM

MELVIN HORWITH, M.D.

There is little doubt that the orthopedist need not know the fine details of bone structure and bone metabolism in order to practice his specialty with full confidence. However, familiarity with the damaged tissue cannot but help give greater satisfaction to the astute surgeon. This material is also being presented to generate interest in bone research among those who may be prone to regard the skeleton simply as an inert supportive structure. Sufficient evidence exists to suggest that bone assists in homeostasis and is a reservoir for buffer substances which aid the body in maintaining electrolyte balance. There is dispute as to the specific or adventitious occurrence of some of these ions in bone. It should be pointed out that bone may also, because of its great surface area, take up a great volume of a given ion and hence cause electrolyte difficulty. It has been demonstrated by use of radio sodium that old bone is relatively inactive metabolically. The continuous remodelling of bone haversian systems provides the body with a constantly available active bone surface. It is not the intent in this chapter to present a consideration of the theories on bone mineralization, crystal growth, composition of ground substance, etc. We shall not attempt to discuss the various achondroplasias, osteogenesis imperfecta or renal tubular pathology, if only because of lack of significant achievement in these areas. Bone structure and metabolism have recently been extensively reviewed by McLean and Urist (1955), Neuman and Neuman (1956), and Bourne (1956). Recently acquired knowledge about bone physiology and metabolic bone diseases will receive the major attention. Because of space limitations we have taken the liberty of selecting the metabolic disturbances that deserve emphasis in a symposium of this sort.

Recent advances in technology have permitted considerable increase in our knowledge of bone structure and physiology; however, there still remain significant voids in our concepts of fundamental bone structure. It would be advantageous to list for our purposes the unequivocal facts as opposed to those concepts that still must be considered tenuous. This division is immediately precluded by the great uncertainty that exists throughout this field. This is especially true of the so-called "ground substance" — the connective tissue of bone. It is likely that many of the metabolic bone diseases will, when resolved, turn out to be pathology of the "ground substance." Unfortunately our present knowledge of the role of glucuronic acid, the hexosamines, etc., is inadequate. The very likely possibility that some of the hereditary diseases of bone will eventually prove to be biochemical abnormalities of enzyme systems has already been suggested by Dent (1957).

The availability of the bone-seeking radioisotopes has permitted investigations heretofore not possible. The radioisotopes of calcium and strontium have enabled localization of these cations in osteones, measurement of rates of uptake and turnover of the mineral phase, and significant understanding of the physiology of calcium absorption and utilization. The intriguing concepts of "accretion and resorption" of bone mineral as measured by Bauer, Carlson and Lindquist have been possible since the advent of these radioisotopes. It is of interest to us that evidence is accumulating to indicate that the protein portion of bone has relatively little turnover once laid down. This will be discussed again under osteoporosis. Of special interest to the orthopedist is the approach to bone physiology as a problem in mechanical engineering as reviewed by Bell in Bourne (1956). A recent review by Neuman and Neuman (1956) on chemistry and structure of bone provides the reader with an excellent discussion of current thinking regarding the mineralization process.

Various etiologies of osteoporosis have been offered; however, to date we do not know the reason for this bone atrophy. Recent studies of gastrointestinal absorption in patients of the older age group do not lend credence to the theory that osteoporosis is caused by inadequate absorption of proteins and minerals. Immobilization, although certainly able to complicate an already existing osteoporosis, is not the etiologic factor in the great majority of cases. The knowledge that the absence of sex hormones is an important factor stems from the osteoporosis that we know occurs subsequent to castration and also from the beneficial effects of substitution hormonal therapy in the treatment of this bone disease. Regarding the pathophysiology of osteoporosis, it has always seemed unfortunate that a definition of "protein disease rather than mineral deficiency" has been applied to this condition. The evidence does not support this clear-cut distinction. On the contrary, metabolic balance data from our laboratory clearly indicate that patients with osteoporosis receive very real benefits from treatment with nothing but increased calcium intake. This is important evidence suggesting that osteoporosis is not simply a disease of the protein matrix as claimed by some authors. On the other hand, it is questionable as to whether pure osteoporosis or osteomalacia can exist independently.

Although the great majority of patients with osteoporosis are postmenopausal women or aged men, we must also expect this condition in the young individual castrated at any age, in patients treated with the adrenal cortical steroids, and in patients of any age who are immobilized for a protracted period. Only recently we have seen a number of middle-aged individuals with so-called "idiopathic" osteoporosis. We have also recently studied a patient with severe osteoporosis coming on soon after the third pregnancy in a three-and-a-half-year period. One should also be aware that endocrine diseases such as hyperthyroidism, acromegaly and especially Cushing's syndrome may be accompanied by considerable osteoporosis. Some of the most severely demineralized skeletons we have seen at this institution have been associated with adrenal cortical hyperfunction.

Regarding the osteoporosis of the older age group, there are a number of points worthy of emphasis. We know that the frequency of occurrence is certainly not easily estimated because of the relatively asymptomatic nature of this condition. We are certainly aware of our relatively poor ability to diagnose this condition early. Since all blood and urine studies are invariably normal in this condition, it is only a combination of complaints plus a roentgenogram showing demineralization that enable us to make the diagnosis. When one attempts to assess changes in bone structure or mineralization, one is confronted with problems involving sensitivity of roentgen technique, ability to duplicate technic on repetitive exposures, and also a question of which bones are best to examine. Although the vertebral column is the most frequent site of complaint, evidence seems to indicate that the ends of long bones (such as the femur) change earlier. This is certainly true in osteoporosis associated with immobilization. Those who have attempted to evaluate bone remineralization with consecutive films are conversant with the inadequacy of this technic.

We have employed the calcium tolerance test during the last few years to help establish the diagnosis of osteoporosis. Briefly, this test measures the ability of the skeleton to hold on to a load of calcium ion (normal — greater than 60 per cent) presented intravenously by slow infusion. Our results confirm those of Laszlo et al, and in general this test has been of value. It should, however, be pointed out that the greatest value for this test appears to be in establishing the diagnosis of primary hyperparathyroidism, which will be discussed subsequently. The necessity for a controlled diet and quantitative urinary calcium determinations unfortunately precludes this test from being performed where these conditions cannot be met. Present studies suggest that within a short time we will be able to establish this diagnosis by tracer studies with a new short-lived radioisotope of calcium.

It cannot be overemphasized that the mere appearance of demineralized bones does not in itself mean osteoporosis. In our clinic we do not consider treating a patient for osteoporosis until malignancy and multiple myeloma have been ruled out as decisively as possible. The differential diagnosis may be extremely difficult and in some cases only time has provided the answer.

The treatment of osteoporosis will be considered at this time (Shorr, 1957). Two therapeutic agents, calcium and protein, have already been alluded to. Although NRC recommendations are for 800 mg. ca./day, we have found that patients with osteoporosis may not be in significant calcium balance until the calcium intake is raised to 1,500 to 2,000 mg./day. This may be accomplished by diet alone, or in older people where diet presents a problem, calcium lactate may be added in tablet form. Since calcium is only about 13 per cent of calcium lactate by weight, this calls for substantial dosage. It is only during prolonged immobilization that the high calcium intake is not recommended since urinary calcium may be increased and renal calculi induced.

The remarks questioning the primary importance of protein deficit in osteoporosis should not be interpreted as implying that adequate protein intake is of no importance in the treatment of the disease. It has been our experience that 70 to 85 Gm./day of protein are necessary for the adult patient. Upon careful questioning one quickly becomes aware that older folks do not really eat as well as they claim. The obvious economic factors plus a natural inclination to avoid protein foods in this older age group militate against adequate nitrogen intake. The physician's ingenuity is often taxed in attempting to induce these patients to eat properly.

The role of the sex steroids in the treatment of osteoporosis is well established. Metabolic balance studies from this institution and from other metabolic units attest to the marked increase in nitrogen, calcium, and phosphorus storage obtainable with the addition to the regimen of the sex steroids in therapeutic dosage. We treat our female osteoporotic patient with conjugated estrogens, usually in the form of Premarin (2.5 mg. = 1,600 R. U.); 5,000 to 10,000 R. U. per day are necessary for adequate metabolic effects. In women with intact uteri the physician should be aware, and so inform his patient, of the inevitable uterine bleeding with protracted estrogen treatment. It is recommended that these patients receive a progesterone substance orally for five days of every month along with the estrogen. We use the oral anhydrohydroxyprogesterone (ethisterone) 100 mg. each day for the last five days of the month. This permits adequate but moderate shedding of the endometrium in cyclical fashion. Another technic is to prescribe the estrogen for 21 days and to omit it for 10 days. Slight breast fullness may be disturbing to some patients on this regimen. Water retention is a rare complication but it may occur. These side effects are infrequent and when controlled with dosage adjustment are of little consequence, considering the benefit derived.

Male patients with osteoporosis are treated with adequate amounts of testosterone, either as long-acting injectable preparations or as orally active methyltestosterone. The recommended dose is the equivalent of 25 mg. of testosterone propionate intramuscularly per day or 100 mg. of methyltestosterone orally.

The use of androgens in the female and estrogens in the male is indicated when the physician deems the severity of the bone disease indicative of such treatment. The side effects, if one chooses to call them such, of opposite sex steroids in the human are sometimes of such significant psychologic import as to contraindicate their use. The physician must consider each situation individually with the knowledge that the use of combined androgens and estrogens may, but does not always lead to additive metabolic effects. However, there is not always cancellation of all of the biological effects of each sex steroid. A special word of caution is justified in relation to patients who are on protracted courses of adrenal cortical steroids. It is our opinion that this treatment is beneficial if it permits a previously immobilized patient to regain some normal motility. This activity will play a major role in strengthening the skeleton. In addition it is wise to supplement the adrenal steroid with the sex steroids in order to provide as much prophylaxis as possible against the known antianabolic action of the adrenal corticoids.

Along with an adequate calcium intake, we have also employed strontium as an adjuvant to calcium in the remineralization process. Strontium ion is extremely similar to calcium ion in physiologic processes. We know that strontium can substitute for calcium in bone remineralization as well as in a number of other biologic systems such as neuromuscular excitability and blood clotting. A dose of 6.4 Gm. of strontium lactate, equivalent to 1.75 Gm. of strontium, is administered orally in capsule form. This amount of strontium has been taken continuously by some patients for as long as nine years without evidence of toxicity as judged clinically and by laboratory study. Metabolic balance studies reveal a number of interesting facts that are as yet not clearly explained. For example, not only is strontium stored better than calcium in some individuals with depleted skeletons but strontium is also stored after a ceiling on calcium retention has been reached. This is not an invariable finding. However, in most cases there is substantial storage of strontium after calcium is no longer stored. The total cation stored is thus significantly greater than the retention of calcium no matter how high the calcium intake. Rarely a metabolic study has revealed very minimal reduction in calcium storage during strontium administration, but in no instance was there significant reduction of calcium storage while strontium was given. It was also learned that strontium storage is affected by vitamin D, estrogens, and androgens in the same manner that these substances affect calcium storage. It is thus possible in severe osteoporosis to combine these therapeutic agents with assurance that there is no incompatability. The manner in which strontium exerts its beneficial action is not known. Originally it was believed that strontium ion acted as an osteoblastic agent. This idea has never adequately been confirmed. It is now suggested that strontium ion may inhibit the resorption phase of bone remodelling. Studies are now under way in this laboratory employing strontium [85] to measure bone accretion and resorption.

The most frequent question asked by the physician faced with the problem of treating osteoporosis relates to the place of vitamin D in the therapeutic regimen. There are a number of statements in the literature implying, some rather forcibly, that vitamin D has no place in the treatment of osteoporosis. The two arguments used against vitamin D treatment are the normal concentration of calcium and phosphorus in the serum and the belief that osteoporosis is purely a disease of the protein matrix. To these arguments one might conceivably add the recently acquired evidence that vitamin D under some conditions actually accelerates bone resorption. These arguments notwithstanding, there is good evidence that in the human with a skeleton depleted of mineral, vitamin D in proper dosage may greatly augment calcium storage. It would be ideal if all patients to be treated with vitamin D could first be evaluated by balance study. This being impossible, we recommend no more than 50,000 units daily in patients who are severely demineralized and who do not respond to the usual therapy. Patients receiving vitamin D should have frequent serum calcium determinations and occasional quantitative urinary calcium determinations to be certain that hypercalcemia and hypercalcuria are not induced by the vitamin D. Qualitative urinary calcium determinations, such as the Sulkowitch test, are insufficient protection for patients receiving vitamin D over a protracted period.

The orthopedist's association with primary hyperparathyroidism is not now nearly as common as is the urologist's frequent encounter with this disease. The prophesy of Fuller Albright that primary hyperparathyroidism would in the future be manifested by renal involvement rather than skeletal involvement has, of course, come true. It has generally been accepted that the protection of the skeleton and the frequency of renal calculi. This does not the protection of the skeleton and he frequency of renal calculi. This does not mean that none of the current patients with parathyroid disease have skeletal demineralization. In all recently published series, including our own group, more patients present with renal calculi than with bone pain. After extensive roentgenographic examination of the entire skeleton, these patients are often found to have "some generalized demineralization" but none of the characteristic bone changes we previously saw with primary hyperparathyroidism. In our group of patients with primary hyperparathyroidism, 50 per cent had renal complications without bone disease while 19 per cent had skeletal involvement only.

Diagnostic criteria for primary hyperparathyroidism have been liberalized during the past few years. We no longer wait for the advanced case with classical hypercalcemia, hypophosphatemia, and elevation of the alkaline phosphatase. A good number of the cases seen today have borderline blood chemistries suggestive of hyperparathyroidism. These patients usually present with renal calculi and suggestive signs such as hypercalcuria and an occasional abnormal calcium or phosphate on frequent serum determinations. I would like to emphasize the need for multiple blood calcium and phosphate determinations since we know that this is not a static disease. Urinary calcium determinations on varying calcium intakes are of considerable help in establishing the diagnosis. A shift in calcium intake will not change the urinary calcium significantly in the normal individual. With an increase in calcium intake, patients with hyperparathyroidism will have a considerable increase in an already elevated urinary calcium excretion. There are three conditions that may present with hypercalcemia that must be differentiated from primary hyperparathyroidism. Metastatic bone disease may mimic primary hyperparathyroidism with a similar blood chemistry picture. The urine calcium excretion may or may not be elevated and may show the same degree of shift in calcium excretion with changes in calcium intake. Sarcoidosis is now commonly associated with hypercalcemia. A therapeutic trial with cortisone, in the range of 300 mg. daily for five days, should lead to a fall in the serum and urinary calcium in the presence of sarcoidosis. Generally in sarcoidosis and in metastatic bone disease the serum phosphate is not depressed; however, we know that this is not an absolute rule. Milk-alkali syndrome, which should also be considered in the differential diagnosis, is best diagnosed by taking a very thorough history. If this condition is suspected the patient should be placed on an extremely low or calcium-free diet. The serum calcium should fall within approximately one month after calcium restriction, but there are instances where it has taken longer. The milk-alkali syndrome may also be distinguished from primary hyperparathyroidism by the normal serum phosphate and usually normal urinary calcium. Other conditions leading to hypercalcemia are hypervitaminosis D, multiple myeloma, and also the collagen diseases. Here again, a thorough medical investigation should preclude an incorrect diagnosis. Not infrequently one is presented with the problem of differentiating between primary and secondary hyperparathyroidism. History is significant if one can document antecedent renal impairment. The presence of normal or elevated serum calcium in the presence of marked renal insufficiency militate against secondary hyperparathyroidism and suggests primary parathyroid disease. In a recent review in this laboratory we were able to show a linear relationship between the serum phosphate and blood urea nitrogen when the latter is above 30 mg. per cent. Before this point of renal impairment, one should not expect retention of phosphate. Although it is commonly held that one does not see bone cysts in secondary hyperparathyroidism, this is not always true. Bone cysts are more common in primary hyperparathyroidism where bone disease exists; however, cysts may occur in hyperparathyroidism secondary to renal disease. Soft tissue calcifications are more likely found in secondary hyperparathyroidism.

The response to a calcium load given intravenously has been of great help in diagnosing primary hyperparathyroidism. We have found that induced hypercalcemia leads to a more profound depression of the urinary phosphate in normal and osteoporotic patients than in patients with primary hyperparathyroidism. Patients with primary parathyroid hyperfunction do not appear to have suppression of the abnormal parathyroid tissue by the calcium infusion. A change of less than 20 per cent from average daily phosphate excretion on the day of the calcium infusion suggests primary hyperparathyroidism. It has also been observed that these abnormal patients will not have as great a rise in the serum phosphate at the end of the calcium infusion as occurs in the normal patient. The dietary preparation for this calcium load test is of great importance. The patient must be on a constant 150 mg. calcium and 600 mg. phosphate intake for at least five days prior to the infusion. This permits a true average urinary phosphate excretion value to be obtained. The calcium retention value for patients with primary hyperparathyroidism does not fall into any pattern. Following removal of the adenoma, there is increased retention of the infused calcium load as well as a very marked depression of urinary phosphate excretion.

Osteomalacia (or rickets) is now rare in this country. We do, however, see representative cases of osteomalacia among patients with the malabsorption syndrome due to gastrointestinal or pancreatic disease. Inherent lack of vitamin D or apparent resistance to vitamin D is not seen in the adult unless one considers very special circumstances. For example Milkman's syndrome, which is now accepted as a form of osteomalacia, requires large amounts of vitamin D for successful treatment. This diagnosis is suggested by the bilateral, symmetric zones of radiolucency within the bone. Some authors have explained these pseudofractures as sites at which muscles exert pull, and others offer the suggestion that these areas represent sites of blood vessel expansion against the bone. In all varieties of osteomalacia the chemical finding that is most helpful is the elevated alkaline phosphatase.

Vitamin D in doses of 50,000 to 100,000 units per day is necessary to cure most osteomalacias. This must, of course, be accompanied by adequate calcium intake. It is vital to remember that these patients may also develop vitamin D toxicity; therefore, frequent blood calcium determinations and checks of renal function are in order. One may get a pretty good idea of the efficiency of calcium absorption by quantitative studies of urinary calcium if balance studies are not available. A very low urinary calcium excretion would obviously rule out renal loss and also suggest poor intestinal absorption of calcium if calcium is being ingested in good quantities. Fat absorption studies or the vitamin A tolerance test also is of aid in determining whether or not vitamin D is absorbable. The phenomenally large doses of vitamin D (sometime more than a million units per day) necessary in so-called "renal rickets" lend support to those who believe that there is a biochemical aberration leading to D resistance or anti-D effect.

References

[1] ALBRIGHT, F., and REIFENSTLIN, E. C.: Parathyroid Glands and Metabolic Bone Disease. Baltimore, Williams and Wilkins Co, 1948.

[2] BAUER, G. C. H., CARLSSON, A., and LINDQUIST, B.: Evaluation of Accretion, Resorbtion, and Exchange Reactions in the Skeleton, Kungl. Fysiografiska Sällskapets Lund Förhandlingar, 25, 1—16, 1955.

[3] BOURNE, G. H., Ed.: The Biochemistry and Physiology of Bone. New York, Academic Press, Inc., 1956.

[4] DENT, C. E.: Symposium on Inborn Errors of Metabolism, Am. J. Med., 22, 671—675, 1957.

[5] McLEAN, F. C., AND URIST, M. R.: Bone: An Introduction to the Physiology of Skeletal Tissue. Chicago, University of Chicago Press, 1955.

[6] NEUMAN, W. F., and NEUMAN, M. W.: Emerging concepts of the structure and metabolic functions of bone. Am. J. Med. 22: 123—131, 1957.

[7] SHORR, E.: Panel discussion on osteoporosis. J. Am. Geriatrics Soc. 5: 4, 363—384, 1957.

CHAPTER 3

THE METABOLIC RESPONSE TO INJURY

JAMES A. NICHOLAS, M.D.

Introduction

It has been known for many years that shortly after the infliction of trauma, the body loses nitrogen, sulfur and phosphorus. These observations have been extended to include the relationship between water, electrolyte and caloric behavior and trauma.

Although the means by which these changes occur is not clearly understood, the pituitary-adrenocortical system plays an essential part. It has been repeatedly demonstrated that some of the characteristic changes which comprise the *metabolic response to trauma* may be reproduced by *sham operation* and the administration of ACTH. Nevertheless, since trauma to adrenalectomized animals and humans on a very low maintenance dose of corticosteroids may also produce these changes, it is felt that there are other equally important and less understood factors at work.

General Considerations

Following trauma, and conditioned to some extent by the previous health of the patient, events occur which can be classified into two main types, nonspecific and specific.

Specific effects are those which are produced by the trauma on the specific tissue, such as a fracture to the femoral neck.

Nonspecific Effects

Nonspecific effects are produced by the metabolic interrelations which exist between the patient and injury. The nonspecific effects produce changes through two channels, systemic participation and organ participation.

Systemic participation relates to the clinically evident effects of injury. It consists of the patient's pain, apprehension, loss of appetite and fluid intake, and the need for sedation and analgesics. Increasing temperature, respiration, and pulse, so commonly associated with injury, reflect in part the complicated biochemical responses evoked by trauma.

Organ participation: The response to trauma includes a hypothalamic central nervous system discharge, with pituitary ACTH and adrenocortical stimulation. In addition, there is increased activity of the posterior pituitary gland as well as the thyroid and reticulo-endothelial system. Undoubtedly, immunological factors, not understood at this time, are also involved.

Homeostatic mechanisms exist in all of these systems. Organs of especial importance are the brain, endocrines, cardiorespiratory system, liver, kidney, and gastrointestinal tract. Following trauma, the ability to maintain homeostasis is lost to a varying degree. Some organs, however, apparently have a profound ability to maintain homeostasis within very narrow limits. Such an example is the remarkably constant preservation of blood pH, controlled largely by the kidney and respiration.

Specific Effects

Although Selye carefully pointed out the nonspecific triad of gastro-intestinal ulcers, thymicolymphatic involution and adrenocortical enlargement in rats, regardless of the specific stress, less understood have been the changes occurring at the site of trauma.

There are several different areas of damage at the site of an injury. Thus, in the case of a wound, a central zone of cellular necrosis, a peripheral area of damaged cells which, though surviving, are altered in that they are not able to reconstitute themselves, and a zone of reconstituting cells may be noted. Extravasation of fluids, exudation and invasion of elements of the reticuloendothelial system may be seen. Of equal importance are histochemical changes in which evidence of increased oxidation and phosphorylation may be noted. Materials necessary for repair of the matrix and cellular regeneration are in the fluids bathing the damaged site, brought by blood from distant regions of the body. This whole complex gradually proceeds to maturity by means of repair if (1) homeostatic mechanisms have not been impaired and (2) if injury is not lethal.

Convalescence

Repair also occurs beginning with the injury. The specific and nonspecific effects intertwine to produce the convalescence which is dependent on many factors. Within a short time, particularly with early treatment, pain is quieted, fluid and caloric intake restored, and the profound stimulation to the participating organs is decreased.

There are various degrees of metabolic stimulation. In the case of some types of injury such as a sprain, the patient is able to continue his activities without being aware to a large extent of the fundamental disturbances which have been evoked by his trauma. In the case of a fracture, however, requiring definitive treatment such as operation, restoration of continuity of bone, internal fixation, plaster cast immobilization and long disuse, fundamental metabolic responses are prolonged. The patient is painfully aware of his injury and loss of well-being for some time. The response continues in gradually waning fashion so that within the first week the systemic component has subsided. The stimulus which at one time involved almost the entire body is now localized to the site of injury which, to a large extent, has become "autonomous."

However, the fate of repair is dependent on the absence of infection, the maintenance of nutrition and adequate blood supply to the injured region. Still other factors must be considered in the ultimate repair of the site of damage. The physiologic age of the patient and his previous health are important. A fractured hip in a young, vigorous athlete in a car accident is a problem totally different from the fractured hip in the patient who has carcinomatosis. The homeostatic mechanisms in the former case are sharply developed, sensitive and efficient. In the latter case, the same stimulus occurs, but depending on the reserve of the participating organs, failure may occur in any of the homeostatic mechanisms at any time. Thus, anoxia and hypoxia may ensue. Acidosis, electrolyte imbalance, dehydration and shock are then more likely to complicate the convalescence.

Relation of the Metabolic Response to Injury to the Clinical Management of the Patient

Any surgeon dealing with trauma has a number of factors to consider in selecting the appropriate treatment for the injured part. These include (1) locale of damage, (2) extent of damage, (3) type of damage and (4) health and age of the patient.

Although these general principles may seem self-evident, insofar as the treatment of a specifically injured area is concerned, the metabolic inter-relationship may be hidden from the surface. For example, reflex sympathetic dystrophy, painful and disabling for months, which has occurred as a result of a simple fracture of the fifth toe, has been observed to trigger a whole sequence of complications in a middle-aged person. Some injuries are potentially far more dangerous than others. All of us have worried about the crushing tissue injury, about burns, compound fractures and long-bone fractures. Definitive treatment is required early in these injuries as complications are more apt to ensue because of the increased stimulation of other areas in the metabolic response. Nevertheless, one must remember, simple injuries may also trigger a chain of events which leads to loss of homeostasis. Early operation usually will lessen the load on other systems and should thus be encouraged. Relief of pain, apprehension and edema will also cut down the load on the patient.

Complications

Many limiting mechanisms influence the treatment of any injury, depending on the particular patient. Additional loads on cardiac and renal function, for example, have produced death in instances where the injuries themselves were not particularly noxious. Aged people who have chest and spinal injuries, for example, are particularly vulnerable to pulmonary infection and ileus. Early attention by means of adequate airway and gastrointestinal lavage sometimes will effectively block other vicious metabolic effects triggered by such injuries. Kidney shutdown and malnutrition are other dangerous complications which are apt to ensue in the aged and will render an innocent injury particularly devastating. Concomitant liver disease or active gastrointestinal ulcers present in patients who undergo injuries, will produce complications with increased frequency, including bleeding, hepatic insufficiency and kidney shutdown. In addition, the electrolyte and feeding problems which exist in some of these people bear some degree of importance in the ultimate repair of tissue, as patients in marked negative nitrogen balance are apt to repair more slowly.

Relation of Trauma to Risk

The most important assessment of the effect of trauma on the individual first is whether there is an *adequate oxygen supply*. This includes adequate airways for respiratory exchange and relief of pain to permit rib cage expansion. Once this has been established, pain and shock must be combated. This done, the relationship of the injury and the appropriate treatment, and the metabolic interrelationships should be simultaneously assessed. The following factors are important and should be kept in mind:

1. Infants and the very aged may rapidly suffer complications in the participating organs so that within 24 hours after injury, the problem of treatment may shift from the injured area to other organs which have been taxed by the additional load. In the very young, the problem is usually one of acidosis or alkalosis, depending on whether there is vomiting and dehydration incidental to high fever. Infants are particularly susceptible to extrarenal losses, and their electrolyte imbalances may very rapidly become irreversible. In the very old, the problem is usually one of pulmonary edema and congestive heart failure with myocardial and cerebral hypoxia. Dehydration is usually not an early problem.

Therefore, injury to these two classes of patients demands early, vigilant, definitive treatment.

2. Other patients who have unrecognized cardiac and renal disease and who, at the time of injury, are reasonably well, may develop complications within a short time after injury. Therefore, early treatment should particularly be sought despite the fact that the patient may seemingly be in good condition.

3. Injury to the chronically ill patient is more likely to produce shock, infection and dehydration. In such cases, simultaneous replacement of the specific deficits, whether they be blood or electrolytes, should be urgently undertaken.

4. The extent and type of reparative surgery contemplated is important. Long anesthesia, prolonged exposure, wide dissection, hematoma, poor closure, concomitant infection and profound pain will so stress the metabolic responses that a chain of events may occur which invokes distant organ failure.

5. Concomitant and pre-existing medical therapy should be carefully evaluated. By the use of digitalis, oxygen and diuretics, patients may be rendered suitable for surgery at a much earlier time than if one waits. In such cases the loads are lessened rather than increased by early operation.

6. The psyche of the aged and chronically ill may require attention in long-term complications. The use of tonics such as wines, tranquilizers, and amphetamine compounds have helped ward off senile changes in the aged who are disinterested in their surroundings. This is of more importance than

one might suspect at first. The highly anabolic area of repair, autonomous though it may be to some extent, requires material for repair. The provisions for adequate diet, vitamins, rest, as well as the stimulus of physical and psychic activity is important.

Because of these factors, one should not delay necessary surgery, as long as there is reasonable certainty that there is no serious inadequacy of heart, lung, or kidney function. The aged should not be deprived of the opportunity to get well by an attitude of "poor risk." The optimistic approach is to try to do the best job one can do on that particular patient. One should not rush to surgery and do an incomplete operation or reduction or poor fixation of fracture simply to save 15 or 20 minutes of anesthesia. Aged people in the seventh and eighth decades may have a good expectancy despite their ages. It has been well established that these people will tolerate surgery, and mortality is very low in carefully prepared patients. Mortality rises only when the prolonged stressing metabolic effects of injury and surgery with their effects on the participating systems are ignored.

Surgeons and orthopedic surgeons interested in trauma should be able to use the laboratory aids with confidence in order to help them make decisions about when and how to treat the patient. All surgeons interested in the treatment of trauma should have some fingertip knowledge of the meaning of acidosis and alkalosis. The appropriate treatment for the common problems of dehydration, overhydration, salt retention, and extreme salt loss and potassium depletion should be at the surgeon's fingertips. The use of the hematocrit, total eosinophile and blood count should be intelligently assessed, and deficiency should not be permitted to exist. Nonprotein nitrogen and urea determinations are helpful in assessing renal function. While assessing the blood loss in these people, one should appreciate that in most cases where trauma is considerable, there is rather marked hemodilution in two to three days. The stethoscope is still the best instrument for the detection of poor respiratory function, and even where legs are injured, the chest should be carefully evaluated. The significance of depleted protein reservoirs should be realized and corrected. Early ambulation, the mobilization of areas not involved by injury, and early feeding of the patient should be emphasized. Careful evaluation of the wound from day to day, the amount of fluid in the tissues about the wound, the character of the urinary output and the fluid intake, should be automatically recorded in one's mind as he watches the postoperative patient. The surgeon should be aware of the significance of pretreatment with steroid or other hormones, the use of these hormones if indicated and their possible adverse effects. The prevention of shock, the significance of a rapid pulse in convalescence after the third day when not explained by cardiac disease, should be carefully investigated. The recognition of complications early in the first hours rather than the first few days and the institution of appropriate treatment will be very rewarding. The aim should be for as little blood loss as possible. The value of a tourniquet where it helps to attain this aim and to permit clean dissection should be recognized. When infection occurs aspiration should be intelligently used, bacterial cultures collected and sensitivity tests performed. The haphazard use of anti-biotics is condemned. All these points should be almost automatically assessed in the surgeon's mind as he manages the patient in convalescense.

These factors are important in reducing stress. A violation of the principle at any time may lead to consequences which are irreversible. In the ensuing chapters, you will read about trauma to the various systems. In these articles the fundamental over-all appreciation of the metabolic effects imposed by these injuries must be kept in mind. With this, mortality will decrease, morbidity will improve, more patients will be operated on earlier and more definitively, and the salvage rate will be higher.

CHAPTER 4

TRAUMATIC SHOCK

JOHN M. BEAL, M.D.

Shock which is associated with traumatic injury belongs in the category of hypovolemic shock. It is a condition that results from the loss of an effective circulating blood volume. Shock and hypotensive states may result from a wide variety of causes, discussion of which is beyond the scope of this chapter. It is thus necessary that the present observations be limited to consideration of the shock of blood volume deficiency.

Even by such restriction, it becomes apparent that several factors may play a role in the development of hypovolemic shock. A review of these factors is indicated because restoration of the patient to a normal, stable cardiovascular status depends on prompt replacement of the elements which have been lost and have thus led to a hypotensive state. These factors have been listed as general categories in table 1. A combination of these factors may occur in various types of injury, depending on the type of trauma, and internal losses as well as external losses may occur in the same patient. This is not infrequent in automobile injuries where lacerations with external bleeding are often associated with fractures, a source of internal bleeding. Detection of these combinations of factors and types of losses may lead to more effective replacement therapy.

TABLE 1.—*Factors in the Production of Hypovolemic Shock*

WHOLE BLOOD LOSS

    Internal Loss (fractures, rupture of spleen, etc.)
    External Loss (lacerations, etc.)

PLASMA LOSS

    Internal Loss (peritonitis)
    External Loss (burns)

WATER LOSS

    "Internal" Loss (water deprivation)
    External Loss (diarrhea, fistulae, etc.)

Great demands are often placed on the physician who must care for the patient who has suffered a major injury. The type of injury may be complex and injuries are often multiple. The problem of the management of shock in such patients, particularly victims of automobile accidents, may be complicated by the wide variation in ages of the patients and by the lack of information of the condition of the patient before injury.

It should be emphasized that shock is a clinical syndrome and that the diagnosis of shock rests on clinical grounds. The clinical findings in established shock are familiar to all. The diagnosis is apparent where there exist apathy, restlessness, cold and clammy skin, with low blood pressure and tachycardia. However, it is often forgotten that shock has its inception before hypotension develops and that hypotension is preceded by an increase in pulse rate. The loss of blood or plasma results in the immediate action of the compensatory mechanisms. The organism attempts to maintain a stable circulatory status by means of vasoconstriction and an increase in pulse rate as the blood volume decreases. Thus, when a fall in blood pressure occurs, an inability of these compensatory mechanisms to overcome the initial loss of circulating fluid has already occurred whether the loss has been blood, plasma or water.

TABLE 2.—*Dynamic Changes in Shock*

Decreased Circulating Blood Volume _ _ _ _ _ _ _ _ loss of } blood plasma water

↓

Decreased Venous Return
Tachycardia } Initial Phase

↓

Reduced Cardiac Output
Hypotension } Established Shock
Peripheral Vasoconstriction

↓

Hypoxia
Hypocapnia } Transitional Phase

↓

Parenchymal Damage } Decompensating Phase

A summary of the changes in the circulatory dynamics has been outlined in table 2. With the initial loss of circulating fluid, which is usually whole blood in traumatic injury, the venous return to the heart decreases. The heart rate is usually increased in an effort to maintain an effective cardiac output and is associated with peripheral vasoconstriction. If the loss of blood has not been great (less than 1 liter) and if the patient is recumbent, the pulse rate and blood pressure may remain normal. As the cardiac output decreases, the peripheral blood flow becomes decreased. The variability in the fall in blood pressure in the initial period of shock is due to interplay of the compensatory mechanisms. Contraction of the spleen contributes to the general circulation as well as do general peripheral vasoconstriction in the skin, musculature and splanchnic region. Anesthesia and position also influence blood pressure change.

If further losses occur and are not corrected, peripheral circulation decreases and anoxia ensues. The latter is accompanied by a rise in the blood lactate and blood pyruvate concentration. The blood pH tends to decrease. The hypocapnia is a result of decreased pulmonary ventilation.

If the anoxia is not corrected by transfusion therapy, increased capillary permeability occurs. The failure of the circulation in shock thus produces changes in individual organs, such as liver, heart, kidney and central nervous system. Since damage to the parenchymatous tissues results in irreversibility of the state of shock, appropriate therapy must be instituted before these changes occur.

Shock is a clinical syndrome, and therefore the guides to the degree of compensation as well as to treatment rest largely on clinical grounds, supplemented by a few basic laboratory determinations. Frank has stated, "The observations of the recent period have disclosed no new signs or symptoms but have affirmed the usefulness of the standard clinical data." He has also pointed out the usefulness of arterial pressure in assessing the severity of the blood volume deficiency. He stated that when the systolic pressure has dropped below 100 in a normotensive individual as the result of blood loss, that the blood volume has been reduced by about one-third. When the arterial pressure has fallen to less than 70, it has been found that the blood volume has been reduced by 35 to 40 per cent or about 2 liters.

The treatment of shock is based on the concept of restoration of a stable circulatory system as soon as possible after loss of blood or plasma has occurred. The time factor is well established. It can be demonstrated readily by bleeding an experimental animal to shock levels, 40 mm. Hg systolic pressure. If the volume of blood is restored promptly to the animal, recovery is prompt and complete. If a delay ensues after bleeding, recovery may be delayed or a larger volume than that withdrawn may be required to establish a stable circulatory system. If a longer delay occurs in replacement, the animal may succumb despite the return of the lost blood or of increased quantities.

The type of fluid lost should be the principal guide in replacement therapy If the injury has resulted in the loss of whole blood, as in lacerations, rupture of the spleen or fracture of a long bone, transfusion of whole blood is required. Burns and peritonitis require more plasma than blood.

Evaluation of the efficacy of replacement therapy rests on the careful observation of the patient. A drowsy, apathetic patient is suggestive of inadequate or inaccurate fluid replacement. While restoration of the blood pressure to normal levels is indicative of improvement, a continued tachycardia suggests that replacement has not been complete. The hematocrit level is helpful in the evaluation of the patient's course. Urine flow is also a simple and valuable determination. While hourly urinary output is usually followed carefully in the treatment of burned patients, it is often overlooked in the assessment of the patient who is suffering from hemorrhagic shock. Urine flow below 30 cc. per hour is usually indicative of inadequate fluid therapy.

The response to treatment depends in part on the degree of trauma, the adequacy of replacement and the time between injury and replacement. One salient point merits emphasis in this regard. After trauma, therapy may appear to have been adequate for the external losses that the patient has suffered and yet response to treatment has not been satisfactory. In such instances, internal injury must be suspected and exploratory laparotomy must be seriously considered.

In addition to fluid therapy, there are numbers of other measures of considerable importance. The application of splints and the cover of sucking wounds of the chest are examples of necessary supplementary measures in shock therapy.

The maintenance of a patent airway is equal in importance to hemostasis and fluid replacement. Albritten has stated, "The need for the preservation of respiratory function under the difficult circumstances usually encountered concomitant to trauma is equal to the need for control of hemorrhage." This is particularly urgent in those who have multiple injuries with associated trauma to the head and neck. A tracheostomy may be lifesaving in such patients, as well as in those who have a flail chest.

Maintenance of body heat is desirable. This can usually be achieved by adequately covering the patient. At the present time there is considerable controversy over the possible application of hypothermia to the treatment of shock. A number of interesting and provocative reports have appeared, but many of these are at variance. The experimental data often deal with animals in which hypothermia has been induced prior to injury, a situation that is not comparable to most injuries which are encountered in clinical experience. Recent data from Swan and his associates have indicated a deleterious effect of hypothermia in hemorrhagic shock.

There have been numerous attempts to find a drug that would have a specific action in shock; however, specific drug therapy has been disappointing. Adrenal hormone replacement seems to have little use in the treatment of traumatic shock unless one can demonstrate adrenal insufficiency. The circumstances that precipitate the state of shock are sufficient in the vast majority of instances to evoke the maximum adrenal response by the patient. There have been recent studies on the use of l-norepinephrine in shock therapy and, again, the application of this drug has not yielded convincing benefits in this problem. Experimentally, it does not appear to increase survival in animals in which hypotension has been produced by bleeding. Norepinephrine must be considered to be of symptomatic use but under certain circumstances may be beneficial clinically if used to maintain blood pressure while whole blood or other specific replacement therapy is made ready.

The role of infection in the production of irreversible shock has been emphasized by Fine. In those cases in which infection can prove to be a real hazard, broad spectrum antibiotics may be employed with benefit. This is particularly applicable to abdominal injuries and severe burns. When open wounds exist and the débridement of the wounds is carried out, with or without closure, it is advisable to obtain cultures of the wound so that specific antibiotic therapy may be initiated if infection becomes a problem later.

More recently the possibility of the application of chlorpromazine to the treatment of shock has been studied. In therapeutic dose range, this drug has an adrenolytic effect, and in experimental studies it has seemed to prolong survival when administration was initiated before injury. However, some patients respond in an unpredictable manner to trauma after chlorpromazine has been given. Further investigation is necessary before this type of drug can be recommended in conjunction with the treatment of shock.

The essential factor in the treatment of hemorrhagic or hypovolemic shock remains prompt restitution of the circulating blood volume to normal levels by the administration of the proper replacement therapy, be it whole blood, plasma or other fluid.

References

[1] ALBRITTEN, F. F., JR., and FREDERICKSON, E. L.: Maintenance of Respiratory Function Following Injury. Philadelphia, W. B. Saunders Co., (Oct. 1956), p. 1221.

[2] FINE, J.: Relation of bacteria to the failure of blood-volume therapy in traumatic shock. New England. J. Med. *250:* 889, 1954.

[3] FRANK, H. A.: Present day concepts of shock. New England. J. Med. *249:* 445, 1953.

[4] WILSON, J. N., MARSHALL, S. B., BERESFORD, V., MONTGOMERY, V., JENKINS, D., and SWAN, H.: Experimental hemorrhage: The deleterious effect of hypothermia on survival and a comparative evaluation of plasma volume changes. Ann. Surg. *144:* 696, 1956.

CHAPTER 5

THE PRINCIPLES OF FIRST AID TREATMENT

Preston A. Wade, M.D.

First aid is the care afforded an injured patient from the time he is first discovered at the site of the accident until he comes under the supervision of a physician for definitive treatment. In many instances, the eventual outcome of the case may depend entirely on what is done during this period, and a life or limb may be saved if the individuals responsible for first aid treatment have a knowledge of the general principles involved. In the great majority of cases the first aid is administered by a layman, and it is the duty of the medical profession to see that the principles of such treatment are made generally known, particularly in view of the possibility of large numbers of casualties which might result from atom bomb attacks, tornados, earthquakes, explosions and other major catastrophes. As a result of sporadic attempts to teach large numbers of laymen the principles of first aid, a great deal of misinformation has been repeatedly printed and passed on from one generation to the other. The most glaring examples of this misinformation have been the absurd "pressure-point" treatment for hemorrhage and the constant advice as to the application of a tight tourniquet. Many first aid manuals still advise that patients be given large amounts of warm water to drink and advocate the routine administration of morphine for shock.

There is very little that can be done for an injured person at the scene of the accident, but some things are exceedingly important and may save the patient's life or prevent a permanent disability. It is probably more important to know what should not be done, and it is just as important to teach these principles to a first aid group as to instruct them in positive steps to be taken.

There are certain important steps to be taken, and in order of their priority these are (1) maintenance of open airway, (2) control of hemorrhage, (3) prevention of shock, (4) splinting of fractures and (5) transportation.

Maintenance of Open Airway

This is the primary consideration in first aid treatment. Interference with normal respiration in the traumatized patient is usually the result of accumulated blood, mucus or vomitus in the mouth and pharynx, and these should be removed as soon as possible, and the patient turned on his side. Face injuries in which the jaws are broken often allow the tongue to fall back, blocking the pharynx. This can easily be corrected by pulling the tongue forward, a safety pin inserted through the tip of the tongue often helps in maintaining traction on it. The safety pin may be attached to the clothing while the patient is being transported, thus assuring a free airway.

31

Open wounds (sucking wounds) of the chest wall are usually quite apparent to the observer and can be temporarily treated by applying a compression dressing to the area. The larger the opening the more serious the difficulty, as the negative intrapleural pressure is replaced by atmospheric pressure. If it is possible to apply one, a vaseline gauze dressing to the wound is more apt to be air-tight.

Tension Pneumothorax. The respiratory difficulty as a result of tension pneumothorax cannot be treated by the usual layman attempting first aid, but if a physican is present the condition may be corrected by means of needle aspiration.

The Control of Hemorrhage

It has been traditional for years in first aid instruction to associate the tourniquet with hemorrhage, and any bleeding, however slight, was thought to require the application of a tourniquet. During World War II it became fashionable to teach first aid students the areas in which "pressure-points" could be expected to stop a severe hemorrhage. Any loss of blood, even in small amounts, seems critical to the patient and to the untrained observer, so one can never qualify instructions to use a tourniquet by a warning that it is necessary only in "severe hemorrhage." It has been said that a great deal more harm than good has been done by the application of tourniquets to injured people. It would seem that Sir Reginald Watson-Jones was wise in his admonition that no first aid kit should include a tourniquet so as not to tempt the first aider to apply it at the first sight of blood. The only disadvantage of this advice is that the first aider is so imbued with the value of the tourniquet that he is apt to apply a tight rope or wire in place of a rubber tourniquet if the latter is not available.

In our first aid courses we are teaching that a tourniquet is rarely necessary to stop hemorrhage. *Hemorrhage is best controlled by the application of a pressure dressing.* The dressing is placed directly over the bleeding area and firm but not tight compression is applied. Patients are often admitted to a hospital with a tourniquet in place applied so loosely that only the venous return is impeded, and removal of the tourniquet is all that is necessary to stop a hemorrhage. Even if the limb be completely severed, as by a propeller blade or a train wheel, the spasm of the divided vessel usually prevents fatal hemorrhage.

The Prevention of Shock

There is very little that the untrained person can do to treat shock at the scene of the accident, but if he handles the patient gently, splints his fracture and stops the hemorrhage by the application of a pressure dressing, the severity of the shock may be lessened.

There has been considerable discussion as to the advisability of using intravenous fluids in the field in the time of war and in mass casualties, but the experience of civilian disasters would indicate that this form of treatment should not be advised. In one tornado disaster it was found that efforts to administer intravenous fluid resulted only in a waste of valuable time. Most of the needles slipped out, the fluid infiltrated the tissues, and the patient derived no benefit from the treatment. Furthermore, there was considerable waste of effort on the part of the personnel and delay in the transportation of the patient.

Many textbooks still advocate that the patient in shock be wrapped in warm blankets and that heat be applied externally. The patient should be covered and protected from rain and excessive cold but no external heat should be applied. It is also unwise to give any fluids or stimulants of any kind by mouth to the injured patient. One standard textbook urges that the patient be given large amounts of warm water to prevent shock. It is obvious that if the patient's stomach is filled with fluid the administration of an anesthetic, if needed on arrival at the hospital, will be dangerous.

Morphine should not be given indiscriminately to the injured patient. Ordinarily the severely injured is not in pain, and the administration of morphine subcutaneously or intramuscularly may only be harmful, since the drug may not be absorbed while the patient is in shock. If he is then given another injection of morphine when he reaches the hospital, and perhaps a third preoperatively, he may then absorb the total dosage of the three injections at once. It is unwise to administer morphine except when the patient is in severe pain, and if he is in shock, the drug should be given intravenously. It is also essential that when the patient arrives at the hospital information about any drugs that have been given be made known immediately to the admitting officer.

Splinting of Fractures

One of the greatest contributions made by the Trauma Committee of the American College of Surgeons has been the teaching of transportation of the injured. The emphasis on the splinting of fractures at the site of the accident as indicated by the aphorism, "splint 'em where they lie," has done a great deal to teach the medical profession the necessity of the early splinting of fractures. Not only does the splinting protect the fractured bone fragments and adjacent soft parts from further injuries, but it is also helpful in preventing blood loss and in alleviating pain. Proper splinting of fractures is one of the most important steps in the prevention and treatment of shock, particularly at the scene of the accident.

Any limbs suspected of being fractured should be splinted before the patient is transported, and the simplest type of splinting is the best.

In the upper extremity, the humerus may be strapped to the body for support and bound by means of a Velpeau bandage or by means of a sling and swathe. It is not necessary to apply a board or splint to the arm. Many years ago it was advocated that a Murray-Jones traction splint be applied to fractured upper extremities, but this has since been discredited because of the danger to axillary structures and the resulting nerve and blood vessel injury.

The forearm may be splinted by means of a board, a magazine, or heavy cardboard. The arm should then be placed in a sling as the patient is being transported.

Injuries to the hip and thigh are best splinted by means of the Thomas splint with moderate traction (fig. 1). The splint is easily applied, but is not often at hand when the patient is first seen, and since we may expect large numbers of injuries in time of war or mass casualties, one must know the simpler means of splinting the lower extremity. A very simple method is to make use of a board about two feet longer than the affected limb. This is inserted into the folds of a perineal sling made of cloth or bandage (fig. 2). A cloth sling is then attached to the padded foot and tied over the end of the board. This cloth sling can then be tighthened by means of a Spanish

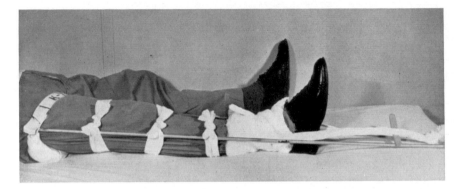

Fig. 1—Thomas splint for transportation of fractures of the femur. Note padding about ankle. Traction by means of Spanish windlass.

windlass maneuver with a stick, and traction applied to the limb. The limb is then bandaged firmly to the board as the patient is transported.

If no other means of splinting is available, the injured limb may be bandaged to its fellow.

The lower leg may be splinted by means of a so-called "board and pillow" splint, such as is illustrated in fig. 3. This is the simplest and most efficient type of splint for fractures of the leg and even those involving the knee. It is also the best means of splinting fractures of the ankle.

The application of traction to fractures of the leg and ankle may cause damage to circulation, and since it is usually unnecessary, its use is not recommended.

Fractures of the Spine: If a fracture of the cervical spine is suspected, the patient should be transported in the supine position with support to either side of the head. It is unwise to attempt traction because of the danger of injury to the cervical cord. If a simple cervical collar is available it makes an effective splint.

If the patient is suspected of having a fracture of the dorsal or lumbar spine, he is best transported in the supine position on a firm board or litter.

Formerly it was suggested that patients with injuries to the back be transported only by means of a blanket in the prone position, thus insuring hyper-extension of the spine. It has been found that this is not practical, and in fact it may be dangerous, as the patient has to be turned onto his abdomen.

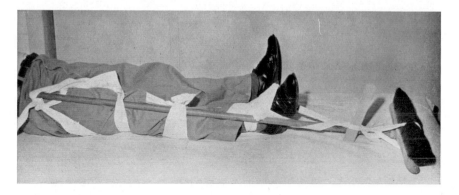

Fig. 2—Broomstick traction for fracture of femur. Broom handle inserted into fold of sling in groin. Traction by Spanish windlass over end of broom.

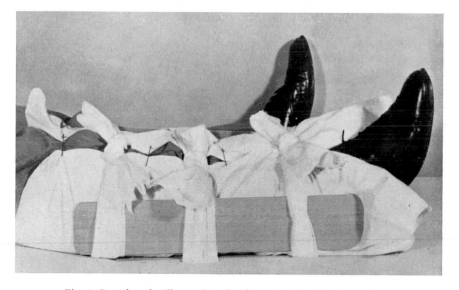

Fig. 3—Board and pillow splint for fracture of ankle, leg or knee.

Transportation of the Injured

In the panic and hysteria which may follow an accident, the injured patient is often rushed to a hospital without proper consideration as to the care of his injuries. It is most important that the measures just mentioned be carried out and that the patient be transported as gently and carefully as possible.

Extreme haste in transportation is rarely necessary to save a life and is seldom an aid in treatment. It is quite possible that speeding ambulances cost more lives and more injuries than they save. It is never necessary for an ambulance to exceed speed limits or to break traffic laws in order to transport a patient to a hospital, and there should be strict laws to make sure that drivers obey all traffic regulations.

References

1 BÖHLER, L.: Treatment of Fractures. New York, Grune & Stratton, 1956, vol. 1.

2 BOWERS, W. F., Col. M. C., U. S. A. F.: Surgery of Trauma. Philadelphia, J. B. Lippincott Co., 1953.

3 First Aid Textbook, American Red Cross. Philadelphia, Blakiston Co., 1945.

4 HAMPTON, O. P., JR.: Wounds of the Extremities in Military Surgery. St. Louis, C. V. Mosby Co., 1951.

5 WATSON-JONES, R.: Fractures and Joint Injuries. Edinburgh, E. & S. Livingstone, Ltd., 1955.

CHAPTER 6

ANESTHESIA FOR THE SURGERY OF TRAUMA

JOSEPH F. ARTUSIO, JR., M.D.

The patient who has suffered a major trauma must frequently be evaluated and operated on under emergency conditions. If the trauma occurs during wartime or during a civilian catastrophe, time is an important factor in the preparation of the patient. However, if the trauma occurs as a single incident following an accident, there is usually sufficient time to prepare the patient for surgery and anesthesia.

The history and physical examination must be as complete as possible. Our knowledge of pre-existing diseases of the patient may be limited, but one must strive for as much completeness in this respect as possible. Extensive laboratory examinations may not be possible, but at a minimum there should be a hemoglobin and a urine analysis before anesthesia or surgery.

There are many dangers in operating under emergency conditions, for we only have secondhand evidence as to how much blood has been lost at the time of trauma, how much food is in the stomach and how much narcotic has been administered in an attempt to alleviate pain.

The Use of Narcotics

It is quite interesting to observe a large number of patients who have suffered major trauma and to find that as a group they have less pain than one would expect. In spite of large wounds and multiple fractures, pain may be minimal. In an attempt to relieve suffering of the patient who has experienced trauma, morphine or other opiates are used liberally and at the slightest provocation. In evaluating the amount of pain, it is important to distinguish real pain from the restlessness, irritability and anxiety that come from cerebral hypoxia. Frequently, these patients have suffered traumatic as well as hypovolemic shock and have low blood pressures and rapid pulses. This state of inadequate circulation decreases cerebral blood flow, or if flow is sufficient, the blood has insufficient oxygen-carrying capacity owing to the anemia of acute blood loss. Therefore it is most important that one distinguish early between real pain and the restlessness and anxiety of hypoxia. If one mistakes the manifestations of hypoxia for pain and gives an opiate, the hypoxic state will be intensified because of the peripheral dilatation caused by the opiate. However, if one gives oxygen for the restlessness and anxiety of hypoxia, the patient becomes remarkably calm and easy to manage and a better evaluation of the amount of his pain can be made at that time. If opiates have to be given shortly following trauma, it is preferable to give them by the intravenous route in small doses (for example, 10 mg. of morphine sulphate diluted in 5 to 10 cc. of any physiologic solution) and slowly, with careful observation of respiration. This produces an immediate effect without the danger of a depot injection. During states of inadequate circulation, a subcutaneous injection will not release the opiate from the depot; however, when circulation has been restored, the opiate may flood the circulation and signs of opiate overdose may become apparent. If large doses of morphine have been given and the patient has become severely depressed, one can use the effective antagonist, Nalline (N-allylnormophine), which will effectively combat the respiratory depression of opiate overdosage. Nalline is used in 5 to 10 mg. doses and can be repeated in 5 minutes if the antagonism has not been adequate.

Premedication before anesthesia must be strictly individualized because there may be opiate action from preceding doses used for pain. If these patients need psychic sedation because of fear and anxiety of contemplated surgery, barbiturates are excellent drugs. Pentobarbital or amytal sodium in doses of 100 to 200 mg. can be given for psychic sedation without fear of respiratory or circulatory depression.

The Full Stomach

One never knows how much food or what type of food or liquid remains in the stomach of a traumatized patient. It is safer to consider that the stomach does contain food and treat the patient accordingly. When a major trauma is experienced, gastric motility stops almost at once, and thus food taken many hours before the injury may still be in the stomach. To be impressed with the importance of emptying the stomach, one has only to see a patient vomit or regurgitate large particles of food, aspirate them into his tracheobronchial tree, asphyxiate and die. When this happens, suction, bronchoscopy or any other maneuver is of little avail. Therefore, it is mandatory that before general anesthesia the patient's stomach be emptied. This may be an extremely difficult task, especially if he is unconscious. However, if the patient is able to co-operate, he must be encouraged to vomit either by placing a catheter against his posterior pharyngeal wall or by using a tongue blade to cause a retching response. There are no tubes available that will effectively empty the stomach of solid particles. They will remove the liquid contents but will soon become plugged with solid particles. It is therefore most important that careful preparation by the anesthesiologist be made before the beginning of anesthesia. He must have an adequate and well functioning suction apparatus nearby; oxygen and a means of artificial ventilation must be close at hand, and the patient should be anesthetized on a table that can be placed immediately in an extreme head-down position.

On the induction of anesthesia, as soon as consciousness is lost, the patient may vomit or regurgitate, and therefore one must protect the tracheobronchial tree from aspiration. This is done preferably before the anesthesia begins. Under any suitable topical anesthetic, an endotracheal tube with an inflatable cuff should be passed, and upon passage into the trachea the cuff inflated to seal off the tracheobronchial tree from gastric secretions. At the moment we are using a 2 per cent Xylocaine (Lidocaine) spray. The anesthesia can then be begun immediately without the dangers of aspiration.

The so-called crash induction of anesthesia with the use of a rapidly acting barbiturate and a muscle relaxant has been used in emergency situations. However, the technic is fraught with danger in that if there is difficulty during the rapid induction, regurgitated gastric contents may spill into the tracheobronchial tree during the flaccid apneic period.

Catastrophes from gastric aspiration usually occur during an extremely simple procedure in which one uses just a small amount of anesthetic for a very short duration and has not paid sufficient attention to the simple details of adequate preparation. The surgery to be accomplished may be minimal in nature, but anesthesia under any circumstances is indeed major.

Hypovolemic Shock in Anesthesia

Patients who have suffered major blood loss and thus have developed hypovolemia will use their compensating mechanisms to maintain an effective circulating blood volume. Before an anesthetic is given, it is wise to replace lost whole blood with whole blood if it is available. However, if whole blood is not immediately available, plasma expanders or plasma may be used in the interval. However, a blood pressure that is buoyed up by plasma expanders or by plasma will not survive the induction of anesthesia. For example, a patient may come to you with a blood pressure of 100/70 and a pulse rate of approximately 100, and upon the induction of anesthesia you may find that the pressure has fallen to 70/50 and the pulse rate has increased to 120 or 140. Thus the anesthetic agent or the anesthetic state itself has unmasked the state of incipient shock, acting much the same as the morphine for the treatment of wound pain under these circumstances. The anesthetic agents themselves tend to dilate the peripheral vascular bed that was just maintaining circulatory compensation.

If active bleeding is present, attempts to bring the blood pressure back to normotensive levels before anesthesia is begun are probably not wise. Under these circumstances blood should be given until it is quite evident that the blood pressure is rising and then the anesthesia should be begun. If one waits until the blood pressure has returned to normotensive levels, massive bleeding may recur and profound hypovolemic shock ensue.

Acidosis

If acidosis is present in the traumatized patient and immediate surgery is indicated, one need not wait until the acidosis is completely cleared. However, treatment for acidosis should be started before the anesthesia is begun. The anesthetic state and the anesthetic drugs themselves may produce a metabolic acidosis, depressed ventilation may produce respiratory acidosis, and both may aggravate the acidosis present before anesthesia. If treatment for acidosis has begun and careful attention has been paid to respiratory exchange, the surgery need not be delayed.

The Anesthesia

With the wide variety of anesthetic agents available today, any specific agent or technic recommended would not be suitable for a particular anesthesiologist in a particular institution. The most important aspect of anesthesia is the competence of the individual administering the anesthetic, and it is mandatory that he maintain the anesthetic state in the lightest degree possible compatible with the surgical procedure. As was pointed out before, these patients may be suffering from traumatic and hypovolemic shock which is aggravated with increasing depth of anesthesia. However, these patients usually withstand light levels of anesthesia well. The lighter the level of anesthesia, the more easily tolerated will be extreme positions on the operating table, change of position on the operating table and further blood loss during the surgical procedure.

Wherever it is possible, a regional form of anesthesia is to be preferred in this type of patient, whether it be local infiltration anesthesia or nerve block anesthesia. Injuries to the extremities can be handled ideally with regional procedures by means of brachial plexus blocks of the upper extremities and sciatic femoral blocks for the lower extremities.

Generally speaking, one can say that spinal anesthesia has little place in the traumatized patient. Because of the precarious circulatory status of these individuals, they do not tolerate well the sympathetic paralysis that accompanies spinal anesthesia. Although one can use appropriate vaso-constrictors in situations of hypotension due to spinal anesthesia, one may be constricting vascular beds simultaneously while attempting to retain circulatory adequacy by means of peripheral arteriolar constriction. Of all the general anesthetic agents, the intravenous barbiturates appear to be the least desirable in the traumatized patient, as they are severely depressant to circulations that are barely maintaining compensation.

Among the gaseous or volatile vapors, the choice is relatively unimportant as long as one maintains extremely light levels of anesthesia.

Anesthesia for Trauma

Head Trauma: In patients who have suffered major trauma to the head with loss of consciousness for a brief interval of time no doubt some brain trauma has occurred. It is my present feeling that these patients may die quite suddenly under general anesthesia for reasons still unknown. Therefore, wherever possible, anesthesia for such patients should be by local infiltration unless one is going to operate on the brain itself.

Trauma About the Face and Neck: Trauma in the area of the face and neck, with its associated bleeding and edema, frequently makes the establishment of an unobstructed airway extremely difficult. Endotracheal anesthesia produces operating conditions which provide the patient with good respiratory exchange during the surgery. However, with the removal of the endotracheal tube, asphyxia may ensue immediately or in the early postoperative period. Therefore, I would recommend without question the early performance of an elective tracheostomy before the endotracheal tube is removed. Despite the fact that this may be fraught with complications, it is still a safer procedure than a period of watchful waiting followed by emergency tracheostomy.

Trauma of the Thorax: Trauma of the thorax associated with fractured ribs and possible perforation of the lung itself presents many anesthetic problems. Multiple fractures of the chest wall may frequently produce a state in which there is inadequate ventilation which allows the accumulation of carbon dioxide and ensuing respiratory acidosis. These patients may be helped by simple inhalation of high concentrations of oxygen. However, assisted ventilation may be necessary to maintain an adequate tidal exchange. The inspiratory positive pressure breathing apparatus (I. P. P. B.) is of great value in this situation and the ventilation can be regulated so that there is not only oxygenation but adequate removal of carbon dioxide.

Trauma to the chest may result not only in fractures of the bony cave but also in lung rupture with the creation of a bronchopleural fistula and tension pneumothorax. The immediate problem is solved by removing the air from the chest, either intermittently or by low pressure suction. However, a closed bronchopleural fistula may be reopened during the induction of anesthesia and one must be prepared to place a needle in the chest to relieve the anesthetic agent or oxygen which is now under tension in the pleural space and which, if unheeded, may produce mediastinal shift and death during the induction of anesthesia.

In summary, it is important to be as thorough as possible in the time allowed in procuring an adequate history and physical examination and in performing minimal laboratory examinations. Second, evaluate the amount of pain the patient has. Do not overtreat him with opiate medication and be acutely aware of the difference between the restlessness of pain and the restlessness of hypoxia. Third, be ever aware of the full stomach and see to it that the tracheobronchial tree is protected from aspiration before the anesthesia is begun. Finally, remember that circulations supported by plasma or plasma expanders will not tolerate conventional levels of surgical anesthesia, and wherever possible whole blood loss should be replaced by whole blood before anesthesia is begun.

CHAPTER 7

ANTIBIOTICS IN TRAUMA

PETER DINEEN, M.D.

The number and diversity of chemotherapeutic agents is so great that it is extremely difficult to keep abreast of the latest developments and indications for usage in this field. Because of this fact it is more appropriate at first to discuss some of the basic principles involved. An understanding of these will allow the surgeon to make a more judicious selection of agents.

The purpose of the antimicrobial drugs is to combat infection. One of the most important factors in the problem of infection is *the nature of the parasite*. Pathogenic bacteria may be classified by their degree of invasiveness. This may be considered as a spectrum. At one end there is botulism, a disease caused purely by the toxin of the *Clostridia botulinus*, in which the parasite does not even enter the host. Next in line is *Clostridia tetani* which causes disease by a small nidus of infection in the host elaborating large quantities of toxin.

The enteric group of organisms are able to invade devitalized tissue, but usually are limited to that area by the host defenses. These gram negative organisms such as *Bacillus coli, Pseudomonas pyocyaneus, Proteus vulgaris, Aerobacter aerogenes*, etc., have no proteolytic enzymes of their own. Consequently, it is necessary for their survival in vivo to have a source of these enzymes. In necrotic tissue these are available from the autolysis of cells, particularly leukocytes. It is for this reason that infections caused by these organisms are seen in association with necrotic material. There is one other source from which these bacteria may gain the needed enzymes — namely, from bacteria that possess them as part of their biochemical makeup. Of these special bacteria, the two most important are the hemolytic *Staphylococcus aureus*, and the *beta hemolytic streptococcus*. These two organisms rank high on the spectrum of invasiveness, and in the wake of their infection the enteric organisms may come — almost like camp-followers.

The *Staphylococcus aureus* is capable of invading living tissue, of surviving in living tissue, and even destroying it. This, then, obviously is a much more formidable opponent than the enteric organism. The characteristic behavior of this organism is to bring about a local inflammatory response.

The *beta hemolytic Streptococcus* is probably one of the most virulent of all organisms. It can do everything that the *Staphylococcus* can and usually is very little hampered by the host's attempts to limit the area of infection. Within a few hours a few bacteria can cause an overwhelming infection.

Therefore, a knowledge of the various organism potentialities suggests which ones should be given first priority in treatment or prophylaxis.

Another important principle which should be considered is the response of the host to trauma and infection. When chemotherapy is started in the presence of an established infection, the drugs may be of little efficacy because they either cannot reach the organisms or because the organisms are able to elaborate protective enzymes. For example, in a subphrenic abscess the fibrin and organization of the walls often prevent the drugs from reaching the cavity in adequate titres. However, in the case of a sudden trauma where organisms have recently been inoculated, there is no barrier to the drugs. Therefore, while the bacteria are going through the lag phase in their growth curve (a matter of a few hours usually), adequate blood and tissue levels of chemotherapeutic agents can be obtained. It has been established experimentally and observed clinically that trauma (or stress) per se has a deleterious effect on the host's ability to combat infection. If, for example, a group of mice are challenged with a certain strain of *Klebsiella pneumoniae*, about half will die in seven days. If these animals are subjected to any stress before infection or at the time of infection, all animals will die within 24 hours. In uninfected mice, the stress used is not lethal. Usually a laparotomy is used as the standard trauma.

Thus, since it is known that trauma reduces the body's capacity to combat infection, and since the parasite initially is not protected from the blood-borne drugs, early chemoprophylaxis is definitely indicated.

The *phenomenon of persistence* should be mentioned. It has become increasingly clear to careful observers in the field of infectious diseases that organisms can remain dormant in the tissues for years without causing clinical disease. Experimentation in the laboratories of this Center has shown that certain stresses or certain bacterial products can cause an evocation of the dormant infection. This is true of the *Staphylococcus*. This type of situation is seen clinically on occasion when a patient with a history of osteomyelitis suddenly has an exacerbation following a remote trauma.

While there is a definite place for *drug sensitivity tests* their limitation should be constantly recalled. These tests are made on single organisms living in vitro. The environment is entirely artificial. The in vivo situation, in which several organisms are present simultaneously, is not reflected in the sensitivity tests. These procedures are of value in some staphylococcal infections. The trend is away from a slavish reliance on sensitivity studies. One is best guided by the clinical course of the patient and by a knowledge of the basic principles.

For all practical purposes it may be stated that the *beta hemolytic Streptococcus* is invariably highly sensitive to penicillin and, to a slightly lesser degree, to all the other drugs. The *Staphylococcus aureus* may be drug susceptible, or may be resistant. As a general rule penicillin and streptomycin act synergistically against most staphylococcal strains, even though in vitro tests may indicate that either drug alone may be ineffectual. The Gram-negative enteric organisms are usually quite susceptible to streptomycin or tetracycline. These organisms can grow out resistant variants but by the time they do, the body defenses are prepared. Occasional organisms may be present in a wound that are resistant to all agents known; for example, certain forms of *Proteus vulgaris* or *Pseudomonas pyocyaneus*. Although these organisms are low grade pathogens, they can cause serious difficulty. This is best prevented by removing all necrotic debris which these organisms need as pablum.

The clostridia require two things to cause either gas gangrene or tetanus. The first requirement is complete anaerobiasis, and the second is necrotic tissue. If these two factors are present, obviously no blood is being delivered to the part. Thus débridement, which removes necrotic material and unroofs anaerobic cavities, accomplishes more in clostridial infections than chemotherapeutic drugs. These bacteria are sensitive to penicillin in large doses.

In any trauma the organisms that have been inoculated remain unknown until the culture is reported. (Every wound and débridement should be cultured). Therefore, one must work on the assumption that any one or all of the types mentioned may be present.

The chemotherapeutic agents that are most commonly used are penicillin, streptomycin, tetracycline, erythromycin, chloramphenicol, neomycin and novobiocin. Besides these there are several others that are very occasionally used for specific indications. A few examples will serve to elucidate how these drugs (and the principles behind their use) can be put to practical application.

A patient suffers an open fracture of the femur with much devitalized tissue and gross contamination. He is brought to the accident room. The treatment of shock, immobilization and preparation for débridement are under way. Tetanus antitoxin is given. Since it is known that trauma of any kind reduces the patient's capacity to combat infection, it is imperative to start antimicrobial drugs. The organisms in the wound are unknown. The worst that could be present would be *beta hemolytic Streptococci,* or *hemolytic Staphylococci.* Since clinical experience has shown that penicillin and streptomycin are most effective agents against these organisms, it is the practice here to give 600,000 units of penicillin and 1 Gm. of streptomycin intramuscularly immediately. If the state of shock is profound, tetracycline, 500 mg. intravenously in 5 per cent glucose, gives a more rapid blood level.

At the time of surgical débridement, a 1 per cent solution of neomycin sulfate is applied to the wound after debriding. This is allowed to remain in place for 15 to 20 minutes. At this concentration, neomycin is bacteriocidal to almost all organisms. No more than one gram should be used.

The prophylaxis with penicillin and streptomycin or with tetracycline should be continued for a minimum of five days, and if any fever or local manifestations warrant, it should be continued longer.

If there is reason to suspect that penicillin, streptomycin, and tetracycline may be ineffective, as, for example, in trauma occurring in a hospital worker, chloramphenicol can be given. The dosage is usually about 2 Gm. a day, either by mouth or parenterally.

In abdominal trauma the same principles obtain. Early blood levels of drug are the best protection. Again, penicillin and streptomycin are preferred. Local intraperitoneal neomycin is definitely of value. The same dosage is used. If neomycin is used intraluminally before suturing a perforation, 2 or

5 per cent solutions may be used, as this drug is not absorbed from the intestinal tract.

In trauma to the chest, head, or neck the same principles apply.

It has been the experience of this Center that penicillin and streptomycin in combination are the best general bacterial prophylactic drugs. The use of tetracycline in combination with these two often causes drug antagonism. Such a practice, therefore, is not recommended.

Tetracycline alone is a good prophylactic agent and should be used if penicillin allergy is present or if the penicillin-streptomycin combination is apparently clinically ineffective after a few days.

Novobiocin, erythromycin, bacitracin, etc., should be reserved for specific indications, usually resistant staphylococcal infections.

One final point should be emphasized. The bacteria that patients bring into the hospital are usually drug susceptible. Infections that arise in open fractures and other injuries are very frequently drug resistant staphylococci. *The Staphylococcus does not become drug resistant under treatment.* The resistant organism comes from the environment and personnel of the hospital and replaces the drug susceptible one in the wound. Therefore, every precaution should be taken from the moment the patient is seen to prevent contamination. This includes keeping the wound covered and wearing masks at all times while examining the wound.

CHAPTER 8

THE CARE OF MULTIPLE INJURIES

Preston G. Wade, M.D.

The problem of the seriously injured patient has never assumed as great importance at it has in the present generation. In this age of rapid transportation made possible by the combination of excellent highways and high-powered motor cars, there is an increasing number of civilian casualties, so that even the smallest hospitals are continually faced with the problem of the treatment of patients with multiple injuries. On an ordinary holiday week end, there may be three or four hundred fatalities and thousands of serious casualties which cause long, painful and costly disabilities. It is well known that the number of civilian casualties arising from motor car injuries in one year is considerably greater than the combined number of casualties suffered during all the wars in which the United States has been involved. On the other hand, the ominous threat of an atomic war makes us realize that in another conflict most of the casualties will occur in our cities, will involve civilians, and will need to be taken care of by our present medical facilities. Even though the threat of war may be more remote than it was a few years ago when civilian defense plans were first initiated, it is essential that we bear these facts in mind and that we be prepared in every community.

Although most hospitals have plans on paper for disasters, when faced with an unexpected catastrophe, they may find that the plans fall short, and it is from the actual experience of hospitals in catastrophes that we may learn important lessons.

It is interesting to read the reports of the three tornadoes which occurred several years ago in Waco, Texas [8]; in Worcester, Massachusetts [7]; and in Flint, Michigan. [5] These were similar in that each had about the same number of fatalities and casualties, and that the difficulties encountered seemed to parallel each other. In Waco, there were 113 deaths and in Worcester 114 deaths. In one there were 1,500 casualties and in the other 950 casualties. In each instance the failure of proper organization caused some of the most serious difficulties. Each report stresses the necessity of preparedness and organization to control fear, panic, confusion and chaos. Communication and transportation seemed to be stumbling blocks in all of these disasters. In the Worcester report, particularly, the reporter was impressed by the difficulty in properly receiving patients and in sorting the injured in hospitals, so that the seriously injured might receive prompt and efficient care. In all these cases the medical services and supplies seemed to be adequate, but there was need for faster communication to the personnel and better transportation to the hospital. In all of these the emphasis was on a small group of well trained and well organized personnel.

Another lesson learned in the disasters mentioned above was the high infection rate of the sutured wounds. This is a lesson which must be emphasized to the young surgeon who is accustomed to laborious suturing of open wounds in civilian practice. We must emphasize the fact that battle wounds and those sustained in civilian catastrophes *should never be closed primarily*.

Accident Room Care

The result of the treatment of a patient with multiple injuries may be determined by the treatment he receives in the accident room. If, on admission, the patient is examined by a competent observer and a proper course of treatment instituted, many serious disabilities may be avoided and many fatalities prevented.

A patient entering the hospital with a single injury, such as a fracture of the shaft of the femur or a fractured skull, will usually be assigned immediately to a special department, and his care will be directed by one surgeon who is responsible for his treatment. There is usually no problem in assigning the responsibility in the case of a single injury. However, if the patient enters the hospital with a combination of various injuries, each of which may be in the domain of a very specialized department, it may be quite difficult to be assured that he will receive proper care. This failure to co-ordinate several surgical specialities in the severely injured patient is too often the cause of neglect in many hospitals.

In most instances the first individual to examine the seriously injured patient is the least experienced member of the staff. He may be an intern or a junior resident, or a substitute medical student. He must then decide who should be called to direct the care of the patient. In many cases the assignment of the case does not constitute a problem if the most severe injury is obvious and is in the province of one specialty. However, the problem may be a very serious one if, for example, the patient has a neurologic condition and an abdominal injury in addition to multiple fractures. In such a case, one surgeon should be assigned to take charge of the case, and he must take the responsibility for the care of the patient regardless of what serious injuries involve other surgical specialties. It is not important whether the surgeon in charge be the neurologic surgeon, general surgeon, chest surgeon or the orthopedic surgeon, but it is essential that whoever is responsible assume his responsibility and see to it that the patient is not neglected because of the lack of co-ordinated care.

In many hospitals the administration assigns the direction of the treatment of the severely injured patient to one individual, and it is his responsibility to see to it that other consultants are called and perform their functions at the proper time. It is most important that the responsible surgeon see the patient immediately, examine him carefully and direct his immediate treatment. Telephone consultation and direction of the case without examination often leads to disaster. Too often, particularly in the late hours of the night, the responsible surgeon will take the diagnosis and observation of an untrained or inexperienced intern and neglect his most important duty, which is the complete and thorough examination of the patient as soon as possible after his admission.

When a patient is admitted to the accident room, the first duty of the surgeon is to make a complete and thorough examination, removing all of the clothes from the patient and examining every part of the body. The most obvious serious conditions must be considered first. An open airway and satisfactory respiratory exchange are essential for survival, and all mucus, blood and vomitus must be removed from the mouth and pharynx, sucked from the bronchial passages, and if necessary, a tracheostomy performed,

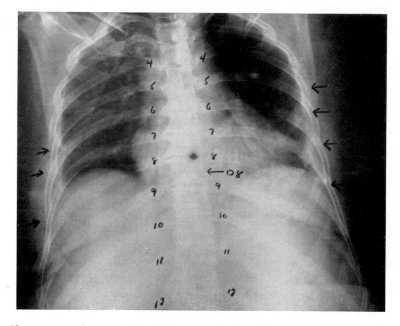

Fig. 1—Chest x-rays show multiple fractures of ribs on both sides. Transverse fracture of body of D8 vertebra.

particularly if there is paradoxic respiration from a crush injury to the chest. Open (sucking) wounds of the chest must be controlled by compression dressing, and hemothorax or pneumothorax should be evaluated and adequate decompression carried out immediately.

The next most important considerations are the treatment of hemorrhage and the treatment and prevention of shock. Every patient who arrives at a hospital after serious injury must be considered a good candidate for shock, if he is not actually in shock. He must be observed for internal hemorrhage. He must immediately have blood drawn for grouping and crossmatching, and sufficient blood of the proper type should be made available when necessary. External hemorrhage should be controlled by pressure bandages if they have not been applied before admission to the hospital. It is rarely necessary to apply a tourniquet in the accident room. It is often necessary to remove a tourniquet if the bleeding continues because the tourniquet has been applied too loosely, causing venous hemorrhage. If a tourniquet has been applied tightly to an injured extremity and the bleeding has ceased, it is better to leave it in place until proper preparation is made for the prevention and treatment of shock, because sudden removal of a tourniquet from an injured limb may suddenly send the patient into shock. The patient should be left in the emergency room until such a time as his condition is stabilized. X-rays should be taken in the emergency room by means of a portable machine, so that

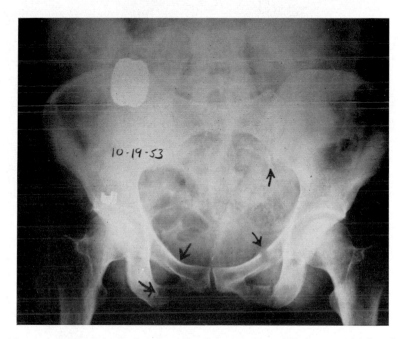

Fig. 2—X-ray showing multiple fractures of pelvis. Fracture of both rami of left pubic bone and fracture through left sacroiliac joint.

the patient does not have to undergo the transfer from accident room to x-ray and return. It is wise to be reasonable about x-ray examination immediately after admission of the patient. Unnecessary x-rays, such as multiple examination of the skull and spine, should not be taken until after the patient has been properly evaluated and his treatment instituted. If it is necessary that the patient be operated on immediately, he should be sent to the operating room in which he can be observed, prepared, and the proper time chosen for operation. He should not be sent to his ward and then be transferred again to the operating room. To transfer an injured patient from stretcher to bed and bed to stretcher is harmful. The use of modern stretchers, through which x-rays can be taken, are helpful in serious cases.

The indiscriminate use of morphine in shock is to be condemned. Morphine should be given only for pain and not routinely for the treatment of shock.

The danger in morphine administration is that it may not be absorbed when the patient is in shock, and when a second dose is given later, the peripheral circulation picks up the multiple doses of morphine which then cause dangerous poisoning.

If the patient has an actual or a suspected fracture, and no splints have been applied before transfer to the hospital, proper immobilization must

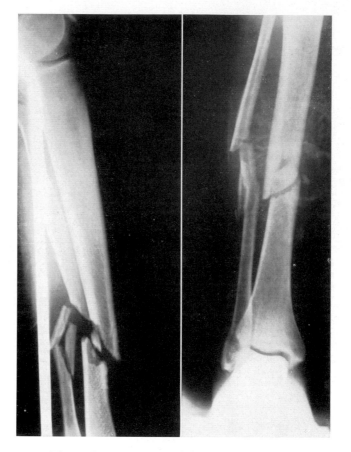

Fig. 3—Open comminuted fractures of left leg.

be instituted in the accident room. If the immobilization was improperly applied before admission, this must be corrected in the accident room.

It may be pointed out that while the examination and correction of the serious conditions of interference of respiration, shock and hemorrhage are being taken care of, blood is drawn for grouping and crossmatching, and tetanus antitoxin (3,000 to 6,000 units) or a booster dose of tetanus toxoid (1 cc.) is administered in the case of open wounds. The initial doses of a broad spectrum of antibiotics are also given in the accident room (see Chapter 7).

After the emergency and urgent problems have been evaluated, a plan of priority for the treatment of other injuries should be formulated. The patient must be evaluated as to every possible area in which an injury might have been sustained.

It has been found in the statistics of the Auto-Crash Injury Research Program at Cornell [2] and verified by study of admissions to The New York Hospital that there is a very definite pattern of frequency of injury to various areas of the body, particularly as the result of automobile accidents.

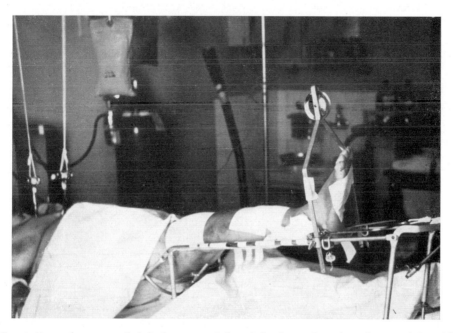

Fig. 4—Open fractures of left leg treated by skeletal traction through os calcis with suspension on Braun-Böhler frame.

The head was found to be most frequently injured, and these injuries could usually be ascertained or suspected because of external evidence or the state of consciousness. The evaluation of the head injury is an important factor in determining whether or not the patient can be expected to withstand operative procedures for injuries to other systems. It is most important that this evaluation be made within as short a time as possible after admission to the hospital.

The next area most frequently involved in injuries in automobile accidents was the lower extremities. Here again the injuries to the lower leg and thigh were quite obvious if only a single area was involved, but injury to the hip, in particular, was often masked by the other lower extremity injuries, and even an x-ray examination, often inadequate as an emergency procedure, would fail to disclose the posterior dislocation with or without fractures of the posterior lip of the acetabulum.

The third most frequently injured areas were the chest and dorsal spine. As mentioned above, injuries to the chest were often obvious owing to the interference with respiration, and crushing injuries to the chest often necessitate a tracheostomy. This procedure has been used much more frequently in recent years even in multiple fractures of the ribs without actual interference with the physiology of respiration. Certainly in paradoxic respiration, it is often a life-saving measure, and this procedure alone may be enough to take care of the interference with the respiration and obviate the necessity

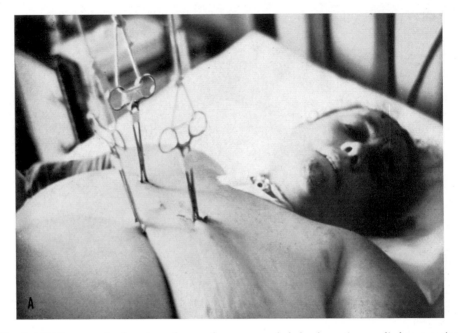

Fig. 5—(A) Photograph of patient after tracheostomy and skeletal traction applied to anterior chest wall.

of traction to the chest wall or internal fixation of the segmental fractures of the ribs. The tracheostomy, although a simple operation, has certain complications and should never be done as an emergency per se but should be performed in the operating room with careful preparation and with careful technic. There are certain precautions which should be taken, particularly in the use of a long enough tube with a large enough diameter so that the full benefit of a airway may be obtained. A transverse incision is to be preferred over a vertical one because the latter leaves a disfiguring scar.

One of the frequently missed injuries in this area is the fracture of the dorsal spine; because in the patient having multiple injuries, this area may not produce immediate symptoms, and unless the injury is suspected and adequate x-rays taken, serious damage may be done to the spinal cord by improper movement of the patient.

The next area found to be injured most frequently was the upper extremities, and often the injuries were minor and missed for several days because of more serious injuries elsewhere. Injuries to the pelvis and bladder were of less frequency than those mentioned, but often were not discovered because of inadequate investigations. If an injury to the bladder is suspected, immediate catheterization should be performed if possible, and if the catheterization is difficult, injury to the urethra may be suspected or discovered, and proper steps taken to treat it. X-ray examination of the bladder and kidneys

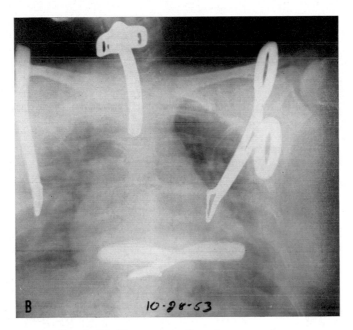

Fig. 5—(B) Chest x-ray after above procedures.

may be done, and considerable information gathered from the catheterized specimen. Abdominal injuries occur less often, but they must always be suspected. They are often masked, and the symptoms may develop hours after admission to the hospital. Frequent observations of the suspected injured abdomen should be made, and although there is considerable difference of opinion as to the efficacy of the abdominal tap, it is very helpful in making a diagnosis of intra-abdominal hemorrhage, when positive.

Care of Fractures in Multiple Injuries

Even though the patient may have multiple injuries of a serious nature, it is essential that the fracture be treated as soon as possible. If one of the injuries is an open fracture, the surgeon should be alert to the fact that early operation is essential, and he must seize the first opportunity to take care of the fracture so as to prevent loss of limb or late disability. Too often, the patient with a suspected head or abdominal injury may be allowed to lie in bed for days before proper disposition is made of an obvious open fracture which should be treated immediately. This is a question of surgical judgment, and the patient's life should not be endangered by any operative procedure in which delay could be tolerated. However, a débridement can often be done in the presence of head injury. The anesthesia can be local, but general anesthesia is not necessarily contraindicated in a head injury. Co-operation between specialists and sympathetic understanding of the pro-

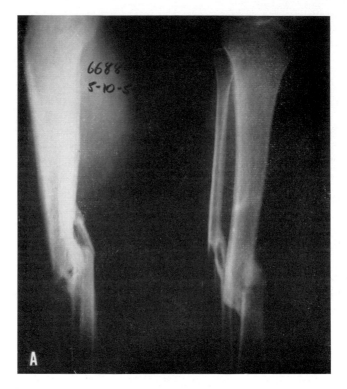

Fig. 6—(A) End result of fractured left lower extremity. Fracture healed with displacement but alignment excellent.

blems of multiple injuries are necessary in any hospital where large numbers of seriously injured patients are received. Fortunately, it is relatively uncommon in present day hospital care to encounter specialists who demand treatment of injuries in their own field at the expense of other necessary treatment. A neurologic surgeon is often concerned only with the result of the injury to the central nervous system, and since his patients may die as a result of a head injury, he may consider a fracture as a relatively minor condition. He may order delay in the treatment of a fracture on the grounds that anesthesia, anoxia or an operative procedure on a bone might cause an aggravation of an intracranial lesion. If, in his opinion, such other treatment might jeopardize the patient's life, he is quite justified in not permitting further treatment. However, the neurologic surgeon does not always recognize that fractures need emergency treatment, and occasionally a bad result in a fracture is due to his unnecessary delay in treatment. The same may be said for the chest surgeon and for the abdominal surgeon, although error in treatment is much less apt to occur as the result of an abdominal injury or chest injury than it is with a head injury.

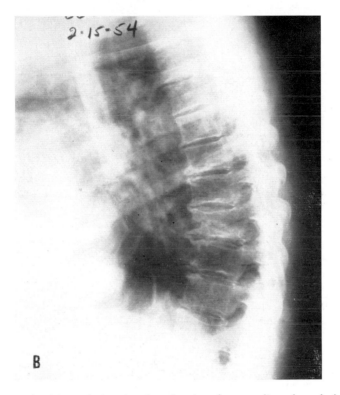

Fig. 6—(B) Lateral vision of dorsal spine showing fracture line through body of D8 4 months post injury.

If the responsible surgeon in charge of the multiple injury case has a broad knowledge of trauma, he will make sure that the patient receives proper treatment regardless of the specialty involved.

The following case will serve to illustrate some of the general principles discussed.

Case of Mary K.: At the age of 55, Mary K. was admitted to The New York Hospital after having been injured in an automobile accident when a car which was being driven by her husband struck a light post going at a high speed. Her husband was killed, and she was brought in with multiple injuries.

She was semiconscious but could be aroused. She was restless and was in acute respiratory distress, breathing rapidly with short gasps, but was not cyanotic.

There were multiple wounds of the head and face with obvious fractures of the jaws and bleeding from the mouth and ears. There were multiple lacerations of both upper extremities and multiple injuries to the chest with obvious paradoxic respiration due to multiple fractures on both sides of the chest. There were abrasions of the abdomen and abrasions of the back in the region of the lower dorsal spine.

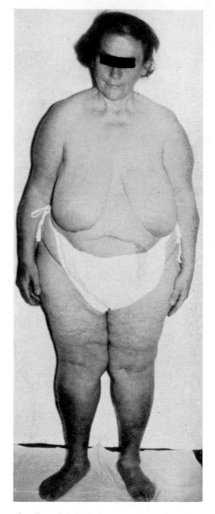

Fig. 7—Follow up photograph of multiple injury patient showing good alignment of left leg.

There were multiple contusions over the lower abdomen and many lacerations of both lower extremities. There was a deep laceration of the lower right extremity extending to the bone, but there was no apparent fracture. There was a markedly displaced open fracture of the left lower extremity with extrusion of the bone fragments and a considerable contamination of the wound. Blood pressure was 100/70, pulse was 120, and respirations were 36 to 40.

Immediately after admission, blood was drawn for grouping and crossmatching, and intravenous fluid was administered until blood was available for transfusion. Oxygen was administered, and within a short time a tracheostomy was performed. Immediately after the tracheostomy, the patient's respirations became much less labored, and her condition rapidly improved greatly. During her stay in the accident room, x-rays were taken of the chest, dorsal spine, pelvis, and lower extremities (figs. 1, 2 and 3). No x-ray was taken of the skull, although at a later time a fracture of the skull was discovered.

While in the accident room, the wound of the right lower extremity was débrided under local anesthesia, and the wound edges closed loosely. At the same time the wound of the left lower extremity was débrided and left open because of the contamination. A Steinmann pin was inserted through the os calcis and the left lower extremity put in a Braun-Böhler frame with six pounds of traction over the end of the frame (fig. 4). These measures were taken in the emergency room before the patient was transferred to her bed. She was then taken to the operating room, and three Lahey clamps were inserted into the ribs of the anterior chest wall for overhead traction. The patient was then transferred to her bed in the ward and overhead traction applied to the chest wall (fig. 5A and B). A tracheostomy alone would have been expected to be enough to take care of the respiratory difficulty, but because of large, pendulous breasts it was thought that skeletal traction would be necessary.

During the first week the patient had frequent episodes of disorientation and restlessness, and there was considerable difficulty with the respiration. Bilateral, pleural effusions appeared, and frequent suctioning was necessary through the tracheostomy. Allevaire spray helped to liquefy the secretions.

X-rays of the chest (fig. 1) showed fractures of five ribs on each side; of the pelvis (fig. 3) fractures of both superior and inferior rami on both sides; and of the spine a transverse fracture of the eighth thoracic vertebra without displacement (fig. 2).

The patient was kept flat in bed with the leg in continuous traction.

Since investigation showed no evidence of injury to the bladder or urethra, and the small amount of blood in the urine shortly disappeared, it was thought that there was no injury to the kidney.

The abdominal symptoms were not sufficient to warrant suspicion of intra-abdominal injury and none developed.

After twelve days, the skeletal traction on the chest wall was discontinued. Two of the traction sites needed treatment for some time because of infection.

The left lower extremity was dressed daily and it gradually closed. Thirty-seven days after admission, the tracheostomy tube was removed. The patient made a complete recovery with good function of the lower extremity and healing of the fracture of the dorsal vertebrae without symptoms (figs. 6 and 7).

This case illustrates the necessity for co-operation between neurosurgeon, abdominal surgeon, chest surgeon, urologic surgeon and fracture surgeon. The most important consideration in the admission of the patient was the respiratory difficulty; the next, the head injury; and finally, the multiple wounds and fractures of the pelvis and the lower extremity.

Summary

In view of the rapidly increasing number of multiple injuries as a result of auto-crash injuries and the mass casualties that war may bring, it is wise for each hospital to investigate its facilities for the care of a large number of seriously injured patients and to organize a program based on the experiences of the minor catastrophes reported at the various hospitals in this country.

The care of the patient with multiple injuries in the accident rooms of most hospitals can be greatly improved. Concerted effort to fix the responsibility of the patient in the hands of one surgeon and to recognize the multiplicity of observations and treatment which are necessary to preserve life and limb and to prevent disabilities may result in improving our care of these patients.

References

[1] Böhler, L.: Treatment of Fractures. New York, Grune and Stratton, 1956, vol. 1.

[2] Braunstein, P. W., Moore, J. O., and Wade, P. A.: Preliminary findings of the effect of automotive safety design on injury patterns. Surg. Gynec. & Obst. *105*: 257—263, 1957.

[3] Committee on Trauma, American College of Surgeons: An Outline of the Treatment of Fractures. Chicago, 1956.

[4] —: Early Care of Acute Soft Tissue Injuries, Chicago, 1956.

[5] Curry, G. J.: The Flint tornado. Am. J. Surg. *87*: 489, 1954.

[6] —, and Lyttle, S. N.: The treatment of multiple severe complex injuries. Am. J. Surg. *83*: 703—710, 1952.

[7] Dunlop, G. R.: The Worcester tornado Am. J. Surg. *87*: 487, 1954.

[8] Jaworski, H. L.: The Waco tornado disaster. Am. J. Surg. *87*: 484, 1954.

[9] Kennedy, R. H.: The appraisal and management of patients with multiple injuries. Surg. Clin. North Am. (Dec.) 1958, 1661—1673.

[10] Watson-Jones, R.: Fractures and Joint Injuries. Edinburgh, E. & S. Livingstone, Ltd., 1955.

CHAPTER 9

THE TREATMENT OF MASS CASUALTIES

Paul W. Braunstein, M.D.

At present there is no definite plan concerning the best way to handle large numbers of casualties. The ideas presented in this chapter are based on the experiences of the military services and on the study of previous civilian disasters. Warren Bowers of the U. S. Army Medical Corps states:

"In this field where none of us can speak from experience, it is too easy for false leaders to arise and becloud the issue. In a subject as complicated and potentially serious as that of surgery for mass casualties, it is especially necessary to define our terms, speak accurately, avoid emotionalism, calm the evangelists, reassure the defeatists, silence the crackpots, stir up interest in the lethargic, do all in our power to arrive at a proper estimate of the probable situation and make adequate flexible plans on such a basis."

The first table records the number of casualties that occurred in recent civilian disasters in the United States from 1947 to 1953 (table 1). The cities listed were struck by blasts or tornados, with the casualty figures running up to 500 killed and 3000 injured. These casualties are relatively large compared to the normal burden of a community and its hospitals. 2000 to 3000 casualties was the greatest patient-load handled by an institution in a relatively unwarned situation. In handling these disasters, there were several

TABLE 1—*Toll in Famous Disasters*

The more serious disasters in the last ten years are recorded with their casualty tolls. In none do the fatalities exceed 600 killed.

YEAR	PLACE	KILLED	INJURED
1947	Texas City Blast	563	3,000
1952	Arkansas Tornadoes	231	1,829
1942	Cocoanut Grove Fire, Boston	181	Severe Burns
1953	Worcester Tornado	94	1,305
1953	Waco, Texas, Tornado	114	1,223
1953	Warner-Robbins Tornado	19	350

obvious defects. The first was lack of disaster plans among the participating hospitals. Frequently no field hospitals or first aid stations were set up, so hospital facilities were immediately swamped with casualties. There was little or no triage, which is the system whereby the greatest number of injured will receive the best care under mass casualty situations. This lack of triage existed despite the fact that there were many physicians with previous military experience who had great knowledge of patient care in such situations. The trained surgeons were not at triage points, where their presence is most necessary. Many of the basic principles of traumatic surgery in treatment of mass casualties were violated. This can best be illustrated by the following: (1) There was no careful appraisal of the over-all situation for stocking of blood donations. The several hundred units of blood secured in the Worcester disaster were usually drawn under questionable aseptic conditions and were finally discarded. (2) There was no communication system to facilitate patient dispersal to different hospitals. The hospital closest to the impact point of the tornado in North Worcester was immediately swamped and nonhospital facilities were also overworked while other well staffed hospitals nearby received only occasional major injuries and only a few other minor injuries. Community hospitals always want to care for *all* patients arriving at their door. This is impractical. For example, during the Worcester tornado a small community hospital northwest of Worcester took care of all patients arriving at its door and ended up doing an inadequate job of over-all patient care. Attempts at triage and dispersal of patients to nearby community hospitals were fought by the hospital administrator, and thus several institutions within easy reach of available transportation for patients with minor injuries were left unused. (3) Inefficiency of patient care even after hospital admission is another serious problem. On entering a first aid and triage point, the patient would frequently be sent to far distant reaches of the hospital where provision for immediate care and close observation were lacking. It is most important to set up shock wards and to provide arrangements whereby the medical personnel can function with a minimum of travel between patients. (4) The primary closure of wounds was carried out with inadequate sterile supplies and without regard to adequate débridement. Some six weeks after the tornado, over 600 patients were still receiving treatment for wounds that had not healed. (5) It is impracticable to use parenteral fluid therapy in the field under emergency conditions. The military has worked out methods of treating severe shock in the field, but in civilian practice it is quite impractical either to administer fluids or to keep them running.

What provisions can we make for the treating of mass casualties? An important one, which always proves tedious to the physician and to the lay person himself, is first aid instruction. In the event of mass casualties, it will be impossible for the physician to reach all the injured. It will therefore fall to the lot of the layman to care for those who cannot be handled by a doctor. Second, every hospital should have a carefully prepared disaster unit which provides for the destruction of neighboring hospitals and for overwhelming patient loads. Doctors should have specifically assigned duties. They should be in a position where they can help the largest number of casualties. While an operating room with one trained surgeon can handle approximately 24 patients a day, a triage point with a similarly trained surgeon can handle hundreds. One trained surgeon should be at the triage point, and another should oversee operations, not be immobilized at one table. Ancillary personnel should be trained to obtain blood and to carry out physicians' requests. The triage system is of utmost importance and decisions there should be made by the most experienced surgeon available. All walking patients and all those with minor injuries should be very rapidly removed from the hospital to make way for sicker patients. Communications should be rapidly established so that the burden can be distributed over a larger geographic area. The medical situation should be frequently appraised by a trained observer who can make rapid decisions concerning further care in that area. Time-tested surgical principles cannot be ignored. Wound débridement without closure is the treatment of choice in any situation involving more than 10 to 20 people at one time. It is most important to apportion available supplies in such a manner that as many people as possible are helped. This is not accomplished by "treating women and children first" nor by favoring those with a higher financial or social background, but rather by duly considering the need for maximal versus minimal to moderate care. For example, if 10 moderately injured patients may have an excellent chance of recovery if one pint of blood is used for each, while there is one seriously injured person who may not survive despite the administration of 10 pints of blood it is obvious that the 10 available transfusion should be distributed among those who are most likely to obtain lasting benefit from them.

TABLE 2—*Man-made Disasters*

The staggering loss of life inflicted by atomic attack is well illustrated.

	KILLED	INJURED
Nagasaki	36,000	40,000
Hiroshima	80,000	80,000—100,000

What difference is there between a thermonuclear or atomic disaster and a natural disaster? First, do they differ (table 2)? As it has been experienced by civilian populations up to this time, the atomic disaster differs from the other disaster primarily in extent. Eighty thousand persons were killed, and approximately 100,000 persons were wounded in each of the atomic attacks on Japan. Note the difference in the number of people involved between the atomic disasters and the previously mentioned civilian disasters. Aside from radiation, the types of injury-producing forces associated with atomic disaster are identical with those that take effect in other holocausts, i.e., blast, heat and debris impact.

In the atomic disaster the first of these is the blast effect. Figure 1 shows that for one second there is a positive pressure blast which is immediately followed by a suction phase which lasts approximately three seconds. It is during these two phases that the severe blast injuries are incurred both from the immediate positive blast and from the secondary reversal suction phase when the rising fireball of the atomic bomb sucks back the atmosphere into the point of impact. Second, there are the effects caused by intense heat. Two types of burns are experienced: the flash burns and those caused by "fire storms." The flash burn is caused by the flash of the fireball, where central temperature measures millions of degrees. This flash burn is usually one-sided, affecting only that side of the patient which faced the impact point. Many fires are started within a sizeable area surrounding the impact point, and these lead to the so-called "fire storms," which are responsible for many burns of the conventional type. Third, the masses of debris hurled through the air by explosive forces contribute many impact injuries similar to those produced by more conventional weapons, i.e., bombs, shells, etc. Fourth, there are the injuries caused by radiation. The "air burst" presents a minimal problem because the radiation is probably effectively diminished over a one and one-half minute period. However, ground or water bursts

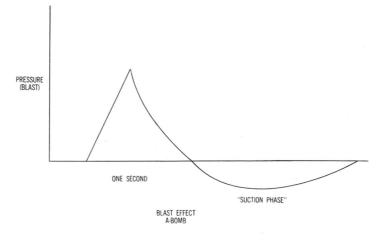

Fig. 1—This well illustrates the positive and negative blast effects of an atomic explosion. Because of the diphasic pressure effect casualties are exposed doubly to missile injuries.

cause a large fallout where the degree of radiation may remain hazardous for a period of days or weeks.

Is an atomic disaster possible in the United States? Most opinion on this question falls into two groups. The first maintains that an atomic disaster will never occur. Because poison gas has never been used on a large scale since World War I, can we assume that an atomic bomb will never be

TABLE 3—*Atomic Casualties with Estimated Severity of Injury*

Note that well over half of all injured patients will require hospitalization for varied periods of time.

Minor	10%	Self Care
Light	25%	Out-Patient
Severe	15%	Hospitalization Needed
Moribund	50%	

employed? Two Japanese cities have already suffered atomic destruction. The second group contends that if an atomic disaster does occur, there is nothing we can do. We, at Cornell, strongly suggest that the following attitude should be accepted. If there is an atomic disaster, it will be a catastrophe. If it does occur, some good can be done; but only by planning, can this good be accomplished.

What would be the probable destruction caused by dropping a very small A-bomb on New York City or Hartford, Connecticut (fig. 2)? If a 20 kiloton bomb were exploded over Hartford, the total metropolitan area including all major hospital facilities would be destroyed. A similar bomb dropped on Manhattan would destroy all of that island as well as a large portion of the other boroughs of the city. Figure 3 shows the four zones of destruction

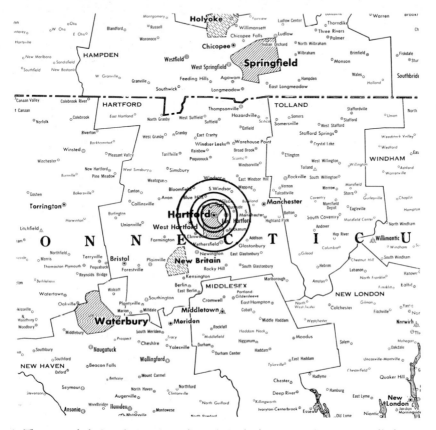

Fig. 2—The overwhelming destruction of a relatively large American metropolis by a small atomic bomb (20 Kt.) is diagrammatically portrayed.

that are created by the explosion of an A-bomb or other thermonuclear weapon. Note that the large area of complete destruction is surrounded by smaller areas of severe destruction and even larger areas of moderate to mild destruction. We have no knowledge of what an H-bomb would do to a civilian population. We do know, however, that on an island on which one H-bomb was detonated the resultant crater was over one mile in diameter with complete disappearance of all land in this area. There is no straight line relationship between the size of the bomb and the area of destruction. An estimate of casualties must be only a random guess at this time. A theoretic example of injury to a known population caused by a small A-bomb is shown

TABLE 4—*Estimated Casualties 20 KT A-bomb City Density Population 5200/Sq. Mile*

The number of casualties is an extremely high percentage of a populace covered by an atomic blast. When one realized that hospital facilities are destroyed by the blast the over-all medical problem is increased many fold.

ZONE	AREA (Sq. Mi.)	KILLED	POPULATION	INJURED (All Hospitalized)	UNINJURED
1	12.6	65,500	59,000	6,500	0
2	7	36,400	21,800	10,900	3,600
3	18.8	97,700	34,216	48,900	14,600
4	56.6	294,000	29,432	117,700	147,100

in table 4. This chart gives the estimated casualties caused by a 20 kiloton A-bomb in a city with a population density of 5,200 per square mile. These figures are an estimate of casualties that would be incurred should an A-bomb be dropped on a city the size of San Antonio, Texas.

Should an atomic disaster occur, the previously discussed principles for treatment of mass casualties must be applied. These are extremely well described in the Army's publication, TB Med. # 246, and it is strongly recommended that this manual be studied by all those interested in this problem. If a disaster does occur, a severely realistic philosophy must be applied in caring for the victims. The injured must be categorized according to their priority for treatment. Those requiring minimal treatment should receive the highest priority (table 5). Within this group, patients who can help with the medical care of others should be treated first. This category

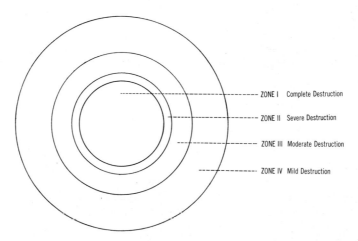

Fig. 3—These zones of destruction are constant in all major atomic blasts, but differ in extent depending on the size of the bomb. Fortunately the size of destructive effect does not increase in linear proportion with increased size of bomb.

includes those with minor closed fractures and superficial injuries. The second group comprises those patients in need of immediate but uncomplicated life-saving treatment. This group should be handled almost simultaneously with the first group. Those with hemorrhage in accessible areas, easily corrected respiratory defects or incomplete amputation should be treated rapidly and then should be evacuated to other areas. The third category is the delayed treatment group. In it are those who require no immediate life-saving

'TABLE 5—*Medical Sorting.* — *Categories of Medical Care in Event of Mass Casualties*

In adopting this severely realistic type of medical sorting in the event of mass casualties the physician must change completely his philosophy of caring for the sickest patient first.

MINIMAL TREATMENT—To be used in support of medical care.
    Minor Closed Fractures, Etc.
    Minor Injuries
IMMEDIATE TREATMENT—Life-saving uncomplicated care.
    Hemorrhage in Accessible Area
    Easily Correctible Respiratory Defects
    Incomplete Amputations
DELAYED TREATMENT—No immediate life-saving measures required.
    Moderate Lacerations
    Closed Fractures Major Bones
EXPECTANT TREATMENT—None under disaster condition — Depends on medical situation.
    Critical Respiratory or CNS Lesions
    Multiple Severe Injuries
    40% Burn or OVER

measures, those with moderately severe lacerations and those with closed fractures of major bones. The fourth or expectant treatment group receive the last priority. This comprises those patients who receive no treatment under disaster conditions until facilities for their complicated care become available. Those with critical respiratory or central nervous system lesions, those with multiple, severe injuries, and those with burns covering 40 per cent or more of their total body surface receive only "expectant therapy" when there are overwhelming patient loads. This is well demonstrated in table 6 where the estimate of fatalities according to burns is summarized. If 900 patients are separated into groups according to what might be expected with a "fire storm," approximately 500 will receive less than 20 per cent burns, 300 will receive 20 to 40 per cent burns and 100 will receive burns of 40 per cent or more. With prompt treatment of burns of 20 per cent or less, the mortality would be 15 in 500. If the treatment were delayed 48 hours, only 10 more would die. Among those with burns of 40 per cent or more, delay in treatment of over 48 hours would result in the death of only 20 more people, though this would be 95 per cent of those burned. However, among those with 20 to 40 per cent burns if no treatment were carried out for 48 hours, 120 people more would die than would die if immediate therapy were administered. According to this formulation, treatment should be administered to those suffering between 20 and 40 per cent burns. Those with less than 20 per cent would receive only superficial

TABLE 6—*Predicted Burn Mortality*

In the group of patients suffering 20—40% body burns a proportionately higher number of people will be lost if medical care is delayed 48 hours. It is therefore this group that will receive priority care of burns under disaster conditions.

% BURN	No. PATIENTS BURNED	MORTALITY	
		PROMPT R	48 HRS. DELAYED R
Less than 20%	500	15	25
20—40%	300	30	150
Worse than 40%	100	75	95

ambulatory care, while those suffering with burns exceeding 40 per cent would fall into the expectant group until such time as heroic therapy could be carried out without denying care to those with a better chance of living.

In time of disaster a staggering amount of blood is required to treat radiation and other injuries. The estimated blood required (table 7) during the first 21 days following thermonuclear disaster is of gigantic proportions. We can estimate that there will be eight million casualties throughout the nation in the event of a surprise thermonuclear attack. 1525 units of blood per 1000 casualties are required. This means that 13 million units of blood must be available during the first 21 days. Actually, with a fair amount of the population unharmed, this could be obtained. It cannot be stored in advance of course, but after disaster those requiring blood could obtain it fairly promptly.

TABLE 7—*Estimated Blood Requirement First 21 Days Following Nuclear Disaster*

While these figures concerning blood requirements are staggering it is a problem which, if prepared beforehand, may be overcome.

1. Estimate — 8,000,000 casualties nationally
2. 1525 units of blood per 1000 casualties
3. 13,000,000 units of blood first 21 days

In summary, thermonuclear attack, atomic casualties and civilian casualties are always a threat to the unwarned population. There is no room for defeatism or lethargy. One must take an active interest in the problem and be prepared as best as possible for any diseaster, either natural or man-made. It is important to teach first aid to the laity, and this instruction must extend into suburban and rural areas, for should a thermonuclear attack occur, the rural areas will have to accept the major share of responsibility for taking care of survivors from metropolitan districts. It is important to observe the time-tested principles of disaster surgery: débridement, open treatment of wounds, triage and other medical and ancillary medical emergency services which have been so well established by the military medical groups. It is necessary to adopt a realistic philosophy of treatment so that medical services may be employed to save the largest number of people with the supplies and services available at the time.

CHAPTER 10

MANAGEMENT OF BURNS

HERBERT CONWAY, M.D., F.A.C.S.

The importance of thermal injury is emphasized by a review of mortality statistics in the United States. In 1937 there were 6,240 deaths due to burns; in 1952 there were 8,814 such deaths. As industrial hazards decrease, a result of attention to safety measures, accidents in homes and in private life appear to be on the increase. In the municipal hospitals of New York City alone, there were 800 major burn cases in 1955. Sixty-eight, or 8.5 per cent, of these succumbed but the entire group of cases required 24,872 hospital days. Thus, it is fitting that the surgeon who is responsible for treating give thought and study to, and be familiar with, the management of burns. This presentation emphasizes the correlation of local and general treatment of the burned patient.

As far back as the history of man can be traced, he has never been found without fire for warmth and cooking. Unquestionably, primitive civilization was plagued by the clinical burn, just as the burns of modern times exact a gruesome toll in death and disability. It is not surprising that improvements and modifications in the management of burns, have followed intensive research precipitated by accidental mass conflagrations and by the holocausts of war. In the year 1925, the clinical care of burns throughout the world was influenced by Davidson's [19] introduction of tannic-acid therapy. The ready and widespread adoption of this technique was based on multiple reports of lowered mortality rates. After nearly 17 years, this once ubiquitous treatment fell into disfavor because of complications such as infection and contracture and because new information showed that tannic acid can cause central necrosis of the liver. [46] The Royal Army Medical Corps of Great Britain, impressed during the early years of World War II with evidence that the eschar of tannic acid delayed healing in wounds of certain locations (finger, face, hand), abandoned this time honored method of therapy. The experiences at the Massachusetts General Hospital with burns from the Cocoanut Grove [33] night-club disaster (1943) demonstrated conclusively that the mortality rate in large numbers of burns could be lowered even further by chemotherapy without tannic acid. Moreover, a new concept of the management of the burned patient had been introduced by Underhill's [43] demonstration (1930) that the chief adverse general effect of the burn, namely a diminution in the plasma content of the blood, is due to the collection of this protein fluid in the burned areas and in the tissues subadjacent to the burns. Allen and Koch [1] emphasized the technic of pressure over the burned area and immobilization of the affected part to limit the exudation of proteins, electrolytes and fluids into the thermally damaged tissues. The concept of correlating the general management of the pathologic physiology of the burned patient and the local care of the burn began to dominate therapy. This correlation stands as the central principle in the treatment of the burned patient. The systemic status of the patient is improved by effective local care of the burn, and this improvement allows for the effective treatment of the local damage.

Superficial and Deep Burns

For practical purposes, burns are classified as superficial or deep. *Superficial burns* include those of first (erythema) and second (blistering) degree, in which the integument of the involved area has not been destroyed, and in which progress to healing with a permanently acceptable cutaneous surface may be expected. These burns are grave only when they involve a large percentage of the total surface of the body. Formerly it was taught that a burn involving only 50 per cent of the surface of the body, and in children, an even lower percentage, doomed the victim to death. The introduction of controlled therapy by administration of fluids, proteins and electrolytes, based on frequent laboratory studies, resulted in an increasing number of reports which showed that patients with superficial burns involving 60—70 per cent of the surface area of the body had survived. While superficial burns do not result in ulceration and contracture, loss of pigmentation may be a significant aftermath in injuries involving the face and hands. This is especially true when the burned individual is of dark complexion or is a Negro.

Superficial burns of first and second degree are important chiefly because the physiologic disturbances which may occur when they involve a sufficiently large surface area of the body may cause death. In such cases death occurs soon after injury from shock in the first 24 hours, and from toxic reaction in 24—72 hours. Seldom can these burns cause death from sepsis, for such mortality is related to the massive infection associated with deep (third degree) burns.

Deep burns (third-degree) are those in which the thermal trauma destroys the entire thickness of the skin and, in some instances, the underlying tissues as well. It is interesting to note that Dupuytren,[15] in the early part of the nineteenth century, explored the pathology of burns and established six types or degrees of burns based on the depth to which the thermal trauma had caused necrosis of tissue. Practical experience through the past century and a half has led clinicians to the widely used classification of first, second and third degree. This is based on the fact that in first and second degree burns therapy is directed primarily toward the general care of the altered physiologic state of the individual, while in third degree burns the clinician must make haste, as well, to separate the necrotic slough to promote the rapid healing which follows the separation of slough due to thermal trauma. More recently, clinicians have been content to classify burns simply as superficial or deep. Deep burns involve complete loss of covering tissue. The success of treatment, i.e., the avoidance of prolonged morbidity and of disabling deformity, depends on early recognition that all layers of the skin have been destroyed and on early institution of measures to remove the devitalized tissue and to overcome the loss. In 1929, Wells [45] called for the treatment of electric burns by immediate excision and skin graft, and in 1942, Young [47]

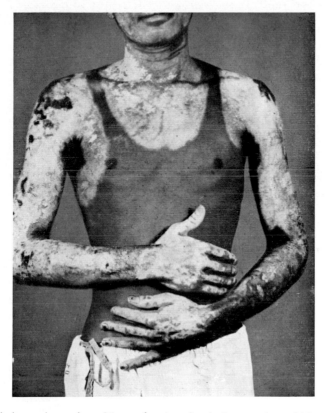

Fig. 1—Second degree burns in a Negro showing the depigmentation which was caused by the burn. The protective effect of clothing also is demonstrated.

reported on one case in which the slough of a deep burn had been excised and the area covered immediately with a skin graft. The fact that improved methods of control of altered fluid balance resulted in the survival of greater numbers of individuals with extensive loss of skin posed problems in surface coverage which taxed the ingenuity of those most experienced in the grafting of skin. History reveals that the plastic surgeon assumed an important position in the forward march of the therapy of burns. Brown [8] has demonstrated the permanent usefulness of thick-split grafts of skin on the surface of the body. Fortunately, improvements in the technic of skin grafting, initiated by Padgett's[36] introduction of the dermatome in 1939, later improved and calibrated precisely by Reese, [38] made the procurement of large sheets of skin for the coverage of extensive areas relatively simple for the average surgeon. Many other mechanical devices (vacutome, [5] electrodermatome [34]) have contributed even further to the facility of skin grafting; however, many plastic surgeons prefer to cut free grafts of skin by hand. A more complicated problem is presented in the patient who may be so extensively burned that there is a paucity of donor sites. To follow the principle of the early removal of the burned tissue, the surgeon must be ready to provide promptly for cutaneous coverage by skin graft. This may mean the cutting of several suc-

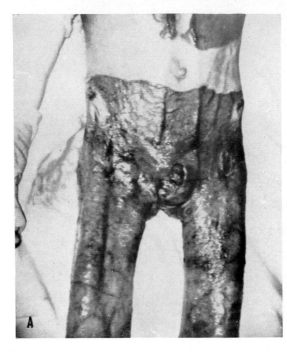

Fig. 2–(A) Unhealthy pale granulations in cachectic 9 year old boy five months after deep burns. Note the subcutaneous atrophy, thinness of the extremities and prominent veins.

cessive crops of skin grafts from the same donor site. With ideal healing, one donor area may be expected to yield successive crops of grafts at three week intervals. But such a plan, although I used it during World War II, has now been replaced by the temporary coverage of burn wounds with homografts of skin. At the United States Naval Hospital, Bethesda, Maryland, the technic of the quick-freezing and vacuumstorage of thick-split skin grafts for such purpose has been worked out. [28] Brown et al. [9] have called attention to the value of grafts obtained immediately post-mortem for this purpose. These homologous skin grafts are of only temporary value. Their period of survival varies from three to five weeks. During this interval, the general state of the patient may be fortified, after which the homologous grafts must be excised and replaced by autogenous skin. Failure to do so will result in chronic granulation with infection, delayed healing of the wound and ultimately extensive fibrosis. D. M. Jackson, following the suggestion of R. Mowlem, has used alternately placed strips of autogenous and homologous skin, toward the end that, as the homoplastic grafts undergo dissolution, epithelization will spread to bridge the interrupted cutaneous defects.

The necrotic tissue of deep burns should be excised just as soon as possible following injury. The surgeon most exercise keen judgment as to just how soon after injury the patient may be safely subjected to operation. Again,

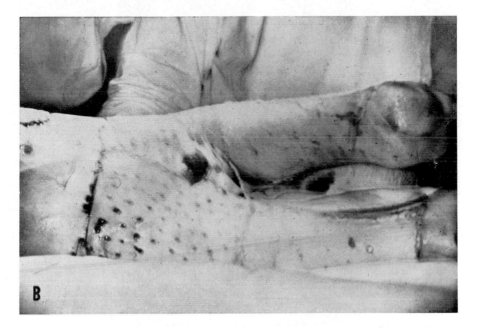

Fig. 2—(B) Because of the paucity of donor sites, this burn of 50 per cent of the body was covered with homoplastic skin grafts.

the principle of the correlation of the local and the general care of the burned patient comes into play. However, the surgeon's most difficult problem may lie in determining which surface areas are the sites of deep burns. Cope[18] and his associates state that "no objective method of determining the depth of destruction of a burn has proven of aid to us." However, there are some aids in the differential diagnosis. Superficial burns usually are exquisitely tender and subjectively painful, whereas sensation is lost and there is anesthesia in the areas of deep burn (Bull, Lennard-Jones sign).[11] Ivory-like pallor of the skin is evidence of its total, thermal destruction. Hypoesthesia may be present in areas of second degree burn. It is of some help to examine the burned area in a dark room under ultraviolet light after the intravenous injection of sodium fluorescein (10 cc. of 20 per cent solution). By this technic (Dingwall and Lord[21]) the circulating red blood corpuscles of the skin appear as yellow bodies, and the portions of the skin which have been killed by heat show a complete absence of this yellow coloration. The fluorescein test is innocuous, but it gives no information as to the exact depth of the deep burn and it is not practical to apply it to patients who are very ill as a result of extensive burns. When uncertainty exists it is wise to err by overestimating rather than underestimating the depth of cutaneous destruction. When the sacrifice of underlying structures such as nerve, tendon or ligament may come under consideration, or where the surface areas of involvement are great, chemical

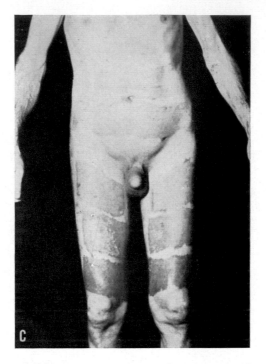

Fig. 2–(C) 22 drums of skin (over 161 square inches) were cut from the boy's father. An inadvertent complication was the development of hematemesis two days after the cutting of the grafts. This could be explained on no basis other than the possibility that Curling's ulcer developed due to the loss of plasma from the donor sites. X-ray failed to demonstrate a gastrointestinal lesion. The wounds healed uneventfully. Experience with this case teaches that it is unwise to take a large number of grafts from a single donor.

débridement, according to the technic of Connor and Harvey, [14] or enzymatic débridement, may be preferable to surgical excision, though it is more time-consuming. The advantage of chemical débridement lies in the fact that organic acids such as phosphoric or pyruvic acid starch paste reduce the pH of tissue to 1.9, a condition favorable for rapid separation of the slough of deep burns.

Emergency Care of the Burned Patient

All those who come into contact with the burned patient should wear masks as long as the wound is exposed. This detail is now especially important because of the current hospital problem of antibiotic resistant staphylococcus. A sterile dressing of fine-mesh gauze (40—44) should be applied to the burned surface immediately. This is preferred to an ointment type of dressing. The patient should receive immediate antibiotic therapy and either tetanus antitoxin or a "booster" dose of toxoid, whichever is indicated. Pain should be controlled by the intravenous administration of morphine. If the patient is in shock, morphine by any other route will not be promptly effective because of peripheral vascular collapse. Repeated intramuscular

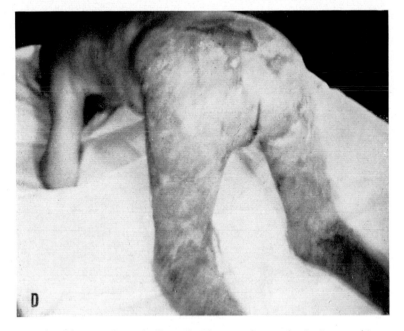

Fig. 2—(D) After three and one-half weeks these grafts are beginning to thin out. After four weeks the child had gained in strength sufficiently that he was able to stand operation for excision of the homoplastic grafts and their replacement by autogenous grafts. The use of homogolous grafts was of distinct value in the management of this neglected deep burn. It is important to excise the grafts before they undergo ulceration because homoplastic grafts provoke extensive fibrous tissue reaction.

injections of morphine, though ineffective while the patient is in shock, may result in overdosage as the patient recovers. The circulating blood volume can be roughly estimated by hematocrit determinations which should be made frequently (every hour) in order to assay the degree of hemoconcentration. These tests may, however, be inaccurate owing to destruction of red blood cells in association with hemoconcentration. A catheter placed in the bladder allows accurate evaluation of the degree of renal function. Fluid therapy should be directed toward the maintenance of urinary output of 50 cc. per hour. Significantly less than this amount of output (25 cc. per hour) indicates a poor prognosis. If large amounts of intravenous fluid are needed, a polyethylene cannula should be secured in the transected antecubital vein. With a catheter in the bladder and a cannula in the vein of the arm, the clinician is equipped to observe accurately and to control effectively the fluid balance and chemical state of the burned patient. Care of the burned area is limited to coverage by gauze until the general condition permits definitive treatment.

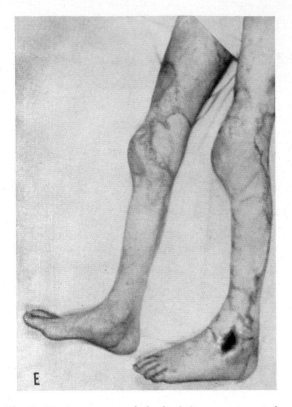

Fig. 2–(E) Appearance of the healed autogenous grafts.

General Care of the Burned Patient

The principles of fluid replacement as promulgated by the late Everett Evans [24] are advocated (table I). The amount of whole blood, plasma or plasma substitute which is required during the first 24 hours after burn is computed by multiplying the body weight (in kilograms), by the percentage of body surface burned, by one cubic centimeter. In addition, Evans theorized that an equal amount of electrolyte solution and 2,000 cc. of 5 per cent glucose in water (for an adult weighing 70 Kg.) also should be given during the first 24 hours.

The New York Hospital Clinic follows the Evans formula for fluid replacement in the severely burned patient. The fluid balance formula of Reiss et al. [39] also is most helpful. In estimating the percentage of body surface burned, Berkow [6] measured the surface area of the various parts of the body and listed them as represented in figure 3. A quick method of estimating of

TABLE 1—*Evans Treatment* *

Plasma, plasma substitute or whole blood = 70 × 35 × 1 cc. = 2,450 cc.
Electrolyte solutions (0.9% NaCl)   = 70 × 35 × 1 cc. = 2,450 cc.
5% glucose in water   —   2,000 cc.

Total to be given first 24 hrs. = 6,900 cc. †

area of involvement is the "Rule of Nines" which states that the leg, the thigh
and the upper extremity each represent approximately 9 per cent of the
body surface. The thorax represents 9 per cent anteriorly and 9 per cent

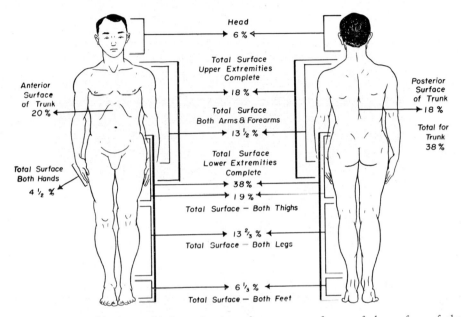

Fig. 3—Berkow's table for rapid determination of percentage of area of the surface of the
body which is involved in a burn.

posteriorly as do the abdominal and lumbar regions. The head and neck also
represent roughly 9 per cent of the surface area of the body.

Once the patient has recovered from shock, attention is directed toward
the local management of the burned areas. If it is certain that the burns are
only superficial, it is correct to apply sterile vaselinized gauze and to leave
such dressings undisturbed for a week or so. However, if there is certainty
that areas of deep burn are present, it is imperative that the clinician adopt
an aggressive plan directed toward the rapid separation of the necrotic tissue.

* For burn of 35% of body of man weighing 70 Kg.

† Half this amount of plasma and/or whole blood and electrolyte (totaling 2,450 cc.)
and the same amount (2,000 cc.) of 5 per cent glucose in water is given the second
24 hours. Calculation will show that should the burn involve 60—75 per cent of body
surface, large amounts of colloid and saline would be required if this formula were strictly
applied. Nevertheless, not more than 4,000 cc. of colloid or 4,000 cc. of saline solution is
given in 24 hours, no matter how extensive the burn.

The slough of deep burns is tenacious and the difficulty of removing it by minor measures coupled with the assurance afforded by the apparent well-being of the patient often tempt the clinician to wait. Such policy can lead only to regrettable deformity, since granulation tissue, the reparative response to destruction of tissue and infection, begins to grow 48 hours after the primary injury. The longer the granulation tissue persists, the more dense the scar and the more crippling the resultant deformity. Thus, the surgeon should act promptly to separate necrotic tissue in deep burns.

Local Care of the Burned Area; Immediate Excision and Skin Grafting of Deep Burns

As emergency covering of the burned area, sterile gauze is recommended. For superficial burns, vaselinized gauze and pressure dressings are the treatment of choice. For deep burns, the same type of dressing may be used

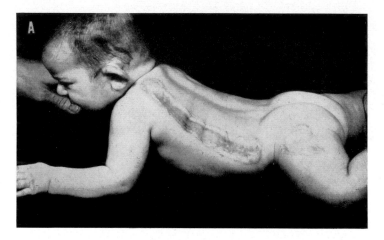

Fig. 4—(A) Primary excision of third-degree burn. This patient slipped out of bed and fell against a radiator.

as for superficial burns, if the condition of the patient does not permit more aggressive therapy. However, if the general condition of the patient is good, immediate excision or chemical (enzymatic) débridement by multiple (q. 48 hours) dressings is the technique of choice.

Limited areas in selected locations lend themselves to primary excision and immediate grafting of skin. Areas uncertain in margin or depth may be brought rapidly to separation of slough by chemical or by enzymatic débridement. It is the experience of this clinic that deep burns of limited area can be excised at once and that the wound can be resurfaced immediately with free, thick-split grafts of skin. This method of management has the following advantages: infection is avoided, the period of morbidity is diminished and complications such as contracture and ulceration are prevented. Application of the method requires that the surgeon exercise keen judgment: he must make a decision at the operating table not only regarding the surface area in which the tissues are completely necrotized but also regarding the depth to which such necrosis extends. Therefore, the method is not practical in burns which are very deep, i.e., those which extend through the subcutaneous tissue into underlying important structures such as the tendons and nerves. However, in the management of electrical burns it may be judicious to sacrifice underlying structures also since if these have been damaged by the thermal trauma, there

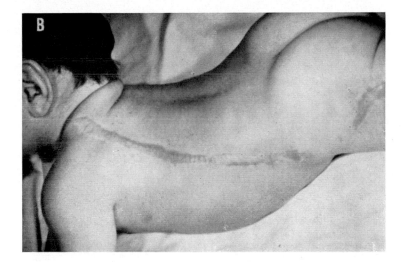

Fig. 4–(B) Dr. Donald Weeks, resident surgeon at The New York Hospital, excised the burned areas and closed by primary suture. The infant was clinically well when he reacted from anesthesia. The hypertrophic aspects of the scar are transient and fortunately are on concealed surfaces of the body.

will be ultimate need for coverage by grafts and by transposition of other tissues to develop acceptable function.

The technic of immediate excision and skin grafting returns many burned patients to useful activity within four weeks after injury. In the opinion of the author, no other method is superior in treating those deep burns to which it applies. MacMillan and Artz [32] reported on 5 cases of deep burn treated by early excision and grafting. No deaths in the early postoperative period could be attributed to operative intervention. The largest area of deep burn excised at one operation was 32 per cent of the surface of the body.

Technic of Chemical (Enzymatic) Débridement of Burns

If the necrotic tissue of deep burns cannot be excised primarily, its separation should be hastened by chemical or enzymatic débridement.[2] Connel, Bowe, and Rousselot [13] evaluated 18 proteolytic enzymes for débridement of eschar and found the most effective one to be a clostridium derivative, unfortunately quite toxic and not available for general use. They reported that less efficient — though less toxic — enzymes require two to five days to effect separation of slough. For this technique Connor and Harvey [14] (1946) suggested the use of an organic chemical, pyruvic acid. The objective of treatment of deep burns is the early achievement of closure of the wound. By reducing the pH of the tissue to 1.9, pyruvic acid was found to be the most effective organic acid in the acceleration of the separation of the slough

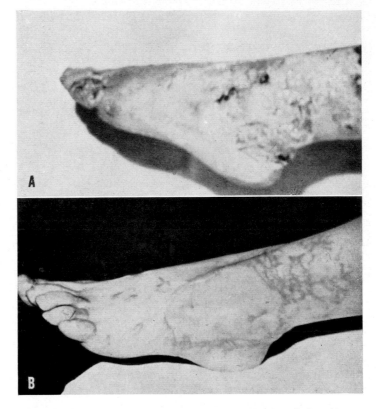

Fig. 5—(A) Deep burn of the foot with necrosis of the skin.

Fig. 5—(B) After five successive applications of pyruvic acid starch paste, the slough had separated completely and skin grafts were applied. This photograph was taken 28 days after the original injury. The objective in deep burns is to get the wound healed and the patient out of the hospital within the calendar month.

of deep burns. It works by releasing enzymes normally present in the tissues (cathepsins). These are the enzymes which ordinarily accomplish the separation of the tenacious necrotic tissue of burns during the fourth to sixth week after injury, often in the presence of already established serious infection. The organic acid serves only to accelerate the rate of release of cathepsins. The wound is kept covered with a one inch layer of pyruvic acid-starch paste (grey in color). In third degree burns not involving important underlying tissues, wounds so treated every 48 hours are ready for grafting in about 10 days. This clinic has utilized pyruvic acid, applying it every 48 hours under light intravenous anesthesia (pentothal sodium). There is some complaint of pain from the dressings though this is not sufficient to be of importance.

The paste is prepared by adding 7 cc. of pyruvic acid C. P. to 1 liter of distilled water. Phosphoric acid is as helpful as pyruvic acid. [40] The pH of the solution will be 1.9. Approximately 200 cc. of the solution is mixed with 10 per cent starch paste so that a thin, cold paste results. The remaining 800 cc. of the solution are heated to just below the boiling point. The 200 cc. of cold starch paste are then added to the 800 cc. of hot, pyruvic acid solution. The mixture must be heated and stirred constantly until a relatively thick, homogeneous jelly results. When cooled the mixture is ready for use. This paste (or jelly) is applied in a one inch layer to the surface of the wound. To prevent drying, it is covered with large sheets of vaseline gauze, around which soft gauze rolls are wrapped. Since pyruvic acid separates the slough by loosening its margins, the process can be hastened further by criss-crossing the slough with the scalpel at the time of each change of dressing. This step greatly increases the margins of slough available for attack by the enzymes.

Exposure Treatment of Burns

In recent years the open-air treatment of burns has been popularized by Wallace, [44] by Blocker et al., [7] and by others. Intensive studies on this method have been reported by the Surgical Research Unit, Brooke Army Hospital, Fort Sam Houston, Texas. [3, 4] We reserve this technic for the management of superficial burns, particularly those of the perineum in children, since the method offers nothing to meet the urgent requirement of removing slough of third degree burns in preparation for adequate surface coverage. Intense interest in the management of mass burn casualties has heightened interest in this treatment. Its advantages are apparent immediately — the greatly diminished work load, and the need for only insignificant amounts of supplies. The Army teams, Artz et al., [4] and Pulaski et al.[37] have come to the following conclusions. Burns involving predominantly one side of the body are suitable for treatment by exposure to the air, but circumferential burns of the trunk have shown infection due to cracking of the crust or failure to form a crust; one week after injury is regarded as the upper limit of applicability of the method, and granulating wounds should never be treated by exposure; crusts formed during the open-air treatment desquamate from superficial burns, whereas in the management of deep burns, eschars must be removed by excision before grafts of skin can be applied.

Bacteriology of Burns

In a controlled series of experimentally produced deep burns in human volunteers, Dingwall and Andrus [20] reported about 14 years ago that the commonest contaminating organism was *Staphylococcus albus*. Widespread use of parenteral therapy with penicillin was at the height of its popularity in 1947 when Langohr, Owen, and Cope [31] reported their exhaustive studies

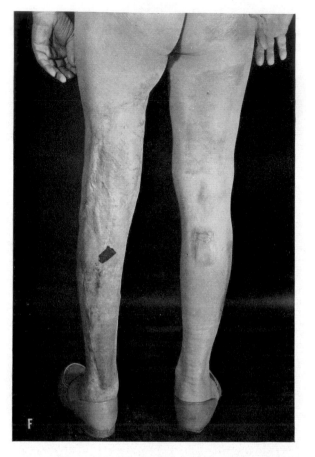

Fig. 6–(F) See legend, facing page.

Burns of the Hand

It is interesting to note that surgeons seldom think of elevating a burned hand. Yet, it is well known that the exudate of protein fluid into the digital joints is the commonest forerunner of ankylosis of the metacarpophalangeal and interphalangeal joints with subsequent atrophy, ankylosis and osteoporosis. The silver fork deformity of the hand with complete crippling is a common sequel of the burned hand. Frank elevation is a *sine qua non* of therapy of the burned hand, to be used in addition to the other principles of general and local treatment. Elevation may be secured by skeletal traction, using a Kirschner wire through the distal ends of both radius and ulva, supporting the hand and fingers in the position of rest by bandaging them loosely to the wicket-shaped Kirschner wire holder. Elevation diminishes the amount of edema and thus the degree of exudation of fluid into the intra-articular spaces. Perhaps in no other anatomical area are immediate excision of thermal slough of deep burn and immediate skin grafting so richly rewarded by accelerated rate of healing and preservation of function. Thick-split grafts are ideally serviceable on the dorsum of the hand and fingers as well as for replacement coverage of small areas of the palm. Larger, deep burns of the palm, where most of the palmar fat pad is destroyed or where tendons and tendon sheaths are exposed, require pedicled tissue for coverage. When a burn destroys the dorsal portions of the joint capsules of the digital joints, there is no hope for preservation of motion. Since ankylosis

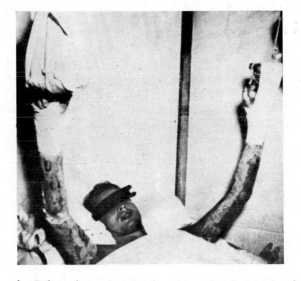

Fig. 7—War wounds. Balanced traction in the treatment of wounds of the extremities. Traction by adhesive or by the use of pins is of extreme value in the treatment of burns of the extremities. Elevation of arms and hands which have been burned is an important point in surgical care. Balanced suspension of the extremities to the overhead struts of a Balkan frame allows for the easy application of wrap-around wet dressings. In this case thick-split grafts have been applied to the granulating wounds. They are secured by the overlay of a thin layer of gauze which is anchored to the adjacent uninvolved skin using collodion. Gauze rolls moistened in saline solution are reapplied to the grafts at four hour intervals. This is the best technic to insure the success of skin grafts applied to infected wounds. The author reported success of skin grafting in 94 per cent of war wounds so treated.

is certain, as soon as the wounds are reasonably clean, the interdigital joints should be fixed by Kirschner wires in partial flexion, i.e., with the hand in the position of rest so that the end result will be a hand which will have pick-up function. No manual deformity is more objectionable than that in which the digits are ankylosed in extension. Burns of the hand should not be treated by the exposure method lest the contractural effect of the digital eschars cause gangrene of the fingers. Moncrief [35] reported that of 21 deep burns of the hands treated by early excision and grafting, 12 regained full range of motion while the remainder showed function which was adequate for all but fine motions.

Care of the Neglected Burn

Too often the surgeon stands idly by, waiting for epithelization of a large burn by ingrowth of epithelium from its margins. Such professional lassitude invites poor healing at best. Wounds which are allowed to heal by epithelization result in unstable surfaces, referred to as scar epithelium. These scars

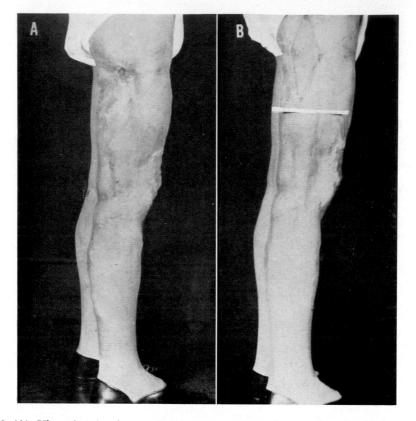

Fig. 8—(A) Ulceration in the annular burn scar of the thigh with obstruction causing varicosities and ulceration. This scar followed a burn sustained 22 years earlier.

Fig. 8—(B) Postoperative photographs taken 30 days after operation at which time the ulcer was excised, relaxation incision was made and whole-thickness graft of skin was placed. The thicker the graft the better its function as an elastic bridge in this particular problem. The ulcer was not malignant.

are not resistant to the ordinary cutaneous trauma of daily life and usually lead eventually to contracture and/or ulceration. Such scars are constantly contracting over a prolonged period of time. It is this characteristic which explains the fact that a given scar may seem satisfactory at first, only to develop ulceration years later. Scar tissue is the end result of granulation tissue, the cellular components of which are the endothelial cell (capillaries) and the fibroblast. Young fibroblasts contain much cytoplasm and little collagen. The latter increases with maturity, causing powerful cellular contraction. To effect healing of the chronic ulceration in scars due to burns, multiple releasing incisions are required to afford new supply of blood. Such incisions should be covered at once with skin grafts. An annular scar of an extremity may not seem important at first, but continued contracture through

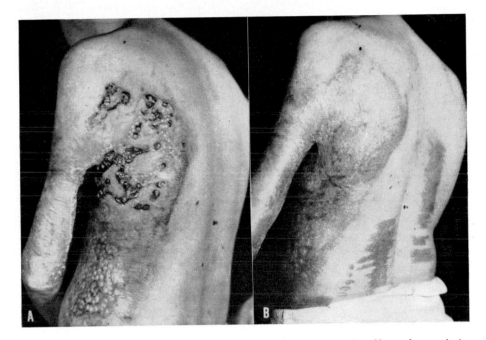

Fig. 9—(A) Ulceration and contracture. The progressive contractile effect of granulation tissue has resulted in adduction, deformity of the shoulder, atrophy of the arm, kyphosis, severe deformity of the torso. In addition, the scar epithelium has broken down so that the open wounds are unhealthy ulcerations with bases consisting of grey, ischemic tissue. The local physician wondered why multiple small grafts applied in the home had not been successful in these areas whereas they had been successful in the lower part of the wound. The answer is that the earlier grafts were done at a time when the contractual effect of the scarred granulation tissue was not sufficiently strong to squeeze the blood supply out of the area. Merely to attain healing of such ulcers presents a formidable problem. Long relaxation incisions are required in order to permit the scarred area to "breathe." Fig. 9—(B) At one operation five vertical insertions were made extending entirely through the scarred area. Thick-split grafts of skin were inserted into the incisions, elliptical in nature by reason of the separation of the margins of the scar.

the years can cause varicosities, lymphedema and atrophy. Such scars, even without ulceration, require relaxation incisions parallel to the long axis of the extremity, with insert of elastic skin, preferably as a whole-thickness graft as described by Conway.[17] In those cases in which release from deformity cannot be achieved by relaxation incisions, the entire scar may be excised and the defect covered with skin grafts.

Marjolin's ulcer is a cutaneous carcinoma which develops in scar tissue following burns. [16] The common denominators in the largest number of cases are the history of slow healing of burn by ingrowth of epithelium from the margins of the wound, the long interval of time (often 15 to 30 years) between healing of the wound and development of malignancy in an ulceration of the scar and the frequency of development of ulceration in scars which are subjected to frequent stress, such as those overlying joints. One must always consider the possibility of Marjolin's ulcer in an ulceration in burn scar. The malignancy may be either basal cell or squamous cell carcinoma. In the pathogenesis of metastases, the growing cancer of Marjolin's ulcer must penetrate its scar-locked barrier in order to get into the lymphatic circulation. Thus only about 20 per cent of cases exhibit metastases. These are to the regional nodes or to the viscera. The therapy of Marjolin's ulcer is as follows: complete surgical excision of the lesion with coverage by skin grafts, amputation in those cases involving the bones of the extremities and resection of regional nodes if palpable. Therapy cannot be discussed without emphasis on prevention. Relief of tension on burn scars by partial or complete excision and replacement by skin grafts is preventive of the condition, as is the appropriate use of skin grafts for the prompt and early closure of wounds of third degree burns. Malignant degeneration of ulceration in scar tissue is a grave complication. Carcinoma of this type can be prevented, even at a date remote from the time of thermal injury, if relaxation incisions are made and fitted with skin grafts, or if the entire scarred area is excised.

Burn Problem in Atomic Warfare

In considering the care of mass casualties resulting from atomic disaster, most planners have concentrated on the problems of triage and evacuation. Intelligent collecting and sorting out of the burned patients is of the utmost importance for efficient management. No accurate estimate of the number of burned individuals to be expected in such a disaster is possible, for this will vary with types of explosive, concentration of population and other factors. While the effects of radiation in such burns are very real, the experiences with the Hiroshima burns indicate that these flash burns resemble those caused by other thermal injuries except that this radiant energy is applied to the surface of the human body in a very rapid, rather than a longer period of time. The late Everett Evans,[22] an astute student of this problem, centered his advice on the following principles; (1) for the *control of pain* he advised morphia, as do I, but others argue against this agent because of the danger of respiratory depression. He also suggests the use of barbiturates. (2) Concerning *the use of closed dressings,* it is likely that this advice would not be practical because of the problems of personnel and surgical supplies. Unquestionably, the thousands of burns due to an atomic explosion would *de facto* be treated by the open-air (exposure) method whether the defense plan called for it or not. (3) *Prevention and treatment of burn shock* is accomplished by oral administration of fluids and electrolytes in patients with burns of less than 20 per cent of the surface area of the body and by intravenous administration of plasma substitutes, fluids and electrolytes in those more gravely burned. (4) *Antibiotic therapy,* now of disputed value, was recommended by Evans.

It is likely that this therapy, even if planned, would not be executed following mass atomic disaster because of the paucity of personnel, drugs and equipment.

Brown and Glover [10] concentrated on the collection, transportation, concentration, and sorting of cases in their recent treatise on this subject. Butterfield, Seager, Dixey and Treadwell [12] of London recently contributed a unique study on the effects of flash burns (infrared and white-light) on volunteer human subjects.

Summary

The management of burns by the correlation of the local treatment of the burned area and the management of the general organic state of the burned patient is outlined. Attention is called to the fact that superficial burns are not important unless they involve such a large percentage of surface area of the body that life is threatened. The exception to this statement is the depigmentation caused by first and second degree burns among Negroes. The principles of fluid balance are set down. Employment of these principles has resulted in the survival of a greater number of individuals with extensive burns of the surface of the body. Deep burns call for early removal of thermal slough by surgical excision or by chemical (enzymatic) débridement (pyruvic acid local therapy) in selected cases. Immediate surgical excision and skin-grafting is the therapy of choice for certain of the deep burns. The survival of a patient with extensive loss of skin presents the serious problem of surgical coverage of the wound by skin-grafting. Improvements in the surgical armamentarium (dermatomes) have facilitated the procurement of thick-split grafts of skin by the surgeon of average experience. Coverage of the wounds of deep burns by thick-split grafts of skin affords permanently useful surfaces. In cases of extensive loss of skin, homologous grafts of skin may be useful in restoring the general condition of the patient to a favorable level in preparation for necessary reparative surgery. Such grafts must be excised and replaced by autogenous skin grafts after a few weeks, before the dissolution of the homologous grafts sets up excessive fibrous tissue reaction, an unfortunate and unfavorable development. Neglected burns result in contractural deformity and ulceration. These complications can be met effectively only by the complete excision of regional scar tissue and coverage of the resultant defect by skin grafts, supplemented by more extensive transplantations of tissue.

Correlation of local and general management of the burned patient and the early replacement of deep burns by skin graft result in lowered mortality, diminished period of morbidity, and freedom from deformity.

References

[1] ALLEN, H. S., and KOCH, S. L.: The treatment of patients with severe burns. Surg. Gynec. & Obst. 74: 914—1024, 1942.

[2] ALTEMEIR, W. A., COITH, R. L., CULBERTSON, W. R., and TYTELL, A.: Enzymatic débridement of burns. Ann. Surg. 134: 581—587, 1951.

[3] ARTZ, C. P., and REISS, E.: The Treatment of Burns. Philadelphia, W. B. Saunders Co., 1957.

[4] DAVIS, J. H., and AMSPACHER, W. H.: The exposure treatment of burns. Ann. Surg. 137: 456—464, 1953.

[5] BARKER, D. E.: Cutting skin grafts with the vacutome. Plast. & Reconstruct. Surg. 5: 188—192, 1950.

[6] BERKOW, S. G.: Value of surface-area proportions in the prognosis of cutaneous burns and scalds. Am. J. Surg. 11: 315—317 (Feb.) 1931.

[7] BLOCKER, T. G., JR., BLOCKER, V., LEWIS, S. R., and SNYDER, C. S.: Experiences with the exposure method of burn therapy. Plast. & Reconstruct. Surg. 8: 87—93, 1951.

[8] BROWN, J. B.: The repair of surface defects with thick-split skin grafts. South. M. J. 28: 408—415, 1935.

[9] FRYER, M. P., RANDALL, P., and LU, M.: Postmortem homografts as "biological dressings" for extensive burns and denuded areas; immediate and preserved homografts as life-saving procedures. Ann. Surg. 138: 618—630, 1953.

[10] BROWN, K. L., and GLOVER, D. M.: Initial treatment of burns in mass casualties. J. A.M. A. 165: 643—646, 1957.

[11] BULL, J. P., and LENNARD-JONES, J. E.: Impairment of sensation in burns and its clinical application as test of depth of skin loss. Clin. Sc. 8: 155—169, 1949.

[12] BUTTERFIELD, O. B. E., SEAGER, E. R. D., DIXEY, J. R. B., and TREADWELL, E. E. E.: Observations on flash burning of human subjects in the laboratory using infrared and predominantly white light source. Surg. Gynec. & Obst. 103: 655—665, 1956.

[13] CONNELL, J. F., BOWE, J. J., DEL GUERCIO, L., and ROUSSELOT, L. M.: Evaluation of present day concepts in the treatment of the severely burned patient. Am. J. Surg. 93: 694—701, 1957.

[14] CONNOR, G. J., and HARVEY, S. C.: The pyruvic acid method in deep clinical burns. Ann. Surg. 124: 799—810, 1946.

[15] Conway, H.: Dupuytren on burns. Am. J. Surg. 87: 101—119, 1954.

[16] —: Marjolin's ulcer. In CONWAY, H.: Tumors of the Skin. Springfield, Ill., Charles C Thomas, 1956, pp. 208—211.

[17] —: Whole-thickness grafts in correction of contractures due to burn scars. Ann. Surg. 109: 286—291, 1939.

[18] COPE, OLIVER, et al.: Expeditious care of full-thickness burn wounds by surgical excision and grafting. Ann Surg. 125: 1—22, 1947.

[19] DAVIDSON, E. C.: Tannic acid in the treatment of burns. Surg., Gynec. & Obst. 41: 202—221, 1925.

[20] DINGWALL, J. A., and ANDRUS, W. DE W.: A comparison of various types of local treatment in a controlled series of experimental burns in human volunteers. Ann. Surg. 120: 377—386, 1944.

[21] — and LORD, J. W.: The fluorescein test in the management of tubed (pedicle) flaps. Bull. Johns Hopkins Hosp. 73: 129—131, 1943.

[22] EVANS, E. I.: The burn problem in atomic warfare. J. A. M. A. 143: 1143—1146, 1950.

[23] —: The early management of the severely burned patient. Surg., Gynec. & Obst. 94: 273—282, 1952.

[24] — et al.: Fluid and electrolyte replacement in severe burns. Ann. Surg. 135: 804—817, 1952.

[25] HARKINS, H. N.: The Treatment of Burns. Springfield, Ill., Charles C Thomas, 1942.

[26] HUMMEL, R. P., Lanchantin, G. F., and ARTZ, C. P.: Clinical experiences and studies in Curling's ulcer. Research Report NR. U. S. Army Surgical Res. Unit, Brooke Army Medical Center, Fort Sam Houston, Texas, 1956.

[27] —, RIVERA, J. A., and ARTZ, C. P.: Evaluation of several antibiotics used locally on granulating burn wounds. Research Report NR. 13—57, U. S. Army Surgical Research Unit, Brooke Army Medical Center, Fort Sam Houston, Texas, Nov. 1957.

[28] HYATT, G. W.: The Navy's wonderful tissue bank. Hosp. Management 81: 41—45, 1956.

[29] JACKSON, D. M.: Pseudomonas pyocyanea in burns. Lancet 2: 137—147, 1951.

[30] —: A clinical study of the use of skin homografts for burns. Brit. J. Plast. Surg. 7: 26—43, 1954 (as suggested by Mowlem—1950).

[31] LANGOHR, J. J., OWEN, C. R., and COPE, O.: Bacteriologic study of burn wounds. Ann. Surg. 125: 452—504, 1947.

[32] MACMILLAN, B. G., and ARTZ, C. P.: A planned evaluation of early excision of more than twenty-five per cent of the body surface in burns. Research Report NR 9—56, U. S. Army Surgical Res. Unit, Brooke Army Medical Center, Fort Sam Houston, Texas, 1956.

[33] —: Management of the Cocoanut Grove burns at the Massachusetts General Hospital. Ann. Surg. 117: 801—965, 1943.

[34] MELOY, W. C., and LETTERMAN, G. S.: The Electro-Dermatome. Plast. & Reconstruct. Surg. 6: 84—87, 1950.

[35] MONCRIEF, J. A.: Third-degree burns of the dorsum of the hand. Research Report NR 5—57, U.S. Army Surgical Res. Unit, Brooke Army Medical Center, Fort Sam Houston, Texas.

[36] PADGETT, E. C.: The calibrated skin graft—a new principle and a new type of graft. Surg., Gynec. & Obst. 69: 779—793, 1939.

[37] PULASKI, E. J., ARTZ, C. P., SHAEFFER, J. R., HUCKABEE, W. E., MITCHELL, R. C. and RUSSELL, J. P.: Exposure (open) treatment of burns. U.S. Armed Forces M. J. 2: 769—776, 1951.

[38] REESE, J. D.: Dermatape: a new method for the management of split-skin grafts. Plast. & Reconstruct. Surg. 1: 98—105, 1946.

[39] REISS, E., STIRMAN, J. A., ARTZ, C. P., DAVIS, J. H., and AMSPACHER, W. H.: Fluid and electrolyte balance in burns. J. A. M. A. 152: 1309—1313, 1953.

[40] SCHWEITZER, R. J., and BRADSHER, J. T., JR.: Acid débridement of burns with phosphoric acid gel. New England J. Med. 244: 705—709, 1951.

[41] SEEGER, S. J.: The treatment of burns. In LEWIS' Practice of Surgery. Hagerstown, Maryland, W. F. Prior Co., 1937, vol. I, chap. 17.

[42] SULZBERGER, M. A., KANOF, A., and BAER, R. L.: Studies on acid débridement of burns. Ann. Surg. 125: 418—430, 1947.

[43] UNDERHILL, F. P., et al.: Studies on the mechanism of water-exchange in animal organisms (superficial burns). Am. J. Physiol. 95: 302—338, 1930.

[44] WALLACE, A. B.: The exposure treatment of burns. Lancet 1: 501—504, 1951.

[45] WELLS, D. B.: The treatment of electric burns by immediate resection and skin graft. Proc. Connecticut M. Soc. (May 22) 1929.

[46] — et al.: Relation of tannic acid to liver necrosis occurring in burns. New England J. Med. 226: 629—636, 1942.

[47] YOUNG, F.: Immediate skin grafting in the treatment of burns. Ann. Surg. 116: 445—451, 1942.

II. FRACTURES — GENERAL CONSIDERATIONS

CHAPTER 11

THE X-RAY IN FRACTURE TREATMENT

Nathaniel Finby, M.D.

The diagnosis of a fracture, a break in the continuity of bone, is usually not difficult with routine radiographic study. Excellent radiographic technic is imperative, however, for the diagnosis of the fine, linear, nondisplaced or impacted fracture, or normal bone (absence of fracture).

The radiograph should show sharp bone texture with fine detail. Motion and underpenetrated films are the chief sources of error requiring re-examination

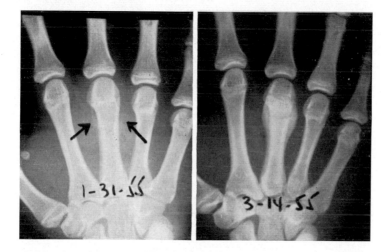

Fig. 1— Stress (fatigue) fracture of third metacarpal. First seen on January 31, 1955 without history of trauma with evidence of early healing. Union seen on March 14, 1955.

with proper technic. The entire bone or the nearest joint should be visualized for proper localization. For medicolegal reasons the film must be identified with date, side and name or number of the patient.

Multiple projections are necessary. In most instances two right angle views will suffice, but oblique films are especially useful in fractures of the carpal scaphoid, tibial shaft, posterior neural arch of the lumbar spine, ankle, skull and face. Special radiographic positions are usually necessary for complete study of the first and second cervical vertebra, patella, knee joint, olecranon, scapula and calcaneus. If good bone detail is obtained, these studies are sufficient to visualize almost all fractures. Rarely, tomography and stereoscopy will allow visualization of an otherwise occult fracture.

Types of Fracture

There are four major types of fracture. These are related to etiology as follows:

1. *Violence* — direct or indirect.

2. *Stress or Insufficiency* (fatigue, march, etc.). Usually transverse, these are seen most commonly in metatarsals, tibia and fibula (fig. 1).

3. *Pathologic* — due to local or generalized disease of bone (fig. 2). Usually transverse or marginal, these fractures are related to minimal trauma.

4. *Milkman's fracture* (Looser's or Umbau Zones). These are symmetric stress fractures in diseased bone undergoing pathologic healing.

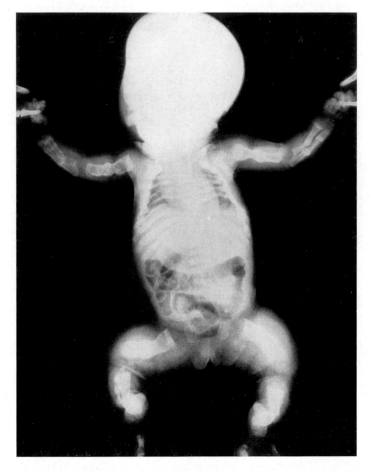

Fig. 2—Pathologic fractures in infant with osteogenesis imperfecta.

Description of Fracture

Apposition and alignment must be clearly described; usually the displacement of the distal fragment is recorded. The appearance of the fracture line may be described (fig. 3) as transverse, oblique, spiral, Y, T, comminuted, epiphyseolysis, impacted, avulsion, greenstick (torus), penetrating, etc.

Changes in the soft tissues such as calcification, swelling, gas shadow or foreign body should be noted. Remember that soft tissues (except for fat) are of unit density and cannot be differentiated. Especially important is the fact that soft tissue density between fracture fragments appears the same whether it be blood, early callus, muscle, periosteum or other soft tissue structure.

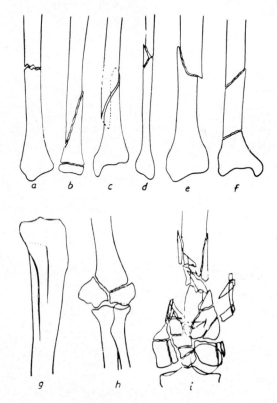

Fig. 3 Appearance of fracture may be described as: (A) transverse, (B) oblique, (C) spiral, (D) triangular, (E) flute mouthpiece, (F) multiple, (G) longitudinal, (H) Y fracture, and (I) severely comminuted fracture. (From Schinz et al.: Roentgen Diagnostics, New York, Grune & Stratton, Inc., Vol. I.)

Errors in Diagnosis

Normal variants are commonly mistaken for fractures. Accessory bones of the ankle, feet (fig. 4), hand and wrist are the most common sources of difficulty. The os acetabuli and os acromiale as well as the bipartite patella or other sesamoids are normal variants simulating fracture. Other common causes of error are Schmorl's nodes in the vertebra, limbus vertebra, (fig. 5), vascular marking (fig. 6) and bifid epiphyses. The clinical picture is extremely important in the diagnosis of fractures and should always be correlated with the radiographic appearance. The opposite side is always available for comparison study (fig. 7) which is helpful in difficult problems. It is good

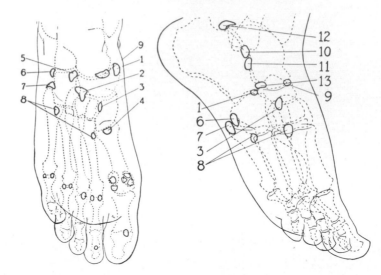

Fig. 4—Schematic diagram to show sesamoid bones and supernumerary bones of the foot. (1) Os tibiale externum; (2) processus uncinatus; (3) intercuneiforme; (4) pars peronea metatarsalis; (5) cuboides secundarium; (6) os peroneum; (7) os vesalianum; (8) intermetatarseum; (9) accessory navicular; (10) talus accessorius; (11) os sustentaculum; (12) os trigonum; (13) calcaneus secundarius. (From McNeill; Roentgen Technique, Springfield, Ill., Charles C. Thomas.) The most common of these are: 1, 6, 7, 9 and 12.

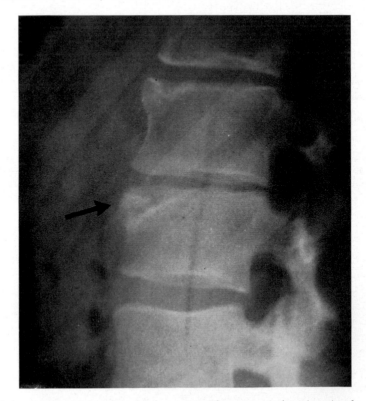

Fig. 5—Limbus vertebra (*arrow*) in lumbar spine. This congenital variant is often mistaken for fracture.

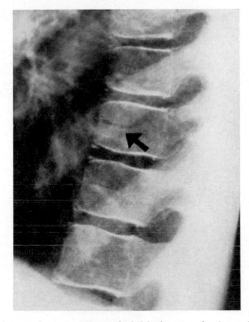

Fig. 6–Lateral view lower thoracic spine of child showing horizontal radiolucent strip in mid portion of the vertebral body. This normal vascular channel may be mistaken for fracture. Note the ossification centers in the annular cartilaginous rings at superior and inferior margins of vertebral body. These may be mistaken for fracture fragments.

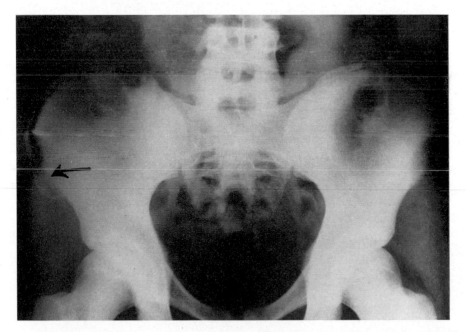

Fig. 7–Fracture of right iliac crest in a young man (*arrow*). Comparison with normal side facilitates diagnosis.

routine to radiograph the opposite extremity of all children after trauma for comparison study. Fresh fracture edges are sharp and serrated in contrast to the smooth, round edge of accessory bones. Of course, a true fracture will show signs of healing and bony callus; a normal variant remains unchanged.

The occult fracture occurs when the thin break in trabecular structure is hidden because of perfect position of the fragments. These are seen chiefly in the carpal scaphoid, os calcis, spiral fracture of tibia with intact fibula in children, femoral or radial necks, vertebral bodies and their processes,

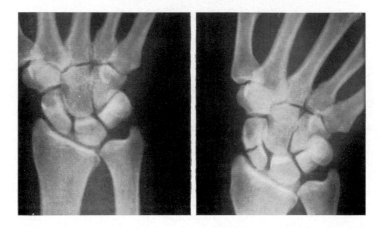

Fig. 8—Fractured scaphoid not seen when hand placed in neutral position (*left*) but demonstrated clearly by traction effected by mild ulnar deviation of the hand (*right*).

condylar fractures about the knee, and insufficiency fractures. Tomography and stereoscopy may be helpful. If the clinical findings are positive for fracture, a negative radiographic study should be disregarded and the patient treated for a fracture. A delayed film will show resorption at fracture site which widens the fracture line. Later there is bony callus. Occasionally traction, performed only by the physician, may aid in diagnosis (fig. 8).

Second fractures are occasionally missed because attention is focused on the more obvious lesion. In any dislocation, check for an avulsion fracture. With a fractured os calcis, check for compression fracture in the spine. With a dislocated radius, check for an upper ulnar shaft (Monteggia) fracture. With a displaced lower tibia (ankle) fracture, check the proximal fibula.

Reduction and Immediate Treatment

Always treat the patient and not the x-ray film. Remember that the soft tissues are not visualized as separate structures — nerves, blood vessels, muscle, etc.

Alignment is of most importance near joints, especially the ankle and knee. Alignment is least important in long bone shaft fractures of children. The normal alignment at the major joints should be known before attempting reduction (fig. 9). The opposite side provides a ready opportunity for comparison.

Apposition is important since a large gap causes slower healing. Impaction thus results in more rapid healing. Rotation of fragments and separate small fragments should be noted.

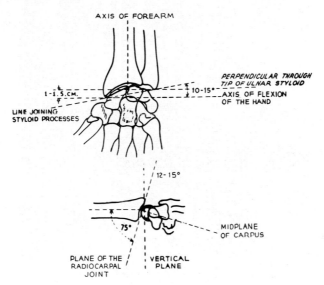

Fig. 9—Axial relations of the wrist. (From Meschan: An Atlas of Normal Radiographic Anatomy, Philadelphia, W. B. Saunders Co.)

The postreduction film, usually in plaster, should be checked for apposition, alignment and joint relationships. Metallic fixation should be described as to type, placement and position (fig. 10).

Course of Fracture Healing

The first radiographic change is a resorptive increase in the width of fracture cleft (in 68 per cent) with associated smoothing of sharp edges. Callus is not seen until calcium salts are deposited (fig. 11). Periosteal callus predominates in shaft fractures; medullary callus predominates in metaphysis, epiphysis and short flat bone fractures (fig. 12), and is often difficult to recognize. The well reduced fracture shows less callus than the disrupted fracture. The fracture cleft sometimes extends into the callus as a radiolucent line.

Healing is rapid with signs of union in one month in the infant, two months in the adolescent and four months in a 50 year old man. The impacted, long oblique or spiral fractures show more rapid union than horizontal fractures. Fractures of long bones near joints, in general, heal more quickly because of a rich blood supply. However, the distal fragment of lower shaft fractures of tibia, humerus and ulna may retard healing because of poor blood supply (distance from nutrient artery).

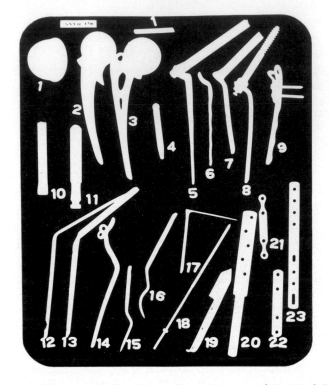

Fig. 10–(A) X-ray surgical appliance chart. (Courtesy of Dr. Fred Deck.)

1. Smith-Peterson vitallium cup.
2. Fred Thompson hip prosthesis.
3. Austin Moore hip prosthesis.
4. Judet acrylic prosthesis (hip).
5. Smith-Peterson nail with McLaughlin bar.
6. McLaughlin bar (obsolete).
7. Jewett nail.
8. Lorenzo screw and plate.
9. Lorenzo plate (obsolete).
10. Smith-Peterson nail.
11. Böhler nail.
12. Moore blade plate.
13. Neufeld nail.
14. Moe plate.
15. Blount plate.
16. Curved Blount plate.
17. Wright knee plate.
18. Austin Moore nail (hip).
19. Bosworth spline (shoulder).
20. Bosworth spline (femur).
21. Sherman plate.
22. Venable plate.
23. Venable coaptation splint.

Union is denoted by a continuous external bridge of callus or uniformly calcified callus of bone density between fragments.

Consolidation means the uniform, uninterrupted calcification and consolidation of external callus with the development of continuous trabeculae across the fracture site.

Dead bone appears more dense than neighboring normal bone. This is occasionally seen with certain fractures of the femoral neck and carpal scaphoid when blood supply of a fragment is lost. The middle fragment of a double fracture or a large isolated fragment may show similar change.

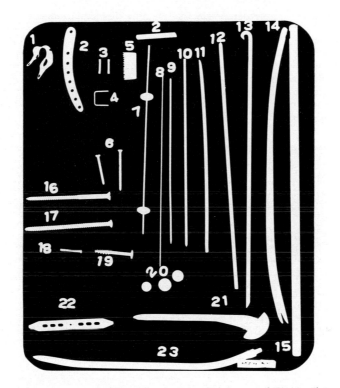

Fig. 10—(B) X-ray surgical appliance chart. (Courtesy of Dr. Fred Deck.)

1. Elbow (trochlear) prosthesis (Wade).
2. Wilson spinal fusion plate.
3. Michel clips.
4. Staple (Downing).
5. Brown corrugated fasteners.
6. Collison screws.
7. Web tibial bolt.
8. Kirschner wire.
9. Guide wire.
10. Steinman pin.
11. Küntscher intramedullary nail (forearm).
12. Hanson-Street diamond shaped nail (intramedullary).
13. Rush intramedullary nail.
14. Küntscher nested intramedullary nail (tibia).
15. Küntscher clover-leaf nail (intramedullary) femur.
16. Arthrodesis wood screw.
17. Arthrodesis full threaded screw.
18. McLaughlin navicular screw.
19. Bosworth acromioclavicular screw.
20. Fett navicular balls.
21. Neer humeral head prosthesis.
22. Livingston intramedullary bar.
23. Lottes intramedullary nail (tibia).

Weight-bearing decisions depend on correlation of clinical and radiographic information. The clinical signs of healing are usually dependable and "weight-bearing" may be permitted in fractures of metatarsals, clavicle and metacarpals before radiographic signs of union appear. The x-ray is of most importance when the blood supply is poor. Radiographic signs of union are essential in femoral neck, carpal scaphoid and long bone shaft fractures. Radiographic study after three weeks of activity will show deossification and some resorption of callus when union is not sound.

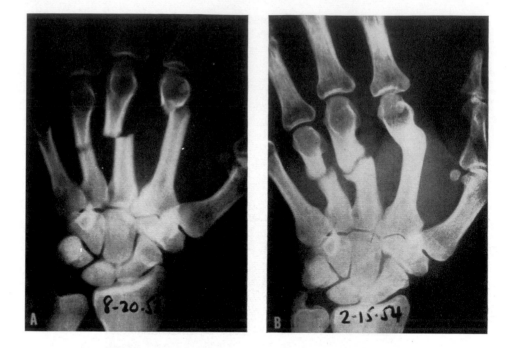

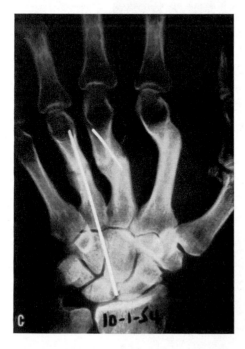

Fig. 13–(A) Fresh fracture of metacarpals 2, 3, 4.

Fig. 13–(B) Six months later there is non-union of fractures in metacarpals 3 and 4. Note smooth fracture margins, persistent gap and marginal sclerosis.

Fig. 13–(C) Union 7½ months later after metallic fixation.

CHAPTER 12

OPEN FRACTURES

ROBERT LEE PATTERSON, JR., M.D.

An open fracture is one with associated damage to the soft parts, producing an opening to the outside. Open fractures (formerly called compound fractures) can be of two types: those occurring from within - out, and those occurring from without - in. The former take place when the force which produces the fracture bruises the undersurface of the skin and the bone extrudes through the soft parts. The latter, which is the common war injury, results from an object such as a bullet penetrating the soft parts, striking the bone and fracturing it, the foreign body either remaining in the body or leaving it. Another example of this second type occurs when an extremity strikes against a fixed object which penetrates the soft parts and bone. The main difference between the two types of fracture is one of contamination. For example, it is probably reasonable to assume that a woman who falls in her own house, having had a bath a short time before, and sustains an open injury, for example, of the ankle joint, will have less contamination and less chance of infection if properly treated, than a man who sustains a gunshot wound or has a brick strike the tibia, the wound being contaminated by clothing, city filth or the bacteria from the ground on which he falls. MacFee [1] and his group did proper débridements on aviators shot by high velocity bullets at about 20,000 feet. These young men had probably had a bath on that morning or the day before and were relatively clean. With primary closure of their wounds, he found about 5 per cent infection. Later Cutler, [2] in studying a group of cases half of whom received penicillin with their surgery and half of whom did not, found on proper evaluation, that on closure of the wound following débridement there was about 9 per cent infection in both groups. This proves that the main factor involved in open fractures is adequate surgical care. The best axiom and dictum is not to underestimate the severity of a fracture or soft part damage associated with an opening outside of the normal body tissues.

Any bone is subject to a fracture and to an open fracture. From the series of cases in the fracture service, the most common areas involved are any site in the tibia including the ankle joints, and the forearm including the wrist.

To cover properly the subject of open fractures, we shall utilize the following sequence:

1. first aid care at scene of accident
2. care in the emergency room
3. definitive care in operating room
4. comments on open joint injuries

109

First Aid Care

It is now unusual for doctors to ride in ambulances. It is also usually impossible for a doctor to be at the scene of the accident. Therefore, every effort should be expended to make the public conscious of the severity of fractures and to teach them what to do until an attendant or other qualified person who knows what to do arrives. These persons may be trained by the Boy Scouts, the Red Cross or by our public services, such as the police and fire departments.

The patient should be made as comfortable as possible. He should be covered with a coat or with anything available, to help to keep him warm until assistance arrives. It is desirable to raise the head off the cement or out of the mud, but before placing something under the head, one must be quite careful that there has not been such an injury as a fracture-dislocation of the cervical spine.

When a person has been hit by a taxi or has fallen off a curbstone, a group gathers in a very short time. Note the fact that air is necessary; everyone wants to help but is usually in the way; people are talking excitedly, which alarms the patient. Often, on the other hand, no one is willing to help and the patient simply lies on the ground. One should try to comfort the patient, wave away the excited people, get rid of the useless bystanders, and then proceed with the job of handling the fracture with its opening and its bleeding. If one sees gross deformity of the extremity, one knows that it is broken. If one sees blood oozing or if the patient says that he is bleeding, the chances are it is an open fracture.

The Splint

All local authorities and public departments and ambulances have Thomas splints, and in fractures of the lower extremity we firmly believe in their use, since this is still one of the best and easiest means of transporting any fracture of the lower extremities. The New York slogan that has spread everywhere, "Splint 'em where they lie," fortunately is known by most people. Do not remove the shoe. It may come in handy as a spot to aid in applying traction. If possible, without moving the patient, rip the trousers and apply the cleanest available object over the protruding ends of the bones. Usually several clean pocket handkerchiefs may be the only things at hand. They are placed directly over the fracture site or the bleeding areas and pressure is applied. If the ends of the bones are grossly contaminated with mud, dirt or filth, it is advisable to apply the Thomas splint with only enough traction to support the bones and to prevent them from moving. It is not advisable to attempt to exert enough traction to reduce them into the wound in the contaminated stage. The only time that we would consider full traction with reduction of dirty and contaminated bone ends is when there is any suspicion or evidence of circulatory embarrassment.

In regard to the care of fractures of the other long bones, the Thomas Splint or traction splint used on the upper extremity usually causes some sort of difficulty and is contraindicated. The proper means of supporting the upper extremity is at the side with any material wrapped around the arm gently and not tightly. When an injury to the upper extremity is obvious, the onlooker usually attempts to stand the patient up. However, there may be some other injury that is far more significant than the one to the arm, and then standing might cause great harm. If the patient has been knocked down by an automobile and one sees a definite open fracture of the upper extremity, whether of the wrist, forearm or humerus, elbow, shoulder or clavicle, the patient is to be treated as if he were in shock. He should be moved carefully to the nearest hospital for treatment.

The Tourniquet

There are extremely few instances in which a tourniquet is justified. As a rule all bleeding can be stopped by local pressure over the area of compounding. The hazards seen in the use of the tourniquet are multiple. For instance, (1) a tourniquet applied too lightly will obliterate venous return but will permit arterial bleeding with resultant blood loss; (2) a tourniquet applied distal to the wound may result in death; (3) the most severe complication arises when a tourniquet is applied too tightly to a limb in which there is already circulatory embarrassment. If, however, a patient arrives in the emergency room with a tourniquet in place, do not immediately remove it unless an operating room, artery forceps and an ample supply of plasma or, preferably, whole blood are available. The escape of even a very small amount of blood on the release of the tourniquet may cause death. It would be unforgivable for anyone to remove a tourniquet without having started proper transfusions and without having proper equipment to control the bleeding.

Care in the Emergency Room

What is most essential when a patient is brought into the hospital with an open fracture is his state as a whole. Any patient who sustains an open fracture of one of the large long bones, such as the humerus or tibia, is in mild shock regardless of how he looks. This shock can be from trauma, or from blood loss, or from both. The shock may be delayed. The blood of a patient with an open fracture of a long bone or a fracture into a joint should be immediately typed and crossmatched regardless of his general condition at the time. In the meantime a complete evaluation of his status must be made. Does he have other associated injuries? Are they more important than the fracture?

The second important factor is the time element following injury. Every hour counts. If we are dealing with a fracture that is compounded, operation is a necessity. Therefore, the operating room should be notified immediately. The operation should be performed only in a sterile operating room. The care of any open wound of the extremities with a fracture is not an outpatient or an emergency room procedure.

X-Ray

X-rays are taken in the emergency room under certain conditions. If the blood has been properly typed and crossmatched, and if there is no gross bleeding at the fracture site, and if the extremity is properly splinted so that in the taking of the x-ray no further soft part damage will be inflicted, then it may be justifiable to take x-rays in order to have some idea of what to plan in the operating room. But if there is any question of shock, delayed shock, improper immobilization or other associated injuries, x-ray examination should be deferred until the patient is on the operating room table where portable x-rays can be taken without futher harm. Circulation in a patient in shock is impaired and any sudden movement may change the whole chain of events.

Dressings

Every change of dressing increases the possibilities of contamination of the wound. However, if one does wish to remove the dressings applied at the scene of the accident in order to look at the bone and the extent of the wound, replace them with sterile dressings without moving the part.

Drugs

If a patient arrives in the emergency room and has been seen previously by his doctor, the latter should have made some notation as to whether or not morphine or a similar drug was administered. If there is no written statement, usually the individual accompanying the patient or the ambulance driver will know if a drug was given. This should then be recorded. Beginning in the middle of World War II, those who studied the problem of drugs radically changed the ideas previously held. Henry K. Beecher [3] has shown that if morphine is to be given to a person bordering on shock or who is in shock, it should be given only for pain. Blocking by procaine, as a method of treating shock, is past. However, when a patient has severe pain, which is unusual, morphine can and should be used, but it should be given in very small doses (8 mg.) intravenously. When there has been blood loss and the peripheral vessels are constricted and the limb is cold, the morphine is very slowly absorbed, if at all. Suddenly the patient receives antishock therapy such as warmth, transfusion, elevation of the feet, etc., and the morphine begins to be absorbed, and if another dose of morphine is now given for pain and restlessness, morphine poisoning may follow. Therefore, it is advisable to appraise the status of a patient in shock as to whether he actually has a tremendous amount of pain or is simply afraid. In the war, most of the wounds were not painful, but the patient was often terribly frightened. In such circumstances it is better to use sodium pentobarbital, $^1/_{10}$ Gm.

Tetanus Antitoxin and Toxoid and Gas Gangrene Serum

In the use of tetanus antitoxin or tetanus toxoid, it is the general feeling that any person who has not had tetanus toxoid within the past eight years, should be given 3,000—5,000 units of tetanus antitoxin after sensitivity has been determined. Stafford and Peterson and their associates have recently shown that in groups tested five and even 10 or 11 years after the booster injection of tetanus toxoid, over one-half have an effective level of circulating antibodies. There has been considerable discussion on this subject and experimental work has been done (Hale and Weiksner [4]) which showed that in the individual not previously immunized, the primary response to tetanus toxoid is inhibited by a high titre of circulating passive antibodies, but also showed that there does not seem to be any significant interference of the effect of the passive antitoxin by simultaneously given tetanus toxoid. It seems to be in keeping with the experimental evidence to wait for two or three weeks after the passive immunization before starting a course of active immunization with the toxoid. Boehler [5] says that it is the adequate cleaning up or débridement of a wound which prevents tetanus, and not the antitoxin. However, he does admit that all patients sustaining an open injury should be given a dose of tetanus toxoid before they leave the hospital.

The Manual of the American College of Surgeons states that antigas gangrene serum should not be used as a prophylactic measure, but only as a therapeutic measure after the diagnosis of gas gangrene has been made. It seems that there can be no question that early surgery is the important means of preventing gas gangrene. There are many spore-forming organisms that simulate *Clostridium welchii*. Amputation should never be performed without a definite diagnosis of gas gangrene. There are two types to consider: edematins and dry forms. Both are accompanied by a sense of apprehension and increased pulse rate out of proportion to the temperature. The character of the wound may either be a localized cellulitis or a definite gross involvement. With the advent of the antibiotics and the recognition of the proper early surgery, gas gangrene should not be too serious a factor.

Antibiotics

Every patient entering the fracture service with an open fracture is immediately placed on one of the broad spectrum antibiotics. Previous to their employment, localized cellulitis, involvement of the lymph system, and bacteremia and septicemia were common in late débridements and massive damage. The organism was usually the *beta hemolytic Streptococcus*. Luckily this organism is sensitive to penicillin and most of the antibiotics, and hence control of it has made for less postoperative infection. Every institution has its own problem with the resistant *Staphylococcus aureus*. Again remembering the work of Cutler, one must always keep in mind that antibiotic therapy is an adjunct only. It is not a substitute for good surgery, and it must not be expected to do the job of the surgeon. For a detailed discussion of antibiotic therapy see Chapter 7.

Care in the Operating Room

Débridement

With the patient properly anesthetized, operation is begun. The word, débridement, brought out in World War I and used extensively in World War II, meant to many surgeons only a simple cleansing of the wound. The word débridement was used so frequently in the last war and in Korea that it is not apt to carry the full impact of what the procedure should imply. It is more than a simple cleansing of the wound. Proper débridement is the opening and the exposure of the area involved, the removal of foreign material, the complete excision of devitalized tissue, and the elimination of blood clots and dead space. There is never any question as to whether débridement should be performed; the only question is the degree to which it should be carried out.

Every attempt should be made to move the extremities as carefully and gently as possible, in order to prevent further soft-part damage. If the bone ends are protruding from the wound, a simple sterile dry dressing is applied. Next, the extremity is shaved, always away from the wound. The dirt or any accumulation on the skin of the patient is now removed. It may be advisable to use ether first, but this should be followed by ordinary soap and water. Antiseptics should not be poured into the wound. Not only are they unable to kill all the bacteria in the wound, but they can also cause a chemical necrosis. The bone ends are then cleansed and freed from any foreign material, after which the area is draped and the operator changes his gloves and proceeds with sterile equipment.

Technic

If one is dealing with a simple penetrating wound or puncture wound, one may proceed by excision of the devitalized skin. There is one axiom that should be followed — that promulgated by Pool[6] in 1917 — to save as much skin as possible. We know that any devitalized skin must be removed, but only that part which is definitely devitalized. Sometimes this may be only a millimeter or two, and sometimes it may be one-eighth inch wide. An incision should be made in the longitudinal axis of the extremity, the proximal end beginning at one edge of the wound and the distal end at the opposite edge. One usually finds that the damage is far more extensive than the external surface would indicate. Use constant irrigation with normal physiologic saline, neither too hot nor too cold. Then remove any foreign bodies or any foreign materials as they are encountered.

An inspection of the character of the tissue damage is most important. Any loose or torn fascia should be excised, as well as any dead or devitalized muscle. Aids in determining viability are that normal muscle is red or pink and shows contractility when squeezed. Arterial supply to the remaining viable muscles must be preserved.

After proper care has been given to the soft parts, the fracture is reduced as nearly anatomically as possible. An anatomic reduction prevents further soft part damage, often makes it possible to cover the areas with normal tissue, and eliminates dead space where underlying infection could easily take place.

Tabulated below are some factors to be avoided:

1. Never remove a piece of bone that has any soft part attachment.

2. Never remove a large fragment even if completely free of soft part attachment.

3. Never ligate large masses of tissue or vessels that can be clamped and squeezed to stop bleeding.

4. Never cause more soft part damage by using extensive retraction with large retractors.

5. Never suture fascia.

6. Never ligate large particles of tissue.

7. Never use harsh antiseptics.

Closure of the Wound

It is impossible to lay down definite rules on the general principles of closing a wound. There are two primary decisions that can be made only by the surgeon after a proper débridement has been performed. The first is how to immobilize the fracture — whether to use internal fixation, traction or plaster. The second is whether to close the skin primarily, to do a primary skin graft or to carry out a delayed primary suture. The decision must rest essentially on the mature judgment of the surgeon. However, there are certain general principles which might be applicable at the time of operation on an individual case. If, in the judgment of the surgeon, he has been able to clean the wound properly and efficiently of all dead and foreign material, and to close dead spaces, if the wound did not appear severe at the outset and the amount of soft part damage was not great, if the accident occurred in the home following a bath and everything was relatively clean, then under these circumstances the use of metal as internal fixation, such as a screw or two screws or even an intramedullary rod, certainly may be indicated. But if there is any suspicion in the surgeon's mind that the wound was grossly contaminated to begin with, or that the soft-part trauma was great, or that there may not have been adequate cleansing, then the surgeon may simply apply plaster or some form of immobilization with or without traction. When wound healing has taken place, providing that everything else is progressing normally, he can proceed to take care of the case in any way his judgment dictates.

There is no question that one of nature's best methods of protection against infection is the closure that allows the soft parts to cover exposed bone. Often, however, it is impossible to do a primary closure, as for instance in the tibia, if the skin defect is large or if there is marked reaction around the area. In many of these cases, a relaxing incision can be made parallel to the exposure incision, thus relieving all the tension at the fracture site and allowing the skin to come together nicely and normally (figs. 1—5). After this procedure, the defect resulting from the relaxing incision may be covered by means of a split thickness graft from the thigh.

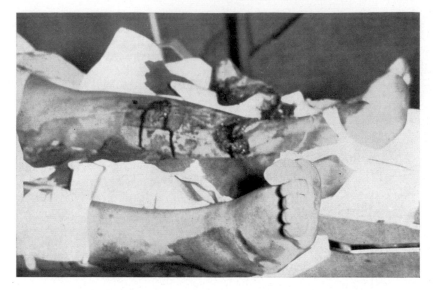

Fig. 1—Patient on arrival in emergency room. Note crescent opening with soft part loss in distal tibia and linear opening in proximal anterior crest.

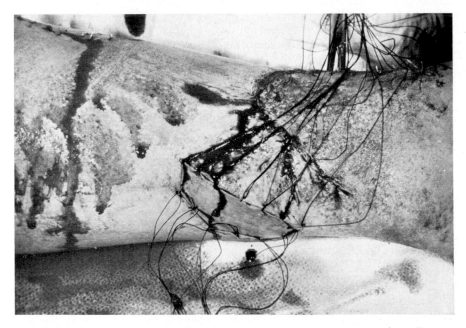

Fig. 2—Closure of distal opening with wire sutures after relaxing incision laterally. Note skin graft over this area. Sutures left very long.

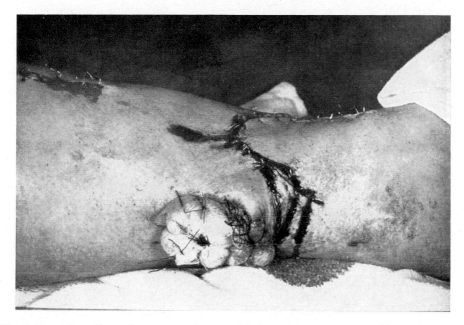

Fig. 3—Pressure puffs applied over graft area with long sutures to prevent floating of graft.

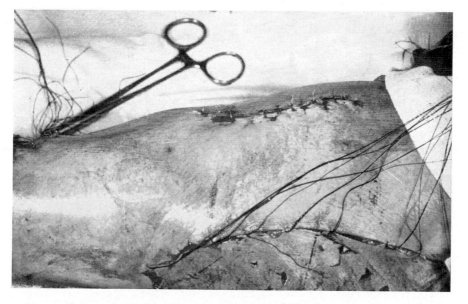

Fig. 4—Closure of proximal wound with relaxing incision covered by skin graft.

Because of the frequency with which this method of closure is used, especially in open fractures of the tibia, it is a standard technic of our Fracture Service to shave, clean, and prepare the skin of the thigh immediately after the fracture area is prepared. The thigh is draped separately. All necessary equipment for removing a skin graft, such as the dermatome, is at hand. We emphasize this additional preparation for two reasons: First,

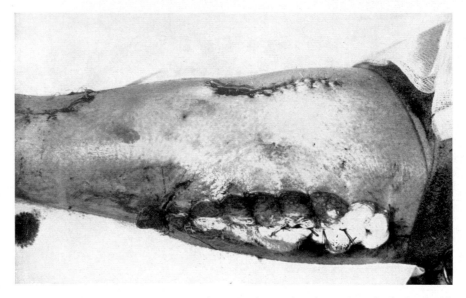

Fig. 5—Again closure with wire sutures of proximal wound and covering of relaxing incision.

when it is found impossible to approximate the skin at the fracture site without tension, the extra time required to prepare for a graft may be dangerous to a patient in or bordering on shock. Second, as a result, the operating surgeon, especially the young or inexperienced one, to save time may decide to put in a few loose sutures or even to approximate the skin edges under tension. Both these procedures are to be condemned. With proper planning, the donor site available and instruments ready, a relaxing incision followed by skin graft can be carried out easily and quickly.

It may be necessary at the time of the operation to do a primary skin graft on the wound. However, if the wound evidences contamination beyond the control of surgery, a secondary delayed primary suture is justifiable. Whether this is pulled together in a suture line or covered with a skin graft at five or seven days, is of little consequence; the main object is to convert an open wound to a closed wound.

Comments on Open Joint Injuries

Open injuries into joints are severe injuries. The fundamental principles laid down in the care of trauma to an extremity are equally if not more applicable when a joint is involved. Though with the aid of antibiotics the mortality rates are far less than during World War I, if infection does take place, a stiff joint is usually to be expected and amputation often results.

The essential factor in the care of an open joint wound is adequate exposure so that all foreign material can be removed. If there are loose pieces of articular cartilage in the wound, they should be removed. If, however, the articular cartilage is associated with a fragment of bone, it is advisable to leave this in place.

A thorough irrigation of the entire wound with normal saline should be carried out, with very gentle manipulation of the joint while irrigation is taking place. Following this, every effort must be made to suture the synovia of the joint. The suturing of the synovia is as important as any part of the operative procedure in that it offers a normal covering for the joint and affords protection by its powers of secretion, absorption and bacteriostatic action. Next, a simple gauze dressing is laid down to the region of the synovia and no attempt made to suture the quadriceps expansion, fascia or the skin. The procedure is concluded by the injection of an antibiotic and the application of plaster of Paris. For open injuries to the knee joint, a $1^1/_2$ plaster spica is advisable.

References

[1] MacFee, W.: The treatment of Air Force combat casualties. Ann. Surg. *120*: 1 (July) 1944.

[2] Cutler, E. C.: Personal communication.

[3] Beecher, H.: The Early Care of the Seriously Wounded Man, American Lecture Series. Springfield Ill., Charles C Thomas, 1952.

[4] Hale, H. W. Jr. and Weiksner, J. F.: Current therapy of tetanus. Am. J. Surg. *91*: 461, 1956.

[5] Boehler, L.: The Treatment of Fractures. New York, Grune & Stratton, Inc., 1956, vol. 1, p. 264.

[6] Pool, E. H.: The Early Treatment of Gunshot Wounds, The Oxford Surgery. London, Oxford University Press, 1921, p. 761.

CHAPTER 13

THE OPERATIVE TREATMENT OF FRACTURES

Preston A. Wade, M.D.

Operative reduction and immobilization of certain fractures are recognized and approved forms of treatment. As a result of improved technics of surgery and anesthesia, the advent of antibiotics, and the introduction of nonelectrolytic metals, many of the objections to operative fracture treatment have been overcome.

In spite of the advances in this field, the surgeon who operates on a fracture must still have adequate knowledge and training and be equipped with proper operative tools. *There is no substitute for sound surgical judgment and meticulous operative technic.* The simplest and most efficient treatment for the treatment of fractures is the "old fashioned" method of manual reduction and immobilization by means of plaster of Paris. In spite of the fact that we use operative methods in our clinic in many cases, the great majority of fractures are treated by manipulation and immobilization in plaster splints. If one embarks on operative treatment of a fracture, he must have very definite and reasonable indications for the operation, and he must weigh the difficulties and possible complications of the operation against the disadvantages of some other form of treatment. We do not consider operative treatment as "radical" or closed methods of treatment as "conservative." It may be that the operative method may be more conservative than a closed method.

The disadvantages of operating on a fracture are primarily those which may result from infection. One must make every effort to prevent infection, and this does not only mean reliance on antibiotics. Judgment as to the time of operation, attention to the condition of the skin and soft parts and the proper preparation of the patient all have a part in the preoperative considerations. At the operating table proper preparation and meticulous draping and covering of the skin about the wound are requirements often overlooked. It is necessary to use properly placed incisions, to handle the tissues gently and to insist on strict hemostasis. A tourniquet is useful and necessary on occasions, but its routine use in order to make the operation easy by neglecting surgical hemostasis is a mark of poor surgical technic. The careful closure of operative wounds and skin coverage of all operative areas are important in preventing the formation of sinuses with ultimate infection. Postoperative care of the limb with proper pressure dressings, elevation and constant observation are also essential in preventing infection.

The use of antibiotics as a prophylactic measure is a debatable question. However, in those cases in which obvious contamination will probably result, due to prolonged operative procedures and extensive exposure of tissue, prophylactic antibiotics are logical and proper. They should not be depended on, however, to prevent infection, in in view of the recent *staphylococcus aureus* hospital infections, one must constantly be on guard to prevent contamination and not depend on the antibiotics to make up for deficiencies in operative technic.

There are other disadvantages associated with operative treatment. The stripping up of periosteum and operative injury to soft parts may result in excessive bone formation, or myositis ossificans. In children the operative trauma may lead to stimulation of epiphyses to overgrowth. Furthermore, one must always bear in mind that plates, screws and rods are foreign bodies and in no way help to stimulate bone-healing. Although the use of intramedullary rods, particularly in the femur, seems to promote a much more rapid and extensive growth of external callus about the fracture site than occurs in any other method of treatment, there is no proof that the rod itself stimulates this growth. In almost every other situation, the presence of metal fixative apparatus actually causes a slowing down of the healing process, and the metal is useful only in maintaining reduction. The use of plates to immobilize a fracture has a very definite objection in that the plate prevents impaction and apposition of the fragments, particularly after the invariable period of bone absorption. This allows the fracture line to widen and makes it necessary for callus and new bone to jump a gap, thus prolonging the healing time. One of the advantages of intramedullary rods is that they allow impaction of fragments.

Indications for Operation

Operation on a fractured bone may be (1) one of necessity or (2) a method of choice.

Operation of Necessity. There are certain fractures in which it is generally recognized that operative treatment is the only effective method of dealing with the lesion, and the operation is therefore considered to be one of necessity. Examples of these fractures will be discussed briefly.

Open Fractures: Débridement should be done as a surgical emergency in all open fractures. The operation should be performed in an operating room under adequate anesthesia with sufficient help and equipment to perform a thorough and painstaking procedure. Delay in the operation or compromise in the details of the surgical technic are justifiable only in the presence of serious complications, such as head injuries, chest injuries or other conditions in which prolonged operation or anesthesia might endanger the patient's life. These complicating conditions must be bona fide contraindications to immediate operation of the fracture. Too often, delay in débridement or improper operative technic is excused on the basis of concomitant complicating injuries which in themselves are not truly contraindications to operation. Proper débridement implies enlargement of the wound, if necessary, along anatomic lines, thus allowing exposure of the involved area. The next step is the meticulous cleaning of the wound to remove all foreign material and obviously devitalized tissue. One must be

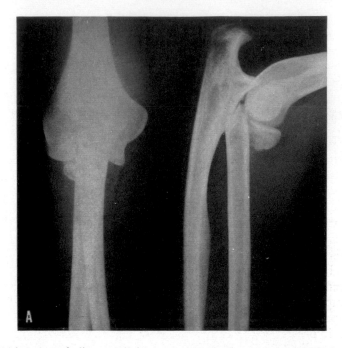

Fig. 1—(A) Dislocation of elbow with fracture of head of radius with marked displacement
in male of 28.

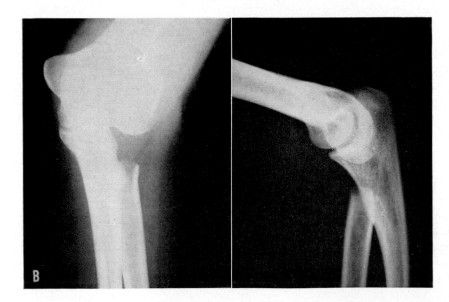

Fig. 1—(B) After reduction of dislocation and operative removal of head of radius.

exceedingly conservative in the treatment of bone and skin. Any sizable bone fragment should be left *in situ* even though it is completely deprived of its blood supply. Skin coverage is essential except in battle wounds or multiple disaster wounds. Preparation for flap coverage and skin shifting should be made before each operative procedure, and plans should be made

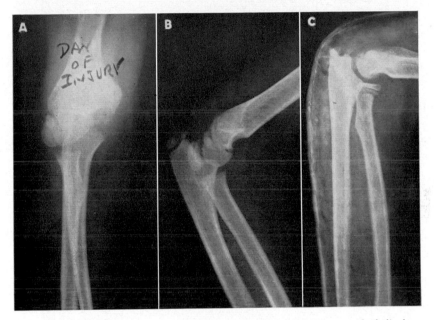

Fig. 2—(A and B) Fracture of head of radius in 8 year old child. Note marked displacement and rotation of radial head. (C) After operative reduction and replacement of head. Fixation by catgut suture.

to skin graft donor areas or defects caused by relaxing incisions. Local antiseptic and local antibiotic treatment of open wounds is not recommended.

Fractures of the Radial Head or Neck with Displacement of the Fragments or Fragment: In a fracture of the radial head or fracture of the neck of the radius with marked displacement of the fragments, a surgical procedure is necessary. In adults, removal of the head and neck just above the bicipital tuberosity is the method of choice (fig. 1). Occasionally, a fragment of the head may be removed, leaving the remainder of the head and neck to function normally.

In children a markedly displaced radial head which cannot be reduced by manual manipulation is one of the few indications for operative treatment. In these cases the radial head is replaced and sutured into position (fig. 2). On occasion the radial head is best fixed by means of a Kirschner wire driven through the lower end of the humerus into the medullary canal of the radius. This wire can be removed in 10 days, after the fragments have become glued together. Under no circumstances should the head of the radius be removed in a child.

Fracture of the Patella with Separation of the Fragments: Fracture of the patella with separation of the fragments must be treated exactly as a divided and separated ligament in any other part of the body (fig. 3 A). The integ-

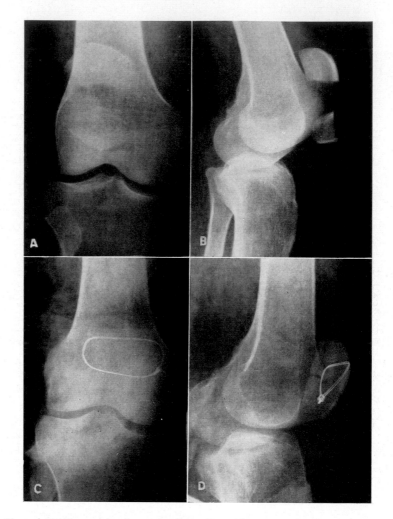

Fig. 3–(A and B) Transverse fracture of patella with separation of fragments. Proximal fragment is pulled upward and lower fragment is rotated anteriorly 90 degrees. This indicates complete tear of extensor mechanism including lateral expansions. (C and D) Lateral expansions have been sutured with silk. Patella sutured with stainless steel circumferential wire.

rity of the extensor mechanism of the knee must be repaired and the essential procedure is the suturing of the lateral expansions of the quadriceps tendon. This may be done with silk, catgut or stainless steel wires. The treatment of the patella itself may be accomplished by circumferential wire (fig. 3 B), making sure that the wire, particularly the knot, does not encroach

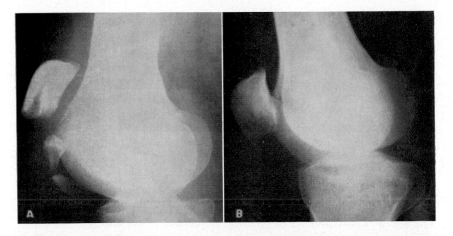

Fig. 4—(A) Fracture of patella with comminution. One large proximal fragment and two smaller distal fragments. (B) After excision of distal fragments, repair of lateral expansion of quadriceps and suture of patellar tendon to patella.

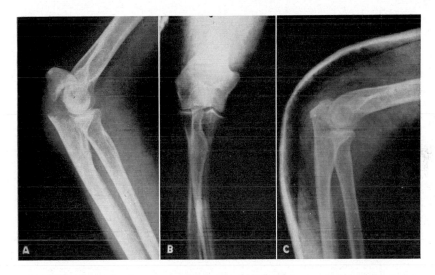

Fig. 5—(A) Fracture of olecranon with upward displacement of proximal fragment. (B) After suture of fragment to ulna by means of circumferential stainless steel wire — anterior-posterior view. (C) Lateral view.

on the articular surface of the patella or that it is not placed subcutaneously over the anterior surface. This method is more useful when the patella is fractured transversely across its middle. If there are one or two smaller fragments, they may be removed and the major fragment sutured to the ligament (fig. 4). Comminuted fractures often necessitate excision of the entire patella.

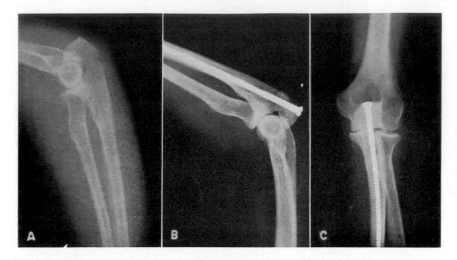

Fig. 6—(A) Fracture of olecranon with upward displacement of proximal fragment. (B) After fixation by means of vitallium malleable screw. Lateral view. (C) Anterior-posterior view.

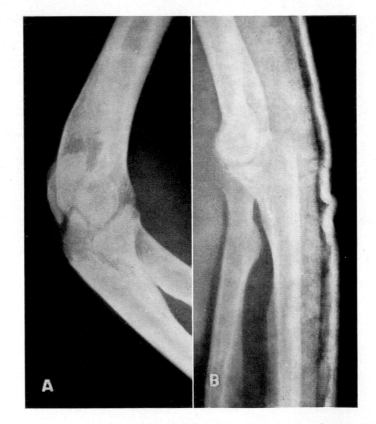

Fig. 7—(A) Fracture of olecranon with displacement. (B) After excision of proximal fragment and suture of triceps to ulna.

Fracture of the Olecranon Process with Separation of the Fragments: Fracture of the olecranon process with separation of the fragments necessitates a repair of the extensor mechanism of the elbow comparable to the procedure employed in repairing a rupture of the extensor mechanism of the knee.

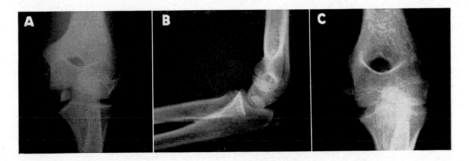

Fig. 8—(A) Fracture of medial epicondyle of humerus, with displacement into joint. Anterior-posterior view. (B) Lateral view. (C) After operative replacement of epicondyle and fixation by suture.

In this instance, the fractured fragment of the olecranon is fixed to the ulna by means of a circumferential wire (fig. 5), being careful to place the wire so that it is neither subcutaneous nor in contact with the articular surface. The wire must be of sufficient strength to withstand the tremendous

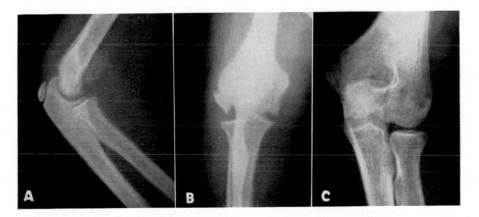

Fig. 9—(A) Fracture of capitellum of humerus with anterior displacement and rotation-lateral view. (B) Anterior-posterior view. Note defect in lower humerus. (C) Six months after operative replacement of fragment.

leverage of flexion of the elbow. The use of an intramedullary screw of sufficient length to secure a firm fixation of the proximal fragment is a useful procedure (fig. 6). Excision of a small proximal fragment of the olecranon is often a desirable method (fig. 7).

Fractures Involving the Joints in which a Loose Fragment Remains within the Joint: One of the best examples of this type of injury is the fracture of the medial epicondyle of the humerus which is often displaced within the joint by the pull of the attached muscles of the forearm (fig. 8). This condition commonly occurs in childhood and is one of the few indications for operating on children. The fragment may be replaced and sutured into position. On occasion it may be excised. It is acceptable to use a removable

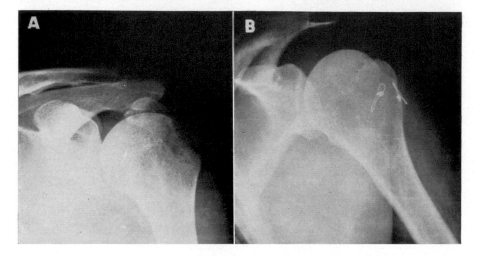

Fig. 10—(A) Fracture of greater tuberosity of humerus with displacement under the acromium. (B) After operative replacement of displaced fragment, sutured in place by means of stainless steel wire.

Kirschner wire to transfix the fragment in position. Another example is seen in the fracture of the capitellum with displacement (fig. 9). A small fragment may be removed or a large fragment replaced and held in position by transfixion with a removable Kirschner wire. The loose fragments within the knee joint often necessitate removal, particularly in the bumper type of fracture.

Fracture of the greater tuberosity of the humerus in which the proximal fragment is drawn under the acromium (fig. 10) also necessitates operative intervention and replacement of the fragment in its proper position.

Fractures of the Lateral Condyle of the Humerus with Marked Rotation, Especially in Children: Displaced fractures of the lateral condyle in children necessitate replacement and fixation by means of catgut suture (fig. 11) or transfixation by means of removable Kirschner wire. If the fragment is not perfectly replaced, there is invariably a growth disturbance of the lower end of the humerus which causes increase in the carrying angle and a cubitus valgus deformity. This does not usually interfere with function but it is an unsightly deformity.

On occasion late ulnar nerve palsy may result when the nerve is stretched because of the deformity. Figure 12 shows cubitus valgus deformity of

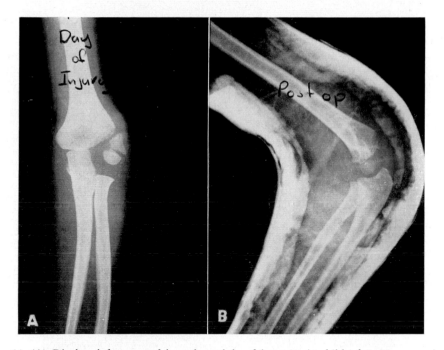

Fig. 11–(A) Displaced fracture of lateral condyle of humerus in child of 5. Note rotation of fragment. (B) After replacement of condyle and fixation by catgut suture.

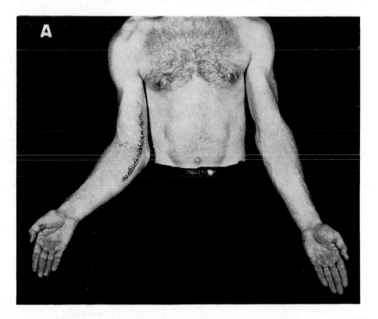

Fig. 12–(A) Male of 28 with increased carrying angle resulting from unreduced fracture of lateral condyle in childhood. Ulnar nerve palsy resulted. Photograph after transplantation of ulnar nerve.

the elbow in a male, 28 years old, who sustained a fracture of the lateral condyle in childhood. Ulnar nerve palsy developed 20 years later.

Intracapsular Fractures of the Neck of the Femur: It is now generally recognized that operative treatment of the intracapsular fractures of the neck of the femur is the only available means of contending with this very difficult problem. As is pointed out in the section on this fracture, the inter-

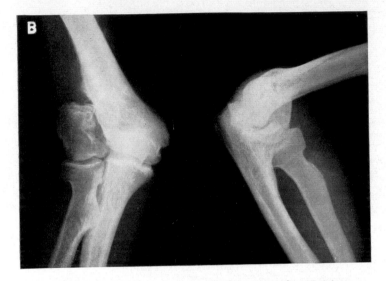

Fig. 12—(B) X-ray of elbow. (Same case as fig. 12 A.)

nal fixation may be accomplished by means of a Smith-Peterson nail, multiple nails or a variation of the nail with plate. There are some cases in which immediate resection of the head and replacement by means of metallic prosthesis is the method of choice.

Fractures in Adults with Interposition of Tissue, Preventing Closed Reduction: There are certain instances in which interposition of soft parts prevents reduction of a fracture, thus necessitating open operation. There is usually no excuse for operation on a child even though there may be interposition of soft tissue between the fragments. In almost every instance these fractures will heal soundly and firmly with sufficient callus bridging the gap between the displaced fragments without operation.

Fractures in Which Other Methods Have Been Tried and Have Failed to Secure Satisfactory Reduction and Immobilization: Operative procedure should be undertaken as soon as possible after the fracture has occurred, since delay may result in swelling due to increased hemorrhage and edema. The skin may break down from pressure of displaced fragments of bone, or fracture blebs may develop over the area through which the operative incision should be made. Therefore, it is unwise to try many so-called "conservative" methods in those cases in which operation is inevitable or seems the method of choice. However, in some instances, closed reduction should be attempted, and if it fails operation may be necessary to obtain a good result.

Nonunion: Operative methods are necessary in established cases of nonunion and in some cases of delayed union. In the treatment of nonunion

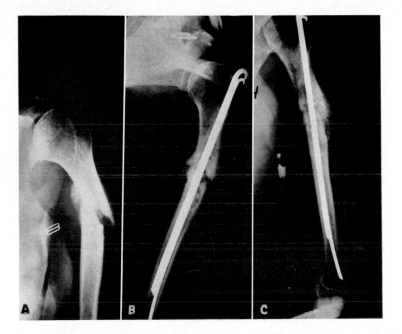

Fig. 13—(A) Nonunion of shaft of humerus nine months after injury. (B and C) After operation with insertion of two Rush nails and use of cancellous bone graft.

there are five essential principles: (1) Healthy skin coverage. It is essential that scar tissue, particularly thin scar tissue over subcutaneous bone, be excised and that the area be covered by healthy skin, sometimes by means of a skin flap. Efforts to operate on an ununited fracture through poor skin invariably lead to failure. (2) In cases of established nonunion the eburnated ends of the bone fragments must be excised to healthy bleeding bone before union can be expected. In cases of delayed union, it may not be necessary to open the fracture site and excise the bone end. (3) The bone ends must be firmly apposed and, if possible, impacted. (4) The fragments must be firmly immobilized, preferably by means of internal fixation. The intramedullary rod (fig. 13) affords the best method of internal fixation of fragments of an ununited fracture since it allows impaction of one fragment on the other. The internal fixation may be accomplished by means of plate and screws or a hard cortical tibial graft immobilizing the fragments by means of metallic screws (fig. 14). On occasion, the onlay graft serves the dual purpose of fixation and osteogenesis. The sliding bone graft serves the same purpose but because of its fragility, it does not serve the purpose of fixation as well as other types of graft. (5) Cancellous bone, preferably from the iliac crest of the patient, is placed about the fracture site as matchstick grafts, or the entire area is packed with cancellous bone chips. Cancellous bone from the bone bank is useful, and there is evidence to support the claim that it is as effective as autogenous bone. In our clinic we prefer autogenous bone.

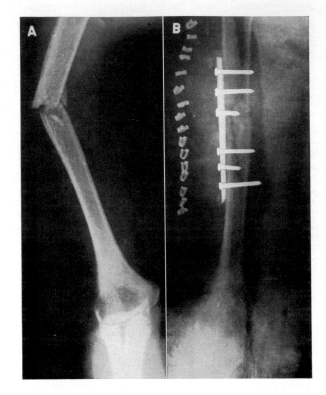

Fig. 14–(A) Nonunion of fracture of humerus ten months after injury. (B) Onlay bone graft fixed by vitallium screws. Cancellous bone grafts packed about fracture area.

Operation as a Method of Choice

There are other fractures in which operative treatment may be the method of choice. It is essential that the complications which may result from the operation be weighed against the advantages one expects to achieve.

There are certain fractures in which union is made more certain by operation. This applies to certain fractures of the tibia and certain fractures of the forearm such as isolated fractures of the ulna or radius.

Operation and internal fixation in many instances allows early ambulation with all of its advantages in preventing postoperative complications. Morbidity is greatly decreased by many operative procedures, and the expense to the patient and to the hospital is greatly decreased. In fractures of the shaft of the femur, intramedullary nailing allows early ambulation and shortens hospitalization.

Operative procedures may allow complete mobilization of contiguous joints or earlier mobilization than treatment by other methods. Intramedullary rod fixation of the femur allows immediate mobilization of the knee and ankle and prevents the stiffness which oftens results from immobilization in plaster or traction. Lag screw fixation of fracture of the navicular bone permits immediate freedom of motion of the hand and wrist. Insertion of the screw is difficult and is not recommended as a routine procedure (fig. 15).

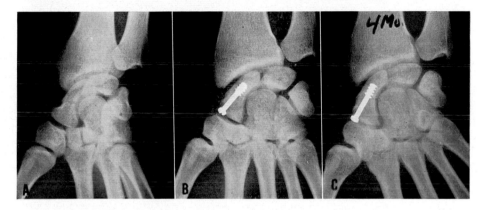

Fig. 15–(A) Fracture of carpal navicular at waist of bone. (B) One month after fixation by means of vitallium lag-screw (McLaughlin). No external immobilization. (C) Four months post operation. Fracture healed. No immobilization was necessary and patient returned to work as secretary 2 weeks after injury.

Early mobilization of the joints is no valid argument for internal fixation in children. Long immobilization of children's joints is well tolerated, and therefore there is no excuse for internal fixation in most instances.

There are certain fractures in which it is conceded that reduction may be difficult and immobilization almost impossible to obtain by external means. In fracture-dislocations of an anatomic head of the humerus (fig. 31), in the posterior lip fracture of the tibia, in cases in which more than 30 per cent of the articular surface is involved (fig 16) and in the unstable fractures of the ankle (fig. 17), operative interference may be the method of choice.

Displaced bumper fractures of the tibia are often best treated by bolt or bolt and plate so as to preserve the integrity of the joint surface (fig. 18).

When injuries to the soft parts, such as laceration of the nerves and tendons, demand operation, the coincident reduction and internal fixation of the accompanying fracture may be the most effective type of treatment. In many instances the repair or grafting of a lacerated artery may necessitate internal fixation of the accompanying bone in order to maintain perfect immobilization for repair of the blood vessel.

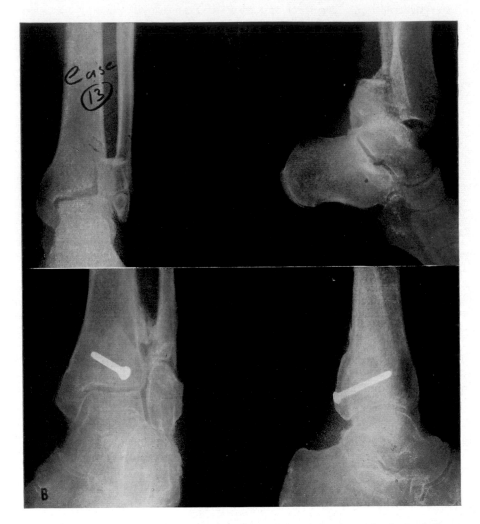

Fig. 16—(A) Fracture of lateral malleolus with posterior dislocation of talus and fracture of large fragment of posterior lip of tibia. (B) Reduction of dislocation and fixation of posterior lip of tibia by means of single screw.

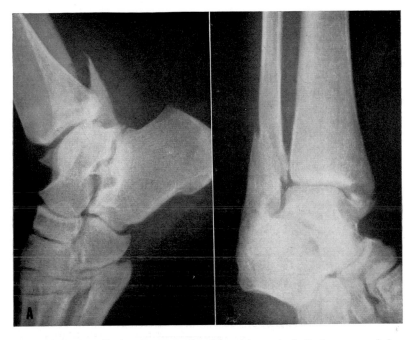

Fig. 17—(A and B) Bimalleolar fracture of ankle with marked displacement of fragments.

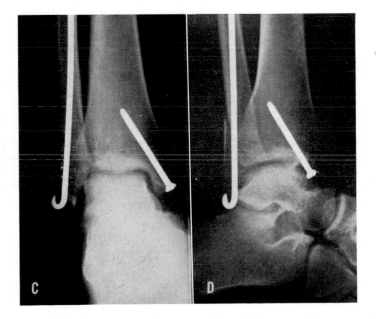

Fig. 17—(C and D) After operative reduction and immobilization of fragments by means of screw medial malleolus and Rush intramedullary nail in fibula.

Screws

In many oblique fractures, adequate fixation by means of two or more transversely placed screws may be all that is necessary to maintain good reduction. The screws should be inserted at right angles to the long axis of the bone (fig. 21) rather than at right angles to the fracture line. In

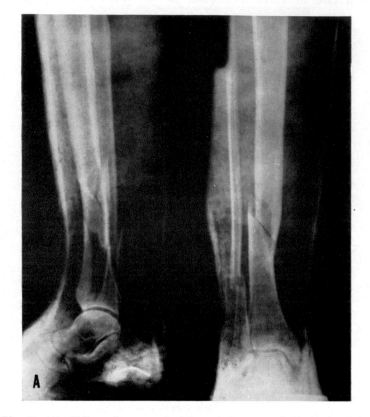

Fig. 21–(A) Oblique fracture of tibia and fracture of fibula in adult.

some instances, in which the obliquity of the fracture line is short, it may not be possible to place the screws at right angles to the long axis of the bone. It is unwise to depend on a single screw to fix an oblique fracture, since this permits rotation of the fragments on the screw. However, fractures of a single condyle and fractures of the medial malleolus are often best secured by means of a single screw (fig. 22).

Intramedullary Nailing

The operative management of long bone fractures has been revolutionized during the past 15 years by the use of medullary nails or rods. Fractures of the shaft of the femur are particularly suitable to this form of treatment. In addition to the femur, other long bones and metacarpals have also been treated by means of intramedullary rods. Intramedullary fixation allows

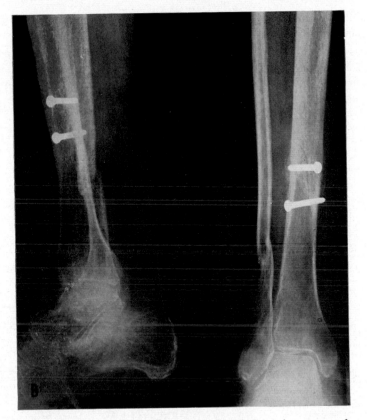

Fig. 21—(B) Six months after operative reduction and fixation by means of two screws. Note screws are placed at right angles to long axis of tibia. Cancellous bone chips have been placed about fracture.

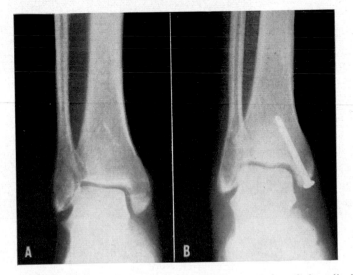

Fig. 22—(A) Bimalleolar fracture of ankle with displacement of medial malleolus. (B) At operation reduction was easily achieved after removal of interposed soft tissue. Fixed by means of single screw.

early joint function and permits impaction of the fragments, which, in turn, promotes healing of the bone.

Various types of nails have been devised. The original Küntscher hollow "clover-leaf," diamond-shaped Hanson-Street, Rush and Lottes' nail have all been used in the management of long bone fractures and all have their place in operative treatment.

Intramedullary Nailing of Femoral Fractures

The ideal femoral shaft fracture to be treated with an intramedullary nail is a transverse or slightly oblique break from approximately 3 inches below the trochanter to approximately 4 inches above the femoral condyles (fig. 23). If the nail is used for fractures above or below these points, stability may be difficult to achieve. Comminuted fractures may be treated with medullary nails but are difficult to stabilize unless circular bands, wires or screws are added (fig. 24). Open fractures have not been treated extensively with medullary nails, but further experience may reveal that there

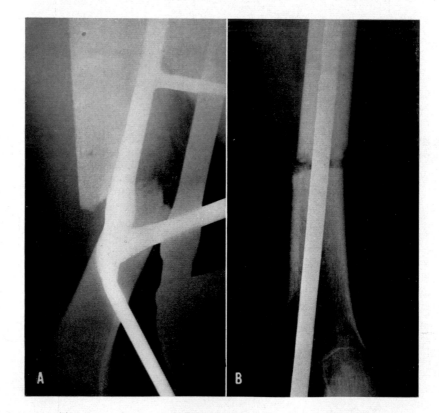

Fig. 23—(A) Transverse fracture of femoral shaft in male of 28. (B) After operative reduction and internal fixation by means of intramedullary Küntscher rod. Patient was ambulated in one week.

is an indication for their use even in the management of some open fractures. The open wound may be sutured and allowed to heal, and the medullary nail inserted ten days to two weeks later.

The surgeon must have adequate training and proper surroundings and assistants. He must be equipped with proper tools, including a complete

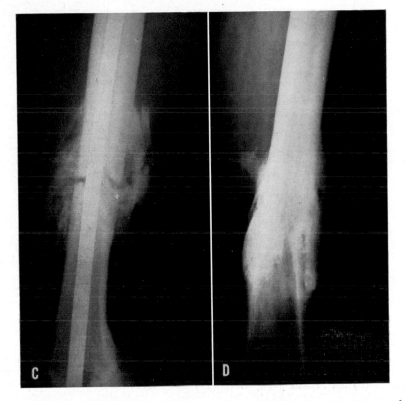

Fig. 23–(C) Eight weeks postoperative. Note abundant external callus. (D) One year follow-up after removal of nail. Solid union.

assortment of nails of varying lengths and diameters. The medullary canal is narrowed at the junction of the upper and middle thirds so that the surgeon chooses a nail which fits snugly at this site. It is wise to use a reamer of proper size so that the medullary canal may be made of the exact size to fit the chosen rods. The nails most frequently used are either 9, 10 or 11 mm. in width. In the younger patient the cortex will be thick and the intramedullary canal narrow, and oftentimes it is necessary to ream out the narrowest part of the intramedullary canal to fit a 9 mm. rod. In the older patient, the intramedullary canal may be 14 or 15 mm. in width, and it is then sometimes necessary to use two nested intramedullary Küntscher "cloverleaf" nails to fill the canal and achieve a good fit. Care should be taken to choose a nail which will give stability but will not bind. It is wise to have a hacksaw at hand so that if the nail becomes fixed on insertion in the bone so that it cannot be removed or driven further, it may be cut off and the patient returned to his bed. After a suitable period of time when the nail becomes loosened, it may be more easily removed. This complication will not occur if the surgeon is meticulous in measuring the size of the rod.

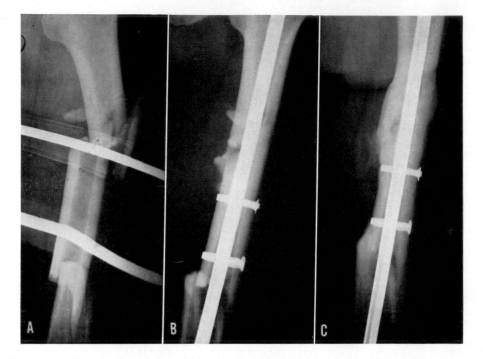

Fig. 24–(A) Segmental comminuted fracture of shaft of femur in male of 44. (B) Immediate postoperative x-ray. Two Parham bands hold central fragment which was split by vertical fracture. (C) Six months postoperative. No external immobilization was necessary.

The patient is placed on the table on his sound side with the injured limb prepared and draped so that it may be freely moved during the operation. The hip and knee are flexed to 90 degrees. The operative approach can be directly lateral, anterolateral, or posterolateral. It is well to use the posterolateral approach for the upper half of the femur and the anterolateral approach for the distal half. The fracture site is exposed, and at this time the surgeon decides on the length and caliber of the nail to be used. When the "clover leaf" nail is to be employed, a guide wire is inserted into the proximal fragment from the fracture site and driven proximally into the shaft of the femur until it makes its exit through the trochanter into the buttock. A stab wound is made over this point to allow for extrusion of the guide rod. The greater trochanter is prepared by means of a suitable bore, and a medullary nail of the proper length with its apex anteriorly placed is driven over the guide rod to the fracture site. When the rod appears at the fracture site, the guide wire is removed and replaced into the rod from above downward. The fracture is then reduced, and the guide wire is driven into the distal fragment. It is wise to use the guide wire to direct the insertion of the nail into the distal fragment so that the cortex of the distal fragment will not be penetrated by the rod. The medullary nail is then driven over the guide rod across the fracture line well into the shaft of the femur to the level of the adductor tubercle. The guide rod is then removed. It is important that the nail project no more than 1 to 2 cm. above the trochanter, but it is also important that it not be driven too deeply into the bone so that it may be easily removed later. X-ray check is necessary during the stages of the operation to be sure the nail is proceeding in the proper direction and that it is placed properly both above and below. The wound is closed in layers, dressing is applied and the leg is placed in suspension for a period of 10 days. Early muscle setting exercises for the quadriceps and hamstring muscles are encouraged. At the end of 10 days, the leg is removed from the splint and the knee motion increased. If good stability has been obtained and when muscle control has been re-established, weight-bearing with crutches is permitted. As soon as possible, the patient is allowed full weight-bearing. There is no fixed rule as to the time of removal of the nail, and if it causes no difficulty it may be allowed to remain in the bone permanently. The chief reason for its removal is discomfort above the trochanter. If the nail is of proper length, there is usually no discomfort to this region. The nail must not be removed, however, until a solid bony union has been established. This usually requires eight months to a year.

The Use of the Intramedullary Nail in Fractures of Other Long Bones

Fractures of the tibia. Intramedullary nails are indicated in certain fractures of both bones of the leg. It is usually necessary to use postoperative plaster immobilization for a considerable period of time because the intramedullary canal of the tibia, with its expanding proximal and distal portions, does not allow for as firm fixation as does the intramedullary canal of the femur. We have used the nested Küntscher nails for intramedullary nailing of the tibia (fig. 25), but we prefer the Lottes' nail (fig. 26) as being more easily inserted and more efficient in stabilization of the fracture. The Lottes' nail is also the best means of immobilization for treatment of nonunion of the tibia (fig. 27).

The nail is inserted through an oblique slot at the upper end of the tibia just medial to the tibial tubercle and is driven down to the exposed fracture site. Occasionally the nail may be inserted blindly without opening the fracture site, but if there is any doubt as to perfect reduction of the fracture, it is better to expose it. If the nailing is to be done blindly, care should be taken as to reduction of the fracture depending upon the site of the fracture line. If the fracture is at the upper third of the tibia it is best to bring the distal fragment posteriorly so that the end of the nail will more readily enter the medullary canal. On the other hand, if the fracture is

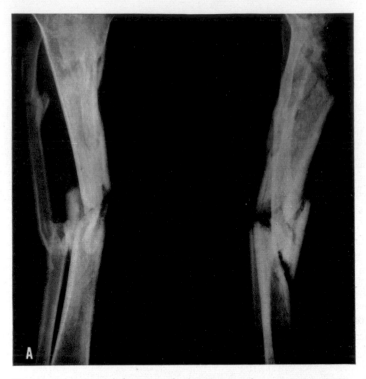

Fig. 25—(A) Comminuted fracture of tibia six months post injury. Nonunion.

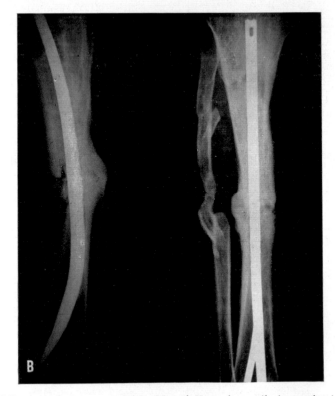

Fig. 25—(B) Nine months post operation. Nested Küntscher nails inserted with cancellous bone grafts.

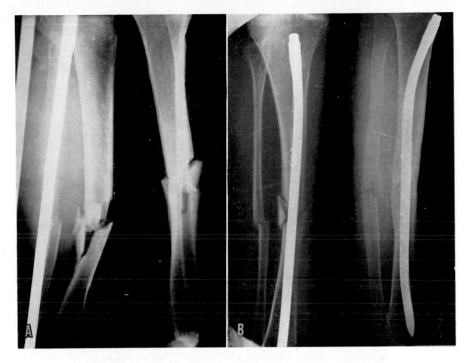

Fig. 26–(A) Fracture of mid shaft of tibia and fibula with comminution of fragments. (B) After insertion of Lottes' nail. Note nail is of proper length, just at cortex distally with proximal end of nail well set into cortex of tibia.

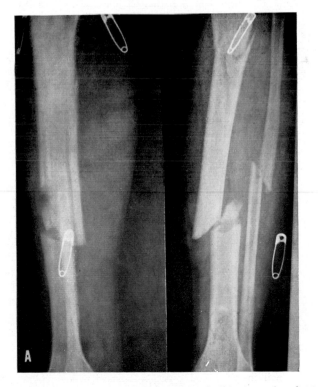

Fig. 27–(A) Open segmental fracture of tibia in male of 32.

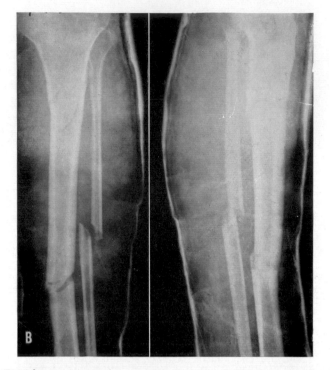

Fig. 27—(B) After treatment by os calcis traction for five weeks, then plaster.

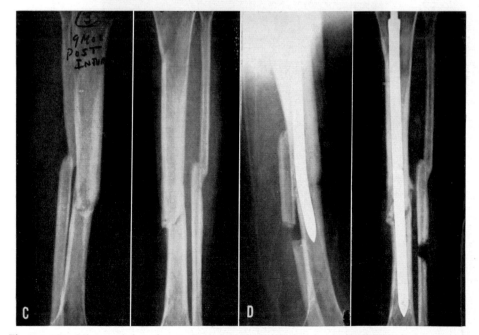

Fig. 27—(C) Nine months after injury. Proximal fracture has healed. Delayed union of distal fracture. (D) At operation, Lottes' nail inserted. At left x-ray shows nail during insertion. At right, nail in place and cancellous grafts packed about fracture. Note a segment of fibula has been excised to insure apposition of fragments of tibia.

in the distal third of the tibia, it is best to displace the distal fragment anteriorly in order that the end of the nail is sure to enter the intramedullary canal of the distal fragment (see Chapter 46). It is essential that proper measurement of the nail be made before the operation, but because of the

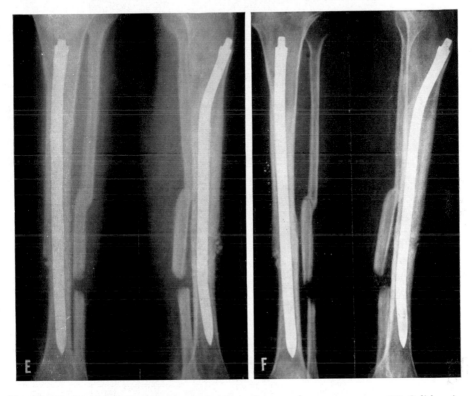

Fig. 27—(E) Two months post operation. Cancellous grafts are apparent. (F) Solid union after 6 months.

fact that 1 and 2 inch extensions can be added to the upper end of the nail, it is better to insert a nail that is too short rather than one that is too long. The nail should not extrude above the cortex at its upper end and should, of course, never penetrate the distal end of the tibia.

Both bones of the forearm. The use of the Rush nail in the treatment of fractures of both bones of the forearm is most helpful in handling these difficult cases (fig. 28). The insertion of the Rush nail is sometimes difficult, and a hole should be drilled into the medullary canal before the nail is inserted. If the fractures of the forearm are at the distal third, the nail should be inserted from the styloid of the radius and the lower end of the ulna. On the other hand, if the fracture is nearer the upper third of the forearm, it is best to insert the ulnar rod through the olecranon process and the radial rod through the radial styloid.

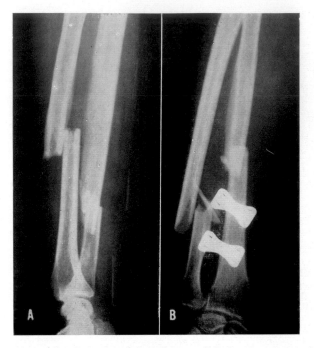

Fig. 28–(A and B) Fracture of both bones of forearm in female of 62.

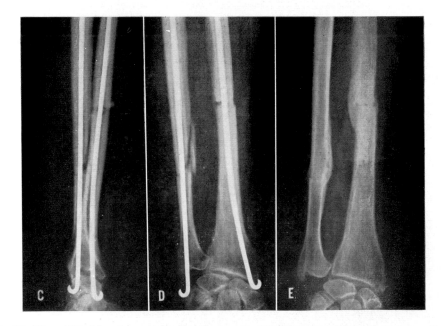

Fig. 28–(C and D) After internal fixation by means of Rush nails and insertion of cancellous bone. (E) Follow-up one year post operation after removal of nails.

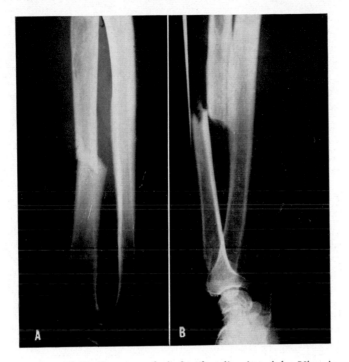

Fig. 29—(A and B) Fracture of shaft of radius in adult. Ulna intact.

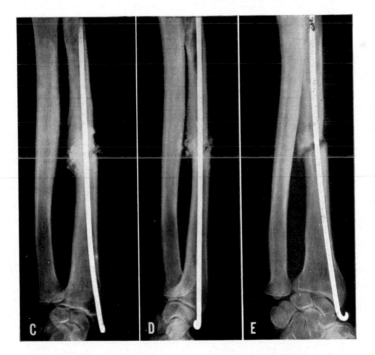

Fig. 29—(C and D) Five days after operative treatment. Intramedullary rod inserted through radial styloid. Note cancellous bone chips packed about fracture.

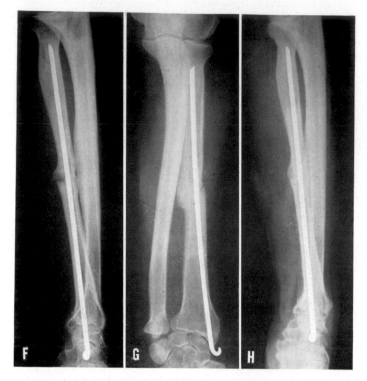

Fig. 29—(E and F) Nine months post operative. Fracture line still apparent.
Fig. 29—(G and H) Twenty-one months follow-up. Solid union. External fixation was never necessary.

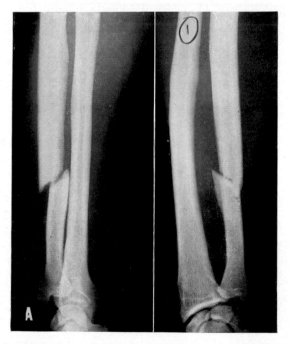

Fig. 30—(A) "Night stick" type of fracture of ulna without injury to radius. Delayed union or nonunion is common in this type of fracture.

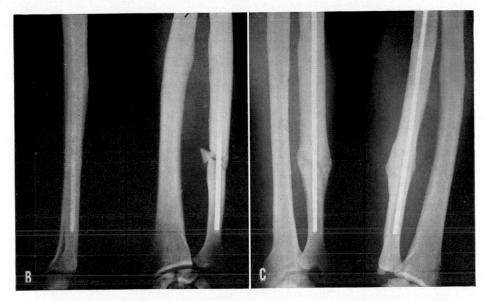

Fig. 30—(B) After insertion of intramedullary rod and cancellous bone chips. (C) Healing was slow but immobilization maintained by rod. Follow-up at one year shows solid union.

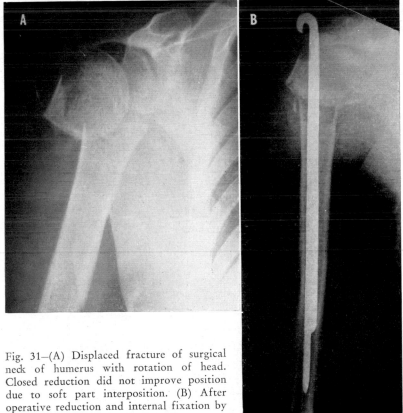

Fig. 31—(A) Displaced fracture of surgical neck of humerus with rotation of head. Closed reduction did not improve position due to soft part interposition. (B) After operative reduction and internal fixation by means of two Rush nails.

If good fixation is obtained by means of the intramedullary rods, external fixation is necessary for only a short time.

Isolated fractures of the radius (fig. 29) or ulna (fig. 30) may be well treated with the intramedullary rod, and external immobilization is not necessary. Fractures of the forearm are slow in healing and often take

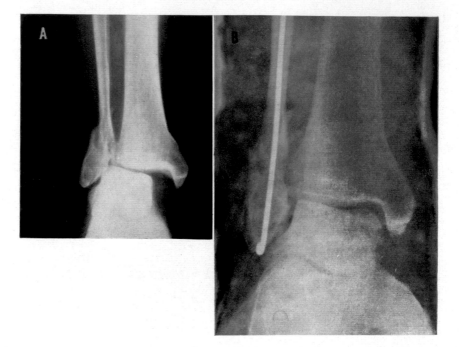

Fig. 32—(A) Abduction fracture of ankle fracture of lateral malleolus, tear of deltoid ligament and disruption of mortise of joint. (B) After reduction, repair of deltoid ligament by silk sutures, and immobilization of external malleolus by intramedullary Rush nail.

10 months to a year for complete consolidation of the fracture line. After this period the intramedullary rods should be removed.

In unstable fractures of the ankle, the use of the Rush nail in the fibula is a most suitable method for maintenance of the reduction. This is particularly useful in fractures involving tear of the deltoid ligament (fig. 32), or in bimalleolar fractures (fig. 17). The Rush nail is also useful in fractures of the clavicle but should not be used as a routine method in this fracture.

Difficult fractures of the humerus are well immobilized by use of the Rush nail. It is sometimes necessary to use two nails in the humerus in order to obtain good stabilization (fig. 31).

Intramedullary fixation of displaced fractures of the metacarpals is most helpful in maintaining perfect reduction in these fractures of the hand. It is also useful in occasional fractures of metatarsals. (See Chapter 14.)

References

1 BÖHLER, L.: Treatment of Fractures. Vol. 1. New York, Grune & Stratton, Inc., 1956, vol. 1.

2 BLOUNT, W. P.: Fractures in Children. Baltimore, Williams & Wilkins Co., 1955.

3 CHARNLEY, J.: Compression Arthrodesis. Edinburgh, E. & S. Livingstone, Ltd., 1953.

4 HAMPTON, O. P., JR.: Wounds of the Extremities in Military Surgery. St. Louis, C. V. Mosby Co., 1951.

5 HENRY, A. K.: Exstensile Exposure Applied to Limb Surgery. Edinburgh, E. & S. Livingstone, Ltd., 1950.

6 KEY and CONWELL: Fractures, Dislocations & Sprains. St. Louis, C. V. Mosby Co., 1956.

7 SMITH, F. M.: Surgery of the Elbow. Springfield, Ill., Charles C Thomas, 1954.

8 VENABLE, C. S. and STUCK, W. G.: Internal Fixation of Fractures. Springfield, Ill., Charles C Thomas, 1947.

9 WATSON-JONES, Sir R.: Fractures and Joint Injuries. Edinburgh, E. & S. Livingstone, Ltd., 1955.

CHAPTER 14

TREATMENT OF NONUNION

PRESTON A. WADE, M.D.

Nonunion of fractures has long intrigued the surgeon, and many experimental and clinical investigations have sought means to prevent it and to improve its treatment. Many factors enter into the etiology of nonunion, but

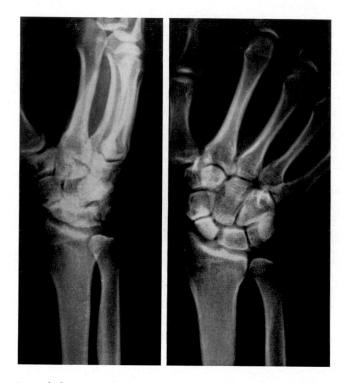

Fig. 1—Nonunion of fracture of carpal navicular 5 years post injury. Note increased density of bone at fracture site.

the most important one is that of drecreased vitality of bone ends of fractured fragments due to faulty blood supply. This may be the result of deficient blood supply in the bone or the isolation of a fragment from its blood supply. Study of a long series of nonunion of fractures makes it quite obvious that the condition occurs most frequently in certain sites of certain bones, particularly in those intra-articular fractures in which a fragment may be isolated from its parent shaft and union must occur across a fracture line within a joint. This is well illustrated in fractures of the neck of the femur, through the anatomic neck of the humerus, the proximal third of the carpal navicular (fig. 1), and the astragalus. These fractures often result in avascular necrosis of the isolated fragment, even after bony union. This indicates that the blood supply is not sufficient to revascularize the detached fragment even if it becomes attached to the viable fragment by bony union.

There are, of course, other factors which influence the development of nonunion, one of the most important being faulty immobilization. No less an authority than Sir Reginald Watson-Jones has stated, "There is only one cause of nonunion of fractures with a continuous hematoma between the fragments — the cause of nonunion is inadequate immobilization." This is undoubtedly true of certain fractures in which nonunion is most apt to occur, but faulty immobilization is not in itself enough to cause nonunion in every fracture. Nor is continuous, efficient immobilization always successful in the prevention or treatment of nonunion. A good example of healing in spite of movement of fragments is seen in fractures of the humerus, now popularly treated by the hanging cast. This treatment in no way immobilizes the fragments of the fractured bone and, as a matter of fact, increases motion at the fractured site, yet in most instances the fracture heals kindly and quickly.

Other factors which enter into the causation of nonunion are infection, interposition of soft parts, and the presence of foreign bodies. In themselves, these conditions do not often cause nonunion, but they have a decided effect on the causation of nonunion when associated with faulty blood supply and improper immobilization.

Fractures of the Shafts of Long Bones

There are certain sites in long bones where fractures result in a considerable percentage of nonunion. These are, of course, the junction of the lower and middle thirds of the tibia (fig. 2), shafts of both bones of the forearm (fig. 3), and some sites in the shaft of the humerus. Fractures of the femur, clavicle and metacarpals also occasionally result in nonunion. The site of nonunion in the tibia is known to be an area of deficient blood supply at the junction of the lower and middle thirds of the bone, and since the medial surface of the tibia is subcutaneous, there is little blood supply from the surrounding soft parts. In fractures of both bones of the forearm, other elements beside blood supply may have something to do with the nonunion, since one bone may unite while the fragments of the other may be held apart. This also occurs in the leg, when the rapid healing of the fibula prevents apposition of tibial fragments, and so helps to prevent union. Fractures of the shaft of the humerus usually heal rapidly and nonunion is not common, but it does occur, particularly when there is a segmental fracture of the shaft which leaves one segment of the bone deficient in blood supply.

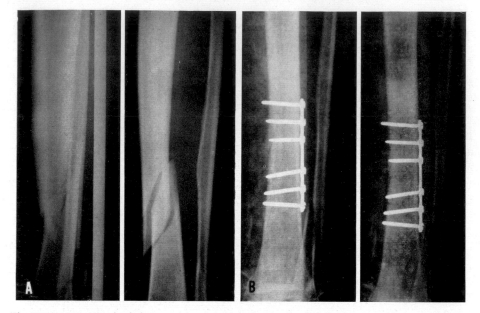

Fig. 2—(A) Fracture both bones of leg — spiral fracture of tibia. (B) After internal fixation with plate and screws.

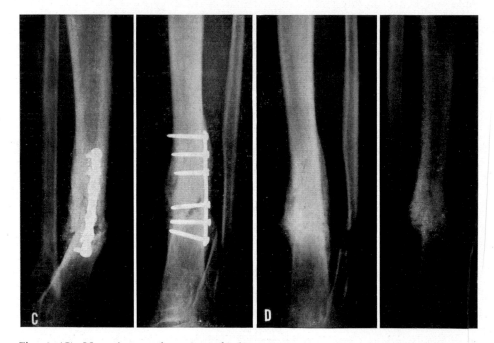

Fig. 2—(C) Nonunion — loosening of plate — angulation 6 months post operation. (D) Seven months after removal of metal. Cancellous bone graft. Solid union.

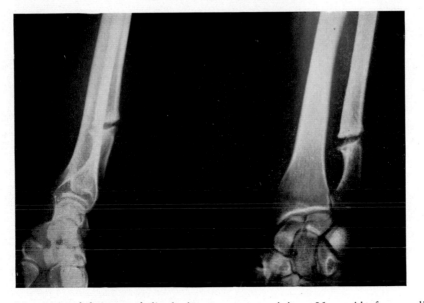

Fig. 3—Nonunion of fracture of distal ulna 4 years post injury. Note wide fracture line, eburnated ends of fragments. The intact radius holds the fragments apart, thus contributing to occurrence of nonunion.

Treatment of Nonunion

Bone Grafting: There are several prerequisites for any bone-grafting operation:

1. There should be no infection.

2. There should be a satisfactory skin covering over the area involved.

3. The operation must remove fibrous tissue between the bone ends, and they must be freshened so that healthy, bleeding bone may be apposed to healthy, bleeding bone.

4. The fragments must be perfectly and continuously immobilized, either by external splinting or by internal fixation.

5. Osteogenesis by means of a graft is an important factor in the operation.

Inlay Grafts

Following World War I, successful bone grafting was based on the concept that healing would result if a segment of normal bone were held in place in a prepared bed in the fragments of an ununited fracture. This was called an inlay graft. When the graft was taken from one of the fragments and slid across the fracture line, it was called a sliding graft. Though these grafts were frequently successful, they were precarious because they were small and weak at the fracture site and therefore apt to fracture. In many instances, they also became completely absorbed, and thus resulted in nonunion. With the inlay or sliding graft, external immobilization was necessary, since the graft could not stabilize the fracture well enough by itself.

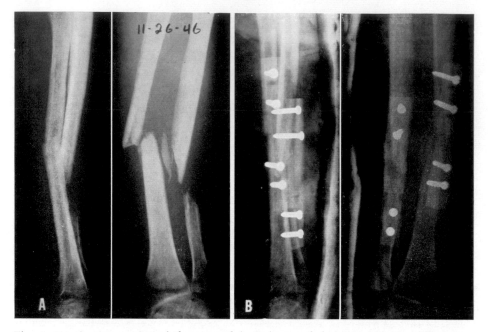

Fig. 4—(A) Open comminuted fracture of both bones of forearm with loss of segment of ulna 6 months post injury after healing of wound and skin grafting. (B) After cortical onlay graft from tibia. Fixation by vitallium screws. Cancellous bone chips packed about fracture.

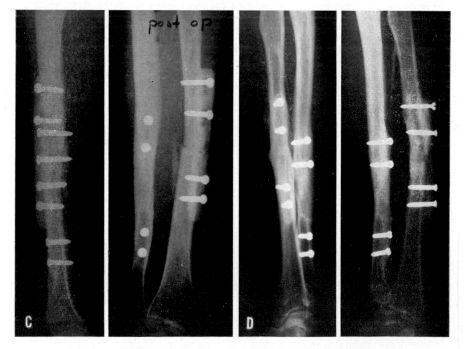

Fig. 4—(C) Six months postoperative — grafts intact. Fractures healed. (D) Eight years postoperative. Bone replacing grafts still evident. Screws loosened slightly. Normal function of arm.

Massive Onlay Bone Grafts

With the advent of nonelectrolytic alloys, other means of immobilization could be accomplished by metallic internal fixation, and the massive onlay cortical bone grafts, taken usually from a sound tibia, were used. These involved taking a large segment of the cortex of the bone and applying it directly to a prepared, freshened cortex of the fractured fragments after the usual preparation of the fracture site. The cortical graft was fixed to the fragments by means of metal screws (fig. 4). In this operation the graft served the dual purpose of immobilizing the fracture and supplying osteogenesis to the fracture site. Bone grafts do not survive as such and must be absorbed and replaced by new bone. This process is a long and precarious one, since the cortical graft tends to break as it is absorbed, and so causes an unsuccessful result. However, this was often more successful than the inlay or sliding graft. Massive onlay graft can be applied in those cases in which there is a loss of substance of a large segment of bone and the graft is used to bridge the gap (fig. 4).

Cancellous Bone Grafts

In recent years we have found that cancellous bone, such as that found in the iliac bone, makes an excellent graft. The vitality of the cancellous graft, with its rapid regeneration is more important than the strength of a compact

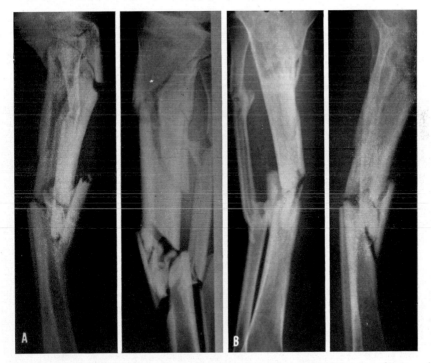

Fig. 5—(A) Open comminuted fracture of both bones of leg. Treated by os calcis traction. (B) Six months later. Wound healed. Nonunion of fracture through middle of tibia. Upper third fractures healed.

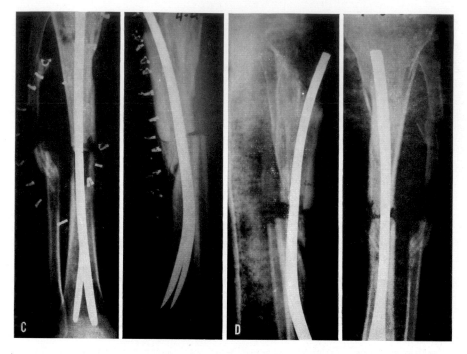

Fig. 5—(C) At operation. Ends of fracture fragments freshened, 2 inches of fibula resected, intramedullary rods inserted and entire area packed with cancellous bone. (D) One week post operation. Distraction at fracture site. Patient allowed to bear weight in long leg plaster.

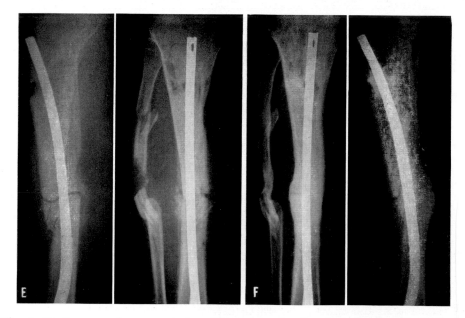

Fig. 5—(E) Seven weeks postoperative. Note external callus. Distraction now minimal. (F) Sixteen months postoperative. Solid union. Note resected area of fibula regenerated.

graft, with its quality of rigid immobilization. Cortical grafts of compact bone have been expected to serve the dual function of providing internal fixation and promoting osteogenesis, but immobilization can often be gained more securely by plates or intramedullary nails, and osteogenesis can be stimulated more certainly by cancellous bone. It is true that bone cells die in a cancellous graft exactly as they die in a compact graft, but dead cancellous bone can be resorbed and regenerated more rapidly than dead compact bone. Thus, the modern treatment of nonunited fractures is to use cancellous transplants (fig. 2) without the use of splints of compact bone and to use cortical bone only when no other method of internal fixation is available or when it is necessary to replace lost bone substance (fig. 4). Even when cortical bone is used, whether it be from the patient's own tibia or borrowed from a bone bank, cancellous bone is used to supplement it.

If it is possible to use a means of internal fixation which allows motion of contiguous joints and, better still, allows weightbearing of the leg or function of the arm, more rapid healing may be expected, and rehabilitation time will be considerably shortened (fig. 5).

Intramedullary Nail and Cancellous Bone Graft

In the case of the tibia, intramedullary nails and cancellous bone grafts provide the necessary immobilization of the fragments and the required osteogenetic conditions (fig. 5). This combination also allows early motion of contiguous joints and early weightbearing. In the humerus, the use of intramedullary nail and cancellous bone graft permits early mobilization of the

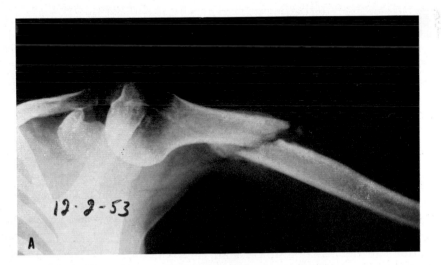

Fig. 6—(A) Nonunion of fracture of upper third of humerus after treated in hanging cast.
6 months post injury.

arm, and prevents the atrophy of bone and soft parts which prolongs convalescence (fig. 6). The same method of intramedullary nailing with cancellous bone graft may be used in the rare case of nonunion of clavicle as shown in figure 7, in the femur in figure 8, and in the metacarpal, figure 9.

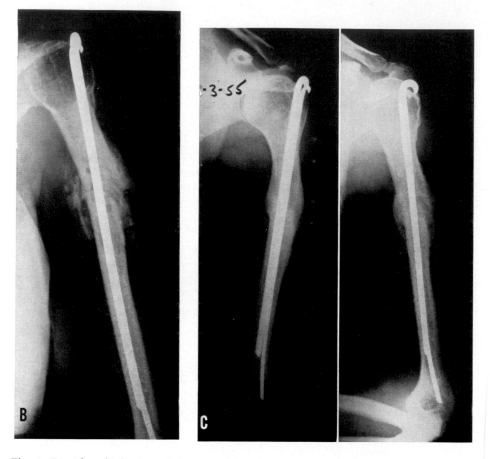

Fig. 6—(B) After freshening of fracture site, insertion of two Rush nails affording firm immobilization. Packed with cancellous graft.

Fig. 6—(C) Solid union — slight restriction of elevation of arm due to prominence of heads of nails.

Certain important precautions must be taken in any of these operations. *There must be no infection.* If any infection is present, the trauma of the operation and the insertion of the bone chips will certainly result in serious aggravation of the infection and failure of the operation. *The skin must be intact over the operative site.* If not, a sinus and infection will certainly result. In view of the fact that the bulk of the limb may be increased by the use of large amounts of cancellous bone, it is necassary to make sure that *there is no tension on the wound*, and in many cases it is essential to use relaxing incisions on one or both sides of the wound. The defects caused by the

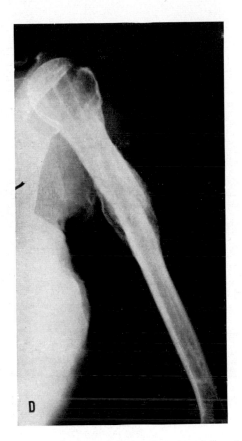

Fig. 6–(D) After removal of nails. Normal function.

relaxing incisions must be covered by a split-thickness graft. This increases the duration of the operation but is nevertheless essential for the success of the procedure.

It must be admitted that the removal of cancellous bone from the iliac crest is not without complications. Many patients complain bitterly of pain after the operation, and on occasion a hematoma develops. We have had one case in which a calcification of the hematoma developed, necessitating removal of a large calcific deposit. Cancellous bone from a bone bank is said to be as effective as autogenous bone, but in cases of nonunion it seems wiser to use the latter.

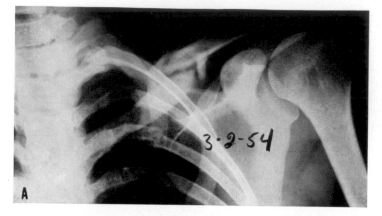

Fig. 7—(A) Nonunion of clavicle 8 months post injury.

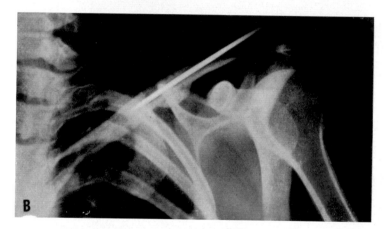

Fig. 7—(B) Four months post operation. Intramedullary nail and cancellous bone graft. Note exuberant external callus.

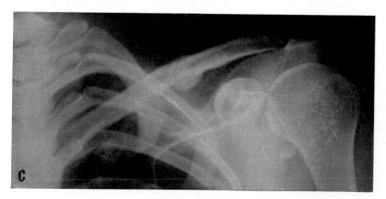

Fig. 7—(C) Seven months follow-up after removal of nail.

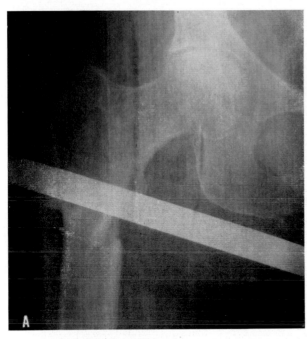

Fig. 8—(A) Fracture of upper third of femoral shaft. This is best treated primarily by intramedullary rod.

Fig. 8—(B) After internal fixation by Jewett nail. Note distraction of fragments. Nonunion after 8 months. (C) After removal of Jewett nail, fixation by means of intramedullary nail, allowing impaction of fragments. Cancellous bone graft.

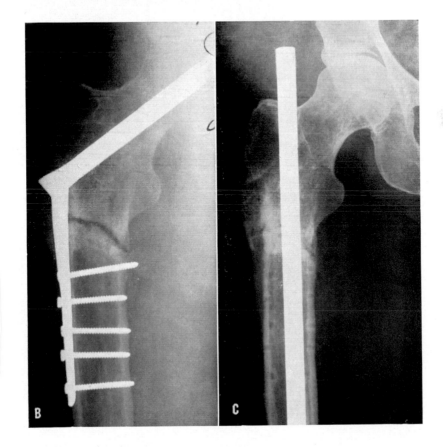

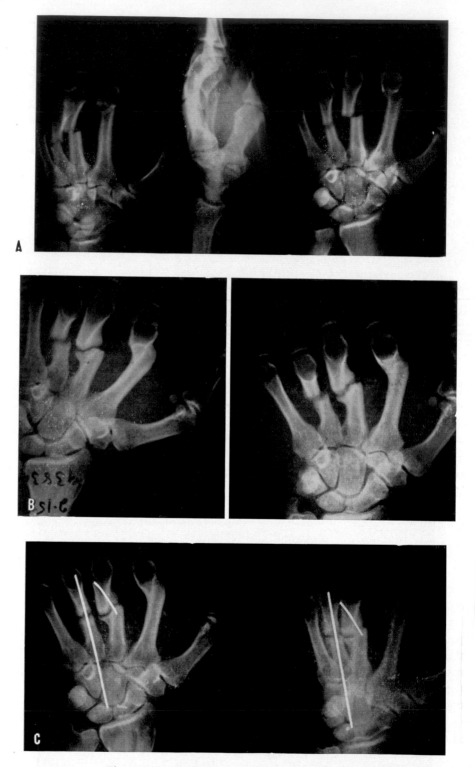

Fig. 9–(A—C) Please see legends on facing page.

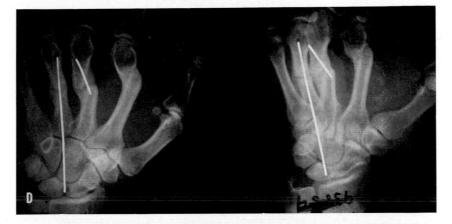

Fig. 9—(A-*top left*) Multiple fracture of shafts of metacarpals. (B-*middle left*) Nonunion of fracture of metacarpals 3 and 4. Fractures of metacarpals 2 and 5 have healed. (C-*bottom left*) After internal fixation by Kirschner wires and application of cancellous bone grafts. (D *above*) One year post operation. Solid union, normal function.

Prevention of Nonunion

Since adequate internal fixation with intramedullary nails and cancellous bone has been successful in the treatment of nonunion, it seems logical that the same method of treatment might be applicable to a fresh fracture in a bone which is known to have a high rate of nonunion. We have, therefore, used the open operation with the application of internal fixation and autogenous bone graft in those cases in which nonunion is feared. Fractures of the junction of the lower and middle thirds of the tibia have a considerable percentage of nonunion, and in these cases we have employed the open operation with internal fixation and the addition of the cancellous bone graft. In these cases precautions must be taken lest the treatment add to the possibility of complications. It is, therefore, exceedingly important that there is no infection, that no sinuses result from the operation and that the skin covering of the operative site is good. Relaxing incisions with skin grafting of the defect are often necessary to prevent tension on wound closure. Since the use of intramedullary nails in the tibia involves difficulties and is attended by a certain risk, we have accomplished immobilization by the use of internal fixation with two or three metal screws (figs. 10 and 11), or if necessary, a plate supplemented by external immobilization in plaster splints. However, the immobilization is not as secure as that achieved with intramedullary nails, and early weight-bearing cannot be allowed as early. We feel, however, that the results are sufficiently satisfactory so that the more extensive operation is seldom justified.

In fractures of both bones of the forearm, or fractures of ulna or radius alone, internal fixation by means of intramedullary nails is the procedure of

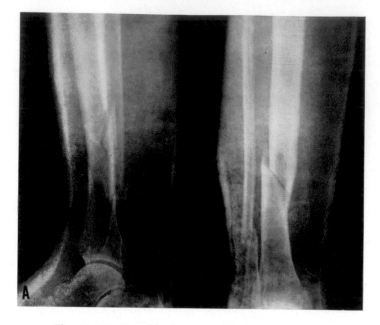

Fig. 10–(A) Unstable fracture of both bones of leg.

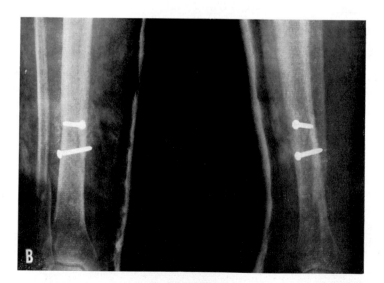

Fig. 10–(B) After open reduction, internal fixation by means of 2 screws and application of cancellous bone graft. Note the screws are placed at right angle to long axis of tibia.

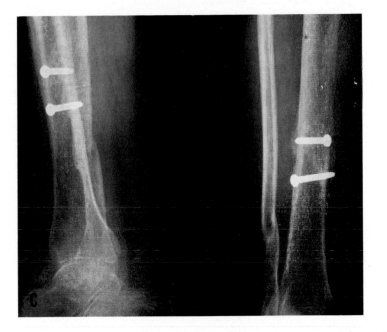

Fig. 10–(C) Six months post operation. Solid union. Note evidence of external callus at site of cancellous graft.

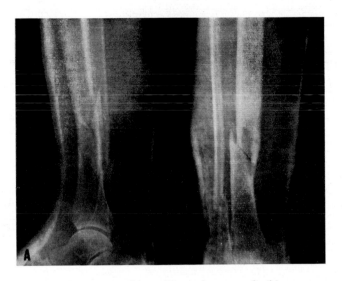

Fig. 11–(A) Short oblique fracture of tibia.

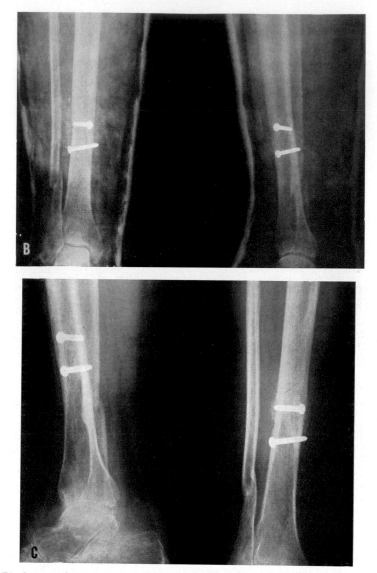

Fig. 11—(B) Open reduction with fixation by two screws. Cancellous bone graft. (C) Six
months follow-up. Solid union.

preference. In these cases cancellous bone graft is also used (fig. 12 and 13),
but great care must be taken that the bulk of the graft does not cause excessive
callus formation so as to cause a cross-union or to prevent proper rotation

Fig. 12—(A) Fracture of radius, midshaft. This fracture is difficult to reduce and immobilize.
Delayed or nonunion is common. (B) After internal fixation with Rush nail and cancellous
bone graft.
Fig. 12—(C) Nine months post operation. Although fracture site is still visible, fixation is
firm and no external fixation is necessary. (D) Twenty-one months post operation. Solid
union. The long continued immobilization possible through the use of the Rush nail
is necessary for eventual healing.

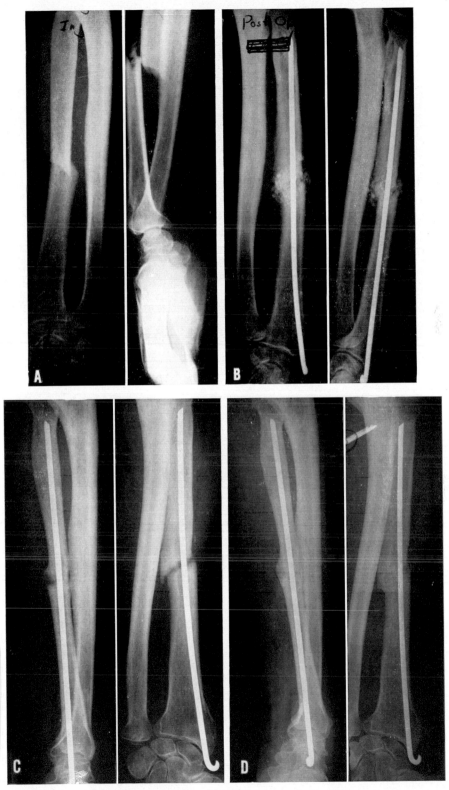

Fig. 12–(A—D). Please see legends on facing page.

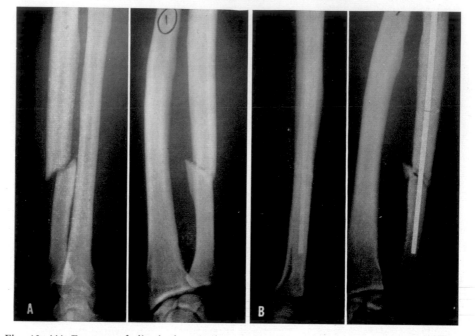

Fig. 13—(A) Fracture of distal ulna similar to that shown in fig. 3. (B) Open reduction immobilization by intramedullary rod. Cancellous bone graft.

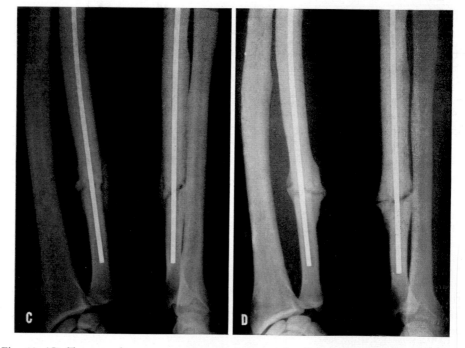

Fig. 13—(C) Two months post operation. Note external callus at site of grafts. (D) Five months post operation. Callus obvious but healing not complete. If immobilization were not firm and continuous, nonunion would result.

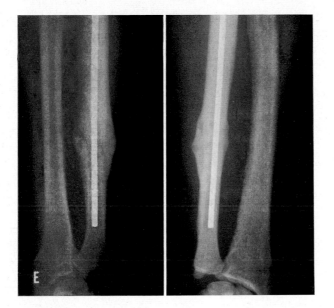

Fig. 13—(E) One year post operation. Solid union. Normal function. Note external callus. If grafts are placed too generously about the fracture site, limitation of rotation may result.

of the forearm. In those cases of fractures of the humerus where open reduction is necessary, cancellous bone graft may also be used.

We have not used cancellous bone in fresh fractures of the femur, since with intramedullary rods nonunion is exceedingly rare and cancellous bone graft is not necessary.

Open Fractures

Although internal fixation may be used in the treatment of open fractures and the wound closed in those cases in which infection is unlikely, it is not wise to insert cancellous bone graft in these cases. We have, therefore, selected cases of fractures of both bones of the leg at the junction of the lower and middle thirds, and have used a delayed method of treatment. In this the internal fixation is applied at the time of the débridement, and after the wound is healed and all danger of infection is past, the wound is reopened and cancellous bone is grafted as a secondary procedure.

Summary

1. The primary cause of nonunion is the decreased vitality of bone ends of fractured fragments, the result of faulty circulation. Poor immobilization, infection, interposition of soft parts and the presence of foreign bodies may be additional causative factors.

2. The treatment of nonunited fractures of shafts of long bones necessitates complete and continuous immobilization with osteogenesis supplied by a graft.

Internal fixation by means of intramedullary rods with autogenous cancellous bone graft most nearly satisfies these requirements.

3. The incidence of nonunion in certain fractures may be decreased by the use of primary internal fixation and cancellous bone grafting.

References

[1] BÖHLER, LORENZ: Treatment of Fractures. New York, Grune & Stratton, Inc., 1953, vol. 1.

[2] KEY and CONWELL: Fractures, Dislocations & Sprains. St. Louis, C. B. Mosby Co., 1956.

[3] VENABLE, C. S. and STARK, W. G.: The Internal Fixation of Fractures. Springfield, Ill. C. C. Thomas, 1947.

[4] WATSON-JONES, R.: Fractures and Joint Injuries. Edinburgh, E. & S. Livingstone, Ltd., 1955.

CHAPTER 15

EARLY MOBILIZATION OF JOINTS IN THE TREATMENT OF FRACTURES

Preston A. Wade, M.D.

The study of end results in the treatment of fractures indicates that the most important and the most common cause of disability is the impairment of joint function. This loss of function is usually the result of joint stiffness, although pain and faulty weight-bearing may also play a part. Nonunion is occasionally a cause of poor result, but in most instances the fractured bone heals and disability is the result of joint stiffness.

A fracture may heal with displacement and shortening, and even with angulation and rotation, and yet from an economic and functional point of view the result may be quite satisfactory. On the other hand, joint stiffness following a fracture will give a poor result with permanent disability in spite of good reduction, perfect healing and perfect anatomic position.

Causes of Joint Stiffness

Joint stiffness may be caused by (1) injury to joint structures, (2) infection or (3) functional inactivity and disuse.

Injury to Joint Structures

It is obvious that fractures through articular surfaces of joints, particularly if there is deformity of the joint-bearing surfaces, will cause a mechanical block to free motion. Also, injuries to the capsule, supporting ligaments, and tendons will cause adhesions and scarring and contracture, resulting in joint stiffness.

In recent years there has been a greater emphasis on the meticulous replacement of displaced joint surfaces, the exploration of injured joints and removal of injured cartilage and menisci and repair of torn ligaments. As a result, the treatment of joint trauma has been greatly improved. This improvement can be said to be due in great measure to advances in open operative procedures and to improvement in the metallurgic design of non-electrolytic metals used in internal fixation. These improved methods have allowed the surgeon to extend the application of operative replacement of injured joints and have permitted early mobilization in many types of fractures that were previously doomed to disability because it was necessary to treat them by old fashioned methods of continued immobilization.

Plates and screws made of the inert, nonelectrolytic metals, vitallium and 18—8 SMO stainless steel, permit the surgeon to use internal fixation to insure maintenance of reduction of displaced fragments of a joint. The fixation can often be depended on to hold the fragments in position while allowing free motion of the joint during the healing period.

Infection

It has long been recognized that the commonest single cause of permanent joint stiffness is infection. The dense scars following infection leave an irreparable stiffness, and the surgeon must take every precaution to prevent infection in or around a joint or fracture. He must use every means in his power to control infection as rapidly and efficiently as possible in order to prevent the scar tissue formation which so stubbornly resists treatment. The antibiotics are, or course, a most useful and effective means of preventing and controlling infection, but the surgeon must realize that even a minimum of sepsis may result in serious joint stiffness, and he must be aware of the fact that antibiotics may only retard the progress of infection, so that sepsis may not be recognized until late — too late on many occasions to prevent impairment of joint function.

Methods of fracture treatment involving transfixion by pins and wires may appear to be advantageous in allowing joint motion, but actually where even minor infection results, or where pins are inserted through muscles, more serious harm may be done by causing stiffness of the nearby joint. Even when properly applied, multiple pin fixation or external skeletal fixation is useful in only a few situations. Some open fractures of both bones of the leg may be best treated by this method, but we believe that it should be used only in this type of fracture and should not be applied to others. Although it may be argued that the criticism of this method is the result of its misuse rather than of the method itself, the fact that it is so easily and widely abused and misused makes it even more vulnerable to criticism.

Continuous traction methods are often excellent for reducing and main-taining position in unstable fractures while allowing some motion of nearby joints. The choice of material for transfixion of bone in skeletal traction is an oft-debated subject. The advocates of wires state that the smaller opening in the skin and bone causes less necrosis, and that infection is less common. Advocates of the Steinmann nail state that it does not rotate in the bone as does the wire, and that the cutting power of the pin is less than that of the wire. Slipping of the Kirschner wire in the bone is one of the objections to its use. This objection is met by the use of the threaded Kirsch-ner wire which is preferable to the unthreaded type. Either nail or wire may be used, but the more important consideration is the site of insertion of the material.

If the pin or wire is inserted too near a joint, even a minor infection may result in severe disability. If a nail is inserted through muscles, such as the vastus lateralis or medialis, pinning them to the bone, joint function may be even further impaired. If wires are placed through the supracondylar region of the femur, the resulting contracture and adhesion formation may cause permanent stiffening of the knee joint. The pin tracts are apt to cause infection, and the muscles impaled by the wire become adherent and lose their function. In the author's opinion, the Kirschner wire is preferable if skeletal traction must be applied to the supracondylar region.

The tibial tubercle is much safer as a site for traction, since it is farther removed from the joint and from the site of fracture, and since no muscles are pierced by the nail or wire.

The os calcis may also be safely used as a site of skeletal traction in those cases where traction is necessary in fractures of the lower leg.

In fractures of the elbow, the olecranon may be safely used for skeletal traction, and in severely comminuted fractures not suitable for open operation, only this method may make early motion possible.

Functional Inactivity and Disuse

In the latest edition of his book, Watson-Jones[1] gives the following as the first principle of fracture treatment: "Every fracture must be treated by complete and continuous immobilization until union is sound." He states that the principle applies to every type of fracture, whether complicated or simple, infected or noninfected, recent or old, treated by manipulation or operation. He further states that complete and continuous immobilization of the fractured bone involves immobilization of the joints above and below the fracture, and that failure to obey this law of treatment is a source of delayed recovery and may be responsible for nonunion.

Unfortunately, as a result of the literal interpretation of this commonly quoted principle, most laymen and many surgeons believe that "a fracture means a plaster cast." We know, however, that there are many exceptions to this rule and that the literal interpretation will result in harmful prolonged immobilization of joints.

As a matter of fact, many fractures are better treated without any form of immobilization and heal more successfully when motion of the injured limb is encouraged. The most striking example of this form of treatment is the so-called "hanging cast" treatment of fractures of the shaft of the humerus. With this method, not only is no effort made to immobilize the fractured fragment, but motion of the shoulder joint is actually encouraged and motion at the fracture line occurs with every motion of the arm as the patient is urged to move his shoulder as soon as the pain will allow. In most cases union results and at the same time the most disturbing disability, loss of motion of the shoulder joint, is prevented by the simple and important expedient of immediate early active motion. We agree with Watson-Jones[1] and do not recommend the hanging cast, but prefer to use the collar-and-cuff treatment of Sir Robert Jones, which allows immediate shoulder motion. The objection to the hanging cast is that the unnecessary weight of the usual weighted cast provides more traction than is necessary, in spite of the fact that the traction is intermittent. Distraction is common as a result of the routine use of the heavy hanging plaster, and the same principle can be more successfully carried out by using the collar-and-cuff "hanging arm" treatment with a minimum amount of local immolization afforded by sugar-tong or lateral splints. The application of the lateral splints not only affords some immobilization but also satisfies the patient in that he is more apt to feel that treatment is adequate, than as if no plaster is applied. In any case, the fact remains that in this fracture, as in some others, immobilization of the fracture is not necessary to insure healing, and immobilization of the elbow and the shoulder is not only unnecessary but undesirable and harmful.

Another false conception of fracture treatment is that all fractures need immobilization by some form of external splinting or internal fixation to prevent movement of fragments. As a matter of fact, many fracture fragments will not change position in spite of movement of contiguous joints, and will proceed to heal promptly and perfectly while the contiguous joints are moving freely and normally and while, in many instances in the lower extremity, the bones may be bearing weight as well.

In the case of impaction of one fragment into the other, as is well illustrated by the impacted fracture of the surgical neck of the humerus, the immobilization is achieved by the force of the trauma which drives one fragment firmly into the other thus allowing early motion of the shoulder joint. There are many other fractures in which no form of immobilization is necessary, and in which early active motion of joints may be instituted immediately. This group of fractures includes fractures of the fibula, in which immobilization is achieved by the intact tibia; and fracture of the ribs, in which the fragments move together with respiration and are prevented from moving apart by the attached muscles. Compression fractures of the dorsal spine and some mild compression fractures of the lumbar spine need no immobilization and are best treated by active motion and regular exercise. Many fractures need no immobilization because the amount of motion at the fracture site is not enough to prevent sound healing, even where nearby joints are mobilized. Fractures of phalanges, some carpal, metacarpal and metatarsal bones, the pelvis, and the clavicle and scapula, as well as some fractures of the os calcis are examples of injuries best treated by early mobilization, in spite of a limited degree of motion at the fracture site.

It is not necessary to immobilize both joints above and below the fracture in all cases. In some cases, only one joint near a fracture must be immobilized to insure healing. The Colles' is a good example of the fracture which, theoretically, needs immobilization of both elbow and wrist joint, but usually necessitates immobilization of the wrist joint only. In the comminuted type of Colles' fracture in the elderly, it is necessary to immobilize the joints above and below the fracture line.

It is obvious that the surgeon must interpret the general principles of fracture treatment in such a way as to insure the healing of the fracture without unnecessary and harmful immobilization of the joints about it.

Mobility and Exercise

Watson-Jones'[1] second principle of fracture treatment is, "Every joint which does not need to be immobilized must be exercised actively from the first day of injury." There are no exceptions to this rule, but it is often disregarded. Many fractures and both their contiguous joints need to be immobilized continuously for a prolonged period, but if during this time the patient is advised, encouraged and directed to move his body, exercise his muscles, and move all his movable joints, those that are immobilized will regain their motion in the minimum time with the least permanent restriction.

If an injured limb is immobilized in plaster and no effort is made to encourage motion of all nearby muscles and joints, all of the factors that cause joint stiffness operate to cause permanent damage to the joints. The muscles become weakened and atrophied, and some become contracted, while the opposing groups become stretched. The circulation is impaired, and edema develops with the infiltration of soft parts and consequent adhesions about the joint. Because of disuse and inactivity, the uninjured joints also become stiff, so that, when the limb is released from the immobilizing apparatus, it is crippled and useless. At this point, the patient feels that any attempts at motion will be harmful and painful, and it is with the greatest difficulty that he can be encouraged to use the only valuable therapeutic measure at his command, namely, active motion. Attempts to force motion in these stiffened joints only cause further damage, further scarring, and restriction of motion, and when passive stretching is combined with heat and massage, the vicious cycle is complete. Further edema and infiltration result, more stiffening takes place, and it is only because of the remarkable ability of the human joint to withstand abuse that many more permanent disabilities do not occur.

This unhappy sequence of events can, in large measure, be prevented by intelligent direction of the patient in the functional activity of all of his muscles and joints, as well as of the injured limb insofar as the immobilizing apparatus will permit. The patient should be encouraged to use all of his muscles. If he is ambulatory, he should not be allowed to sit in a chair all day but should be made to walk in spite of obvious difficulties. If he is confined to bed he should be given regular exercises so that he does not suffer the atrophies and weaknesses of disuse. He should be made to move all of the joints about an immobilized fracture because such motion not only prevents circulatory stasis, but movement of the structures about an immobilized joint, no matter how slight, helps to prevent "gluing" together of the soft parts. Furthermore, there is considerable evidence to indicate that motion of muscles about a fracture does, in fact, stimulate the formation of external callus and actually accelerates bonehealing.

One of the earliest and strongest advocates of early functional activity was Lorenz Böhler.[2] In his clinic, there is little emphasis on post-immobilization physiotherapy or special rehabilitation, because he believes that a patient should be able to walk out of his plaster with no disability if rehabilitation in plaster has been effectively carried out. Charnley[3] states; "When a decision is made to remove a plaster, it is unwise to do so if the patient is not by this time already capable of good function in the plaster."

Treatment of fractures of the lower extremity in walking plaster, as advocated by Böhler,[2] is an effective means of continuing the functional activity so essential to the prevention of joint disabilities. One may not agree with Böhler's theory that contact compression of fractured fragments promotes bone-healing, but the weight-bearing does allow use of the limb and hastens return to normal function after removal of plaster.

Early Mobilization

Another aphorism of fracture treatment is, "Never immobilize a joint one day longer than is absolutely necessary." In children and young adults, one may expect a rapid return to joint function in the absence of infection, in spite of unnecessarily prolonged immobilization. However, in adults such an error may lead to permanent disability. There is a mistaken notion that before a fracture can be released from immobilization, the fracture line in the x-ray must be obliterated. Obviously, there are other factors involved in deciding whether a fracture is healed. One is the clinical examination of the part, an evaluation of pain, tenderness and false motion. The other is the experience of the surgeon, which may prevent immobilization of certain fractures longer than is necessary. The surgeon must know which fractures must be judged as healed only by x-ray appearance, such as those of the neck of the femur and the carpal navicular. He must know that in other fractures the radiographic evidence of calcification of the callus does not appear until weeks after the fracture is clinically united, and that dependence on the x-ray reading only will lead to prolonged and harmful immobilization. Fractures of both bones of the leg are commonly immobilized for a much longer period than is necessary because the surgeon waits for complete ossification of the fracture line before he permits weight-bearing and removal of the plaster.

Early mobilization of joints may be achieved by the newer methods of internal fixation, which sometimes allow immediate mobilization of joints and even weight-bearing as well. In the past few years, the use of newer nonelectrolytic metals has enabled the surgeon to extend the application of internal fixation to many fractures previously treated by long periods of immobilization. The use of plates and screws in long bones will allow the mobilization of a limb in suspension during the period of healing. The newest and most striking example of the value of internal fixation in early joint motion is the use of the intramedullary nail in treating fractures of the shaft of the femur. In this method, all of the requirements for the preservation of joint function are present. The patient is ambulatory almost immediately, there is no immobilization of any joint, weight bearing is allowed early and functional activity may be instituted as soon as the patient awakens from his anesthetic. Böhler has recently published comparative figures of morbidity, disability, and insurance company costs of a case treated by traction and one treated by the intramedullary nail. He found that in the case of a femoral fracture treated by closed reduction, the hospitalization time was 172 days as compared to 28 days in the case treated by the intramedullary nail; the expense to the insurance company was 160 times greater. Furthermore, in cases in which intramedullary nails are used, joint motions in knee and ankle are greatly increased and more rapidly achieved. Although the operation does carry a risk of infection, as well as other less serious complications, it is a definite advance in fracture treatment and is entirely justifiable, particularly because of the reduction of morbidity and disability, as well as the economic advantage of decreased expense of treatment and disability.

Massage and Passive Motion

The treatment of joints after removal of immobilizing apparatus is still misunderstood by many surgeons and by many physiotherapists. If proper care has been taken to follow the principles just outlined, there is a minimum

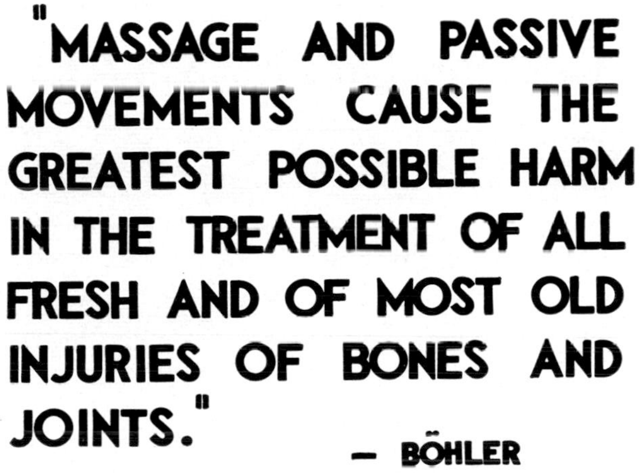

"MASSAGE AND PASSIVE MOVEMENTS CAUSE THE GREATEST POSSIBLE HARM IN THE TREATMENT OF ALL FRESH AND OF MOST OLD INJURIES OF BONES AND JOINTS."
— BÖHLER

Fig. 1–Placard posted in the fracture clinic to emphasize joint care after removal of plaster.

of disability and treatment is rarely prolonged. Unfortunately, the patient who is in greatest need of good treatment, having had no instruction in exercise during immobilization, is often apt to receive the worst possible late treatment: heat, massage and passive stretching of his joints. In our fracture clinic we have copied a placard (fig. 1) posted in Böhler's[2] clinic which we feel is important in teaching the care of our cases after removal of plaster. Companion placards, shown in figure 2, are added to indicate the importance of active motion.

If a stiffened joint is forcibly stretched, trauma is inflicted, the muscles and ligaments are torn, and new scars are formed during healing. There is further contraction, and the joint becomes stiffer after each manipulation. The elbow is the joint most susceptible to passive manipulation, and to emphasize the importance of this fact we have copied an instructive drawing which recently appeared in a publication entitled, "Position of Hands of Physiotherapist During Treatment of Stiff Elbow" (fig. 3). We have followed Watson-Jones' advice and do not send elbow cases to the physiotherapy departement, but take on the responsibility in the fracture clinic. Watson-Jones feels that physiotherapy technicians should not be tempted to stretch elbows, so he does not refer them to his massage department. He undertakes the instruction of active motion himself.

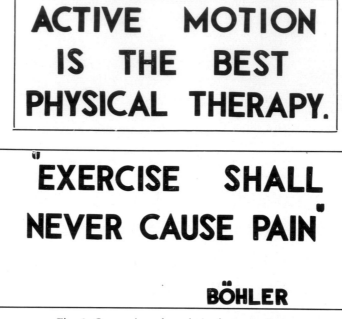

Fig. 2–Companion placards in fracture clinic.

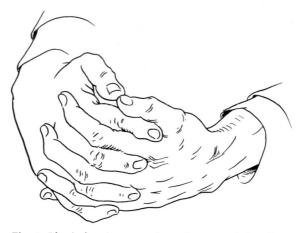

Fig. 3–Physiotherpist at work on fracture of the elbow.

Rehabilitation

Recent overemphasis on rehabilitation has created grave tendency to consider rehabilitation as a specialty or a distinct phase or stage in the treatment of trauma. There is an impression in many industrial circles that after a patient has had his fracture reduced, immobilized and the plaster removed, he should then be transferred to a rehabilitation department, where, by certain mysterious treatment by a specialist, he is returned to normal. Rehabilitation should begin the moment the patient is injured, and represents all we do for a patient from the time he sustains his fracture until he returns to his work, cured. If there is a dividing line where rehabilitation begins after other treatment leaves off, the early treatment has not been satisfactory. A good fracture surgeon is the best rehabilitation expert the patient can have. The surgeon who needs a specialist in rehabilitation to achieve a good result is not a good fracture surgeon.

If, during the course of our treatment, we consider the patient and the muscles and joints about his fracture, and encourage him to mobilize his body, to move all of his joints that are not immobilized, to move his muscles within the immobilization apparatus in so far as it is possible, to walk in walking plaster, to move his fingers when the wrist is immobilized and to exercise his quadriceps regularly when the knee is immobilized, we can then expect that the recovery period will be greatly shortened. The patient will be more contented, the cost of treatment will be decreased and the result will more nearly approach the ideal we wish to achieve – the complete return to normal joint function.

References

1 BÖHLER, L.: The Treatment of Fractures, ed. 5. New York, Grune & Stratton, 1956.

2 CHARNLEY, J.: The Closed Treatment of Common Fractures. Baltimore, Williams and Wilkins Co., 1950.

3 WATSON-JONES, R.: Fractures and Joint Injuries, ed. 4. Baltimore, Williams and Wilkins Co., 1952.

CHAPTER 16

PATHOLOGIC FRACTURES

Robert Lee Patterson, Jr., M.D., and Sidney N. Eichenholtz, M.D.

It has become increasingly apparent that pathologic fractures occurring in metastatic lesions from primary carcinoma elsewhere, are not an infrequent occurrence in any fair sized general hospital. The literature has been scarce on this subject. The handling of these fractures has been based on hopelessness. Jones [6] has amply stated that "death of a patient does not constitute failure and salvage of an additional period of useful, symptom-free life, is a major success." We do not know of any condition associated with fracture work that requires such care and demands such a high degree of attention to the physiologic and psychologic status of the patient than a fracture occurring in a metastasis. We shall limit ourselves to the management of these fractures.

There are certain things that we should keep in mind when dealing with a patient with a pathologic fracture in a metastasis: (1) They are not all hopeless. These patients may live for years after the fracture has been properly treated, lead a useful life and die from some other cause. (2) Fractures through a metastasis can heal. (3) The pain connected with a fracture of a long bone in a metastasis is far greater than that of the average fracture. You cannot treat these patients as you do the ordinary patient with a fracture. (4) They have a prodromal time or symptoms; they have a sense of heaviness or ache in the extremity, as we shall bring out, before the fracture occurs. (5) If one is able to x-ray them and find this condition and give prophylactic treatment, one can save a tremendous amount of pain and disability, hospitalization, etc.

Source

The metastatic lesions are most common from the lung, kidney, breast, prostate and thyroid, not necessarily in the order of their relative frequency. Bone involvement from the solid lymphomata and leukemias, of course, can but rarely have produced pathologic fractures in our experience. Osseus metastases from malignancies of the gastrointestinal tract, and of the lower genitourinary tract with the exception of the prostate, are relatively rare in our series.

Symptoms

Symptoms of localized pain and swelling were always present prior to the time of fracture in long bones, and in every case the patient was cognizant of a specific time of increased pain and disability when fracture occurred. This was equally true in those instances in which significant displacement of the fracture fragments did not occur. The ensuing pain was frequently

188

far in excess of that seen with similar fractures in normal bones. In those patients with involvement of the vertebral bodies or the innominate bones, local pain of deep, boring nature was usually present with no gross change in the intensity of pain when fracture occurred.

Definitive Care

Such factors as surgical accessibility, extent, and location of tumor tissue at the fracture site, the specific bone involved (whether weight-bearing or not), the presence and location of other lesions, are all vitally important in selecting the treatment of choice. We suggest that, unless *in extremis*, the patient's general condition as a poor surgical risk must not interfere with any reasonable procedure which will provide comfort and solace to him. It should be emphasized that regardless of the source of primary tumor and multiplicity of metastatic lesions, immediate definitive care for the pathological fracture is indicated.

Specific procedures recommended may be classified as follows:

ABLATION

Excision: Excision of a pathologic fracture with the surrounding tumor may be possible in such areas as the clavicle, proximal fibula and radius, distal ulna, phalanges, and metacarpal or metatarsal bones (fig. 1 A and B).

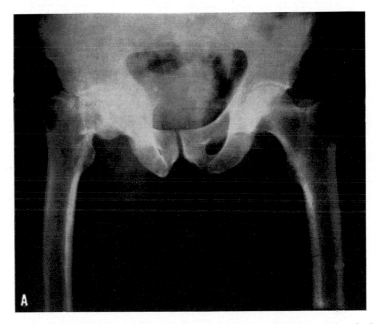

Fig. 1–(A) Proven bronchogenic carcinoma with metastases to the neck of the femur. Patient was at home when fracture occurred and had excruciating pain, requiring anesthesia to move him to the hospital. Attempts at closed reduction prior to internal fixation were grossly unsatisfactory. On exposure of fracture site, it was obvious that tumor tissue had replaced most of the head, neck and trochanteric regions. Internal fixation or replacement was not possible.

Excision and Reconstruction: In other areas excision of fracture and tumor may be accompanied by major reconstructive surgery when life expectancy is exceptionally good.

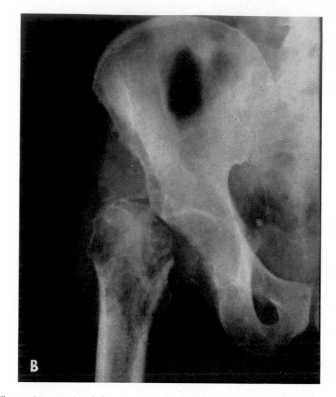

Fig. 1—(B) The entire proximal fragment was excised and this patient remained comfortable until he died months later.

Amputation: This is definitely indicated in certain instances, that is, when the metastatic lesion has also involved the adjacent soft tissues, making adequate local excision impossible (fig. 2 A and B).

EXTERNAL IMMOBILIZATION

Simple immobilization either with plaster or with splint. The use of plaster or splints for immobilization of pathologic fractures has been quite unsatisfactory in our experience. A one and onehalf spica plaster for a fracture through the femoral mid-shaft not only failed to relieve the extreme pain in one of our patients, but also failed to prevent fracture (fig. 3 A and B). In the nonweight-bearing long bones, the use of plaster or splints has proved cumbersome and has not effectively relieved pain.

INTERNAL FIXATION

Fixation with Screws: This method of internal fixation in pathologic fractures is most readily adaptable to those instances of long oblique or spiral fractures at the metaphyseal end of a bone, and more especially a

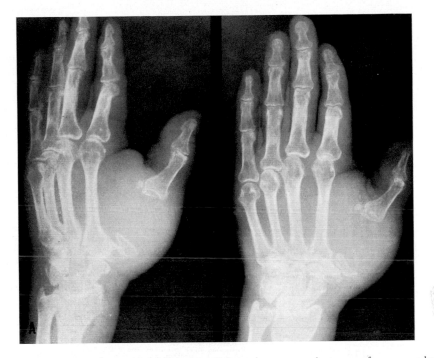

Fig. 2—(A) Gross replacement of metacarpal bone by metastatic tumor from an adeno-carcinoma of the kidney.

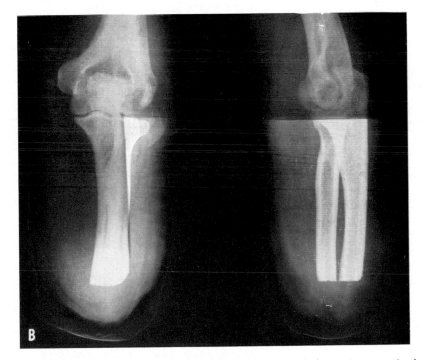

Fig. 2—(B) Pain was relieved by midforearm amputation and the patient remained com-fortable for fifteen months.

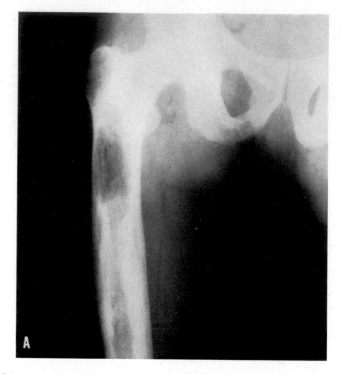

Fig. 3—(A) Proven case of Paget's disease, developed a painful plasma cell myeloma at upper end of right femoral shaft.

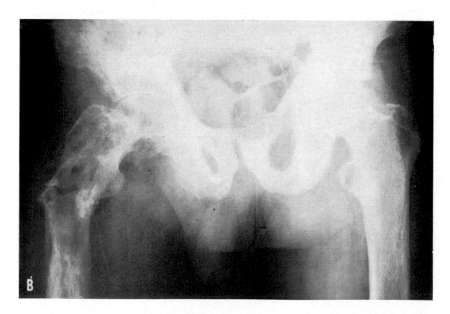

Fig. 3—(B) Placed in a one and one-half spica, but developed fracture while in plaster.

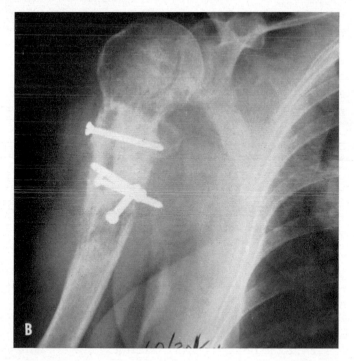

Fig. 4—(A) Type amenable to screw fixation.

Fig. 4—(B) Healing has taken place despite the extension of the tumor tissue distally. Patient lived comfortably for 19 months after original fracture.

nonweight-bearing bone. Healing occurs readily in these instances (fig. 4 A and B).

Fixation with Plates, Nails, or Combination of these: A very common area for metastases is the subtrochanteric region of the femur, and not infrequently the femoral neck itself. The appropriate appliance for internal fixation has proven to be most satisfactory where the extent of the metastatic lesion and the degree of bone destruction have not contraindicated this type of fixation (fig. 5).

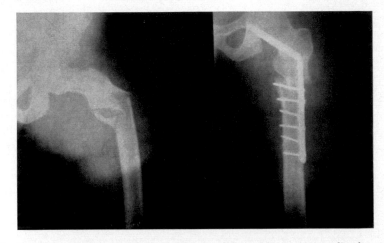

Fig. 5—Pathologic fracture secondary to carcinoma of the breast. Patient lived comfortably for seven months following operation.

Intramedullary Fixation. Whenever feasible, fixation of the long bones by means of an intramedullary appliance is the procedure of choice for the following reasons:

(1) In many instances this is relatively simple to accomplish and frequently can be performed without exposure of the tumor at the fracture site, using 1 per cent procaine for local anesthesia with very little discomfort to the patient (fig. 6 A—D).

(2) This, of course, permits early return of function and does not interfere with subsequent use of x-ray therapy. In most instances we have found that, following the procedure of intramedullary fixation, the relief of pain is phenomenal.

(3) Healing occurs rapidly in the same manner as that occurring in the long bones in normal fractures that have been fixed by intramedullary nailing. Open reduction for insertion of an intramedullary appliance should be avoided whenever possible, since this may permit extrusion of tumor tissue into the adjacent soft parts and indeed may result in the development of a fungating lesion at the operative site. Nevertheless, if reduction and intramedullary fixation cannot be accomplished without exposure of the fracture site, such exposure is not contraindicated.

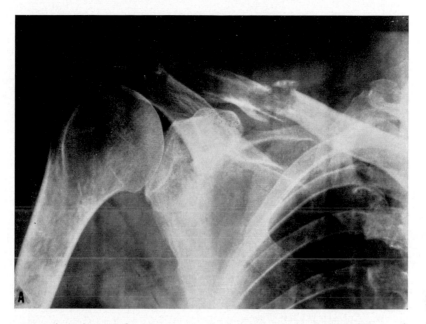

Fig. 6—(A) Relatively pain-free metastases of adeno carcinoma of the kidney to the right clavicle. Note the evidence of metastatic involvement of the upper humerus, for which intramedullary fixation was advised and refused.

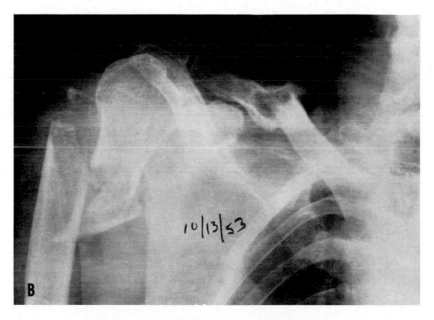

Fig. 6—(B) Same case. Note fracture displacement accompanied by excruciating pain. Fracture of clavicle is healed.

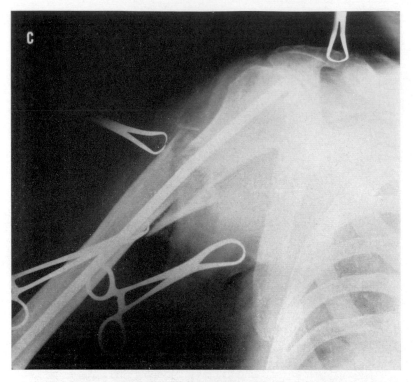

Fig. 6—(C) Intramedullary fixation.

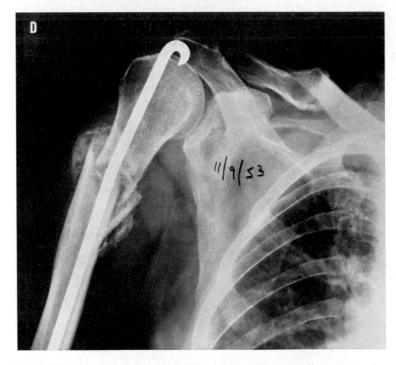

Fig. 6—(D) Three weeks postoperative. Note exuberant callous. No pain.

Prophylactic Use of Intramedullary Fixation

It has been our practice to advise intramedullary fixation of the involved long bones prior to fracture when it becomes apparent that fracture is imminent or even likely in the near future (figs. 7 A and B, 8 A and B).

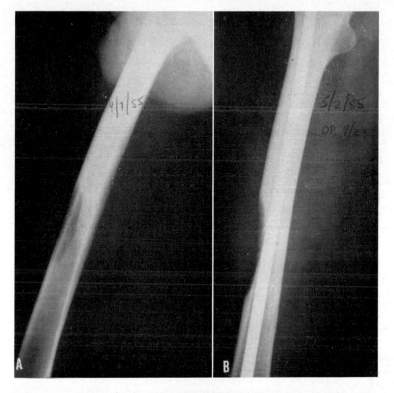

Fig. 7-(A) Metastases from adeno carcinoma of the kidney. (B) Prophylactic intramedullary nailing.

In such instances, the insertion of the intramedullary appliance is relatively simple, the site of the metastasis is not exposed and minimal anesthesia is required. This procedure is frequently quite rewarding in producing complete relief from the pain which was present at the site of the pathologic process despite the absence of fracture. Fracture may occur after nailing, but absence of displacement and telescoping of the fracture fragments minimizes pain and disability (fig. 9 A and B). It should be pointed out that in no instance in which an intramedullary appliance was inserted, has repeated x-ray examination disclosed an additional destructive lesion along the nail tract. Fitts et al. [2] have also reported no "evidence of secondary growths along the medullary cavity" by the insertion of an intramedullary nail (figs. 10 A—C).

On completion of the definitive orthopedic procedure, the physician continues a planned program of management. If an accurate and unequivocal

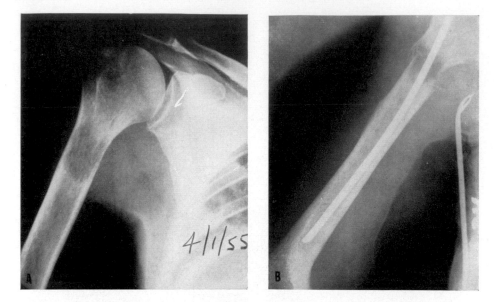

Fig. 8–(A) Epidermoid carcinoma of the larynx with metastases.
Fig. 8–(B) Prophylactic nailing upper extremity.

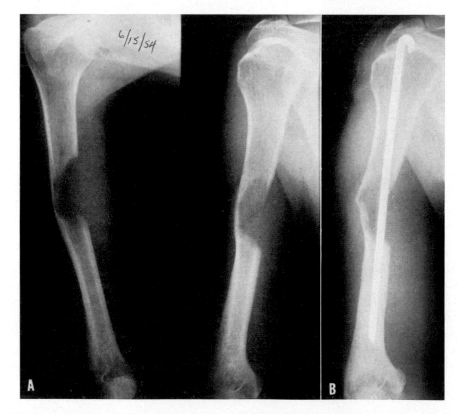

Fig. 9–(A) Metastases from epidermoid carcinoma of the lung. (B) Fracture occurred
17 days after prophylactic nailing without appreciable pain.

histologic identification has not yet been established, then further diagnostic studies must be pursued in order to determine the nature and site of origin of the lesion. After all other means have failed, one should not hesitate to utilize biopsy.

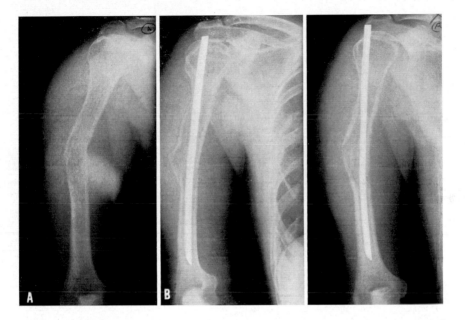

Fig. 10—(A) Fracture through area involved by Hodgkin's Disease. 10(B) Intramedullary nailing. Fracture site not opened. Pain completely relieved.

The importance of positive specific identification of the lesion lies in the availability of specific palliative (but not curative) therapeutic agents. Such agents are currently available for the treatment of carcinoma of the male and female breasts, carcinoma of the prostate and thyroid, bronchogenic carcinoma, certain carcinomas of the genital tract, Hodgkin's disease, lymphosarcoma, plasma cell (multiple) myeloma, and some others (table 1).

The cytotoxic alkylating agents have been found effective in the palliative treatment of tumors arising from the reticuloendothelial system and in bronchogenic carcinoma. The most common of these is nitrogen mustard. Therapeutic effectiveness with this and most of the other chemotherapeutic agents depends on the difference in sensitivity of tumor cells and normal cells to damage by the drug (table 1). Accordingly, dosage must be carefully controlled up to the point of maximum tolerance. All of the therapeutic agents have definite undesirable side effects requiring a close familiarity with dosage schedules and pharmacologic action. Androgenic and/or estrogenic hormones have a distinct place in the therapeutic armamentarium of cancer management. The mechanism of their action is unknown, but the clinical response is usually readily apparent. Androgens produce an anabolic effect with nitrogen retention, protein synthesis, accompanied by increased appetite and a sense of well-being. The same clinical response may be achieved with the adrenal cortical hormones or ACTH.

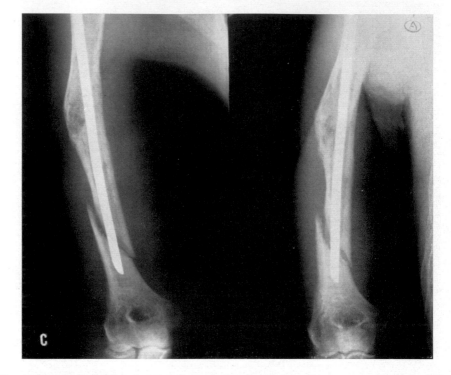

Fig. 10–(C) Patient tripped and fell on the outstretched hand seven months after nailing, fracturing the involved humerus at a lower level. However, pain was minimal and relieved by a sling. There is still no evidence of bone destruction along the nail track and the patient lived for an additional five months with comfort.

Radiation therapy for local lesions is most effective where surgical excision is not feasible. Radioresistance is relative, and with the new technics and more efficient equipment it is now possible to deliver extremely high doses to tumor masses without destroying adjacent normal tissues. This procedure can be applied to many portals of different areas of involvement. With the advent of the atomic pile, a variety of radioactive elements are readily available for specific palliative treatment. And finally, the use of various neurosurgical procedures for specific and clear-cut indications offer the patient additional protection against intractable pain. Rhizotomy, unilateral chordotomy, prefrontal lobotomy or topectomy, and hypophysectomy each has its place in the control of pain.

Table 1—PALLIATIVE AGENTS

	CHEMO-THERAPEUTIC (SELECTIVE TOXICITY)	SEX HORMONES (MECHANISM UNKNOWN)	ADRENAL CORTICAL HORMONES	X-RAY THERAPY
Bronchogenic Carcinoma	Nitrogen Mustard	Androgen-(Anabolic) Nitrogen retention Protein synthesis Improved appetite Well being	Cmp. E & F ACTH Increased appetite Euphoria	Local deep therapy Moderately resistant
Carcinoma Kidney		Androgen	Cmp. E & F ACTH	Radio resistant High dosage therapy
Carcinoma Breast		Estrogen for a) Male breast Ca. b) Female after menopause Androgen for Female antemenopausal c) Castration	Bilateral adrenalectomy Cmp. E & F Hypophysectomy	Local Therapy X-ray Castration after menopause
Carcinoma Prostate		Estrogens Castration (most effective)	Cmp. E & F Bilateral adrenalectomy	Final palliative Deep therapy
Carcinoma Thyroid		Androgen (Limited value)	Cmp. E & F	I^{131} Beta rays Gamma rays $1/2$ life 8 days 15% of cases relieved Thyroidectomy and/or Thiouracil plus I^{131} additional 10-15% Local deep therapy
Solid Lymphomata Hodgkins Reticulum cell Large > cell Small Lymphosarcoma	Disseminated HN₂ TEM TEPA THIO-TEPA		Cmp. E & F	Local Deep Therapy Radio-sensitive for localized disease
Plasma Cell Myeloma	Urethane	Androgen Estrogen Increased appetite Euphoria	Cmp. E & F	Deep therapy
Primary Bone Tumors Ewing's Sa.			Cmp. E & F	Deep therapy Radio-sensitive

Code HN₂ — Nitrogen Mustard
  TEM — Triethylene Melanine
  TEPA — Triethylene Phosphoramide

THIO-TEPA — Thioethylene Phosphoramide
I^{131} — Radioactive Iodine

Summary

1. Definitive care of pathologic fractures is both successful and rewarding in terms of patient comfort.

2. Basic principles of fracture treatment may be applied.

3. "Prophylactic" management of osseous metastases must be considered whenever feasible to prevent disabling and painful fracture displacement.

4. Fracture healing may be expected in many instances of pathological fractures.

5. The intramedullary nail has not produced additional "seeding" foci along the nail track.

6. The "medical team" approach to the management of these patients provides maximum assurance of best results.

References

[1] CHAMBERLAIN, R. H.: Modern therapeutic measures in cancer and their effectiveness. Bull. New York, Acad. Med. *31:* 746—749, (Oct.) 1955.

[2] FITTS, W. T., JR., ROBERTS, B. and RAVDIN, I.: Fractures in metastatic carcinoma. Am. J. Surg. *85:* 282—289 (April) 1953.

[3] GELHORN, A.: Cancer chemotherapy. Bull. New York, Acad. Med. *31:* 750—756, (Oct.) 1955.

[4] GRAHN, H.: Use of ad-amphetamine — amobarbital combination as an adjunct to the treatment of carcinoma. J. Am. Geriatrics Soc. *11:* (Sept.) 1954.

[5] HUGGINS, C., JR., and TAYLOR, G. W.: Carcinoma of the male breast. Arch. Surg. *70:* 303—308, (Feb.) 1955.

[6] JONES, R., JR.: Medical management of patients with incurable cancer. V. A. Technical Bull., Dept. Med. and Surg, TB 10—107.

[7] LEVINE, B., and WEISBERGER, A. S.: The response of various types of bronchogenic carcinoma to nitrogen mustard. Ann. Int. Med. *42:* 1089—1096, (May) 1955.

CHAPTER 17

FRACTURES IN CHILDREN

PRESTON A. WADE, M.D.

The general principles of fracture treatment in adults are familiar to most physicians and even to the laity. Early and accurate reduction of fractures, followed by immobilization in splints, plaster or traction, are procedures well known. Of late years new operative methods and internal fixation by means of screws, plates and intramedullary rods have been publicized in the medical as well as lay literature, so that even those who have no actual part in treating fractures feel they have a very good idea of how one should be managed. However, the laity, and even a large segment of the medical profession, are not aware that the treatment of fractures in children is based on different principles. As a result, unnecessary operations or other harmful therapy may be used, and disaster sometimes results.

Several good reasons explain the fact that children's fractures cannot be treated by methods based on the general principles which apply to adults. First, younger bones are softer and more pliable than older ones and do not fracture as easily. They are very apt to break incompletely in a greenstick fashion, without complete displacement of the fragments. This fact aids in maintaining satisfactory postreduction positions and, on occasion, even makes immobilization unnecessary. The tough periosteum of children's bones often remains intact after fracture, thus helping to prevent displacements and to maintain reductions. In forearm or leg, one bone may fracture while the other remains intact and helps to immobolize its companion bone.

Although the thick periosteum and the abundant blood supply of adolescent bones make nonunion an almost unknown complication, some fractures in children do fail to unite. Fracture of the neck of the femur in the child, fortunately a rare occurence, has no better prognosis than in the adult. Fractures of the navicular bones in older children also may fail to unite. Fracture of the head of the radius occasionally goes on to nonunion even after perfect reduction (fig. 1 A—E). Otherwise, nonunion is rarely encountered in the treatment of children's fractures.

The second and perhaps most important difference between fractures in children and adults has to do with the growth potential of the bones. In the epiphyses at either end of the long bones, this potential is very important in correcting shortening in children's fractures; the ability of the bone to grow in width as well as in length helps to correct lateral displacements and to reshape and remold deformed bone, even correcting certain degrees of angulation. Because of these factors, considerable degrees of shortening and lateral displacements can be accepted, and healing without fear of nonunion or permanent deformity can be expected even if the fragments are not in

203

contact. As a matter of fact, it is an advantage to have some overriding of fragments of long bones, since this shortens the healing time, and the stimulus to the epiphysis allows for overgrowth of the broken limb so eventually it becomes as long as the unbroken one (fig. 2 A—C). If a fracture is too

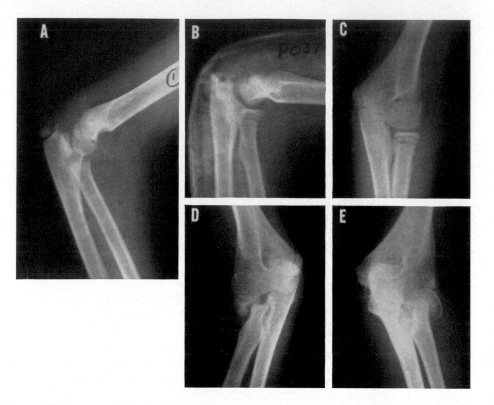

Fig. 1–(A) Fracture of head of radius in 6 year old child. Note marked displacement and 90 degrees rotation of head. (B) After open reduction and replacement. Catgut fixation. (C) After 6 weeks fracture line distal to epiphysis is still visible. (D) One year follow up. Nonunion. (E) Five year follow-up. Nonunion of fracture with displacement of head. Note overgrowth of head.

accurately reduced, the fractured limb will sometimes outgrow its fellow (fig. 3). In younger children especially, up to 20 degrees of angulation may be completely corrected by the callus which is laid down in the concavity of the angulation and which reshapes the bone to normal contour (fig. 4). However, correction of marked degrees of angulation cannot be expected, especially in older children, nor will rotation deformities always return to normal. When faced with apparent malposition of a fracture, the physician who is unaware of these facts may not await nature's kindly help, but to play safe may try frequent manipulations or unnecessary operative procedures with internal fixation to obtain a more acceptable immediate x-ray correction of the displaced fragments.

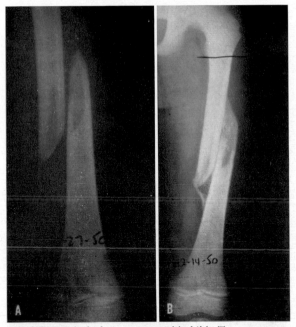

Fig. 2—(A) Fracture of femoral shaft in 5 year old child. Two cm. over riding. "Bayonet position." (B) After 7 weeks. Treated in Bryant's traction. Over riding unchanged.

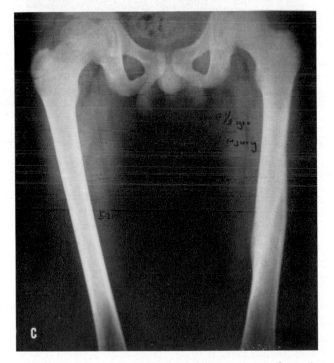

Fig. 2—(C) Four and one half year follow up. No shortening.

The third factor also concerns the epiphyses. While their growth potential is a great help in correcting deformities, anything that interferes with this growth will cause shortenings or deformities. Therefore, any injury which involves the epiphyses must be considered with great respect. Most fractures

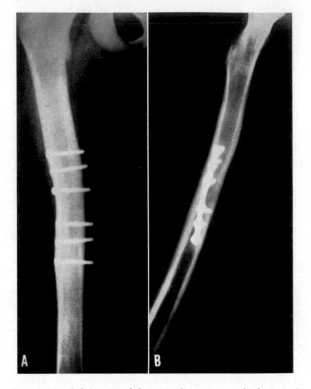

Fig. 3—(A) Boy of 9 sustained fracture of femur. Plate was applied. Anterior posterior view postoperatively. (B) Lateral view.

through epiphyses do not cause any change in the normal growth of the bone, but in some fortunately rare cases, the epiphyses may become prematurely closed thus causing serious degrees of shortening, or there may be partial closing of an epiphysis which may cause even greater deformity through the unnatural growth of one portion of the single bone. When the epiphysis of one of two companion bones becomes prematurely fused, the continuing normal growth of the opposite bone will cause a deformity such as the deviation of the hand due to a shortened radius (fig. 5), deviation at the ankle due to a fused tibial epiphysis, or an increased carrying angle such as is seen in the elbow when the lateral condyle is injured. Certain epiphyseal displacements must be corrected by open operation and internal fixation to assure normal growth. The capitellum of the humerus (fig. 6) and the displaced radial head (fig. 1) are examples of sites needing operative intervention.

The probability or the extent of a deformity following any epiphyseal injury cannot always be predicted, but the physician must always be on the alert for its development. The degree of displacement at the epiphysis is not a measure of epiphyseal injury. As a matter of fact, normal growth after

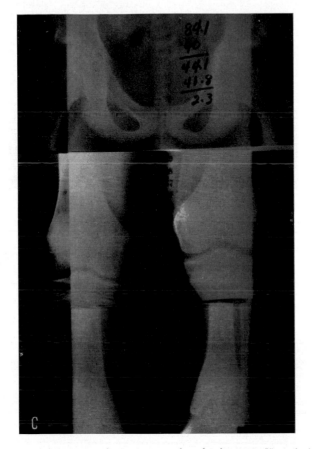

Fig. 3–(C) Five years later, 2.3 cm. lengthening on affected side.

epiphyseal dislocation is as common as it is after only slight displacement. If the fracture line crosses the epiphyseal plate and causes injury to the epiphyseal side, growth is more apt to be disturbed than if the injury is to the diaphyseal side only. Only one constant factor can be noted in cases of growth disturbance, and that has to do with the trauma of treatment. Cases subjected to repeated and forceful attempts at reduction are more likely to result in growth changes than those treated by gentle manipulation, even though com-

The elbow is the one area in a child where complications are most apt to follow a fracture. The first complication involves the circulation. Nowhere else does the rapid swelling and embarrassment of circulation cause as much worry as in impending Volkmann's ischemic paralysis in the elbow. The loss of radial pulse, cold limb, continued pain and loss of motion of fingers call for immediate release of all constricting bandages, release of flexion of elbow and elevation of the limb, often by skeletal suspension. Decompression of the cubital space by incising the lacertus fibrosis fascia may be necessary.

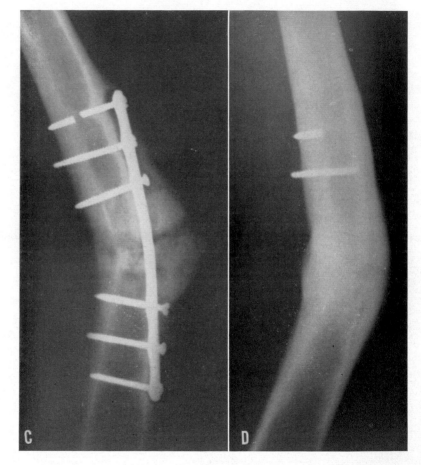

Fig. 7—(C) After 18 months in plaster. Nonunion with angulation and breaking of screws. (D) Three months after removal of metal. Prompt union.

A late complication of elbow injuries may be the rare but tragic stiffening of the elbow by myositis ossificans. This condition is the result of ossification of a subperiosteal hematoma in the cubital region. The most serious damage that can be done in an impending case of myositis ossificans is caused by the pernicious practice of passive, forceful motion of a child's stiff

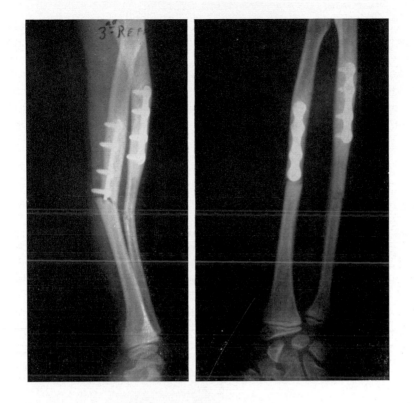

Fig. 8—Boy of 9, three years after internal fixation by plates with screws of fracture of both bones of arm. This is the third refracture this boy had sustained since original operation. Note that the plates are embedded in the bones and cannot be removed.

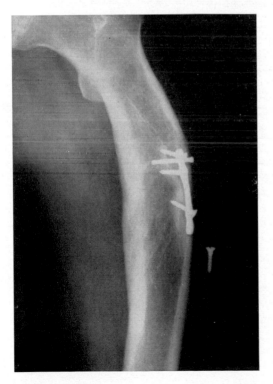

Fig. 9—This man of 43 had a plate applied to his fractured femur at the age of four. The result is marked angulation, bowing and shortening of 4½ inches.

elbow. Forced motion of any joint in a child or adult is the most harmful therapeutic method that can be employed and should always be carefully avoided.

General Considerations

Anesthesia: The reduction of fractures in children may be accomplished under either local or general anesthesia. It is often said that local anesthesia is too frightening to a child and causes more psychic trauma than general anesthesia. However, a single injection of procaine into a fracture hematoma may be less traumatic than a general anesthetic. Local anesthesia may also be more suitable when the child has recently eaten, and there is doubt as to amount of food retained in the stomach. It is, however, a good rule to insist on general anesthesia wherever reduction of the fracture may be difficult. In these instances, complete relaxation and painless manipulation are necessary to assure the minimum of trauma. It is essential that all epiphyseal separations be reduced under general anesthesia so that the procedure may be accomplished by as gentle maneuvers as possible.

Parents: It is the duty of the surgeon undertaking the treatment of a fracture in a child to take into consideration the exaggerated fears of the parents and to explain the situation thoroughly in an effort to spare them unnecessary suffering. It is also necessary that the surgeon explain the possibility of growth disturbance in those cases of epiphyseal injury where complications may ensue. This must be done with considerable tact so that the parents may not be alarmed but still may understand that observation must be continued over a long period of time.

Removals of Splints and Casts: Splints and casts should be removed without causing the child unnecessary fear and discomfort. The electric saw is often dangerous and should always be used with great care to avoid cutting the skin, particularly over a bony prominence. When the cast is removed, the child is often disturbed because of the appearance of the limb and the unusual sensation of lightness. When removing plaster, it is wise to have the child supine on an examining table rather than sitting in a chair so that he may not fall if he suddenly becomes faint. After removal of plaster from a lower limb a child will undoubtedly exhibit a limp, and will walk with the foot everted. This temporary gait must be explained to the parents so that they will not be unduly alarmed.

Massage and Passive Motion: Böhler has stated; "Massage and passive motion cause the greatest possible harm to all fresh fractures and most old fractures." Nowhere is this dictum more applicable than in children's fractures, and baking, massage and diathermy are not only contraindicated because they are unnecessary but also because they are definitely harmful. The child soon regains normal function of his limb by gradually increasing its use, and he will seldom go beyond the limits of pain in moving his joints. Particularly in the region of the elbow, return to normal function is slow, and both the parents and the physician must exercise considerable patience in allowing nature to take its course. Any attempts to hasten motion in the elbow joint are apt to delay the return to normal function.

Birth Fractures: Fractures occuring as a result of trauma at delivery are most commonly found in the shaft of the humerus. Next in frequency are fractures of the clavicles and the femur, depressed fracture of the skull and epiphyseal injuries of the humerus or femur. The fracture is usually markedly displaced (fig. 10), and may even be unrecognized until the rapid callus formation presents a palpable or visible swelling at the fracture site fig. 10 B).

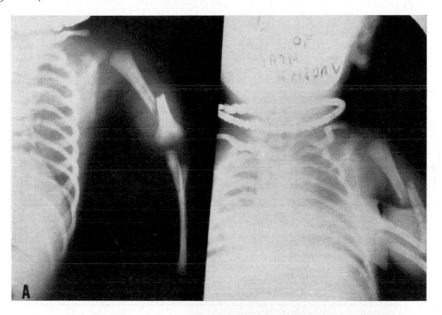

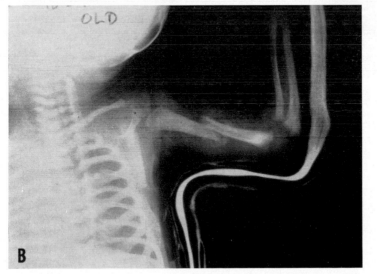

Fig. 10—(A, *top*) Birth fracture with usual displacement and overiding. (B, *bottom*) At six days — note the obvious abundant callus at fracture site.

The simplest methods possible should be employed in the effort to reduce and immobilize these fractures, since nature provides perfect restoration of a deformed bone regardless of the amount of displacement or angulation. Bandaging of the arm to the chest is sufficient in fractures of the clavicle or humerus, and a week or 10 days in a suspension frame or abduction splint is usually sufficient in the treatment of fractures of the femur. The callus forms rapidly about the fracture site, the break is usually solid within 10 days and perfectly healed within three weeks, and in a few months the normal anatomy of the bone is restored (fig. 10 C).

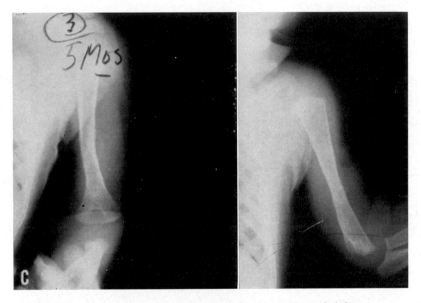

Fig. 10–(C) At 5 months. Almost complete correction of deformity.

Open Fractures: The open fracture in a child is as serious a surgical emergency as it is in the adult, and prompt débridement is necessary. The details of this procedure are described in Chapter 12. In treating the open fracture in a child, the principles and technics are different because internal fixation is never justifiable.

The wound should be closed loosely by means of through-and-through sutures and the fracture then treated with plaster immobilization as though it were a closed fracture.

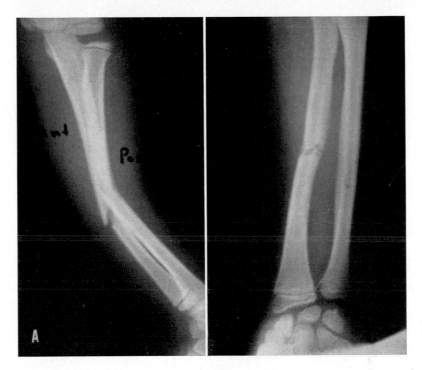

Fig. 11–(A) Fracture of both bones of arm in child of 8 with usual volar angulation. Greenstick fracture of both bones. (B) After reduction. Volar angulation has not been corrected completely. It is necessary to break through dorsal cortex completely to achieve full reduction.

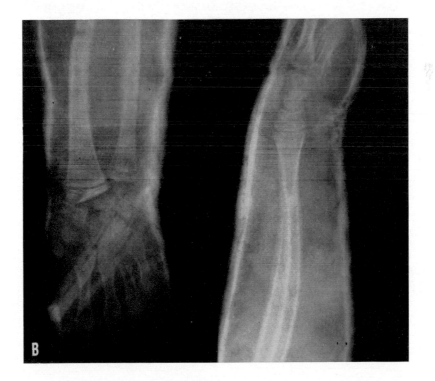

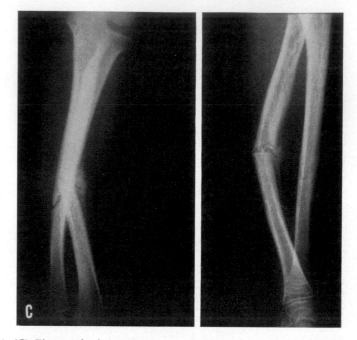

Fig. 11–(C) Five weeks later. Recurrence of angulation of radius within plaster.

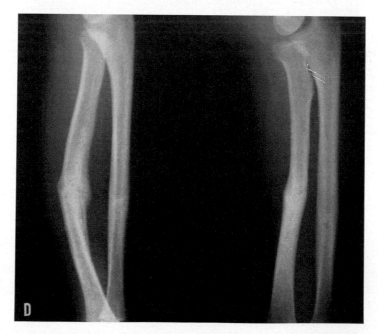

Fig. 11–(D) Ten weeks later. Note callus being laid down on concave side of fracture
correcting angulation.

Specific Fractures: Fractures of specific bones will usually be described in the section of the book devoted to the pertinent area. However, a few of the more common fractures will be discussed here.

Fractures of the Wrist and Forearm: The most common fracture in children is one involving both bones of the arm. It usually is caused by a fall on the extended arm. There is usually a volar angulation (fig. 11 A) at the

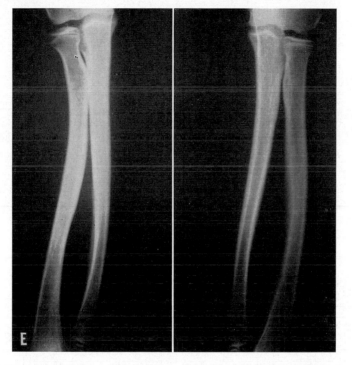

Fig. 11—(E) Five year follow-up. Slight bowing remains. Clinically no deformity. Function normal.

fracture site with a moderate displacement of the fragments. Often the fracture is of the greenstick variety. The reduction may be accomplished under local or general anesthesia, and in the greenstick type it is often necessary to complete the fracture by breaking through the cortex to achieve satisfactory alignment. If this is not done, the volar angulation may recur. Though this is usually not permanent, it may cause a deformity for a long time. Even after perfect alignment and completion of the fracture (fig. 11 B), there may be a recurrence of the volar alignment (fig. 11 C), but this does not warrant repeated efforts at reduction since nature will invariably correct the angulation (fig. 11 D—E).

Fractures of the midforearm are often associated with considerable displacement of the fracture fragments so that the inexperienced surgeon may fear crossunion of the two bones (fig. 12). It is not necessary to achieve perfect

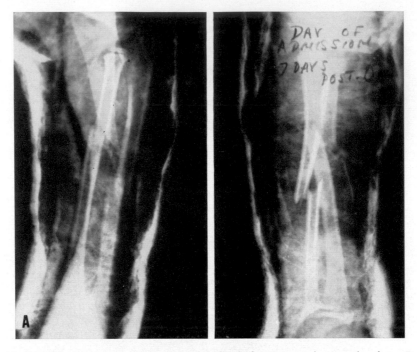

Fig. 12—(A) This 6 year old child admitted 7 days after open reduction elsewhere. Parents had been advised a second operation was necessary.

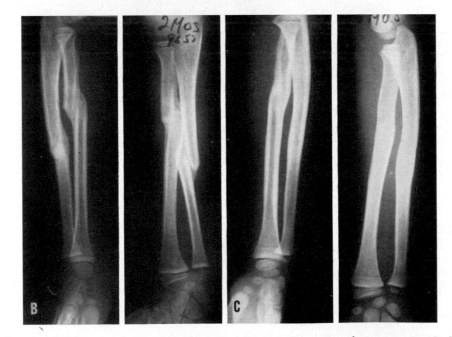

Fig. 12—(B) After two months — in plaster in original position. No other treatment. (C) Six months follow up. Correction of deformity and normal function.

reduction of the fragments of both bones of the forearm since crossunion never occurs except in the presence of an open fracture or after operative intervention. If the arm is aligned in a fairly satisfactory manner even though there may be some displacement at the fracture site, a full return of function with the normal anatomy may be expected (fig. 12 C). If one unwisely operates on this type of fracture, it is often difficult to maintain reduction. The operator is then forced to use internal fixation by means of plates or other material which causes refractures of the forearm (fig. 9), and which may become embedded within the bone.

Fractures of both bones of the forearm may heal within five or six weeks and may seem clinically solid and show sufficient callus by x-ray to allow removal of the plaster. For 10 or 12 weeks after the original fracture, however, they are very apt to be the site of refracture even after a relatively minor trauma. The rigid callus, which does not allow for normal bending as does the resilient normal one, is apt to snap in the center. This site is the most common area for refracture of children's bones. It is rare to see a refracture in other bones. For this reason, it may be necessary to treat the fracture of both bones of the forearm for 8 and 10 weeks in a cast immobilizing both elbow and wrist. The child's joints rapidly return to normal function, and the increased immobilization period will prevent most of the refractures which occur in this area.

Fractures About the Elbow: Fractures near the elbow in children have caused difficulties in treatment and show a higher rate of complications than any other type. The dangers of Volkmann's ischemic paralysis and myositis ossificans have already been discussed.

There are four important fractures about the elbow, each of which may result in a permanent deformity if proper treatment is not instituted.

1. Supracondylar Fractures. The common supracondylar fracture with posterior displacement of the distal fragment is caused by a fall on the extended arm with the elbow in hyperextension. There may be considerable swelling and deformity and interference with circulation, and the most important consideration is prompt reduction and maintenance of circulation to the hands and fingers.

If manipulation and reduction of the fracture with simple elevation do not suffice to restore circulation in the hand, suspension in an overhead frame by means of a wire through the olecranon is usually successful in treating the impending circulatory disturbance.

Commonly there is a rotation of the distal fragments, which gives the so-called "fish-tail" apearance in the x-ray (fig. 13). Reduction is accomplished by traction on the distal fragment with the elbow extended and the arm supinated, and immobilization is applied by means of a plaster splint with the arm in flexion. Flexion of the elbow tightens the triceps over the lower fragment, and it acts as a very satisfactory splint in maintaining reduction. It is essential that these cases be observed carefully after immobilization to prevent circulatory complications.

2. Fractures of the head of the radius with marked displacement of the head (fig. 1) should be operated on an open reduction accomplished if manipulation will not replace the displaced head. The head of the bone should never be removed. Occasionally, these fractures go on to nonunion as illustrated in figure 1.

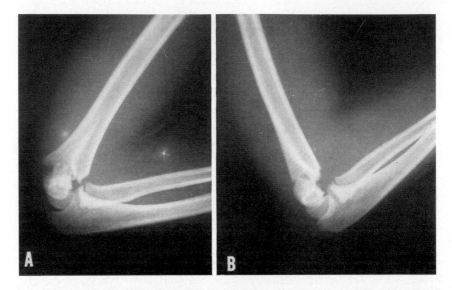

Fig. 13–(A) Supracondylar fracture with typical "fish tail" appearance. (B) After correction of rotation.

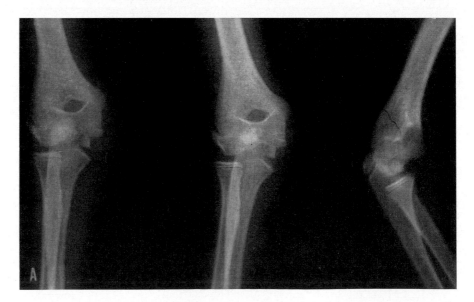

Fig. 14–(A) Fracture of medial epicondyle with displacement of fragment into joint.

3. Fractures of the medial epicondyle with displacement into the joint need operative intervention and replacement of the medial epicondyle to its normal position (fig. 14). This may be accomplished by means of catgut suture or occasionally by means of a removable pin.

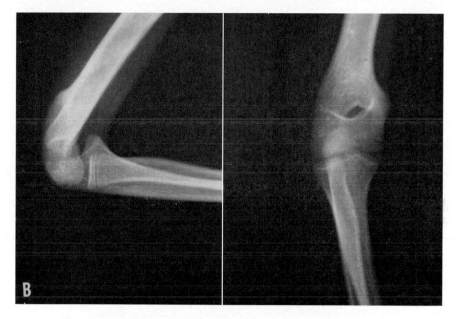

Fig. 14—(B) After operative replacement of epicondylar fragment.

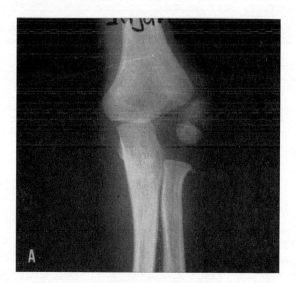

Fig. 15—(A) Fracture of lateral condyle of the humerus with displacement. This must be replaced to prevent deformity.

4. Fractures of the lateral condyle of the humerus often need open reduction for replacement (fig. 15). If the lateral condyle is not perfectly replaced, a growth deformity will occur causing an increase in the carrying angle with marked deformity. It is this deformity which leads to late ulnar palsy due to stretching of the ulnar nerve.

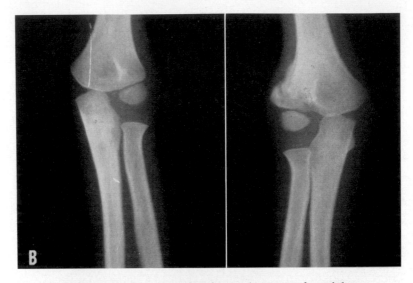

Fig. 15—(B) Three months after replacement of condyle.

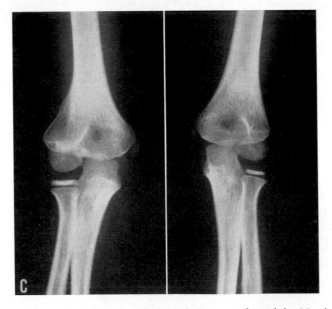

Fig. 15—(C) Three year follow up. Slight enlargement of condyle. No deformity.

Fracture of the shaft of the femur usually occurs in the midportion of the shaft and is often associated with considerable overriding and displacement. Treatment should be directed toward maintaining alignment of the fracture fragments and correction of rotation. It is not only unnecessary but unwise to correct the overriding since the displaced fragment causes a stimulation of the epiphyses with increased growth of the shortened limb, so that perfect correction of the overriding will usually lead to overgrowth and permanent lengthening on the affected side.

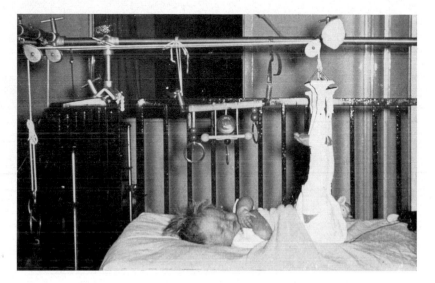

Fig. 16—Bryant's traction for fracture of femur in infant. Note adhesive traction is applied as high on thigh as possible. Circulation of feet must be carefully watched.

The "bayonet position" (fig. 2 A–C) is the desired one to maintain, since the fracture will heal more rapidly and 1–2 cm. of shortening with young child will be corrected by growth.

Maintenance of alignment and correction of rotation may be best accomplished in the infant by means of a pillow splint.

In the child from 1 to 5 years of age, the Bryant's traction (fig. 16) is the best method of treatment. The adhesive traction is applied high on the thigh and circumferential bandaging is carefully applied so as not to interfere with circulation. The circulation of the limbs must be carefully watched since cases have been reported in which Volkmann's ischemic paralysis, and even gangrene, have resulted from improper application of traction. The child is usually active in the bed and need not be confined too closely, since union with good alignment of the limb occurs in every case. After four to five weeks in the traction, the child may be allowed to move about in the bed, and at the end of six weeks he may be allowed full weight-bearing.

The child above 5 is best treated in Russell traction with attention paid primarily to alignment and correction of rotation. No attempt should be made to apply enough traction to reduce completely the overriding of the displaced fracture (fig. 17).

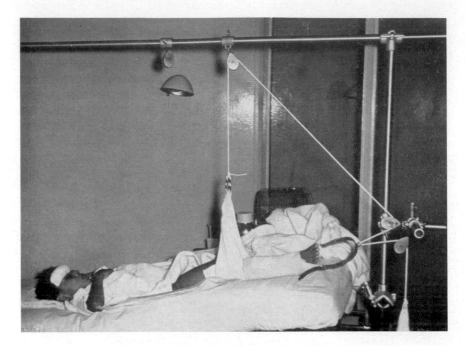

Fig. 17—Russell traction in older child.

Fractures of the upper third of the femur often result in an abduction, flexion, external rotation deformity of the upper fragment and are often difficult to hold in traction. In spite of these deformities, complete restoration of normal anatomy and function can be expected even in the presence of considerable angulation (fig. 4).

Reduction of the fracture and application of plaster are perfectly suitable methods of treatment and allow the patient to leave the hospital and be treated at home.

Injuries to the Distal Femoral Epiphysis: Epiphyseal separations often result in severe displacements, and when they cannot be reduced even by manipulation under anesthesia, operation is necessary. Internal fixation should never be used to maintain reduction of the distal femoral epiphysis (fig. 18). The reduction can usually be accomplished by means of traction and flexion of the knee. The limb is kept in plaster for four weeks, after which full function may be expected in the knee joint.

Fractures of the Shafts of Both of the Leg Bones. Fractures of the tibia and fibula are often greenstick in variety, and because of the thick periosteum,

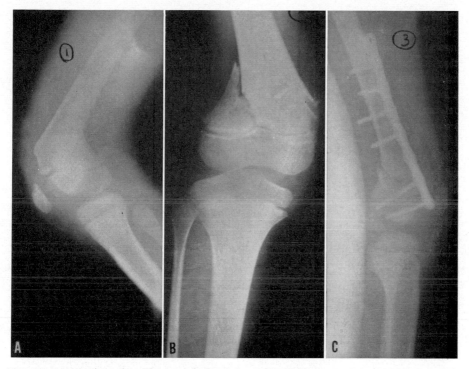

Fig. 18–(A) Epiphyseal separation of distal femoral epiphysis. Lateral view. (B) Anterior-posterior view. (C) Unwise operative reduction performed elsewhere. Note epiphysis effectively stapled by internal fixation. This was promptly removed in 7 weeks and fortunately no growth disturbance occurred.

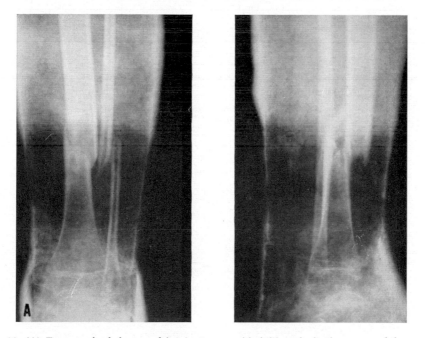

Fig. 19–(A) Fracture both bones of leg in 8 year old child with displacement of fragments.

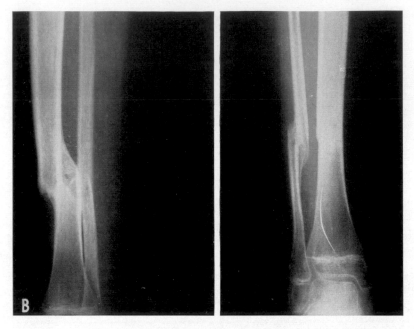

Fig. 19—(B) Rapid healing $2^1/_2$ months later.

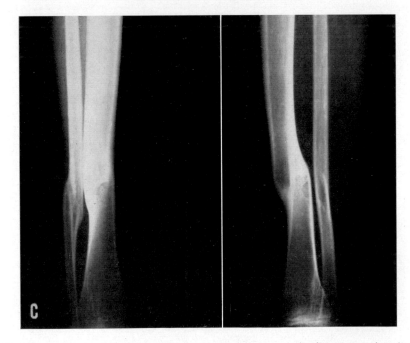

Fig. 19—(C) One year follow-up. Displacement almost completely corrected. Clinically no deformity.

displacements are not common. The fracture can usually be easily reduced and immobilized in a long leg plaster. The fracture is usually well healed within six weeks (fig. 19) when full weight-bearing may be allowed. Refracture of both bones of the leg is exceedingly rare. This is in contradistinction to fractures of both bones of the forearm, where it is quite common even after six to eight weeks of immobilization and apparent clinical and roentgen ray evidence of union.

References

[1] BLOUNT, P.: Fractures in Children. Baltimore, Williams and Wilkins co., 1955.

[2] BÖHLER, L.: Treatment of Fractures. New York, Grune & Stratton, 1956, vol. 1.

[3] KEY, J. A., and CONWELL, H. E.: The Management of Fractures, Dislocations and Sprains, ed. 6. St. Louis, C. V. Mosby Company, 1956.

[4] SMITH, F. M.: Surgery of the Elbow. Springfield, Ill., Charles C Thomas, 1954.

[5] WATSON-JONES, R.: Fractures and Joint Injuries. Edinburgh, E. & S. Livingstone, Ltd., 1955.

III. HEAD, NECK AND SPINE

CHAPTER 18

MANAGEMENT OF HEAD INJURIES

Bronson S. Ray M.D.

Over a quarter of a million serious head injuries occur annually in our country according to conservative estimate. The mortality rate has not been accurately determined, but it is believed that one-fourth of the deaths could be prevented by appropriate care of the patient. Whether such estimates are correct or not, the fact is that head injuries are common and potentially fatal, and that survival often depends on alert, intelligent management.

The majority of these injuries are cared for by physicians not specializing in neurology or neurosurgery, and this is not only understandable, but as it should be. However, the physician who accepts the responsibility must understand the principles of good management and recognize – even anticipate – the complications that may require assistance from those better equipped to deal with them. Fortunately, the majority of the injured recover without special treatment and possibly some recover despite poor care; some die even though the best methods are employed; the remainder constitute the group in which preservation of life and useful function is the obligation of the nonspecialist physician.

Immediate Observations

It may seem trite to remind practicing physicians of the importance of an accurate history, but the circumstances and nature of the injury and the patient's reactions up until the doctor sees him, can provide invaluable information. Loss of consciousness, its degree, and duration are clues to the seriousness of the injury, and much confusion and embarrassment in legal matters can be avoided if there is no delay in obtaining pertinent information before it becomes garbled and inaccurate.

Since the degree of injury to the brain is the principal concern, the state of consciousness is the most important observation to make in the initial examination and to observe thereafter. Simple methods suffice. Note the degree of restlessness, or lack of it, the presence of purposeful movements, the degree of lethargy or alertness, the response to question or command, the degree of orientation and ability to recall. Subsequent improvement in such responses provides reassurance, while deterioration is a warning of impending complications.

Every patient with a potentially serious injury deserves to have a record of vital signs kept for a period of 12–24 hours. Though it may not always be practical to do so, if this rule were observed, the occasional disaster could be avoided.

Soon after the injury, particularly if it has been painful or accompanied by much blood loss, there will be some degree of shock, evidenced by rapid pulse, low blood pressure, and altered respirations. But unless bleeding continues, or there is some injury of significance to other parts of the body, the element of shock is not serious and can be expected to respond to warmth, quiet, and intravenous infusion of fluids. Two methods commonly employed in treatment of shock are to be avoided in these cases: lowering of the head and administration of narcotics. The former will increase intracranial pressure and promote bleeding, while the latter will depress respirations, diminish the cerebral responses and alter pupillary reactions.

Evaluation of the state of the pupils is invaluable. The presence of equal pupils of average size and normal response to light is highly reassuring. Unilateral enlargement and fixation of a pupil usually implies damage to the oculomotor nerve, and in particular, indicates the possibility of hemorrhage in the meningeal spaces or laceration, swelling or hemorrhage involving a cerebral hemisphere. Although the large pupil is usually on the same side, as the hemorrhage or swelling, occasionally it may be contralateral. While symmetrically constricted pupils speak for probable injury to the brain stem but do not signify irreversible damage, dilated, fixed pupils in a patient who gives other evidence of serious injury almost always indicate irreversible and fatal damage. The latter sign assumes importance as a usual contraindication to any proposed "life-saving" operations. Under no circumstances should mydriatics be used to dilate the pupils to facilitate opthalmoscopic examination of the ocular fundi, at least during the first 2 days. No useful purpose will be served, and pupillary responses, so important to watch, will be altered for many hours.

When possible, voluntary motor responses in moving the face and extremities should be tested and retested periodically. Evaluation of sensation is less important. In less co-operative patients motor responses can be tested by some painful stimulus. Reflexes are also important, but less so than movements. Babinski signs on plantar stimulation are commonly present even in the absence of other motor or reflex abnormalities, and at times after relatively minor injuries. Alone, the positive Babinski sign does not imply a serious prognosis. Convulsions in the early period after injury usually mean a laceration of the cerebrum, and seizures restricted to one side of the body will usually serve to localize the injury. The presence of aphasia reflecting injury to the speech centers (predominately on the left side of the cerebrum) can be easily missed by regarding it as mental confusion, but in an even partially co-operative patient, aphasia can often be identified merely by asking for the names of common objects. Progression or change in some or any of these symptoms and signs may be strong indication of the need for surgical intervention.

Roentgenograms of the head are said by some to be of little or no value, since the concern is with the degree of damage to the intracranial structures. Certainly a critically injured patient, or restless and unco-operative one, should not have the rigors of a complete radiological examination imposed on him. But there are distinct advantages to knowing whether there has been a fracture, and if so whether it is linear or comminuted or depressed, and where it is located, particularly if it traverses the regions of the middle meningeal arteries, the major dural venous sinuses, the mastoid cells or the paranasal sinuses. Some types of fractures predispose to specific complications; to be forewarned by adequate roentgenograms is to be forearmed. In addition, the case may later present embarrassing medicolegal aspects to the physician who has neglected to obtain roentgenograms.

The place of spinal puncture in the evaluation and treatment of head injuries is also controversial, but there are advantages and disadvantages to the procedure which depend on the circumstances. Three advantages can be listed: (1) In an alcoholic, or one addicted to narcotic or sedative drugs, clinical signs of a head injury may be masked, in which case, the demonstration of bloody spinal fluid can be expected to accompany any head injury of sufficient degree to be of concern. (2) Measurement of the intracranial pressure by spinal puncture at times provides needed information, both in the initial period and during the progress of treatment. It can also have therapeutic value, particularly in the early days after the injury, as an adjunct to other methods employed for controlling increased intracranial pressure. (3) Repeated spinal drainage (up to 30 cc. at a time), usually between the third to the eight day, in patients with heavily blood-stained fluid can have a salutary effect in decreasing headache, fever, and restlessness. Three principal disadvantages can be listed: (1) Spinal puncture can be inconvenient or harmful if performed with difficulty on a combative patient, or on one whose other injuries do not permit easy positioning for the puncture. (2) The withdrawal of spinal fluid in the presence of a hematoma in the meningeal spaces or in the parenchyma of the brain, is attended by the same risk of producing serious herniation of the brain at the tentorium or foramen magnum as exists in the presence of a brain tumor. Thus, clinical signs suggesting the possible presence of an intracranial blood clot contraindicate spinal puncture. (3) The reduction of intracranial pressure by spinal puncture in the presence of a compound fracture, or of one which traverses the mastoid cells or paranasal sinuses, is attended by serious risk of introducing meningeal infection from these potentially infected sites. There is no justification for concern that spinal lumbar puncture will otherwise produce meningitis or irreparably damage nerve roots of the cauda equina.

Supportive Treatment

The first and by far the most important consideration in early treatment is to provide an adequate airway. An obstructed airway not only results in a degree of hypoxia, but also causes venous congestion and elevation of intracranial pressure. The existence of these dangerous conditions, even for a short time, in a patient with a serious head injury and a small margin of safety can make the difference between survival and death, or between complete recovery and serious neurologic deficits. Usually sufficient are such simple measures as placing the patient on his side and aspirating mucus and blood from the mouth and pharynx. But if this is not obviously effective, or if there is doubt of its adequacy, an intratracheal tube should be passed, or a tracheostomy performed. Of the two procedures, the latter is usually the easier and quicker to perform. It is far better to perform a tracheostomy needlessly than to permit any extended period of obstruction. The administration of oxygen is no substitute for poor aeration, and it is not necessary if the airway is open.

The control of extreme restlessness is a common problem in management in the early period after injury. Mechanical restraint is of limited value and at times intensifies the activity. It is better to permit some movement and to rely for a while on having a bedside attendent guard the patient. Occasionally, evacuation of a full bladder by catheterization will make a difference. If it is necessary to resort to sedation by drugs, a short acting one, such as paraldehyde or chloral, is preferable to a barbiturate. Exceptions to the use of morphine may sometimes be made, and particularly if other injuries are the principal source of the patient's distress. At such times it is better to administer the morphine in doses as small as 5 mg. at a time and to repeat as required.

Other measures must be considered in the supportive care of the patient. If he remains unconscious, an indwelling urethral catheter is advisable, and if he continues so after the first two days, it is desirable to add to the parenteral administration of fluids, an adequate caloric supply via nasal tube passed into the stomach. There is no justification for restricting the normal fluid intake for the purpose of counteracting increased intracranial pressure. The enthusiasm for the use of hypertonic infusions to reduce intracranial pressure is a thing of the past, but occasionally their judicious use is helpful in reducing pressure for short periods. Although induced hypothermia as a means of providing protection to the brain by reducing its metabolic requirements is still being investigated, the method is known to have some drawbacks and has yet to prove its usefulness. Fever is always a deterrent to recovery of damaged nerve function and should be diligently combated by antipyretics, cold sponges, and rectal irrigations. The use of antibiotics is ill-advised unless there are distinct risks of meningitis or some supervening infection. Care of the skin in those long unconscious is a nursing problem and is greatly facilitated by the use of an alternating pressure mattress.

Surgical Treatment of Special Types and Complications of Head Injuries
Depressed Fractures

Depressed fracture of the skull results from a direct blow, usually by a relatively sharp object or projection, whereas linear fracture characteristically results when the head strikes a flat surface, or is struck by a blunt object. The type of injury producing a depression often lacerates the scalp, thus producing a compound fracture attended by possible contamination of subgaleal structures. In the repair of a laceration of the scalp, the possibility of an underlying depressed fracture must always be kept in mind.

It may be possible to detect the depression by exploring through the laceration, but early roentgenography is particularly advantageous in the detection of such fractures. The best rule is to explore surgically and to repair all depressed fractures. There may be occasion to take exception to the rule, but the risk of overlooking an intracranial hematoma, the danger of cranial and intracranial infection and of late convulsions, make early operation important. Even if the scalp is not lacerated and the depression is located over the poles of the cerebral hemispheres, away from the motor cortex, it is unwise to neglect repair. Rontgenograms cannot be relied on to demonstrate the damage occurring to tissues underlying bone.

In the repair of a depressed fracture, bone fragments that may be contaminated should be removed. though for cosmetic reasons it may be appropriate on occasion, to replace large fragments after they have been boiled for three minutes. Contaminated and devitalized meninges and brain tissue should be débrided, hematomas evacuated by suction, and particular attention given to the removal of in-driven fragments of bone or foreign material. Wounds should be closed without drains, and antibiotics should be administered systemically if the fracture has been compound. Special caution must be exercised in repairing a depressed fracture that overlies the saggital or transverse dural sinuses. The torn walls of the sinus may be supported by a depressed fragment of bone and serious bleeding may result as the fragment is elevated. This danger can be met by raising the head to equalize the venous pressure and by sealing the opening with some material such as muscle, fascia or one of the proprietary hemostatic materials. If it seems desirable to repair a defect in the skull, the placement of a prosthesis is usually better delayed until reaction of tissues has subsided. In case of infection, such repair should be delayed at least six months after all evidence of infection has subsided.

Penetrating Wounds Of The Brain

This type of injury, though more common in wartime, must occasionally be dealt with in civil life. The same principles obtain in the management of a penetrating wound as in a compound depressed fracture. Particular attention must be given to débridement of devitalized brain tissue and removal of easily accessible fragments of foreign material, though there is usually no need to pursue metal fragments in remote parts of the brain.

Extradural Hemorrhage

Hemorrhage in the extradural space is nearly always the result of bleeding from a torn middle meningeal artery or major dural venous sinus. It is one of the early and serious complications of head injury. Failure to recognize its presence and to evacuate the blood promptly may lead to death. Roentgenographic evidence of a fracture traversing the groove for the middle meningeal artery, or the regions of the dural venous sinuses, should suggest the possibility of this complication. If there are no severe associated injuries to confuse the picture, the symptoms and signs of extradural bleeding should be readily recognized. Characteristically, the patient gives evidence of recovering shortly after injury but, within one to several hours, has a waning of consciousness, and develops a dilated pupil on the side of the hemorrhage and weakness on the opposite side of the body. While the dilated pupil is usually on the side of the hemorrhage, occasionally the reverse may be true. The important thing to remember is that lessening of the conscious state and appearance of unequal pupils should alert the physician to the imminence of this possibility. On rare occasions the hemorrhage may be less severe and the clinical changes less rapid, possibly requiring one to several days to make their appearance.

No time should be wasted in evacuating an extradural hemorrhage. In cases with fulminating signs, if a neurosurgeon is not available, any surgeon may save a life if he is merely capable of making an opening in the temporal bone to permit evacuation of the blood.

While it is impracticable to retain all patients who receive a head injury under 24 hour observation, some protection will be provided if relatives or friends of the patient who is allowed to go home are warned to return the patient quickly if he develops stupor, coma, paralysis or fits within a week.

Acute Subdural Hemorrhage

After head injury, persistent venous bleeding occasionally occurs from tears in cerebral veins that traverse the space in their course from the surface of the brain to the dural venous sinuses. The rapidly progressing signs may be indistinguishable from those of the acute extradural hemorrhage, but the surgical approach is the same. Thus, if symptoms and signs lead the surgeon to expect an extradural hemorrhage but none is found on opening the skull in the temporal region, he should open the dura, for the hematoma may occupy this next meningeal space.

On release of freshly accumulated blood from the subdural space, there may be continued bleeding from unidentifiable regions. Patient and gentle irrigation of the space will usually stop the bleeding as the brain expands and obliterates the space. If this fails to occur, a useful measure is to inject saline under pressure into the lumbar subarachnoid space. If the arachnoid is intact, the subdural space will be obliterated and the bleeding controlled by a tamponade effect of the filled cerebrospinal fluid spaces.

With the more severe injuries that cause laceration of the brain and its vessels, there is commonly some degree of bleeding into the subdural space, but small amounts of blood in the space are of no consequence and little is gained by trephining the skull in such cases.

The chronic subdural hematoma produces a different syndrome which will be discussed hereafter.

Intracerebral Hematoma

While localized collections of significant amounts of blood in the parenchyma of the brain occur infrequently as a result of trauma, they may occasionally produce clinical changes much like those caused by the expanding hematomas that occur in the meningeal spaces. This is particularly true of hematomas that occur in the temporal lobes. It is therefore the usual practice at the time of temporal craniotomy to open the dura if extradural blood is not encountered, and if there is an insignificant amount of blood in the subdural space; also, to pass a blunt exploratory needle into the temporal or frontal lobe. In case a hematoma is thus encountered, it is better not to rely on aspiration by needle alone, but to pass a small sucker into the cavity or even to make a larger opening directly into the cavity.

The evacuation of large-sized hematomas, particularly in a temporal lobe, may be a life-saving measure. Blood is not likely to recollect and the wound should be closed without drainage, though an ample subtemporal decompression is of added advantage.

Cerebrospinal Fluid Leak

Linear fractures through the petrous portion of the temporal bone commonly result in meningeal tears and leakage of cerebrospinal fluid into the middle ear. If the drum has also been torn, the fluid as well as blood runs from the ear canal. If the drum remains intact, the fluid passes down the eustachean tube, often unrecognized, and is swallowed. Fortunately, these fistulae can be expected to close spontaneously, but they are a potential source of meningeal infection and there must be careful avoidance of irrigation or introduction of any medications into the external ear canal. Antibiotics should be administered systemically.

When there is a meningeal tear along with a fracture into the paranasal sinuses, particularly the frontal and ethmoid cells, the fistula may be more persistent and hazardous. At times careful search must be made for the fluid leak, since the patient may swallow the fluid, especially if he lies on his back, or the fluid coming from the nose may be masked by blood or mistaken for mucus. Cerebrospinal fluid can be distinguished from mucus by the presence of sugar in the former.

In case of persistent fluid fistula in the frontal region, blowing of the nose must be guarded against lest infected material be forced into the meningeal spaces. The presence of intracranial air, visible on a roentgenogram, constitutes a warning of the presence of such a fistula and is a matter of particular concern because it raises the possibility of infection.

With the relative safeguards provided by antibiotics, it is permissible to wait up to 10 days for the fistula to close, and in most cases, no further treatment is required. If the fluid leak persists, the opening must be closed, and this is usually accomplished by placing a patch such as fascia lata or periosteum from inside the skull, over the dural defect through a frontal craniotomy.

Chronic Subdural Hematoma

The infrequency of collections of blood in the subdural space causing acute symptoms soon after head injury has already been mentioned. More common are smaller but unresorbed collections of blood in this space. They frequently follow a relatively minor injury to the head, often so slight that the patient may have been unimpressed with its importance or even forgotten it temporarily.

The bleeding comes from torn cerebral veins. The blood in an amount too large to permit resorption becomes partially clotted, and a neomembrane forms about the clot. With time, more blood may accumulate or fluid may be added through osmosis. The increasing displacement of the brain causes progressive symptoms and signs which are often subtle for some days or weeks, but which eventually provide definite clues to the presence of the lesion. Among the common symptoms and signs are inequality of the pupils, moderate headache, mental confusion, varying degrees of somnolence (sometimes with transient periods of stupor), hemiparesis, aphasia, and occasionally, hemaniopsia or convulsions. Papilledema is exceptional. In most cases, there will be a persistence of some symptoms, particularly headache, giddiness and mental confusion, between the time of the injury and the appearance of more definite symptoms.

In treating chronic subdural hematomas it is well to remember that the subdural spaces over the two cerebral hemispheres are confluent beneath the falx cerebri, and therefore, bilateral clots may be present even though signs indicate that only one side is affected. Evacuation of blood and soft clots through one or more burr holes is sometimes adequate, but particularly if there is much organization of the clot and thick vascularized neomembranes, it is much safter to employ a larger craniotomy.

Subdural Hygroma

Subdural hygroma is a relatively rare condition, presumed to result from trapping of cerebrospinal fluid which leaks into the subdural space through a tear in the arachnoid. The accompanying clinical manifestations are much like those of chronic subdural hematoma, though usually less pronounced. Treatment consists of simple evacuation of the fluid through a burr hole.

Osteomyelitis and Intracranial Abcess

Osteomyelitis may result from unrecognized or improperly treated compound fractures of the skull. Fortunately, the osteomyelitis that develops under these circumstances is not likely to be of the fulminating and widely spreading kind that complicates a purulent frontal sinusitis. The treatment is local excision of the infected bone and drainage of the wound.

Untreated osteomyelitis is attended by a particular risk of spread of infection to the meningeal spaces or to the brain itself. Subdural abscess or empyema may become unmanageable if not dealt with by prompt drainage early in its development.

Brain abscess more often results from infected foreign matter carried into the brain by penetrating wounds or in-driven fragments of bone. The pos-

sibility of an abscess developing is greatly minimized by appropriate débridement of the wound soon after it is inflicted. Of the numerous methods
of dealing with brain abscess, the most successful, if it can be accomplished,
is complete excision of the infected material including the abscess wall, with
closure of the wound overlying it.

Carotid Artery-Cavernous Sinus Fistula

Fractures passing through the base of the skull may tear the internal carotid
in that portion which traverses the cavernous sinus, thus causing an arterio-
venous fistula. The fistulous opening may be so small at first that the
symptoms of its presence are meager and easily overlooked. Enlargement
of the opening in the next few days produces tell-tale symptoms and signs
which permit easy diagnosis. The eye becomes prominent and pulsating with
engorgement of the conjunctival veins, chemosis and swollen lids. Extraocular movements of the eye are impaired and vision begins to recede. The
patient is aware of a bruit, which can also be heard by the examiner at all
points over the head but is loudest over the involved eye. Compression of
the carotid artery in the neck on the involved side will usually abolish or
diminish the bruit.

It is appropriate to wait a few days to see if the fistula will close spontaneously or possibly with the aid of repeated compression of the carotid
artery in the neck. If the fistula persists, the procedure of choice to save the
eye and prevent further complications is to "trap" the fistula by occlusion
of the carotid artery on each side of the opening. This is accomplished by
ligating the common carotid first; occasionally, this will be enough to slow
the circulation and permit spontaneous closure of the fistula. If not, the
internal carotid in the neck is ligated within a few days and followed
promptly by occlusion with a metal clip of the intracranial segment of the
internal carotid at its point of emergency from the dural wall of the cavernous
sinus. Occasionally, it is also necessary to occlude the ophthalmic artery in
its proximal portion.

Post-Traumatic Convulsive Seizures

The incidence of seizures after head injury is in direct proportion to the
seriousness of the injury. In "closed" head injuries, the incidence of late
convulsions is 2 to 4 percent. Open and penetrating wounds, on the other
hand, are followed by a relatively high incidence of seizures varying from
10 to 45 percent in reported series. Early and adequate treatment of open
wounds doubtlessly contributes to a lower incidence of late convulsions.

The treatment of post-traumatic convulsions is primarily medical. If this
fails to be adequate and the injury has produced a definite cerebral cortical
scar, the excision of this scarred area can be expected to result in cure in
approximately one-third of the cases, improvement in one-third, and no
benefit in the remainder.

Cranioplasty

Small defects in the skull do not require repair, but larger ones may be unsightly, particularly in the frontal region, and some type of plastic repair is desirable. Occasionally, large defects which permit sudden alterations in intracranial pressure on straining or on changing position from reclining to upright, may cause symptoms of giddiness and headache. In these cases, repair of the defect by a prosthesis is indicated. Of the various materials employed for cranioplasty, tantalum plate has been found the most practical by the author.

The Postconcussion Syndrome

This term has come to be applied to a group of vague complaints which include principally: headaches, giddiness, difficulty in concentrating, feelings of confusion and trouble in focusing vision.

It is understandable that some, or all, of these complaints might exist for a limited time on an organic basis after a serious or relatively serious head injury, but the complaints most often come from patients who have had slight injuries. Most of these patients are concerned about litigation, or for one reason or another, develop a neurotic reaction to their situation.

The postconcussion syndrome could be avoided or greatly reduced in many patients if they were encouraged by early ambulation, early return to work and assurance that it is impossible to injure the head in such a way as to produce permanent headache.

Summary

Head injuries are so common that many physicians other than neurosurgeons must take the responsibility for their management. However, the physician who accepts the responsibility must understand the principles of supportive care and be on the alert for complications which require surgical treatment. If he is incapable of performing the necessary surgery, he must seek skilled assistance.

Surgery is needed in about one-fifth of the cases. The conditions requiring early operations include depressed fracture, open wounds and intracranial hemorrhage into extradural space, the subdural space or the parenchyma of the brain. Somewhat later operations may be necessary for cerebrospinal rhinorrhea, chronic subdural hematoma or hygroma, intracranial abscesses, osteomyelitis, and carotid-cavernous sinus fistula. Still later elective operations include cranioplasty and cortical excision for convulsive seizures.

CHAPTER 19

EYE INJURIES

JOHN M. McLEAN, M.D.

Many physicians who have not had specialized training in ophthalmic surgery are inclined to shy away from treating eye emergencies. In many complicated and delicate situations this tendency is proper, for ill conceived or executed procedures may be disastrous. However, there are situations in which immediate action is imperative, and in which delay may result in irreversible damage. Less frequently, emergencies arise in which the trauma surgeon is forced to act in cases of injury to or about the eye because of the utter unavailability of a skilled eye surgeon. Still other accidents present themselves where the general surgeon feels that trauma about the eye should be part of his general repair. It is to these three types of problems that this chapter is directed. No attempt will be made to discuss the highly specialized techniques of the ophthalmic operating room.

Burns

Most urgent of all ocular injuries are the severe chemical burns. Prompt action may make the difference between recovery of vision and permanent blindness. There is no time to send for expert help. The key to immediate treatment is prompt removal of the offending chemical agent by copious irrigation with the first available bland fluid. Under hospital emergency room conditions or in the physician's office, this fluid may well be physiologic salt solution. In many other cases it will be plain water. The lids must be forced open and large quantities of saline, water or whatever substitute is available must be used to flush out the eye and the cul-de-sacs until all traces of the offending agent are removed by dilution and irrigation. Any bits of particulate matter should be picked out, remembering that chunks may be found wedged under the lids. Then, and not until then, may one take time to investigate the ph of the offending chemical. Attempts at preparing neutralizing solutions result in waste of valuable minutes. In general, the greatest importance of the acidity or alkalinity of the caustic material is in its effect on prognosis. The ocular tissues, particularly the cornea, tend to be more resistant to penetration by acids and more easily invaded by alkalis. It is a fair rule of thumb to say that after removal of the burning material, the damage done by acids can be reasonably estimated. However, the effects of alkaline burns can be expected to be worse than are immediately apparent because of alkaline penetration to the deeper structures. Atropinization of the eyes to combat chemical iritis is usually in order. The immediate topical use of antimicrobial agents is rarely necessary since the burned tissues are usually sterilized by the chemical agent and most antibacterial drugs have some depressant action on the repair processes of corneal epithelium. Adrenal corticosteroids may be indicated to decrease sterile inflammatory reactions, but their use is a complicated matter which is better left to one well equipped to evaluate the overall problem if he will be available to take over management shortly. Local anesthetics to control pain should be used sparingly since they, too, depress corneal repair.

Attention must be given to the conjunctival surfaces lest de-epithelialization result in extensive adhesions and symblepharon. Lubrication with bland oils or greases, protection with mechanical conformers and mucous membrane grafts all have to be considered.

Burns of the skin of the eyelids are handled according to the same general principles applicable to chemical burns of skin in general (see Chapter 10). However, it is to be remembered that lid skin is thinner and more delicate than most other skin, and that the free borders of the lids make them more susceptible to contracture than most other skin sites. Consequently, the indications for skin grafting are rather more liberal.

The principles of treatment of thermal ocular burns from flame, steam and similar agents are the same as those given above except that there is no problem of the removal of chemical materials.

Burns from radiant energy (therapeutic or accidental x-ray, radium or nuclear energy exposure) are slower in taking effect and there is usually ample time to refer such cases for expert ophthalmologic care. Immediate ocular burns from nuclear explosions are rarely severe enough to warrant special measures unless the total exposure is so great as to be potentially fatal.

Exposure to ultraviolet light can result in painful, frightening symptoms which are hard to recognize because of their delay in onset. Much of the ultraviolet is absorbed by the corneal epithelium which undergoes necrosis and sloughs over a period of about 10—12 hours. Desquamation of the epithelium exposes the pain nerve endings of the cornea and results in severe ocular pain, photophobia, lacrimation, and blepharospasm. The last of these may be so severe that the patient is convinced that he is suddenly blind and may therefore go into a severe state of panic. Because of the delay in onset of symptoms, the ultraviolet exposure may well be forgotten or not associated with the immediate condition. Treatment is simple and very satisfactory. The most effective means of allaying the severe apprehension consists of manually forcing the lids open and demonstrating to the patient that he can see. Control of the severe pain and reflex symptoms is achieved at once by simple instillation of a few drops of any topical anesthetic. Thereafter, any bland oil or ointment and cool compresses over the lubricated lids will promote comfort. Total regeneration of the epithelium occurs without scarring, and restoration of function is almost always complete.

Foreign Bodies

Superficial foreign bodies represent the commonest of eye injuries. Their removal is so well understood that space need not be wasted on detailed description. The use of sterile materials, good light and magnification are important factors that need only be mentioned. Most foreign bodies on the

conjunctiva can be removed without anesthesia. Those that are on or imbedded in the cornea present more of a problem. Whenever possible they
should be washed off with a thin, strong stream of physiologic saline without
resort to instrumentation. Topical anesthesia renders this maneuver much
easier. If the foreign body will not wash off, attempts at removal with limp,
moist sterile cotton may next be made, or a small loop of softened gut suture
held in a clamp may be used to drag the foreign body away. Attempts at
removal with sharp instruments must be undertaken with extreme caution
for, except in experienced hands, real damage may be done. Where practical,
it is often better to instil a local anesthetic, apply a sterile dressing, and
get the patient to someone properly equipped to handle the removal.

Contamination is often a potential danger, so it is usually advisable to
instil a broad spectrum antibiotic after removing a particle from the cornea.
The use of steroids is to be avoided as unnecessary and probably dangerous
in the presence of potential virus or fungus infection.

The possibility of ocular penetration by flying particles must never be
forgotten and appropriate search for intraocular foreign bodies by clinical
and radiological methods is an important protection for both the patient
and the physician.

Lacerations

Lacerations of the eyelids which involve only skin may be sutured directly
by any physician, using 5–0 or 6–0 silk (fig. 1). Lacerations which involve
the lid margin or through and through cuts or tears of the lids require much
more careful repair. Simple end-to-end closure with sutures may provide an
approximation which looks satisfactory immediately thereafter, but usually
results in later notching of the margin from scar tissue contracture. This
late failure is serious beyond its cosmetic implications, for exposure keratitis,
corneal ulcer, perforation, panophthalmitis and loss of the eyeball may be

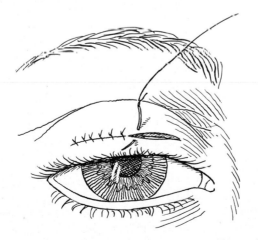

Fig. 1—Simple closure of lid laceration in skin only.

the sequence. Full thickness lacerations of the lid are usually more or less vertical (fig. 2 A). The edges should be adequately débrided (fig. 2 B) and meticulous closure in offset layers provided. The "halving" method of Wheeler is very satisfactory. The lids are divided into two layers; skin,

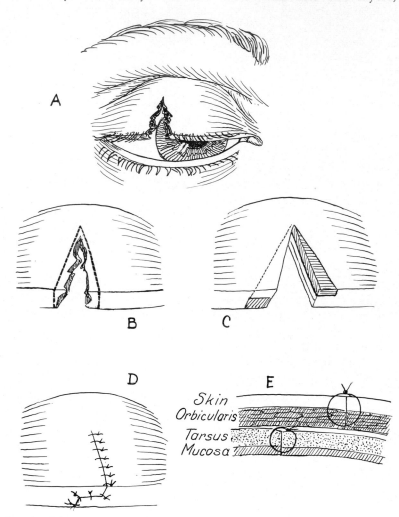

Fig. 2—Repair of laceration involving lid margin. (A) Jagged vertical laceration. (B) Area to be débrided. (C) Preparation for "halving" closure. (D) Suture lines offset. (E) Diagram in cross-section.

subcutaneous tissue and muscle in the outer; tarsus and conjunctiva in the inner (fig. 2 C). Part of one layer is resected on one side, part of the other layer, to the same extent, on the other. The inner layer is closed accurately with absorbable sutures, the knots buried to avoid corneal abrasion. The outer layer is closed with silk or similar material, the knots exposed (fig. 2 D). Fine sutures are used to secure perfect alignment of the lid margins. This type of repair is more trouble to perform but is amply repaid by the excellent lasting cosmetic result and safety.

Lacerations of the lids near the medial canthus require special care if the lacrimal canaliculi are severed. The cut ends should be identified and catheterized with a heavy stiff suture, fine plastic tube or wire (fig. 3). Accurate

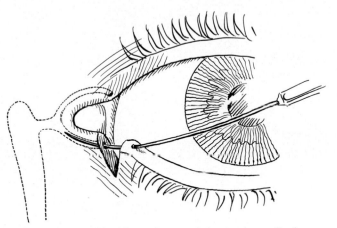

Fig. 3—Reapproximation of severed lacrimal canaliculus.

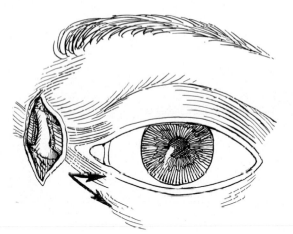

Fig. 4—Severed canthal ligament requiring deep repair (arrows indicate direction of displacement).

approximation around these ends is essential to assure re-establishment of tear flow. If the canthal ligaments are cut at either end of the lids, these structures must be identified and resutured to avoid sagging and lateral displacement of the entire palpebral fissure (fig 4).

Lacerations of the globe itself are much better left to the ophthalmic surgeon. Sterile dressings should be applied and the patient transported carefully. From time to time exigencies of the local situation require that initial

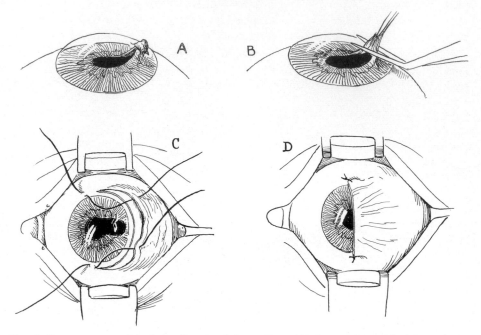

Fig. 5–Emergency repair of small corneal laceration. (A) Laceration with iris prolapse. (B) Prolapsed iris excised. (C) Simple suture closure of conjunctival flap. (D) Completed closure.

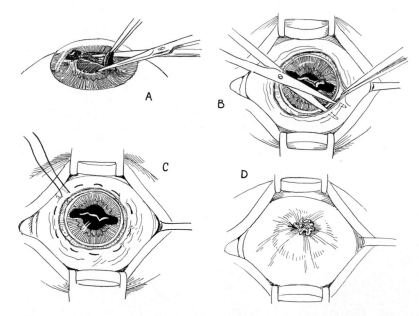

Fig. 6–Emergency closure of large corneal perforation with double iris prolapse. (A) Excision of prolapse. (B) Undermining of conjunctiva. (C) Preparation of purse-string suture. (D) Completed closure.

repair be performed by one who is neither trained nor equipped for specialized ocular surgery. In such emergencies very satisfactory closure of corneal lacerations can be effected by utilizing slidings flaps of conjunctiva, not attempting direct corneal sutures or other forms of keratoplasty. If the laceration is small or well to one side (fig. 5 A) an apron flap may be prepared by undermining conjunctiva from the limbus until an adequate amount is freed to cover the entire wound. Then any prolapsed iris tissue is put on tension and abscised (fig. 5 B). The edges of the previously prepared flap are sutured in place (fig. 5 C) to undisturbed limbal tissue beyond the wound with a satisfactory emergency closure. If the corneal wound is too large or central, it may be necessary to free up conjunctiva and undermine it all around the limbus with a purse-string closure covering the entire cornea (fig. 6).

In all bulbar lacerations, systemic antimicrobial therapy and antitetanic precautions must be used.

Contusions

Blunt trauma to the eye may cause a large variety of intraocular injuries as well as the familiar "black eye." The latter, in itself, is not serious. If it is seen early and there is no damage of the eyeball, pressure and cold applications may be used to minimize extravasation into the loose periorbital tissues. Later heat and, rarely, injections of hyaluronidase may be given to hasten absorption of blood. One must always remember that the ecchymosis may be a sign of skull fracture.

Blunt injuries to the globe may result in ocular rupture, either anteriorly where it can be seen or posteriorly where pain, loss of vision and hypotony are suggestive. Intraocular hemmorrhage either into the anterior or posterior segment may mask damage to the lens, tears of iris, ciliary body, or choroid, or detachment of the retina. Such cases should be given the benefit of the doubt until definitive evaluation can be had and should be treated with rest and binocular bandaging.

Traumatic ptosis of the eyelid and paralysis or pareses of the extraocular muscles and nerves do not require immediate action and are too complicated in their management to be dealt with by nonophthalmologists.

Trauma to the eye and its surrounding structures has so many ramifications and involves, or potentially involves, so many delicate parts of a highly complicated organ that it is essential for the trauma surgeon to recognize when he must step in and take immediate action, when he must stay his hand until the properly equipped expert can be reached, and how to render adequate first aid measures if such an expert is not immediately available.

CHAPTER 20

FRACTURES OF THE MANDIBLE

STANLEY J. BEHRMAN, D.D.S.

The mandible is the tenth most frequently fractured bone in the body and, except for the nose, the most frequently fractured bone of the face. Its integrity is important to respiration, mastication, deglutition, speech and facial appearance. The emotions involved when this bone is fractured are evidenced by the patient's anxious queries, "How will I eat? How will I look?" The objectives of treatment are the re-establishment of normal occlusion of teeth and of masticatory function. This should be done in the simplest manner compatible with the patient's over-all care, permitting a rapid return to his usual life situation and involving minimal facial disfigurement.

Anatomic Considerations

The mandible is a horseshoe-shaped bone suspended from the skull at the temperomandibular joint. Its arch form provides great inherent strength. When it is supported by being held against the maxilla, aided by a boxer's mouthpiece for example, the mandible can withstand considerable direct trauma. Normally, however, it is freely movable and in its prominently exposed position it is frequently fractured. The neurovascular bundle enters the medial aspect of the ramus, travels through the mandibular canal, terminates with branches to the lip and chin and emerges through the mental foramen. This bundle consists of the third division of the fifth cranial nerve, the mandibular branch of the internal maxillary artery, and the associated vein.

The insertion of muscles on the mandible and the direction of their pull are of particular interest in the diagnosis and treatment of fractures. Of principal concern are two groups of muscles of three muscles each, plus one additional muscle. One group is attached to the posterior portion of the mandible, the other to the anterior portion. The three muscles attached to the posterior portion of the jaw close the mouth and, when there is a fracture, tend to displace the posterior fragment upward. These three muscles are the masseter, temporal and internal pterygoid (fig. 1 A and B). The three muscles attached to the anterior portion of the jaw open the mouth and, when there is a fracture, tend to displace the anterior fragment downward and backward. These three muscles are the mylohyoid, geniohyoid and digastric (anterior belly) (fig. 1 B and C). The additional muscle is the external pterygoid. It is attached to the condyle of the mandible and, in function, moves the jaw forward. When there is a fracture of the neck of the condyle, the external pterygoid muscle pulls the superior fragment forward and medially (fig. 1 B). The vertical ramus is suspended between the masseter and internal

252

pterygoid muscles as in a "sling." This minimizes displacement of the fragments when the ramus is fractured. The ramus, however, is quite thin, and just several millimeters of medial or lateral displacement permit overriding of the fragments. The posterior muscle group then pulls the mandible upward,

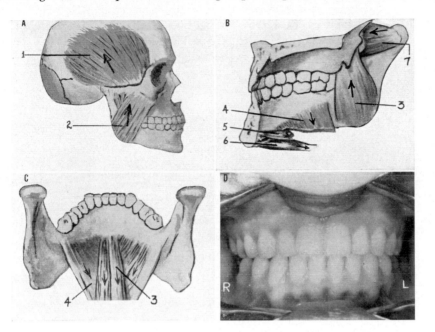

Fig. 1—Anatomy. (A) Two of the three muscles attached to posterior portion of mandible (lateral view) and direction of their pull. *1* Temporal. *2* Masseter. (B) Muscles attached to the mandible (medial view), and direction of their pull. *3* Internal Pterygoid. *4* Mylohyoid. *5* Geniohyoid. *6* Digastric (anterior belly). *7* External Pterygoid. (C) Two of the three muscles attached to the anterior portion of mandible and direction of their pull. *3* Geniohyoid. *4* Mylohyoid. (D) Normal centric occlusion. The intermeshing on the left side is ideal. That on the right side, while not "ideal" (posterior shifting because of missing first molar) is normal for this patient and would have to be re-established in the event of a fracture.

shortening the ramus and pulling the entire mandible to the injured side. This deviation of the midline of the mandible towards the injured side is an important diagnostic finding (fig. 2 C).

Emergency Care

Two conditions requiring immediate attention may result from a fracture of the lower jaw. They are respiratory obstruction and hemorrhage. Bilateral fractures at the angle of mandible with posterior displacement of the anterior segment may carry an edematous tongue against the posterior pharyngeal wall. Relief is immediate when the anterior portion of the jaw is grasped, pulled and held forward. The patient should be placed on his side or in a prone position with his head to the side. If other injuries make a supine position mandatory it may be necessary to perform a tracheostomy.

Most hemorrhage arises from lacerated soft tissues of the mouth. Pressure with a gauze pad generally is sufficient to control bleeding. On occasion vessels in the floor of the mouth will have to be clamped and tied. When severed, the mandibular artery usually retracts and seldom is a source of difficulty. If there is undue bleeding from a fracture site, quick manual reduction and the application of a head-chin bandage usually are adequate to control the hemorrhage. In the rare instances when bleeding still persists, gauze must be packed tightly into the fracture site ($\frac{1}{2}$ or $\frac{1}{4}$ inch packing, if available). If a local anesthetic is at hand (2 per cent procaine or the equivalent), the mandibular nerve should be blocked. When a block is not feasible, the anesthetic solution may be infiltrated about the fracture site. The packing should be removed within 24 to 48 hours after hospitalization.

General Evaluation of the Patient

Trauma to the jaw is transmitted to the skull. There may be loss of consciousness and even fracture of the tympanic plate of the temporal bone by the head of the condyle. The latter occurrence will be manifested by bleeding into the external auditory canal. All fractures of the mandible should be evaluated clinically as skull injuries. In automobile accidents usually there are concomitant injuries; the patient who has been struck by a fist often is inebriated.

Diagnosis

Diagnosis is made on the basis of clinical and roentgenologic findings. The latter are indispensable and even when the clinical examination is unremarkable, a roentgenologic survey of every jaw injury must be made.

Clinical Findings

Change in Occlusion of the Teeth

This may be objective or purely subjective. Check the relationship of the lower teeth to the upper teeth. A fracture of the body of the mandible with displacement will alter the intercusping of the teeth (fig. 2 A and B). An edentulous patient may indicate that his dentures do not fit properly. Fractures of the ramus with displacement will produce deviation of the midline to the injured side and an "open bite" (inability of the anterior teeth to contact). Many people do not exhibit the ideal or "normal" occlusion (fig. 1 D). A cross-bite, "open-bite" or prognathism may have existed prior to the present trauma and be normal for the individual patient. The facets on the canines and bicuspids usually are good indicators of position. The presence of mamelons (developmental tubercles) on the lower incisors of an adult indicate lack of function due to a prognathic or micrognathic jaw relationship or an "open-bite." (Hours have been spent attempting to reduce a "dislocation" of a prognathic mandible when, in fact, the protrusion was normal and the "open bite" due to bilateral fractures of the condylar necks.) The upper and lower central incisors serve as a guide to the midline of the jaw.

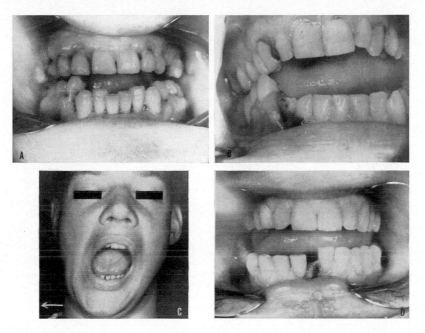

Fig. 2—Diagnosis. (A) Changes in occlusion of the teeth; moderate displacement of fragments. (B) Changes in occlusion; considerable displacement of fragments. (See fig. 7 D for postreduction appearance.) (C) Deviation of mandible toward the injured side. (D) Displacement at fracture site resembling the socket of an evulsed tooth.

Abnormal Jaw Movements

Loss of integrity of the mandible will produce abnormal movements during swallowing, opening, and closing. Points of motion within the body will indicate sites of fractures; fractures of the ramus with displacement will produce deviation of the jaw toward the injured side (fig. 2 C). The absence of movement of the head of the condyle, as determined by preauricular palpation, often will be indicative of fracture of the condylar neck. It is seldom necessary to manipulate the jaw to locate fracture sites.

Swelling and Ecchymosis

Swelling and pain are useful in that they encourage the patient to seek medical attention. Swelling generally is at the site of trauma but often is not extensive at the sites of indirect or secondary fracture. Ecchymosis of the oral mucosa, especially of the floor of the mouth, is a good sign of a fracture in the area. This is particularly helpful in edentulous jaws.

Pain and Tenderness

Pain may occur during deglutition, mastication, and speech. Tenderness is a much more valuable diagnostic aid. The entire mandible, including the head of the condyles, should be palpated both at rest and in motion.

Looseness of Teeth

Teeth often are loosened at a fracture site but seldom evulsed. Wide displacement of the fragments of a mandible fractured in the region of the incisors, canines and biscuspids has been interpreted incorrectly as an evulsed tooth. The teeth always should be identified and counted (fig. 2 D).

Other Signs and Symptoms

Crepitus: As a subjective symptom during jaw movements crepitus may indicate unusual fractures not detected by clinical examination and the usual roentgenologic views. (An example is a fracture of the medial cortical plate in the molar area undetected in a lateral-oblique view but clearly shown in an occlusal film (fig. 3 D, *right*).

Hypesthesia of the lip may be produced by injury to the mandibular nerve. (This is a temporary condition and sensation invariably returns, although occasionally there may be slight residual hypesthesia or paresthesia.)

Bleeding from the ear, as previously described, is produced by a fracture of the tympanic plate of the glenoid fossa and usually is accompanied by fracture of the condylar neck.

Fetor oris, the accumulation of whitish *gingival slough* and *trismus* are other signs which may be present if there is a delay before the patient is seen.

In addition to knowing "what to look for" an essential aspect of diagnosis is knowing "where to look." In the majority of instances the mandible will be fractured at two sites. One of these usually will be detected readily; the other may require more careful clinical and roentgenologic inspection. The most frequent combinations of fracture sites are:

1. Mental foramen area and opposite angle of the jaw
2. Mental foramen area and opposite neck of the condyle
3. Bilateral necks of the condyles
4. Bilateral necks of the condyles and symphysis
5. Mental foramen area and angle on same side

Roentgenologic Examination

The routine roentgenologic examination should include the following four views:

1., 2. Right and left lateral oblique: Two views of each side may be necessary in order to visualize adequately the horizontal body and vertical ramus (fig. 3 A and B).

3. Anteroposterior: This must show the entire vertical ramus from the angle to the condyle head (fig. 3 C).

4. Intra-oral occlusal: This view is essential to visualize the anterior portion of the mandible. This area cannot be seen adequately in the lateral oblique views and always is superimposed on the spine in the anterior-posterior view (fig. 3 D).

Additional films may be necessary in specific instances: temperomandibular joints (fig. 12 C and D), occlusal views of the posterior portion of the body (fig. 3 D, *right*) periapical dental films, modified Waters position to visualize the coronoid process, and others.

It is important to note that the body of the mandible often fractures obliquely in a medial-lateral direction. On the roentgenogram this will appear as if there are two distinct fracture lines with an intervening sequestrum (fig. 3 B).

Another essential factor is revealed by the roentgenograms: the *direction* of the fracture line. The direction of the fracture line determines whether or not the fragments can be displaced by muscle pull. In figures 3 A and 8 C the

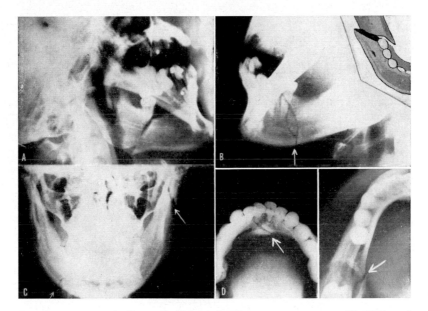

Fig. 3—Roentgenograms. (A) Example of lateral oblique roentgenogram. (B) Oblique fracture in a medial-lateral direction, as shown in inset, appears as a sequestrum in lateral oblique view. (C) Anterior-posterior roentgenogram showing fractures of left condylar neck and right body. (D) *1* Routine intraoral anterior occlusal view demonstrating fracture which could not be seen in anterior-posterior view. *2* Posterior occlusal view demonstrating fracture which could not be seen in lateral-oblique view but which was indicated by subjective symptom of crepitus.

direction of the fracture line permits the posterior fragment to be elevated and the anterior fragment to be depressed. In figure 10 A the direction of the fracture line prevents either upward displacement of the posterior fragment or downward displacement of the anterior fragment. Similarly, the medial-lateral direction of the fracture line, as mentioned in the preceding paragraph, permits or prevents medial displacement of the fragments.

Treatment

All fractures of the body of the mandible should be considered compounded intra-orally. The fracture site is contaminated with mixed organisms, and broad-spectrum antimicrobial therapy should be instituted immediately. Patients with intermaxillary fixation may have difficulty taking capsules of noninjectable antibiotics. If the capsule is placed in the buccal sulcus, it usually can be pushed back behind the last molar into the mouth. Pediatric oral suspensions are well tolerated or the capsules may be opened and the contents mixed with food.

Treatment should be instituted as soon as the patient's general condition permits. Because of other bodily injuries or associated trauma to the head, initial treatment may consist only of the application of a head-chin bandage. (If definitive treatment cannot be instituted immediately a bandage should be applied, if possible. The support will make the patient more comfortable, enable him to swallow more easily, and minimize further muscular displacement of the fragments. Application of the bandage prior to taking x-rays will permit easier positioning of the head.) The Barton bandage, however modified, produces backward pressure on the chin. This can be deleterious, hastening displacement of the anterior segment or interfering with

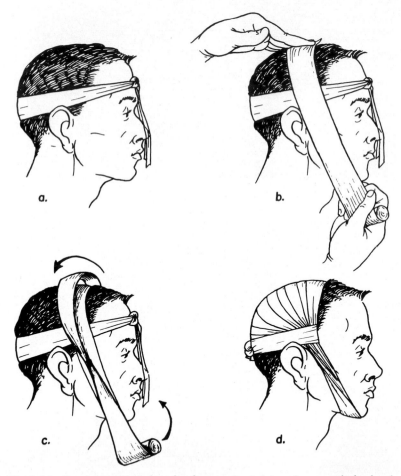

Fig. 4—Head-chin Bandage. (A) A length of gauze is tied loosely around the head. (B) A roller bandage is applied from the vertex around the chin. (C) Repeated, with half-twists in front of each ear, spreading bandage over crown. (D) Initial strip is untied, drawn back and tied behind head.

respiration and swallowing. A simple efficient bandage which can be applied rapidly is placed as follows (fig. 4):

The patient is told to occlude his teeth as best he can; if he has dentures, they should be inserted. A four foot length of two or three inch gauze roller bandage is placed behind the occiput and loosely tied at the forehead. The ends are left dangling, the ears are

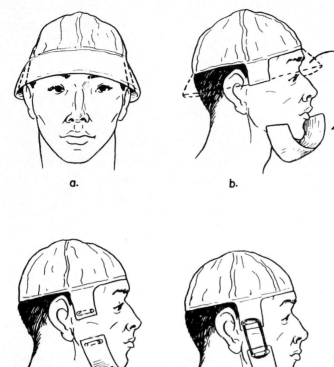

Fig. 5—Head-chin Cap. (A) Sailor's hat with brim turned down. (B) All of brim cut off except 2-inch flap in front of ears. Front portion of brim placed beneath chin. (C) Safety pins in ends of flaps. (D) Rubber bands around pins provide support.

free (fig. 4 A). Starting at the vertex, the roller bandage is brought down in front of the ear and under the chin, passed up in front of the opposite ear and then over the vertex (fig. 4 B). This is repeated, gradually increasing traction in an upward direction. The bandage should be given a half-twist in front of the ear and distributed about the crown (fig. 4 C). The free end is taped at the vertex. The strip which was knotted at the forehead is untied. The ends are brought backward simultaneously, tightening the chin-vertex portion, and are tied beneath the occiput (fig. 4 D). This bandage provides support in an upward direction and will not slip off easily.

A more elaborate head-chin cap can be made from an ordinary sailor's hat (fig. 5). This provides particularly good support after open-reduction of an edentulous jaw and for certain maxillary fractures. The hat is placed on the head and the brim turned down (fig. 5 A). Two lines are marked on each side of the brim, one just in front of the ear and the other two inches anterior to it. The hat is removed and the 2 inch strips of brim between these lines on each side are kept attached to the hat while the remainder of the brim is cut off. The hat is replaced, covering the crown, with the 2 inch flaps of brim in front of each ear (fig. 5 B). That portion of the brim which formerly covered the forehead is now placed beneath the chin. It and the "flaps" should be trimmed so that there is a gap of about 2 inches between them. Large safety pins are then placed in a horizontal direction across the lower end of each flap and the ends of the chinstrap (fig. 5 C). Rubber bands are placed around the safety pins, producing traction on the chin strap (fig. 5 D). A crescent-shaped section may be trimmed from the latter if it impinges against the neck. Sanitary pads placed beneath the chin strap and the flaps make them more comfortable.

Treatment Planning

Development of a proper plan of treatment is critical. Inadequate reduction may produce malocclusion, masticatory inefficiency and facial disfigurement. Inadequate fixation may allow fragment displacement and malunion, encourage infection and result in nonunion. Elaborate surgical procedures may be detrimental to the patient's general condition and may leave avoidable facial scars. Complicated extraoral appliances are uncomfortable, unsightly, and hamper a return to economic and social activities while treatment is underway.

When the fracture sites have been determined, potential displacement of the fragments is evaluated on the basis of present position, direction of fracture lines and direction of muscle pull. Treatment must re-establish the normal position of the fragments and provide fixation adequate to counteract the displacing muscular forces. The presence or absence of infection, the presence of teeth, their position and condition, the age and general health of the patient, are other factors affecting the plan of treatment. Assistance of a dental colleague will be of great value and should be engaged whenever possible.

Treatment Methods

There are basically three methods of treatment:
1. Fixation of the teeth in the mandibular fragments to the maxillary dentition.
2. Application of a splint to the lower dentition.
3. Extraoral surgical procedures.

These methods are employed singly and in combination. Almost invariably there must be some period of intermaxillary fixation.

As a guide in the selection of treatment method, fractures of the mandible may be classified as follows:

Class   I: Teeth present in all fragments (fig. 3 A).
Class II: Edentulous posterior fragment; no displacement (fig. A and B).
Class III: Edentulous posterior fragment; displaced (fig. 9).
Class IV: Edentulous mandible or displaced edentulous anterior fragment (fig. 10).
Class V: Fractures of the ramus and condylar neck (fig. 11 and 12).

If the teeth in a particular fragment have inadequate crowns or alveolar supporting bone, the fragment should be classified as edentulous. (The methods of treatment to be outlined presume the existence of an intact maxilla with adequate dentition. Adaptations for the edentulous or fractured maxilla are outlined later.)

Teeth in line of fracture should be retained whenever possible. Teeth in a posterior segment usually are needed to prevent excessive upward displacement of this segment (fig. 3 A). Removal of a tooth in the line of fracture may increase the amount of displacement. The tooth socket presents a wider area for the healing process to span and the opposing upper tooth may be made unfit for use in reduction or fixation because of potential extrusion. The antimicrobial therapy which is administered routinely usually will hold any dental infection in check. Fracture of the root of a vital tooth does not necessarily produce death of the dental pulp; these teeth may heal. Periodontal membrane reattaches itself rapidly to the denuded tooth and tooth socket surfaces. If a tooth becomes nonvital the root canals can be filled and, if indicated, an apicoectomy performed when union has taken place. The extraction of teeth in the line of fracture usually should be limited to teeth whose crowns are shattered, very loose teeth with no bony support and and teeth preventing the reduction of displaced fragments.

Class I—Teeth in all Fragments

Method of Choice: Interdental Wiring plus Intermaxillary Rubber Band Fixation

Twenty-five gauge stainless steel wire is suggested for all interdental wiring. It is strong, easily manipulated and does not stretch. The position of the wire about the tooth is below the height of contour or widest portion of the crown. On anterior teeth this will be at the junction of the crown and the root — the cemento-enamel junction, or "neck" of the tooth. A constriction at this point prevents the wire from riding up onto the crown where it will be loose. Always wire the upper teeth first and the teeth near the fracture site last. Avoid wiring teeth in line of fracture. Whenever possible, avoid wires on anterior teeth; the traction during fixation may cause them to extrude. All wired teeth that are not in occlusion should be prevented from extruding by opposing them with a plastic or modeling compound block. When tightening wires, the twisted ends should be grasped with a needle holder held in the palm of the hand. The thumb is placed against the tooth around which the wires are being tightened. Firm steady traction is applied against this tooth as the needle holder twists the wire tight. Tightening twists should be made in a clockwise direction.

The patient always should be premedicated. This may include a barbiturate for sedation and for protection against a procaine reaction, meperidine to raise the pain threshhold and atropine or scopolamine to reduce salivary secretion. The choice of drugs and their dosage are governed largely by the patient's over-all condition. Since the wires do not penetrate the gingiva a topical anesthetic usually suffices to prevent discomfort. When wires must be forced beneath the gingiva, procaine 2 per cent, or the equivalent, may be infiltrated about the teeth.

Types of Interdental Wiring

Interdental Loops (for adjacent posterior teeth). A ten inch strand of wire is grasped at the center with the tips of a needle holder. One and one-half tight twists are made to produce an eyelet as shown in figure 6 A. The ends should be cut off evenly. About ten such eyelets should be made before any are placed about the teeth. A large safety pin may be passed through the eyelets for convenience in handling. The wires are sterilized and then handled as "clean."

When the dentition permits, the ideal pairs of teeth for this method of wiring are the first molar and second bicuspid, and the first and second bicuspids. Two pairs of teeth are utilized in each quadrant so that if one wire breaks during the healing period another will be present to provide fixation.

The double strands are grasped with a needle holder about 1 cm. from the ends. The ends are curved with finger pressure to resemble a suture needle. They are passed from buccal to lingual (lateral to medial) through the interdental space between two teeth (fig. 6 A–1).

The wires are separated. One strand is passed around the posterior tooth, through the interdental space, and out to the buccal; the other strand is passed similarly about the anterior tooth (fig. 6 A–2). The posterior strand is brought between the wires medial to the twists (fig. 6 A–3). The anterior and posterior strands are pulled tight and twisted together. The twist is grasped with a needle holder and, with steady traction, the wires are twisted tightly against the tooth. The end is cut 5 mm. away from the tooth. Then it is turned down to form a hook for the placement of rubber bands (fig. 6 C–6) The eyelet is grasped with a needle holder and tightened. It, too, is turned down as a hook.

Multiple Loop (Stout) Wiring (for anterior teeth). Because of their tendency to extrude, when anterior teeth must be wired they should all be wired together and if possible, fixed to a bicuspid on each side. An 18 inch strand of wire is passed from the lingual through the interproximal space between the right first and second bicuspids (fig. 6 B–1). The end is carried along the buccal and labial surfaces of the teeth until it extends 1 cm. beyond the first bicuspid on the left side of the arch. The long end is then passed around the lingual of the right first bicuspid and brought buccally through the interproximal space between the first bicuspid and canine. It is passed gingivally to the wire lying along the buccal surfaces of the teeth. The long end is then carried over the short buccal wire and passed back through the same interproximal space, thus forming a loop encircling the short buccal wire (fig. 6 B–2). This loop should be about 3 or 4 mm in diameter. (A piece of 8 gauge lead wire may be placed through the loop and held parallel to the short buccal wire against the teeth to facilitate loop formation.) The long end is passed lingually around the canine, through the interproximal space between the canine and lateral incisor, under and then over the short wire (and piece of lead), and then back through the same interproximal space, again forming a loop encircling the short wire (Fig. 6 B–3; if the lead is present, the wires may be pulled tightly against it). This process is continued (bringing the lead forward from time to time) until the long end meets the short end at the interproximal space between the left bicuspids. The ends are twisted together tightly. (The lead is removed.) Each loop is then grasped with the needle holder and tightened a bit, moving from loop to loop applying traction and gradually tightening them (fig. 6 B–4).

The wires should be tightened firmly. The twisted end and all the loops are bent gingivally to form hooks for rubber band placement. (If edentulous spaces are encountered, the wire is twisted across the space to the next tooth where the formation of the loops is continued.)

Clove Hitch Twist (for isolated teeth). An eight inch strand of wire is grasped at each end with the fingers. A simple loop is formed by bringing the right hand up and over (fig. 6 C–1). This loop is grasped between the left thumb and forefinger. Again a loop is made by bringing the right hand up and over (fig. 6 C–2). This loop is grasped between the right thumb and forefinger. The loop held by the right fingers is passed *beneath* that held by the left fingers, forming a "clove hitch" (fig. 6 C–3). The left forefinger is

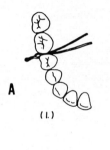
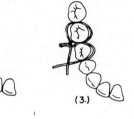
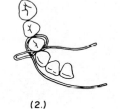

A

(1.)   (2.)   (3.)   (4.)

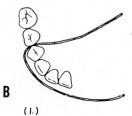
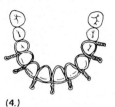
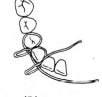

B

(1.)   (2.)   (3.)

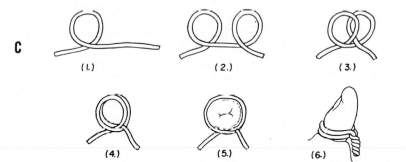

(4.)

C

(1.)   (2.)   (3.)

(4.)   (5.)   (6.)

Fig. 6—Interdental Wiring. (A) Interdental loops — for adjacent posterior teeth (see text). (B) Multiple loop (Stout) wiring — for anterior teeth (see text). (C) Clove-hitch twist — for isolated teeth (see text).

passed up through both loops of the hitch. The ends are pulled gently, tightening the loops about the finger (fig. 6 C–4). The twists are grasped with a needle holder and the loops placed about the single isolated tooth to be wired (fig. 6 C–5). Each end is grasped with a needle holder and traction is applied. As the loops of the clove hitch tighten, be sure they are around the neck of the tooth. The ends then are bent together against the tooth and twisted. The twist is grasped with a needle holder and tightened. The twist is cut, leaving 7 to 8 mm to be turned gingivally to form a hook for rubber bands (fig. 6 C–6).

Arch Bars. When there are insufficient teeth in each fragment to provide adequate fixation with the described methods of wiring, arch bars should be used. They are also used instead of continuous loop wiring when traction is to be placed on anterior teeth (fig. 7 A–C). Arch bars are available commercially and should be kept in supply at the hospital. These malleable bars are contoured to fit snugly against the buccal and labial surfaces of the teeth. The ends are cut and bent behind the last tooth on either side. There are loops or lugs for rubber band traction attached to the bar. They must point gingivally when the bar is positioned. Individual wires are passed around as many teeth as possible and then twisted tightly about the arch bar. The ends are cut short, bent gingivally and tucked under the bar. The upper arch bar is placed first. If there is no displacement of the mandibular fragments, or if the fragments can be reduced manually with ease, the lower arch bar is placed in the usual manner. If there is considerable displacement the lower bar may be cut in sections with one section placed on each fragment.

Intermaxillary Rubber Band Fixation: Rubber bands, not wires, should be used to fix the lower teeth to the upper teeth. The danger of vomiting always is present. When the jaws are wired shut they cannot be opened and the vomitus may be aspirated. In an emergency rubber bands are pulled off readily; the vomiting patient often will be able to open his mouth sufficiently even if none of the rubber bands are removed. Wires have a tendency to stretch and must be tightened periodically to prevent movement of the mandible. Rubber bands require occasional replacement if they break. Number 240 Angle's assorted orthodontic rubber bands are excellent, although bands may be cut from narrow rubber tubing. The bands should be placed around the wire hooks so that the direction of their pull will hold the fragments in position against each other and against the maxillary dentition (fig. 7 C).

When fragments are displaced, rubber bands provide excellent traction for reduction. The bands are placed so that the direction of their pull counteracts the forces of displacement. Stretching a rubber band over several hooks increases the tension it exerts. A few rubber bands will slowly and comfortably reduce fractures that have been displaced for many days. The direction of the pull may have to be adjusted over a period of several hours. Once reduction has been attained the rubber bands are used for fixation (fig. 7 A–C).

Alternate Method for Class I Fractures: Plastic or Metal Splints

An excellent method of treatment which has the advantages of permitting early function of the mandible is the use of sectional plastic (acrylic) splints (fig. 7 D). The services of a dentist are required for this method.

When there is no displacement of the fragments, an impression is taken of the lower dentition using a flexible dental impression material (alginate, hydrocolloid or silicone). If the fragments are displaced but are easily reduced, they may be reduced and held in place by continuous loop wiring with fine 28 or 30 gauge wire. The loops are made very small and forced into the interdental spaces so that they will not tear the impression. The impression is poured in stone to make a model. Another method for displaced fractures is to take an impression of the displaced fragments, cast a model in plaster, cut the model at the fracture site, correctly align the fragments of the model,

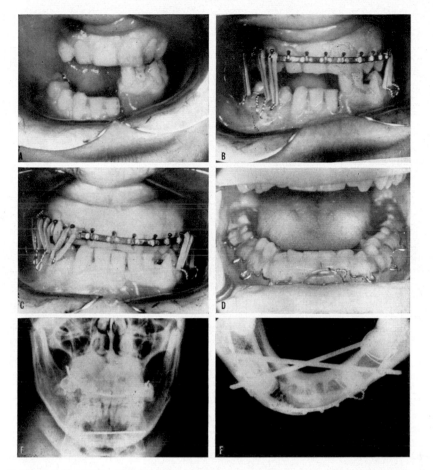

Fig. 7—Class I Fractures. (A) Considerable downward displacement of right anterior fragment. (B) Arch bar on upper teeth, interdental loops on lowers; rubber band traction applied, partial reduction apparent. (C) Reduction completed. (D) Acrylic splint on lower teeth (see fig. 2 B for prereduction appearance) (E) Kirschner pin through anterior portion of body of mandible as a supplementary means of fixation. (F) Occlusal view of another case utilizing Kirschner pins. Two pins were used here because of the thin obliquely fractured fragments.

hold them in position with wax or glue and take an impression of the correctly aligned model. This is poured in stone.

A sectional acrylic splint is prepared on the stone model. (The details of construction are described fully in Ivy et. al.: Manual of Standard Practice of Plastic and Maxillofacial Surgery, pp. 322—338; in Ferris Smith: Plastic and Reconstructive Surgery. W. B. Saunders Co., Philadelphia, pp. 71—87.) One section covers the lingual aspect of all the teeth. By means of a wire behind the neck of the last tooth on each side, the lingual section is connected to the two buccal sections which meet in the midline forming a large button. The splint is placed by positioning the lingual section and then closing the two buccal sections so that they meet in the midline. A single strand of wire is fastened about the button in a clove hitch, pulled and twisted tight. The extensions of the plastic into all the interdental spaces and undercuts hold the splint firmly in place. Quick-cure acrylic resin may be used to fill any defects, assuring a firm fit. Metal loops or plastic buttons may be incorporated in the buccal sections of the splint for rubber band fixation to interdental wires on the upper teeth. After several weeks of immo- bilization the rubber bands may be removed and the mandible mobilized (fig. 7 D). A gradual return to a semisolid diet is permitted.

A splint may be constructed after several weeks of intermaxillary fixation have provided enough union of the originally badly displaced fragments to permit an impression to be taken. They are useful also in the treatment of Class V fractures if early mobilization is necessary, and particularly for fractures in children when the dentition is mixed (deciduous and permanent teeth).

Supplementary Methods

Occasionally fragments are displaced so badly and the muscular displacing forces so strong that intermaxillary fixation alone cannot provide adequate fixation. This occurs most frequently in fractures at the symphysis and with those just anterior to the mental foramen. Sufficient additional support may be provided by looping a wire through an interdental space two or three teeth posterior to the fracture site, around the buccal and lingual surfaces of the teeth, through an interdental space two or three teeth anterior to the fracture site and then twisting it tight. At the symphysis more substantial support often is needed. A simple method of supplying it is to pass a Kirschner pin across the fracture site.

Anesthesia is obtained by bilateral block of the mandibular and lingual nerves, or by infiltration about the mental foramen and the floor of the mouth. The skin over the chin is pulled up taut and a few drops of local anesthesia infiltrated in the area overlying the lower border of the mandible beneath the canine. A small incision is made through the skin and blunt dissection is carried down to the bone. The Kirschner pin is held perpendicular to the outer cortical plate. As penetration begins, it is angulated and directed across the floor of the mouth toward the canine area on the opposite side. When the pin is felt to penetrate the outer cortical plate on the opposite side, drilling is stopped. The pin is cut off as close to the point of insertion as possible (fig. 7 E and F). The overlying soft tissue is closed with a few sutures. This simple supplementary treatment will provide excellent additional support to intermaxillary fixation or a plastic splint. In about ten weeks the pin will have become loose enough so that it can be pushed from side to side beneath the skin. A few drops of local anesthesia are infiltrated over the point of the pin. Pressure is placed at the opposite side to push the point out as far as possible. The overlying skin is pulled up taut and a stab incision made to the pin which then is grasped with a clamp and pulled out. The soft tissue is closed with a suture or two.

Class II—Edentulous Posterior Fragment with No Displacement

Method of Choice: Interdental Wiring, plus "Bite-Block", plus Intermaxillary Rubber Band Fixation

When an edentulous posterior fragment is not displaced (fig. 8 A and B), interdental wires should be placed on the teeth in the anterior fragment. If the direction of the fracture line is unfavorable, permitting displacement of the fragments (fig. 8 C), some substance must be provided to prevent the posterior fragment from being displaced upward. Quick-cure acrylic plastic is excellent for this purpose although dental modeling compound may be substituted. Powder and liquid are mixed to form a putty-like mass. A thin layer of lanolin or petrolatum is applied to the mucosa. The plastic is placed in the mouth and molded over the alveolar ridge of the edentulous fragment. The teeth are brought into occlusion and the upper teeth (or upper edentulous area) closed into the plastic. Irregularities are smoothed with the finger. The plastic is permitted to set for several minutes. (The bite block may be removed from the mouth and irregular areas filed smooth.) Intermaxillary rubber band fixation is then applied. The upward pull of the masseter, temporal and internal pterygoid muscles will keep the posterior fragment in position against the block; the block will prevent upward displacement (fig. 8 D).

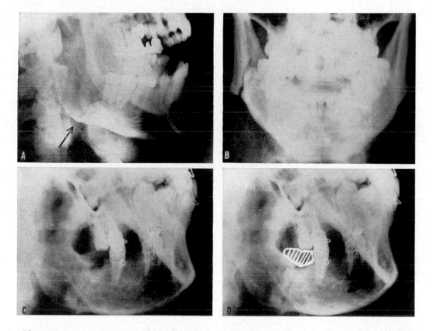

Fig. 8—Class II Fractures. (A and B) Minimal displacement of edentulous posterior fragment. (C) Unfavorable fracture line permitting upward displacement of posterior fragment. (D) Plastic bite-block, shown diagramatically, to maintain posterior fragment in position.

Class III—Edentulous Posterior Fragment with Displacement

Method of Choice: Closed Reduction to Class II

Reduction of a Class III fracture to a Class II often can be done when there is vertical displacement with minimal lateral or medial displacement. Interdental wires are applied. The mouth is opened wide and the posterior fragment pushed down as far as possible. A soft plastic bite-block is placed in position. The mouth is not closed immediately as in the treatment of a Class II fracture, but the plastic is allowed to set with the mouth open. Rubber band traction then is applied to the anterior teeth bringing the anterior fragment up into position. When the displacement is overcome, the bands are adjusted for fixation by relieving as much of the anterior traction as possible.

Alternative Method 1—Open Reduction to Class II: Interosseous Wiring

When the edentulous fragment cannot be reduced sufficiently by aforementioned method, or when there is considerable medial or lateral displacement, open reduction is indicated (fig. 9 A). The open reduction will bring the fragments into a Class II position (fig. 9 B). Control of the posterior fragment by a plastic bite-block and inter-maxillary fixation still will be necessary. All interdental wiring should be done prior to surgery. The plastic bite-block is made in the operating room as soon as the drapes are removed and before the rubber band fixation is applied.

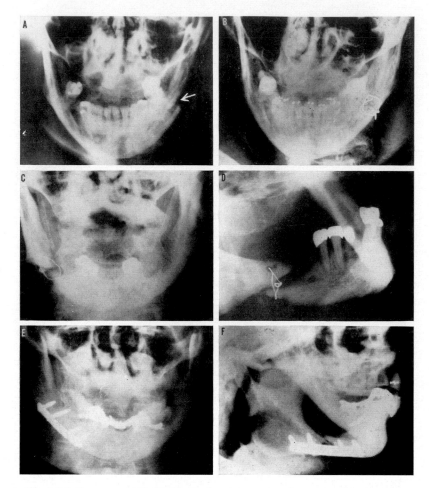

Fig. 9–Class III Fractures. (A) Badly displaced posterior fragment. (B) Appearance after open reduction, interosseous wiring. (C and D) Ununited, badly displaced, edentulous posterior fragment after two unsuccessful attempts at open reduction at another hospital. (E and F) Appearance after open reduction. Plating used for additional support and because of poor condition of ends of fragments as a result of previous procedures.

Local anesthesia is preferred for all of these procedures. General anesthesia greatly increases the incidence of vomiting, making it hazardous to fix the jaws shut in the operating room. When general anesthesia must be used, nasoendotrachael intubation and a preoperatively passed Levin tube are mandatory. The Levin tube should be left in place for at least 24 hours postoperatively. Good preoperative sedation and local anesthesia provide an easily managed, comfortable patient and increase the safety of the procedures. The mandibular nerve should be blocked with 4 cc. of the newer dental local anesthetic agents containing a vasoconstrictor. An intraoral block is preferable, but where displacement or trismus preclude that route, an extraoral block may be given. (Simple extraoral block technic is described by Herd and Weeter: Am. J. Surg. *87*; 74—77 (January) 1954). The same anesthetic agent, without the vasoconstrictor, should be infiltrated in the skin and underlying soft tissue.

The operative site is prepared in the usual manner. Before draping, it is helpful to mark the lower border of the mandible, the facial artery and vein, and the site of the fracture with methylene blue. The drapes are applied; the drape covering the mouth should be sewn to the cheek and the lower lip. An incision about 3 cm. long is made in a skin cleavage line 1 cm. below the lower border of the mandible. Dissection is carried down to the bone, care being taken to preserve fibers of the facial nerve and to retract the facial vessels if encountered. At the lower border of the mandible the periosteum is incised sharply and carefully freed from the lateral and medial aspects of the bone. The periosteum usually is torn at the fracture site and retracting sutures should be placed for ease of identification during closure. The bone fragments should be grasped with Kocher forceps and the fracture reduced. The fracture site probably will have to be debrided of soft tissue to permit precise alignment. A flat, blunt retractor is placed beneath the medial surface of the bone. With a hand or power drill, a small hole is drilled about 5 mm. from the fracture line and 3 mm. from the lower border of the mandible. Another hole is placed 3 or 4 mm. above the first one. Two similarly placed holes are drilled in the other fragment. (A stream of saline should be played against the bone during the drilling.) A piece of 22 gauge stainless steel wire is passed through the upper hole in one fragment and the lower hole in the other. The ends are pulled taut, twisted tight and cut off. Another piece of wire is passed through the unoccupied holes in a similar fashion. Each of the twisted ends is then bent close to the bone and tucked into one of the holes. The periosteum, muscle, fascia and subcutaneous tissue are closed in layers. The skin is closed with interrupted silk or subcuticular 32 gauge wire. A small sterile dressing is applied (fig. 9 B).

The drapes are removed and the plastic bite-block prepared and inserted as described previously for Class II fractures. Intermaxillary rubber bands are placed for fixation. An elastic head-chin bandage is placed and kept on for 24 hours.

Alternative Method 2 — Open Reduction to Class II: Bone Plating

There may be instances when the displacement and displacing forces are so pronounced, or when intermaxillary fixation has to be compromised, that interosseous wiring cannot provide the necessary stability. In these instances a small four-hole metacarpal bone plate can be fixed across the fracture site at the lower border of the mandible in place of the interosseous wires (fig. 9 C—F).

Class IV—Edentulous Mandible or Anterior Edentulous Fragment
Little or no displacement: Circumferential Wiring plus Intermaxillary Fixation

When the fragments are not displaced significantly (fig. 10 A) several strands of 22 gauge wire may be passed under the lower border of the mandible and tightened around the patient's lower denture. (If no denture is available, an impressions taken and a acrylic splint constructed.) The anesthesia and draping are identical to that for bilateral open reduction except that the mouth is included in the field. A small skin incision is made beneath the lower border of the mandible about 1.5 or 2 cm. lateral to the fracture site. A curved trochar-and-cannula is placed in the incision and carried to the lower border of the mandible. Hugging the lingual (medial) aspect of the bone it is carried up into the mouth. A finger should be placed in the mouth to guide it through the mucous membrane.

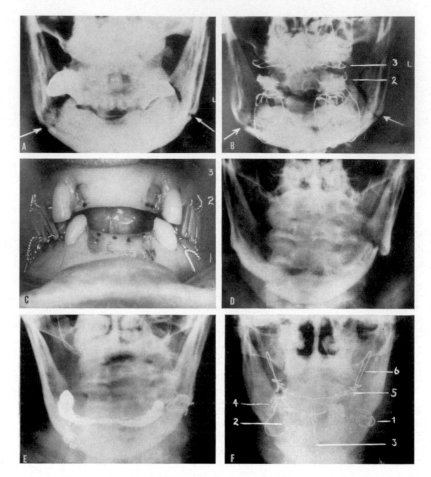

Fig. 10—Class IV Fractures. (A) Minimal displacement of edentulous fragments. (A piece of lead foil has been placed on the undersurface of the patient's denture to determine with roentgenograms whether it overlies both fragments, as on the right, or has to be extended, as on the left.) (B and C) Appearance after circumferential wiring. *1* Circumferential wires around lower denture and mandible. *2* Interdental loops on dentures. *3* Circumferential wires through upper denture and maxillary alveolar bone. (D) Badly displaced edentulous fragments. (E) Appearance after open reduction and interosseous wiring. Metal base lower denture in position. (Intermaxillary fixation by head-chin cap.) (F) Another case demonstrating a combination of techniques. *1* Extra-oral open reduction and interosseous wiring. *2* Intra-oral open reduction and interosseus wiring. *3* Circumferential wiring. *4* Interdental loops around teeth in lower denture. *5* Wire in plastic splint (in lieu of full upper denture) for intermaxillary rubber bands. *6* Upper splint wired to molar process of maxilla.

The trochar is removed and a long strand of wire passed through the cannula. The cannula is removed and the trochar reinserted. Then it is placed in the mucobuccal fold at a point opposite the wire on the lingual surface. Hugging the bone, it is carried down and out through the previous skin incision. The trochar is removed and the wire is passed through the skin incision into the cannula, care being taken to make sure there is no twist. The cannula is removed. The wire is grasped at each end and pulled back and forth until it hugs the lower border of the bone. The skin wound is closed with a suture or two. If the fracture is in the mental foramen area, wires should be placed on either side of the fracture and another on the opposite side of the mandible. The sterilized denture or splint is placed in position and the wires tightened around it. It may help to cut notches or grooves in the border of the denture to keep the wires from slipping (fig. 10 B).

Intermaxillary fixation is achieved by one of several methods. If upper teeth are present, interdental wires may be applied to them and to the teeth on the lower dentures. Intermaxillary rubber bands then are placed in the usual manner. If the upper jaw is edentulous, interdental wires should be placed on the teeth in both dentures (fig. 10 C). If the upper denture (or an acrylic splint if there is no denture) has excellent retention, intermaxillary rubber bands may not displace it. If the denture is not well retained additional support is required:

1. The simplest method is to place the upper denture or splint in the mouth, occlude the circumferentially-wired lower denture to it, and apply a head-chin cap. The previously described head-chin cap made from a sailor hat is excellent for this purpose. Two of these are made for the patient, who wears one constantly except when shaving, washing the hair or replacing it with the clean one. The fixation afforded by a head-chin cap is far from ideal. In addition, it is uncomfortable and unsightly. It should be restricted to the poor-risk patient who cannot undergo one of the following short operative procedures.

2. The upper denture is easily fixed to the malar process of the maxilla. Local anesthetic is infiltrated intraorally about the malar process. The overlying buccal mucosa is incised, care being taken to avoid Stensen's duct. Blunt dissection is carried down to the inferior rim of the malar process. The lateral and medial surfaces are exposed. A retractor is placed medially to protect the underlying structures. A small hole is drilled, lateral-medially, about 3 mm. above the inferior margin. A six inch strand of 22 gauge stainless steel wire is passed through the hole and the ends brought out of the mouth. The soft tissue is closed with interrupted plain gut. The procedure is repeated on the other side. The upper denture, with interdental wires in position, is inserted. The wire from the malar process is passed through one of the interdental loops and twisted tight. This is repeated on the opposite side and the intermaxillary rubber bands applied (figs. 10 F and 11 B–2).

3. The upper denture may be wired intraorally to the piriform aperture margins of the nose or to the alveolar process (fig. 10 B and C). It also may be suspended from the infraorbital rim or zygomatic arch through extraoral procedures (fig. 11 B–3).

Displacement of Fragments: Open reduction, Interosseous Wiring plus Intermaxillary Fixation

Open reduction and interosseous wiring is performed as described previously for Class III fractures. After the drapes are removed, the patient's lower denture is placed in his mouth. If the patient has no denture, an acrylic splint to occlude with the upper arch should be made preoperatively. At insertion, the lower denture or splint may be lined with a rubber-type impression material. This will remain soft for many weeks and minimize the development of sore areas and ulcerations beneath the denture.

A method of intermaxillary fixation is selected from those described above. Any method other than the head-chin cap will require circumferential wiring of the lower denture following the open reduction (fig. 10 F).

Class V—Fractures of the Ramus and Neck of the Condyle

Fractures of the ramus and neck of the condyle usually are accompanied by fractures of the body of the mandible.

A—Fractures of the Ramus

1. When there is no displacement of the ramus, treatment is that for a Class I or Class II fracture. If the patient is edentulous, the dentures (or splints) should be placed in the mouth and appropriate intermaxillary fixation applied (fig. 11 A and B).

2. When the ramus is displaced, there is overriding of the fragments, shortening of the ramus and deviation of the midline to the fractured side. This is overcome by placing

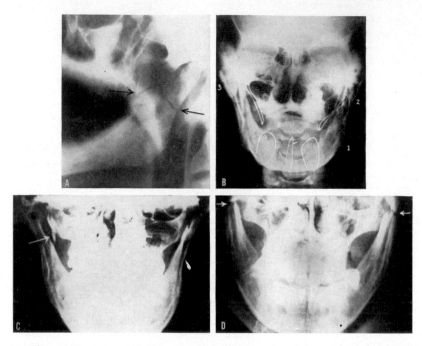

Fig. 11—Class V Fractures. (A) Fracture through ramus just below sigmoid notch. (B) Appearance after reduction and fixation. *1* Circumferential wiring of lower plastic splint (in lieu of denture). *2* Fixation of upper splint to malar process of maxilla (intraorally). *3* Fixation of upper splint to infra-orbital rim (extraorally). (C) Fracture of coronoid process (and zygomatic arch). (D) Bilateral fracture of necks of condyles (and symphysis).

a disc of plastic or modeling compound in the molar region on the involved side to "open the bite", and by putting rubber band traction on the anterior teeth. The disc should be about 3 or 4 mm. thick. It is placed in position just before it has set completely. The patient bites down a bit which forms depressions locking the disc in occlusion. When the plastic has set fully, the traction is begun. Several days of traction may be necessary to overcome pronounced displacement. The disc is removed, but intermaxillary fixation is continued. If the patient is edentulous, the procedures outlined under Class IV—B are adapted to provide the necessary bite-opening and anterior traction.

3. Fractures of the coronoid process are untreated (fig. 11 C).

B—Fractures of the Neck of the Condyle (fig. 11 D)

1. When there is no displacement, the fracture is treated as an ordinary Class I, II or IV case.

2. When there is displacement the fracture is treated the same way as a displaced fracture of the ramus (Class V—A 2). Four or five weeks of immobilization are adequate.

When the mandible is mobilized the patient must be followed carefully while retraining of the jaw movements takes place (fig. 12).

3. When the fractured condylar fragment is dislocated out of the articular fossa, bony union of the fragments is *not* desired. The bite-block is kept in place for about ten days. (Traction is taken off the anterior teeth after several days and kept only on posterior

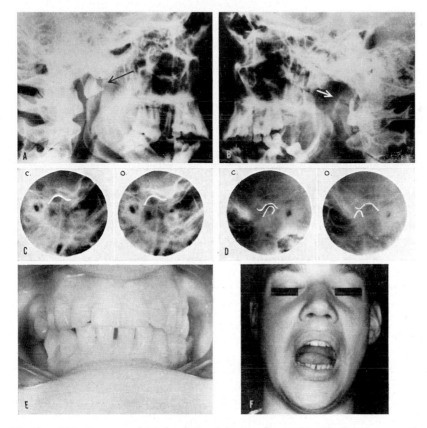

Fig. 12–Class V B–Fracture of Neck of Condyle (see fig. 11 D). (A) Pretreatment: lateral oblique view, right side. Head of condyle is dislocated out of articular fossa. (B) Pretreatment: lateral oblique view, left side. Head of condyle is displaced slightly. (C) Post-treatment: right temperomandibular joint. Dislocated condyle head cannot be seen. (D) Post-treatment: left temperomandibular joint. Condyle head displays normal excursions. (E) Post-treatment: good centric occlusion. (F) Post-treatment: adequate mouth opening. Jaw ex-cursions and function are normal despite only one functioning condyle.

teeth which are blocked from extruding.) This gives the external pterygoid muscle an opportunity to dislocate the fragment further. If the fractured ends are not in apposition, immobilization is continued for four or five weeks. If the fractured ends are in apposition, the mandible is mobilized to prevent union at the fracture site. Muscle training is essential. If an "open-bite" begins to develop, an additional two week period of immobilization may be required. If there are associated fractures of the body, an acrylic splint may be applied which will maintain the body fragments in position yet permit mobilization treatment of the condylar fracture (fig. 12).

Open reduction of a fracture of the neck of the condyle is necessary only when a dislocated fragment prevents the mouth from opening. This rarely will occur if the outlined treatment is carried out.

Length of Time of Intermaxillary Fixation

The length of time intermaxillary fixation will be necessary is determined by an evaluation of many factors: the age and general health of the patient; the length of time between injury and proper fixation; the amount of displacement prior to fixation; the degree of muscle pull to which the fixed fragments are subjected; the presence, extent and duration of infection at the fracture site; the type of supplementary fixation, if any, (e.g., interosseous wiring, Kirschner pin). Eight weeks of fixation should be considered the mean – the proper period for a moderately displaced, well reduced, uninfected fracture in a healthy adult in the third or fourth decade. A similar fracture in a teen-ager requires less fixation; in an older patient, more fixation. Where there has been no initial displacement, and favorable fracture lines prevent subsequent displacement, the period of fixation may be shortened. If the fracture is at the symphysis or canine area, and there is considerable displacement, longer fixation is necessary. The presence of infection at the fracture site increases the period of necessary fixation. It is a good plan to count the weeks from the time clinical signs of infection have disappeared, rather than from when fixation was obtained. You cannot err by keeping the fragments fixed too long; you can err by inadequate length of fixation.

Immediate postreduction roentgenograms always are taken and evaluated. An additional lateral oblique film should be taken two or three weeks later. Teeth in line of fracture may develop periapical abcesses; the fracture site may be infected with low-grade organisms which do not produce clinical manifestations. Anything more than a very slight increase in width of the fracture line must be evaluated carefully.

Callus does not form about fractures of the mandible. After eight weeks of fixation, roentgenograms of the fracture line may appear essentially unchanged from the immediate postreduction films. When consideration of the previously mentioned factors indicates that there probably has been adequate fixation, lateral oblique roentgenograms should be taken. If no increase in width of the fracture line is shown, union of fractures of the body of the mandible should be tested clinically. The intermaxillary rubber bands are removed. The middle finger and forefinger of each hand are placed on the teeth (or alveolar ridge) on either side of the fracture site. The thumbs are placed at the lower border of the jaw. Union is tested with moderate pressure. If movement is discernible, make certain that it is of the jaw itself and not loose teeth. If the jaw fragments move, replace the rubber bands and maintain fixation for two more weeks, at which time union should be tested again. If there is no movement, the intermaxillary rubber bands are left off. The interdental wires (or arch bars) are left in place. Muscle stiffness may make jaw movements uncomfortable for a few days; this will disappear gradually.

The diet may be modified to include soft foods. After two or three days, union is tested again. If the patient is comfortable, and there is no motion of the fragments, the interdental wires are removed. The patient is permitted a gradual return to a normal diet.

Oral Hygiene

Proper hygienic care of the mouth is essential for the patient's comfort and for the maintenance of healthy gingival and dental tissues. Whenever possible, the teeth should be scaled and cleaned by a dentist or dental hygienist before interdental wires are placed. The teeth should be brushed, or the mouth thoroughly rinsed, each time food is ingested. A child's-size toothbrush may be manipulated more easily than a regular brush; occasionally a patient will require a brush as small as an eyelash brush. At least once a day the patient should irrigate around the wires and rubber bands with an irrigating bag. (An enema-bag or douche-bag is filled with warm water to which four tablespoonsful of salt have been added. The bag is suspended high. The patient leans over the sink and directs the stream of solution around the bands and wires.)

When the interdental wires are removed, a dentist or dental hygienist should scale, clean and polish the teeth. Sometimes there is gingival hyperplasia where the rubber bands and wires have produced irritation. After scaling and cleaning, the dentist should instruct the patient in proper gingival massage with a rubber interdental stimulator. This soon will return the gingivae to their prefracture condition.

Diet

When informed that their jaws are to be fastened shut, patients show immediate concern over the problem of eating. They must be reassured that even with a complete dentition and no apparent apertures for the passage of food, they will manage to take a fluid diet very nicely. Fluids can be sucked through the spaces between the teeth with surprisingly little difficulty. If there are edentulous areas, intake is simplified further. (Small removable bridges, when they are not needed for fixation of the fracture, should be left out of the mouth; teeth may be removed from full or partial dentures to provide spaces to facilitate eating) (fig. 10 C). The caloric intake requirement is affected by the patients activity. Patients at rest usually require between 12 and 14 calories per pound of body weight. Working patients need between 16 and 20 calories per pound of body weight, with upward adjustment for the very active.

It is advisable to furnish written instructions with suggested foods and sample meals (fig. 13). Particular attention must be devoted to the patient who is on a special diet, e.g., diabetic, low salt, low cholesterol, etc. Commercially prepared baby foods are available in a wide variety of fruits, vegetables and meats. Mechanical blendors and mixers simplify meal preparation.

Fig. 13—Diet instruction sheet given to patients at The New York Hospital Oral Surgery Clinic.

THE NEW YORK HOSPITAL OUT PATIENT DEPARTMENT
(DENTAL AND ORAL SURGERY CLINIC)

3000 Calorie Liquid Diet

Include the following foods in your diet each day:—

Milk	6 glasses (this can be taken in the form of cream soup, cocoa or milkshakes).
Heavy cream	1 cup (this may be taken in eggnog or milkshakes).
Eggs	4
Cereal	2 tbsp. dry farina, cream of wheat or strained oatmeal made up into gruel.
Citrus fruit juice	1 glass
Fruit juice	1 glass
Tomato juice	$1/_2$ glass
Cocoa	4 tsp.
Butter	4 tsp. (this can be melted in cereal or used in cream soup)
Sugar	4 tsp. (this can be used to sweeten cereal, in milk shakes and eggnogs)
Broth	coffee, tea as desired.

Sample Meal Plan:

Breakfast

1 glass citrus juice
1 serving cereal gruel with butter and cream,
   Coffee with cream and sugar.
Mid morning: 1 glass eggnog
            $1/_2$ glass fruit juice

Lunch

1 serving cream soup
$1/_2$ glass tomato juice
1 glass malted milk with added egg, cocoa with cream.
Mid afternoon: Milk shake with egg

Dinner

1 serving broth
1 glass eggnog
Coffee with cream and sugar
Mid evening: $1/_2$ glass fruit juice

Vitamin supplements are necessary — Take vitamins as directed:
1) New York Hospital Vitamin Capsule   Two daily (Hexovitamin)
2) ACD Liquid 10—12 drops   )   twice
    B Complex liquid 1 teaspoon)   daily

The following may be placed between your lips with a spoon and sucked into your mouth:
   Ice cream, custards, sherbert, gelatin, (without fruit or nuts) and
   Cooked cereals and simple puddings.

Milk and fresh fruit juices are dietary essentials. Additional vitamins must be prescribed. Proprietary dietary supplements are a valuable adjunct. (Meritene, produced by the Dietene Company, is an example of a useful dietary supplement. It is a low-cost, palatable powder which mixes rapidly with milk and which is available in three flavors. Eight ounces [four level tablespoonsful] in a glass of milk taken four times a day satisfies the National Research Council recommendations for protein and essential vitamins and minerals.) The patient should be weighed at each visit and dietary adjustments made when indicated. A fluid diet becomes quite monotonous, and after several weeks a few moments should be taken to check the current intake and to prescribe adjustments and changes. After intermaxillary fixation has been removed, the transition to solid foods should be gradual.

Treatment of Complications

The two most common complications are infection and nonunion. As mentioned previously, all fractures of the body of the mandible are considered compound and a course of broad-spectrum antimicrobials is instituted routinely and maintained for two weeks. The therapy may be continued longer when there is a tooth in line of fracture whose viability is suspect. The specific management of infections is discussed elsewhere in this text. Nonunion is treated best by open reduction. The fracture site is freed of fibrous tissue, the bone ends freshened, and wires or bone plates positioned (fig. 9 C–F). Where there has been substantial loss of bone, a graft may be necessary. When nonunion is complicated by infection, the infection must be controlled and some temporary means of stabilizing the fragments employed. An adequate period of time must elapse after the infection is controlled before operation for reduction and fixation is attempted.

CHAPTER 21

INJURIES OF SOFT TISSUES AND BONES OF THE FACE

HERBERT CONWAY, M.D.

The widespread institution of safety measures has reduced the incidence of injuries caused by industrial accidents, but there has been an actual rise in the incidence of facial injuries due to the increased use of automotive and other forms of transportation. The primary care of such injuries usually must be managed by general practioners or by hospital resident staffs. Since knowledge of a few basic principles of facial surgery and adherence to them are rewarded by primary healing without significant deformity in the majority of cases, these principles should be reiterated and surgical technics which have been developed in recent years should be reviewed. [1, 2]

Wounds of Soft Tissue

When only the soft facial tissues are involved, and there is no need to use specialist help for the management of intracranial, intrathoracic or skeletal injuries, there is no need for haste in the execution of detailed surgery. However, the importance of limiting the time interval between accident and surgical repair must be emphasized. Carelessness or ignorance of the basic principles of facial repair results in excessive cicatrix and deformities of contour which require extensive corrective surgery later or which may never be eradicated completely. Facial repair must be performed unhurriedly and deliberately. The circulatory supply of the facial tissues is so abundant that repair may be carried out effectively after greater lapse of time than, for example, in the management of injuries to the extremities. In the majority of cases the patient with facial injury receives primary care within four hours. However, suture can be executed with little concern for complication as late as 12 or even 16 hours after injury. Injuries to soft tissues may occur either with or without damage to the underlying bony structures or the specialized organs such as the eye and the brain.

In the *emergency care* of injuries to the soft tissues the problem of maintaining the pharyngeal airway is not encountered except in the unusual circumstance in which internal laceration of the mouth may be complicated by brisk hemorrhage into the oral cavity and the pharynx with formation of obstructive clot. Injuries to the soft tissues usually do not require tracheostomy. As in the management of facial fractures, the patient should be transported in the prone position and treated for shock. Hemorrhage from the wound should be controlled by application of hemostats or snug packing. Barton's bandage is the time-honored type of emergency dressing. If the degree of shock or the inadvertent swallowing of large amounts of blood causes nausea, this type of bandage is contraindicated.

Once the patient has arrived at the doctor's surgery or the emergency room of the hospital, definitive management of the injury is undertaken. Shock is combated by conventional therapy, i.e., external warming of the body with

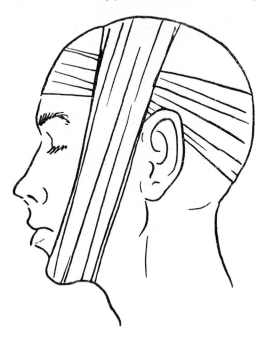

Fig. 1—When properly applied, the Barton's bandage brings the teeth of the upper and lower jaws into occlusion, thus holding the majority of fractures of the mandible and maxilla in fairly accurate reduction. It is a most useful dressing for fractures of the facial bones.

blankets, elevation of the foot of the operating table, intravenous administration of physiologic saline, plasma or whole blood and intramuscular injection of morphine. In severe shock it is well to give a smaller dose of morphine, for the capillary circulation is so inefficient that the drug may not be absorbed promptly. It is a mistake to employ successive full doses of morphine intramuscularly to obtain the desired effect of the opiate, because on recovery from shock rapid uptake of the drug may be followed by signs of overdosage. Antitetanus serum should be given.

Definitive facial repair [1,2] requires that the extent and type of the injury be assayed accurately. Following the cleansing of the skin with soap, water and a detergent, the wound should be irrigated copiously with warm physiologic saline solution. This reduces bacterial contamination, removes clots and loose foreign bodies and allows for the evaluation of the degree and type of trauma. Injuries to the soft tissues of the face are classified as (1) abrasions and contusions, (2) simple lacerations, (3) lacerations with avulsion flaps, (4) laceration with loss of soft tissue, (5) lacerations into the oral cavitiy and (6) lacerations with injury to the eye or with associated fractures of the underlying facial bones. General measures which are necessary include liberal treatment with penicillin, which is very effective against mouth organisms.

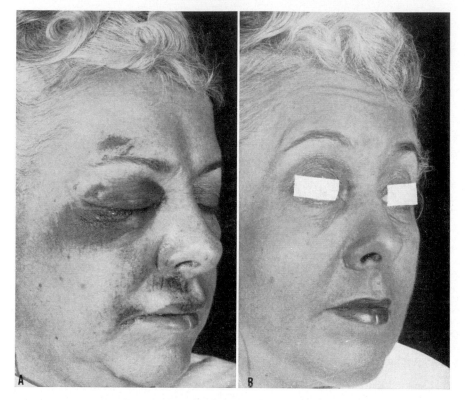

Fig. 2–(A) Severe abrasion of the face suffered when patient tripped on a curbstone and fell against the asphalt pavement. Numerous minute particles of dirt and foreign material were embedded into the dermis. (B) Appearance eight days after emergency treatment by abrasion using novocain injection to the point of tense rigidity of the tissue, the application of the rotary steel brush and vaseline gauze dressings. (Reproduced from Am. J. Surg., vol. 90: December 1955, with permission of author and journal.)

Abrasions and *contusions* formerly were treated with simple cleansing and the application of a vaseline dressing. This treatment failed to take care of the problem of foreign material imbedded in the dermis. Injury by scraping on macadam, brick or similar materials almost invariably results in traumatic tattoo. In such instances it is justifiable and correct to treat the cutaneous area of foreign body embedment by the abrasive technique, using fine sandpaper supported on wooden blocks or the rotary steel brush powered by a dental drill apparatus or a conventional motor. Although this method adds further trauma, the results justify the technic (figs. 1, 2 and 3).

Simple lacerations are treated by strong brushing of the floor of the wound, loose coaptation of fascial structures by fine catgut sutures, and approximation of cutaneous margins with sutures of 6–0 fine silk starting at key

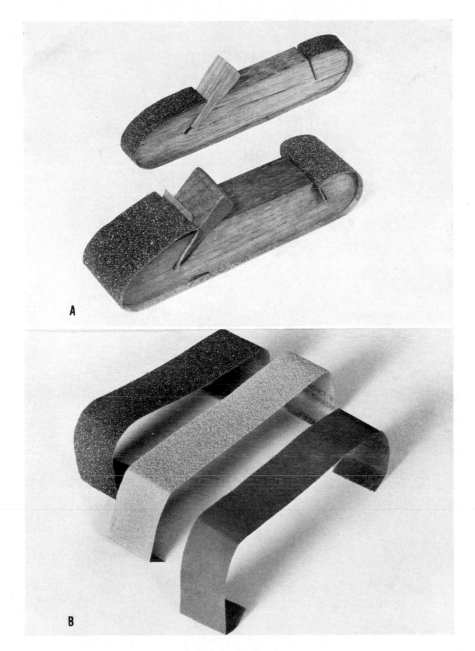

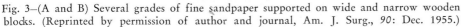

Fig. 3–(A and B) Several grades of fine sandpaper supported on wide and narrow wooden blocks. (Reprinted by permission of author and journal, Am. J. Surg., *90*: Dec. 1955.)

points in an irregular laceration. Margins of eyelids, vermilion of the lips, alae of the nose and curves of the ear serve as guides in repair. Dead space is obliterated by the pressure of firm dressings. Excision of margins of the wound is contraindicated, for facial tissue is precious and the likelihood of complicating infection is remote. There is no authentic case report in the literature of gas gangrene developing in a wound of the face, just as infection by partial tension organisms such as the gonococcus is not encountered in

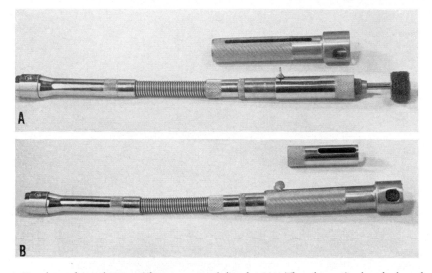

Fig. 4—Buncke safety sleeve with rotary steel brush. (A) The sleeve is detached and the rotary steel brush (which is power driven) is exposed. (B) The safety sleeve is in place so that the bristles of the brush project only through the small opening in the cylindrical sleeve.

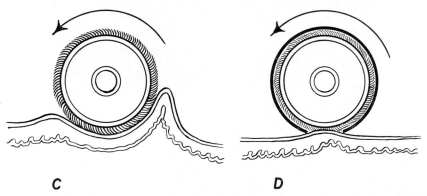

Fig. 4—(C) Without the safety sleeve the bristles of the brush cause heaping up of the skin to one side and there is no protection against penetration of the complete thickness of the skin. (D) With the safety sleeve in place the rotary action of the steel brush does not allow for tenting up of the skin. Moreover, protection is offered against too deep penetration of the dermis and centrifugal spray of blood and cellular material is prevented. (From Buncke, H. J., Plast. & Reconstruct. Surg. *16:* 65, 1955. With permission of author and journal.)

the mouth. The rich oxygenation of facial tissues due to the abundant blood supply protects against infection following trauma except in the very rare instance in which there is massive devitalization of tissue or in which the interval of time between injury and repair is unduly prolonged. If simple facial lacerations are parallel to the wrinkle lines of the skin, primary suture is rewarded with an unnoticeable scar of healing.[4] On the other hand, violent trauma does not always respect laws or lines of physiologic tension, and lacerations may be at right angles to the wrinkle lines or at variance with them. In such cases primary suture results in minimal cicatrix which may be corrected at a later date by excision and revision of the tissue by the Z plastic technic. In this classic procedure two incisions are made at an angle of 60 degrees to the long axis of the scar, which itself forms the oblique line of the Z. The horizontal arms of the Z are created by incision parallel to the wrinkle lines, which always run at right angles to the line of contractile force of the underlying platysma (figs. 4 and 5).

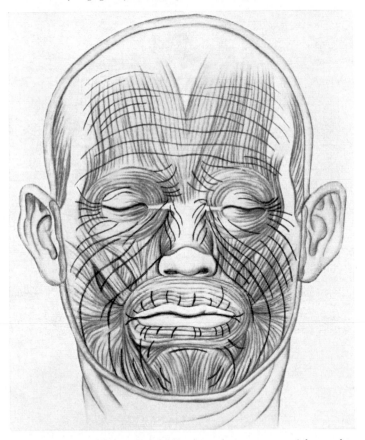

Fig. 5—Wrinkle lines of the face. Note that they always are at right angles to the line of contractile pull of the underlying muscles. Facial lacerations parallel to these lines heal ideally after primary suture. (From Kraissl, C. J. and Conway, H.: Surgery 25: 592, 1949. With permission of author and journal.)

Lacerations with avulsion flap of soft tissue are treated by gentle cleansing with saline sponges, irrigation of the wound, removal of blood clots, meticulous hemostasis, and replacement of the flap by loose fascial suture and minute (6–0 silk) cutaneous sutures even though the flap is significantly

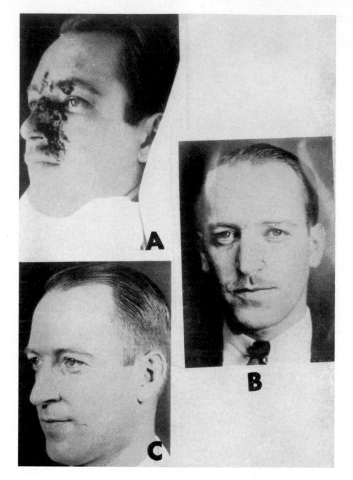

Fig. 6–(A) Severe facial laceration, incurred in automobile accident. (B) After primary suture (without débridement) it was apparent that the vertical hypertrophic scar paralleling the nose on the left was due to the fact that the laceration was not parallel to the wrinkle lines of the face. (C) Appearance after secondary excision of scar and shifting of tissue by the Z plastic technic. (Reprinted from Am. Surg. 90: Dec. 1955, with permission of author and journal.)

cyanotic. It is the rule rather than the exception that because of the abundant vascularity of this anatomic region, post-traumatic, cyanotic flaps of soft facial tissue regain their viability after suture. At any rate, the recovery of circulation invariably saves more of a severely damaged flap than would be saved by conservative débridement or amputation of portions of such flap.

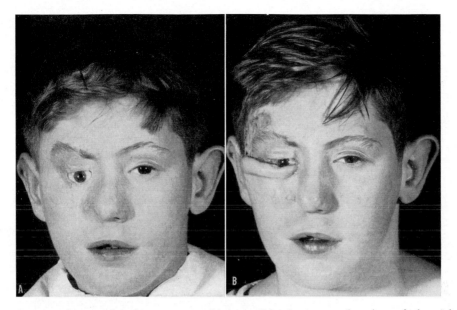

Fig. 7—(A) Photographs of a 14 year old boy with almost complete loss of the right lower eyelid due to trauma at birth as the result of an instrument delivery. Inability of the patient to retain his prosthetic eye indicated that the lower lid should be reconstructed. (B) A temporal flap incorporating the frontal branch of the superficial temporal artery and the inferior branch of the temporal vein was transferred to the lower lid. Provision for lining was made by folding the flap on itself.

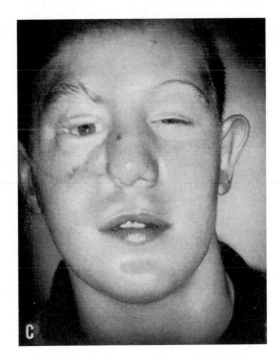

Fig. 7—(C) Pedicle detached after twenty-one days and the base returned to the temporal region.

through loss of tissue from the ear should be treated by suture of the aural remnant down to the skin of the mastoid area. Such a step avoids infection and prepares the defect for correction by subcutaneous burial of cartilage and its subsequent elevation from the mastoid area and backing by skin graft. This method takes the first reconstructive step at the time of repair of primary injury. If only simple suture of cutaneous margins of aural remnant is done, the reconstruction may require four or more operative steps. It is intriguing to consider the possibility of abdominal burial of a completely detached portion of auricular cartilage after excision of the overlying skin if such detached specimen has been saved. Manual carving of cartilage for aural replacement never has been rewarded by a contoural result which is equal to the sculptured effect of the natural auricular cartilage. The only case in which I have had the opportunity to replace the detached auricular cartilage was a late disappointment owing to the excessive formation of fibrous tissue over the cartilaginous transplant.

Lacerations into the oral cavity require thorough cleansing, irrigation with hydrogen peroxide or sodium perborate and loose suture of the mucous membranes. Thereafter the details of closure of musculature and skin are carried out as listed heretofore. If there is sizable loss of tissue, infection can be avoided by the immediate suture of mucous membrane to skin, thus creating a temporary fistula of the cheek. Injury to Stensen's duct must be searched for in lacerations of the cheek. If the duct is divided, its proximal end should be brought into the oral cavity at a position posterior to its normal aperture. If this is not feasible, the duct should be ligated even though parotid atrophy follows. Minor injuries to the duct of the parotid gland may cause localized subcutaneous or submucous accumulation of saliva. Usually this condition responds to successive aspirations.

Lacerations in association with underlying severe fractures of the facial bones are treated just as other injuries to soft tissues, after reduction of the fractures has been accomplished (fig. 15). Injuries to the globe call for care by an ophthalmologist.

Fractures of Facial Bones

In this chapter it is not feasible to go into great detail regarding all aspects of management of injuries to the bones of the face. However, principles of treatment [3] are set down and operative techniques for the common fractures are described.

Shock and *hemorrhage* deserve the most careful consideration in the management of injuries to the facial bones. These states account for the primary mortality not only on the battlefield but also in accidents of civilian life. In fractures of the maxilla especially, tears of the branches of the internal maxillary arteries are followed by copious hemorrhage which may be followed by death either due to loss of blood or to suffocation by collections of large gelatinous clots in the hypopharynx. It is imperative to provide early first aid by simple removal of the clots and the attainment of firm closure of the jaws by Barton's bandage.

Obstruction to the airway, common in sectional fractures of the lower jaw, may also be the cause of death soon after injury. This may be prevented by pulling the tongue forward and securing it to fixed clothing of the chest by suture through the tip. Some first aid manuals advise the use of a safety pin, plunged through the tongue and tied to the clothing. When the continuity of the mandible is interrupted at two points, the tongue and the hyoid bone fall backwards, thus closing the epiglottis. The simple emergency measure as described has saved many lives. When fractures of upper and lower jaws have occurred simultaneously, *tracheostomy* often is imperative.

Associated injuries must be considered. It is not unusual for facial fractures to be associated with injuries to the globe of the eye or to the cranium and intracranial structures. Rhinorrhea is an evidence of the latter, and this often occurs when there is a fracture of the cribriform plate of the ethmoid bone. Downward dislocation of the eyeball occurs frequently when the malar bone is fractured and displaced. In addition, injuries of the extremities and torso must be looked for and evaluated. Particular care of injuries to the orbit, the cranium, the thorax, the abdomen and the extremities is discussed in other chapters.

Once the patient has reached a safety plateau in respect to the states of hemorrhage and shock and has been cleared as to intracranial, intrathoracic, intra-abdominal, ocular and extremity injuries, the surgeon must set about the management of wounds of the face and fractures of the facial bones. Fortunately, there is no need for haste, though too long a delay invites difficulties. Early examination is important because facial edema sets in rapidly and prevents the ready diagnosis of fractures of the zygomatic arch, the malar bone and dislocation of the eyeball. X-ray views are taken when the general condition of the patient permits, and this also is the guide to the correct time for the institution of reduction of fracture of the facial bones. In general, it is safe to wait two, three or four days, but delay of 10 to 14 days means that the operation may have to forcibly open up fracture lines, for the flat bones of the face heal in deformity with remarkable rapidity.

Fractures of the Nasal Bones

Most commonly compounded into the nose, the usual fracture of the nasal bones is one of medial and backward displacement of the bones on one side and lateral displacement of those on the other. It is a mistake to note only the indentation of the side that received the blow, for replacement of these fragments alone gives a disappointing result. It is necessary to anesthetize the area by injecting novocain into the soft tissues and by applying cocain crystals (moistened with 1:10000 solution of adrenalin) to the mucous membranes of the nose. With an instrument inserted through the nostril into the nasopharynx of the depressed side the fractured fragments of nasal bone and maxilla are mobilized. In the majority of cases a small incision within the vestibule of the nostril allows for the insertion of a chisel which may be used to cut through the impaction of the bones on the side opposite

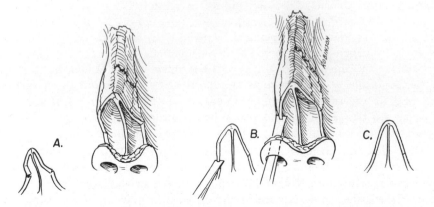

Fig. 10—Nasal fracture. Demonstration of the displacement of bony fragments of nasal bones, maxillae and septum to the side opposite that which received the impact. Simple elevation of the displaced fragments on the side recipient of the impact is not sufficient for accurate reduction. Through an incision inside the nostril, a chisel should be inserted to free the line of impact opposite that which received the blow. This allows for molilization of the nasal bones and accurate reduction of the fracture.

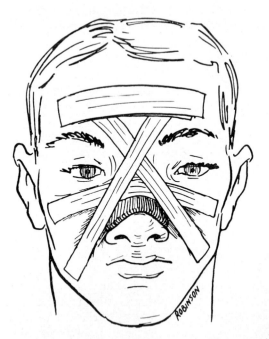

Fig. 11—Dental compound which can be molded accurately after emersion in warm water and which hardens on cooling makes an excellent nasal splint. Intranasal packing may or many not be required for nasal fracture.

that which received the impact. Once this is done the entire bony and soft tissue nasal mass may be moved freely from side to side for accurate midline setting of the fractures. Position may be maintained by intranasal packing with vaselinized gauze and a light pressure dressing kept in place by an external nasal splint fashioned from dental compound. Often the intranasal packing is not necessary. Associated injuries to the nasal septum and to cartilaginous structures of the nasal tip are not uncommon. The quadrilateral plate of the cartilaginous septum may undergo linear fracture just as bony structures do. Correction of cartilaginous displacement by manipulation may result in acceptable nasal contour, though more often injuries to cartilaginous structures result in later obstruction of the nasal airway due to frankly deviated nasal septum. Furthermore, the late result may show an unacceptable deviation of the nasal tip. Both of these conditions often require later operative correction.

Fracture of the Zygomatic Arch

Fracture of the arch composed of the zygomatic process of the temporal bone and the temporal process of the zygoma are important only because, there is a deformity of appearance if they are not reduced accurately. The usual fracture is a V-shaped indentation of the anatomic arch, which is reduced easily by the classic Gillies procedure. Incision is made in the temporal region of the scalp just back of the hair line. The fascia of the masseter is identified and incised so that a long periosteal elevator or other similarly shaped instrument may be bluntly plunged within the temporal musculature down to a point just under the indented fracture of the zygo-

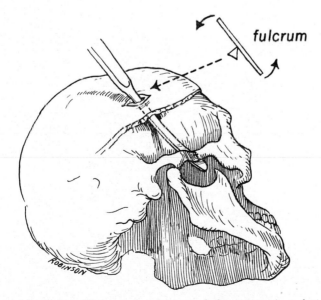

Fig. 12—Fracture of zygoma. Technic of reduction of the zygomatic arch (see description in text).

matic arch. The convergence of the temporal muscle at its insertion into the coronoid process of the mandible assures that the blind end of the instrument will reside just under the zygomatic arch. The instrument is then used as a lever of the first class, the convexity of the temporal and parietal bones of the skull acting as the fulcrum. With sudden forceful pressure the handle of the instrument is moved toward the vertex. This causes the buried end of the instrument to push the indented arch outward, thus restoring its contour. The small incision into the scalp is closed and no dressing or fixation is required.

Fractures of the Malar Bone

The usual injury here is a downward dislocation of the L-shaped bone which makes up part of the lateral and part of the inferior wall of the orbit. If there is extensive comminution, there may be downward dislocation of the eyeball. This complication, which results in diplopia if untreated, may escape the clinician's notice became of the regional edema. Therefore it is of the utmost importance that fractures of the malar bone be reduced. The best approach is an operative one. Through the classic Caldwell-Luc incision, the maxillary antrum is unroofed. Instrumentation within the antrum allows for the upward movement of the fragment with reduction of the fracture.

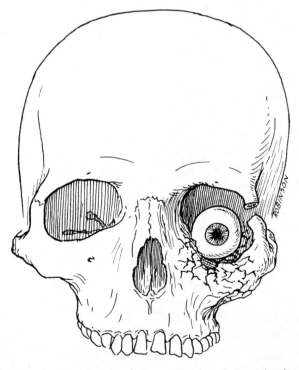

Fig. 13—Fracture of the malar bone is often associated with comminution and downward displacement of the occular globe as is shown in this sketch.

If there is comminution or collapse of the anterior wall of the maxilla due to fracture, packing of the sinus for a period of 3 to 4 days may be indicated. Surprisingly, these injuries, their operative reduction and the packing of the nasal sinus are not followed by interference with the physiology of the maxillary sinus unless there is a purulent infection of the antrum. In severely comminuted fractures, open reduction by wiring at the lateral and inferior margins of the orbit is the procedure of choice. It is well to state here that though the diagnosis of fracture of the malar bone is made by palpation and by x-ray, interpretation of roentgenograms of this area is so difficult that palpation for deformity and tenderness is a more reliable guide. It should be mentioned here that another fracture, an uncommon one, recently has been emphasized as a cause of diplopia due to downward dislocation of the eyeball. This is the comminuted fracture of the inferior wall of the orbit without interruption of the inferior bony orbital margin. This fracture often evades early diagnosis. It is treated effectively in cases of recent injury by the same approach and technique, through the maxillary sinus.

Diplopia due to an old fracture of the malar bone or floor of the orbit is treated fairly easily by the insertion of a block of cartilage. This is done through a small incision at the lateral margin of the eyeball. The cartilage is so carved and inset that it holds the eyeball on a level with its fellow and thereby relieves the symptom.

Fractures of the Maxilla

These are classified as horizontal, pyramidal and transverse facial. They may be unilateral, but more commonly are bilateral. Frequently, these fractures cause excessive hemorrhage due to tear of the internal maxillary arteries

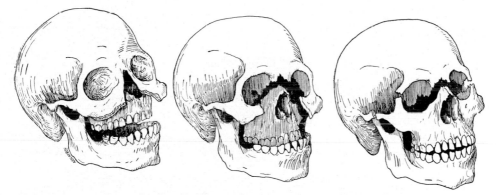

Fig. 14—Three common types of fractures of the maxillae. On the left the most common type, referred to as a horizontal or transverse fracture of the upper jaw in which the majority of the maxilla is as a free floating fragment.
Second type as shown in the middle sketch is referred to as a pyramidal fracture and extends through both antra and up to the base of the nose. The detached fragment is composed of both maxillae together with the nasal bones.
On the right is shown a third type of fracture of the maxilla, relatively rare in occurrence and referred to as a transverse facial fracture. The fracture line extends through the base of the nasal and ethmoid regions and across the orbits to the zygomatic arches.

or their branches. Great accumulations of gelatinous blood clot in the oro-
pharynx and in the hypopharynx are common. Shock, which frequently
accompanies these injuries, may preclude the spontaneous emission of the
clots. Effective first aid is of the utmost importance. This may be accom-

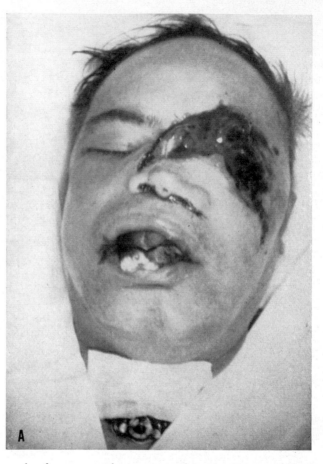

Fig. 15—(A) Example of a severe soft tissue wound in association with horizontal fracture
of the maxilla. Patient had been struck by a taxicab. Emergency care included maintenance
of airway by upward pressure on the upper jaw and the institution of tracheostomy.
Blood transfusion was required as an emergency procedure. (From Conway, H.: Am. J.
Surg. *90*: 891, 1955. With the permission of the journal.)

plished easily by manual replacement of the dislocated upper jaw, closure
of the jaws, and the bandaging of the jaws in a closed position by a Barton's
Bandage. Respiratory difficulty when a fractured maxilla occurs in association with other bony injuries of the face may create an emergency in which
tracheostomy is imperative. However, simple fractures of the maxillae
without associated injuries usually are held quite effectively by the Barton's

bandage if the patient has sufficient teeth to allow effective pressure on the maxilla by outer dressings on the lower jaw. The teeth of the upper and lower jaws fit into each other like cams so that this simple maneuver results in accurate reduction. Often the detached bones are forced backward by the impact of the injury so that the upper jaw must be pulled forward manually. Manuals on this subject usually refer to the Kingsley splint and a variety of procedures based on the principle of counterpressure from the

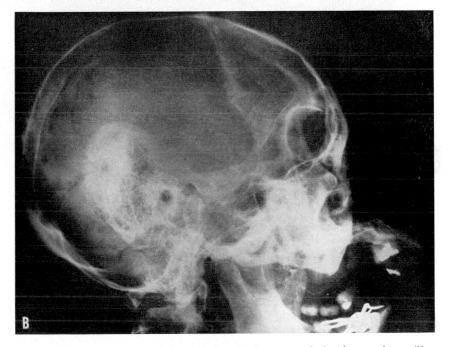

Fig. 15 (B) Lateral x-ray following the displacement of the fractured maxilla.

vertex of the skull, utilizing a plaster head cap. These head caps are notably ineffectual because they tend to slip. Only in those individuals whose skulls have a pronounced occipital protrusion can a plaster head cap be held in place effectively for the necessary fourweek period. When such caps are used, they are applied in combination with an upper dental plate which is connected by an adjustable extraoral rod to the plaster cap. A variation of this principle is to attach the head cap by turnbuckle or wires which are passed through the skin of the malar eminence, the soft tissues of the cheek and then secured to the teeth of the upper jaw. My experience has led to the conclusion that open reduction with direct wiring is the procedure of choice for fractures of the maxilla. This is especially true since there often is an associated fracture of the nasal bones. Secure operative wiring means that the upper jaw is in position effectively and that soft diet may be started

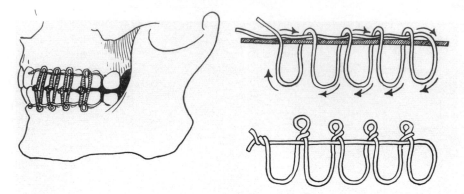

Fig. 16—Diagram of the technic of intradental wiring. Rubber bands are passed around the loops to hold the teeth of the upper and lower jaws in occlusion. This device effectively reduces the majority of fractures of the mandible.

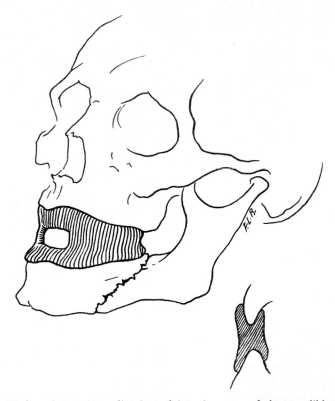

Fig. 17—The H-shaped Gunning splint is useful in fractures of the mandible in edentulous subjects. It must be supplemented with an accurately fitted Barton's bandage. Alternate methods of management of fractures of the mandible in edentulous subjects are open reduction or the use of intramedullary wires.

of reduction, the bony pegs known as teeth, are missing. A Gunning splint may be used, or, intramedullary wires, or open reduction. Fractures of the mandibular condyle are best handled conservatively, i.e., by wiring of the teeth of the lower jaw to those of the upper jaw. Severely displaced condylar fragments may require open reduction, a difficult operative procedure

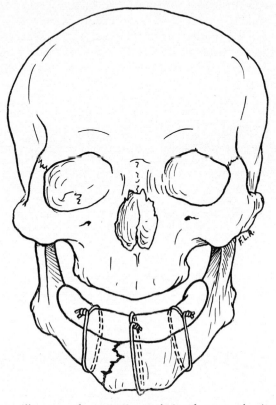

Fig. 18—This diagram illustrates the operative technic of open reduction of the jaw in an edentulous subject by the use of the mandibular splint held securely in position by circumferential wiring passed around the mandible.

because of the problem of obtaining operative exposure without injury to the ramifications of the facial nerve which overlie the operative area. Ideally, anesthesia for reduction of fractures of the mandible is by novocain block of the mandibular nerves. In a recent review of the treatment in 1305 cases of fractures of the facial bones, Walden and Bromberg [5] reported that no anesthesia was required in 137 cases, general anesthesia was employed in 283 cases, while local anesthesia was effective in 885 cases.

Summary

This presentation outlines the principles of the management of soft tissue injuries of the face and emphasizes the value of preservation of tissue rather than sacrifice by débridement. Attention to the basic principles of soft tissue repair at the time of emergency suture avoids the crippling deformities which follow infection of facial wounds or which may, on occasion, be caused by injudicious excision of marginal tissue. In the managnment of facial fractures, the early reduction and immobilization of fractures of the facial bones is the key to suitable cosmetic restoration with minimal functional impairment. In addition, complications are held to the minimum. Tracheostomy is invaluable as a life-saving procedure in severe injuries and also as an effective route of anesthesia. The value of direct operative wiring of fractures of the facial bones is definitely established. This technic utilizes the principle of attaching the loosened facial bones to the nearest, cephalad, solid, bony structure.

References

[1] CONWAY, H.: Injuries of soft tissues of the face. Am J. Surg. *90*: 891—896, 1955.

[2] —: The surgery of major and minor traumatic wounds including burns. Rocky Mount. M. J., August, 1952.

[3] ERICH, J. B., and AUSTIN, L. E.: Traumatic Injuries of Facial Bones. Philadelphia, W. B. Saunders Co., 1944.

[4] KRAISSL, C. J., and CONWAY, H.: Excision of small tumors of the skin of the face with special reference to the wrinkle lines. Surgery *25*: 592—600, (April) 1949.

[5] WALDEN, R. H., and BROMBERG, B. E.: Recent advances in therapy in maxillofacial bony injuries in over 1000 cases. Am. J. Surg. *93*: 508—516, 1957.

CHAPTER 22

TRACHEOTOMY

JAMES A. MOORE, M.D.

Historical Aspects

Tracheotomy, or laryngotomy, as it was first called, is not a new procedure. Galen (130—201 A.D.) and Aretaeus (second to third century A.D.) both referred to cutting the trachea.

Antonio Musa Brasavola (1490–1554) was apparently the first person actually to perform a laryngotomy in 1546. The second was Sanctorius (1561–1636) who made use of a trocar, leaving the cannula in the wound for three days. Then in 1620, Nicholas Halicot reported four successful cases.

The best early description of the operation was written by Hieronymus Fabricius (1537—1619), an Italian surgeon, embryologist and anatomist, pupil and successor of Fallopius and teacher of William Harvey at Padua. He described the operation of opening of the "aspera arteria", as the trachea was called, in patients who were suffocating due to obstruction of respiration. He disputed the former authors as to its utility and stated that the operation was useless when the lungs were affected and the trachea full of material. He pointed out that it was useful only when the obstruction was in the larynx and above the place of incision.

Fabricius was the first to criticize the transverse skin incision, employed up to his time, and advised that the incision should be made vertically over the third and fourth tracheal cartilages. He also recommended the use of a small, straight, short cannula with two wings at its outer ends to prevent it from slipping into the trachea.

It was some time later, around 1627, that Julius Casserius, a pupil of Fabricius, illustrated a more refined technique.

In about 1707, Pierre Dionis wrote that it was wrong to call the operation "laryngotomy," and suggested that "bronchotomy" was the proper word.

In 1718, Lorenz Heister suggested the operation should be called "tracheotomy" and that the other names should be discarded. However, it was not until the beginning of the nineteenth century that the term, tracheotomy, displaced the others.

Emergency Tracheotomy

Our first consideration should be to do as few tracheotomies as an emergency procedure as is possible. Whenever it is feasible, one should convert an emergency procedure into an orderly operation by the insertion of an endotracheal tube, a bronchoscope, or a Mosher life-saver. By preference, tracheotomies should be done in the operating room with proper illumination, suction, hemostats, and other necessary equipment. One should endeavor to

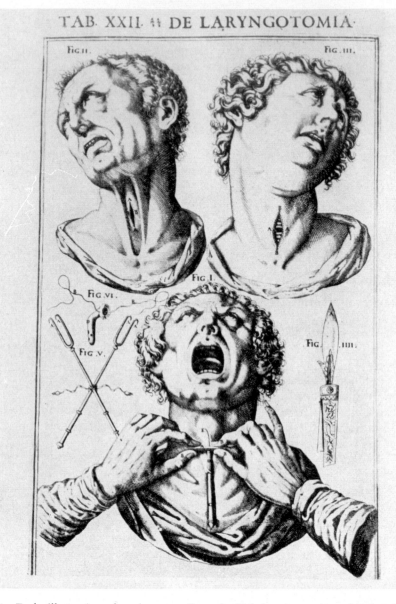

Fig. 1— Early illustration of tracheotomy (from the *Tabulae Anatomicae* of Julius Casserius, 1627).

avoid doing tracheotomies in the treatment room or in the bed, except in real emergencies or under unusual circumstances. When time and conditions permit, anesthesia should consist of local infiltration with procaine and adrenalin solution. Ordinarily, general anesthesia should not be used in a case with severe laryngeal obstruction.

Emergency tracheotomy may be indicated under certain conditions, which include automobile or airplane accidents, attempted suicide, foreign bodies, as a complication of thyroid surgery, acute laryngeal edema and occasionally with certain pedunculated tumors.

Preoperative Medication

In the preoperative preparation of the patient for tracheotomy, one should omit opiates, sedatives and even atropine. Opiates and sedatives are contra-indicated, because they dangerously reduce the effectiveness of the accessory muscles of respiration, which are under voluntary control. It is for this same reason that a general anesthetic is hazardous.

Technic of Tracheotomy

The position of the patient is important. A roll of fabric or a sandbag should be placed under the shoulders, so as to extend and expose the trachea. If necessary, in an emergency, the left knee of the operator can be used in place of the roll of fabric. The trachea should be fixed by the thumb and middle finger of the operator's left hand, leaving the index finger free.

The vertical incision is then made in the midline through the skin and fascia from approximately the suprathyoid notch level to the suprasternal notch. In the elective procedure, with an endotracheal tube or bronchoscope in place, the collar incision may be substituted for the vertical incision where the cosmetic effect is of prime concern. However, as a routine procedure, it is not recommended.

After making the initial incision, the strap muscles are separated in the midline and the trachea identified by inspection or by the index finger. In most cases, the isthmus of the thyroid should be resected and the cut surface of the remaining gland secured by suture ligature.

The first four or five rings of the trachea are exposed in the midline and usually the third and fourth tracheal rings are incised vertically. A small piece of cartilage is removed from either side of at least one tracheal ring to form the so-called "Mosher punch tracheotomy."

The lips of the tracheal incision are then separated by means of the Trousseau dilator, and the tracheal tube is inserted. A curved hemostat, or even the handle of the scalpel, may be used instead of the Trousseau dilator, if necessary.

Hemostasis is of prime importance and should be complete.

The wound should be closed only loosely, taking care to leave space above and below the tube for air to escape on coughing. It is a mistake, all too frequently made, to close the incision too tightly about the tracheal tube.

On completing the procedure, the tracheotomy tape should be tied snugly, so as to hold the tube firmly in position and to prevent the tube from being dislodged by coughing.

Pitfalls in Emergency Tracheotomy

There are many pitfalls in emergency tracheotomy. The more common ones will be enumerated and discussed.

Perhaps the most common of all pitfalls in this procedure is "panic." Occasionally, a tracheotomy must be done on the spot and in a matter of two or three minutes. However, fortunately, this is a rare occurrence. One should do as few tracheotomies as possible in the patient's bed or in the treatment room.

General anesthesia is contraindicated in a patient with severe laryngeal obstruction. The obstructed patient is using his accessory muscles of respiration under voluntary control. If general anesthesia is induced, then, with the loss of consciousness, the patient ceases to breathe and a real emergency ensues.

Opiates are contraindicated for the same reasons that dictate against a general anesthetic.

An unduly short incision may make the operation more difficult. An adequate incision should always be used.

Too tight a closure may lead to subcutaneous and/or mediastinal emphysema, or even to a pneumothorax. Occasionally ill advised packing may be used, with the same result.

Attempts to change the outer cannula too soon after tracheotomy may lead to the formation of a false passage and an inadequate or blocked airway.

Postoperative hemorrhage may develop if bleeding points are not secured, particularly in a hypertensive patient, or in one with a blood dyscrasia. Occasionally an anomalous artery crosses the trachea in the area of the isthmus of the thyroid.

Another complication which may arise is postoperative obstructive atelectasis, which can be relieved by bronchoscopic aspiration.

Occasionally failure to obtain a free airway may result from using a cannula which may be too short or may have the wrong curve. When in doubt, a lateral x-ray will help to reveal the difficulty.

After-Care

The proper after care of a patient with a tracheotomy should include a special nurse, trained in tracheotomy care, and such care should be provided around the clock. The nursing care will include special suction technic, effective but atraumatic. Moist warm air should be provided, usually by means of a croup kettle. Alevaire inhalation may be indicated. As a rule, no opiates or sedatives should be given. Good postoperative care includes the use of a suitable antibiotic agent for four to five days.

At the time the patient leaves the operating room, the tracheotomy tube tape should be checked to make sure the tube is securely held. Then the outer cannula should not be changed for approximately 72 hours.

Summary

In summary, one should avoid a hurried emergency tracheotomy by converting the emergency into an elective procedure wherever this is possible, by the insertion of an endotracheal tube, a bronchoscope, or a Mosher lifesaver. Once the airway is established, an orderly tracheotomy can be done, and usually in the operating room.

A general anesthetic and preoperative opiates or sedation should be avoided.

If one is forced to do a high tracheotomy (above the third and fourth tracheal rings) as an emergency, it should be converted into a low tracheotomy as soon as practical.

As a rule, the first tracheal ring should not be incised.

The outer cannula should remain in place for approximately 72 hours before changing.

When the above precautions are carried out, the procedure carries a relatively low mortality and fewer complications are encountered.

CHAPTER 23

FRACTURES AND DISLOCATIONS OF CERVICAL SPINE

P. D. WILSON, JR., M.D., and J. PAUL HARVEY, JR., M.D.

Cervical spine fractures and dislocations are important chiefly because of the neurologic damage that might ensue either immediately at time of injury, subsequently when moving the patient from scene of injury or even during phases of treatment.

Neurologic symptoms run the gamut from instantaneous death, particularly in high complete transections, down through quadriplegia in lower cervical levels, to signs of root injury only. Many cervical injuries cause no neurologic damage but result only in stiffness of neck muscles and perhaps some rotation of head and neck. The latter may be the only symptoms, even in cases with severe bony disruption at any level. However, the threat of neurologic damage is always present in any cervical spine injury and at any time until definite, permanent fixation and healing have taken place. Occasionally, long after an injury one may see neurologic signs. These may be secondary to pressure from herniated discs or to osteophyte formation with decreasing size of the foramen between laminae or even with decreasing size of neural canal, because the bony excrescences form along the inferior or superior margins of injured vertebral bodies.

Because of this constant threat, any case where cervical area damage or injury exists, or is suspected, must be handled with extreme care. The cervical spine must be carefully immobilized without flexion or extension until extent of damage can be ascertained and proper treatment instituted.

Initially, in moving the patient from the scene of injury, the attendants can use their hands to support the head, holding it in straight line of body, or, if it is held firmly by the patient in some degree of rotation, then supporting it in this position. However, no flexion or extension should be permitted. On arrival at a place where therapy can be instituted, a Sayre head sling with 8 pounds of traction can be applied whereupon x-rays can be taken easily, the damage assessed, and definitive therapy started. Ingenuity and care must be shown in manipulation of x-ray tube and film about the patient, since it is important not to move the patient. No matter what degree of nerve damage exists, extensive or minor, extreme care should be taken, since further damage can occur at any moment.

Treatment of cervical spine injuries consists in immobilization of this area until sufficient healing of damaged tissue takes place to prevent instability. As stated initially, attendant's hand will immobilize the area; and then a Sayre head sling can be used. However, once definitive diagnosis has been made and long-term heavy traction therapy necessary for reduction of a dislocation has been instituted, other means must be used. The Sayre head sling presses against chin and occiput and prevents easy opening of mouth for eating. Heavy weights applied through this means cause severe pain, and prolonged use of this method results in ulceration of the skin.

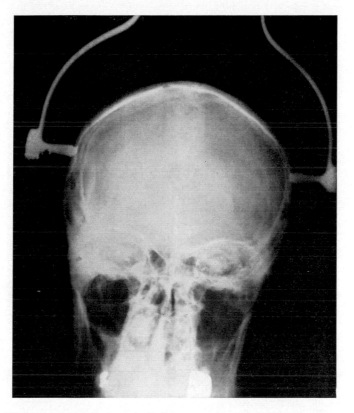

Fig. 1—Winke tongs applied to skull flange to prevent slipping evident on right.

The introduction of Crutchfield [6] tongs was a definite advance in this field. These metal tongs are inserted obliquely into the parietal region of the skull under local anesthesia. Holes are drilled through the outer table only, just in line of the cervical spine. This line can be determined by the coronal plane through the auditory meatus. Modifications of this type of skeletal traction have been suggested, each with some advantages and some disadvantages. Winke tongs, used in this institution, (fig. 1), are applied in similar fashion, but on the temporal region. These offer greater security in fixation than do the Crutchfield tongs but have many more parts and are more complicated to apply. Barton [2] has devised tongs which allegedly combine the simplicity of the Crutchfield type with the advantages of the Winke type. Dr. T. Hoen [10] devised a method utilizing two burr holes in each parietal area, one 2 or 3 cm. anterior to the other. Wire is inserted from one hole to the other on the same side beneath the calvarium and above the dura. This wire can then be tied to a spreader and traction applied easily. Heavy stainless steel wire must be used.

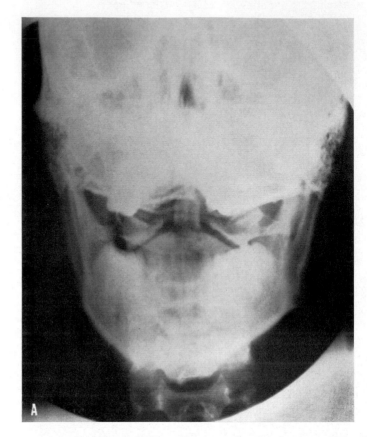

Fig. 2–B. C. July 1952. Fell off ladder. Pain in neck. Negative neurologic. Two weeks traction, then Minerva jacket. In October, persistent dislocation; therefore, fusion of 1st and 2nd cervical vertebrae. 1957 check showed broken wire and no fusion in spinous processes, but odontoid process has healed. Full activity.

Fig. 2–(A) AP through mouth, time of injury, fracture odontoid.

With any of the above procedures care should be taken and frequent observations made. Finally, traction, particularly with heavy weights, should not be continued longer than necessary to obtain the desired result. Aseptic necrosis of bone may occur after five to six weeks, and even sooner with continuous heavy traction; thus, the tongs, which must be constantly adjusted, may pull out. In an effort to keep tongs in place, pressure is applied to inner table (particularly with Crutchfield tongs) and they have been known to penetrate it and project into the brain substance. Also, infection has been known to occur in the bone at the site of the application of the apparatus. [12]

Another method has been introduced elsewhere and used occasionally in this institution – the introduction of fishhooklike apparatus through skin and muscle, attached under the zygomatic arch. This method is useful where scalp or head injuries preclude the use of traction in calvarium, but there is slight

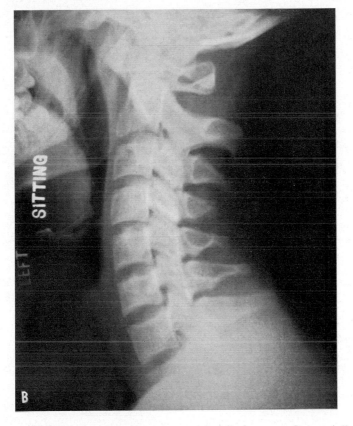

Fig. 2–(B) Lateral at time of injury, anterior displacement C–1 ond C–2.

irritation of masseter muscle and care must be taken to prevent injury to skin by pressure of the apparatus.

With skeletal traction, heavy weights can be applied. With the weight of the body in bed as countertraction, weights up to 35 pounds have been suggested by Crutchfield for reduction of dislocation with overriding articular facets. The author has seen 50 pounds applied for a short time. Once reduction has been obtained, the weight applied can be reduced to about 8 pounds, which seems sufficient to keep good, firm traction on the cervical spine and to maintain reduction.

The cervical spine is very well immobilized by a Minerva plaster jacket. This cast rests on the pelvic crest; thus, the weight is carried by the lower extremities rather than hanging on the shoulders. The plaster jacket extends up around the occiput and chin, where it must be carefully molded and padded. Also, a strap must extend from the occipital portion above the ears around the forehead, thus gripping the head and preventing rotation.

For prolonged immobilization of the neck where it is possible occasionally to remove the apparatus, a leather collar molded to the chin, neck and occiput,

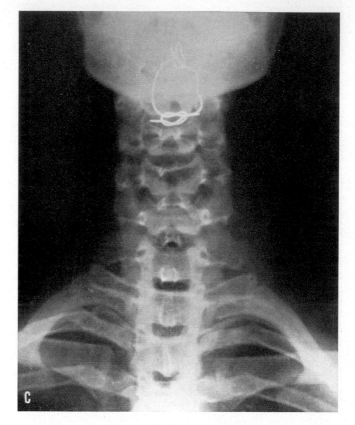

Fig. 2–(C) AP post wiring.

and braced by metal bands, offers the firmest type of fixation. This molded leather collar is somewhat unsightly and bulky.

A Thomas collar offers good but less firms support than preceding types. This collar consists of two plates, one resting on the chest and one on the back and connected by straps over the shoulder. Adjustable uprights from these plates go to a chin piece and to the occiput piece, and these are also connected by straps.

Finally, the simplest device is a Shanz collar. This consists of a heavy roll of cloth wound over a cardboard form, covered with stockinette, and wrapped around the neck between the chin, occiput and cervicothoracic junction. This offers moderate immobilization. These collars have also been made of plastic and leather.

The first thing to determine in a patient with a cervical spine injury is the extent and cause of neurologic damage. If the bony defect which injured the cord is present, this must be taken care of. Dislocation with loss of neural canal should be reduced, preferably by traction but by open surgery if neces-

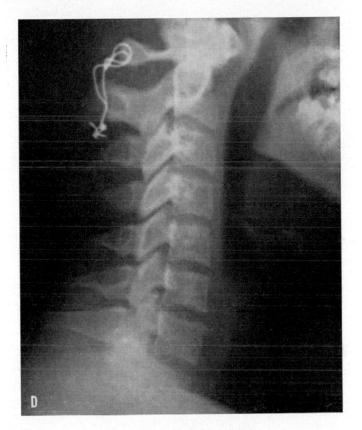

Fig. 2–(D) Lateral post fusion.

sary. If there is a crush injury and pressure on the cord by bony fragments, laminotomy and removal of this pressure must be done at once. In cases of severe damage with marked paralysis and loss of sensation, a Stryker frame, constant nursing care and tidal drainage of bladder will be necessary. In high cord lesions with quadriplegia, death, if not instantaneous, usually supervenes with hyperpyrexia and convulsions.

Cervical injuries have not been seen in sufficient numbers to allow ready classifications. [7, 14] However, we believe that when these are associated with pain with or without sign of neurologic damage, they indicate injury somewhere in the cervical spine, from C-1 to C-7. Since the absence or presence or even the amount of nerve damage does not necessarily indicate the type or

extent of bony damage and joint dislocation, we prefer to make our classification on an anatomic basis. [8]

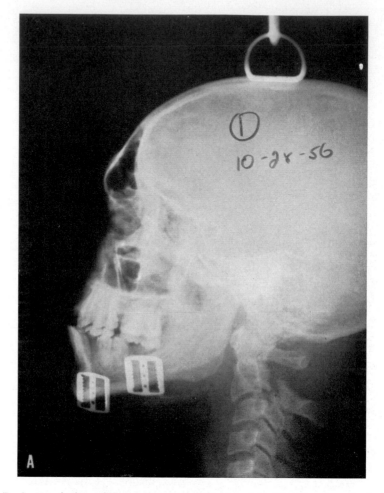

Fig. 3—E. S. Knocked to floor and kicked. Pain in neck. Negative neurologic findings.
Traction, but pulled out two times. Therefore, five months in Minerva jacket. Ambulatory.
Post-treatment comfortable. No pain.

Fig. 3—(A) X-ray at time of injury fracture through pedicle C–2.

Fracture of C-1 usually takes place through small weak portions of the
ring on either side of the articular processes. These fractures usually increase
the size of the neural canal. If the transverse ligament providing stability of
C-1 on the odontoid process of C-2 is torn or atrophied, as may occur with
pharyngeal infections in children, dislocation of occiput on C-2 can occur and
some loss of neural canal space takes place. [9] The head must be supported
until healing of injury takes place, or, if there is persistent instability, the

occiput must be fused to C-2. This type of fusion is quite disabling and is rarely necessary.

The second cervical vertebra with the odontoid process thrust up as a pivot for C-1 presents many problems not found elsewhere. This process, with weight of head transmitted through C-1, can be fractured and displaced in

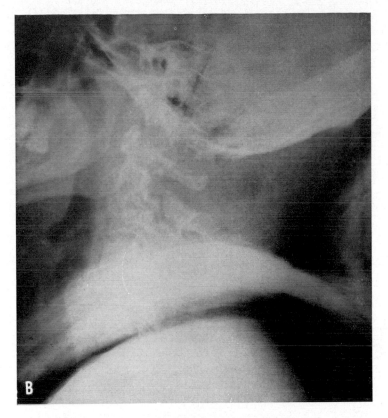

Fig. 3—(B) Treated in Minerva jacket.

any direction. A hyperextension injury where the patient falls on his face may cause this, particularly since a great deal of extension takes place at the junction of occiput and first and second cervical vertebrae. The neural canal is wide here, but any extremes of displacement will cause neurologic damage. This, however, is fortunately not the usual result. Once fracture in this area has been ascertained and this is best done by x-raying the odontoid process through the open mouth, the best treatment, we believe, is fusion of C-1 to C-2 (fig. 2). The spinous processes can be wired and bone chips laid down over laminae. This is both for the purpose of preventing odontoid displacement and also to give maximum chance for bony healing since non-union of the odontoid has been reported. However, conservative therapy of six weeks in traction and then six weeks in plaster Minerva jacket to allow firm healing has been advised by some authorities. [3]

Occasionally, fracture through pedicles of C-2 is seen (fig. 3). This fracture should permit widening of the neural canal, but if there is complete disruption,

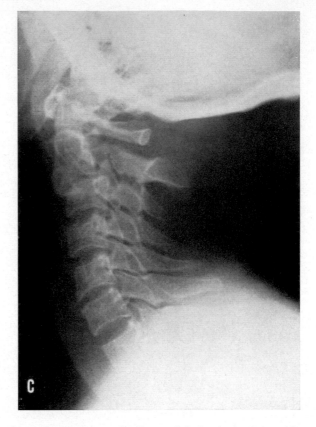

Fig. 3—(C) Last x-ray healing and fusion body C–2 to C–3.

the cord may be stretched and death ensue, as reported by Grogono. [9] This lesion with wide separation of fragments is the one desired in hangings, since it will obviously produce instantaneous death.

From C-3 to C-7, the vertebrae show similar anatomic form and we would therefore expect similar types of lesions. In cases where acute flexion occurs, we would first expect a compression of the vertebral body or a chipping off a piece of that body (fig. 4). Conceivably, severe compression might cause an intervertebral disc to be forced backward into the canal. This could cause neurologic signs, but with negative x-ray findings. Although there might not be any neurologic finding initially, eventually signs of osteoarthritis and alternately neurologic sequelae may present themselves.

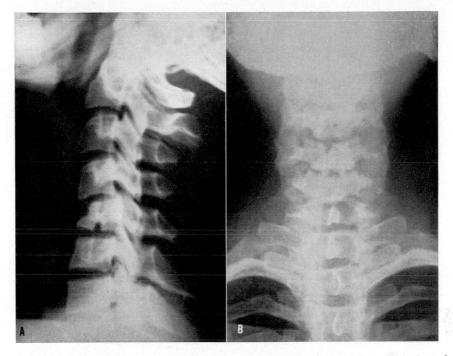

Fig. 4—W. C. June 1954. Dived into shallow pool. Struck head. Sensation of paralysis for 15 seconds. Weakness and pain in hand. Stiffness in neck. Bed rest, traction three weeks. Then Minerva jacket. No neurological sequelae found. However, subluxation evident. Fusion December 1954. One year post-op; no complaints; full activity.

Fig. 4—(A) Lateral at time of injury traction applied. (B) AP at time of injury traction applied.

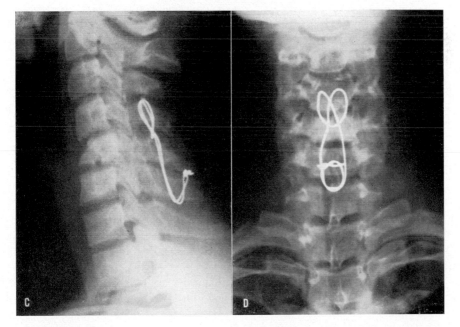

Fig. 4—(C) Lateral at time of wiring and fusion (note wire around Lamnae) (D) AP at time of wiring and fusion.

During flexion the articular facets of the cervical vertebrae from the inferior aspect of C-2 to C-7 slide forward over the facets of the lower vertebrae. Occasionally, the inferior facet of the superior vertebra dislocates forward, so that the facet from superior vertebrae catches anteriorly over the facet

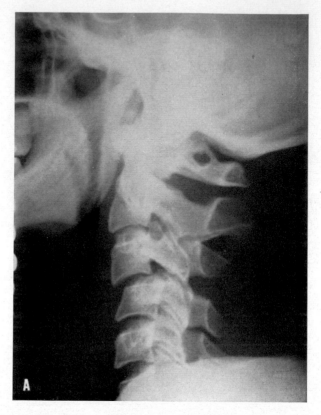

Fig. 5—J. F. Auto accident November 1951 — pain in neck. Attempted reduction of neck injury by traction, then put in Minerva jacket and transported. No neurologic symptoms. Open reduction C–3 on C–4. The left lower facet of C-3 locked anterior to left upper facet of C-4. Post-op 6 years. Moderate limitation of neck motion. Normal neurological. No pain.
Fig. 5—(A) Lateral after injury.

from inferior vertebrae. This dislocation may occur with a compression fracture of a vertebral body. In this instance, early use of strong traction up to 50 pounds is very effective. If reduction does not occur after a period of several hours with maximum weight, and particularly if compression of spinal cord is suspected, open reduction can be done, rongeuring away the superior tip of the facet or else gently levering the superior facet up and over the inferior one (fig. 5). Although manipulations have been devised, particularly in unilateral dislocation, straight, firm traction should suffice. If this proves unsuccessful, open reduction while traction is continued will be most successful, and wiring and fusion with bone chips can be done later. Severe forward dislocation, i.e., where superior vertebrae overly inferior vertebrae by more than one-half the diameter of body, will usually result in severe neurological injury, if not in transection of the cord. However, if the pedicles or laminae fracture during this process, the canal may remain widely opened and there may be less neurologic damage than one might expect with such a severe anatomical disturbance. Strong ligaments surround the vertebral bodies

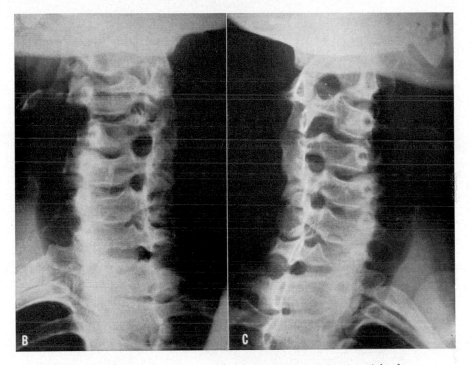

Fig. 5—(B) Oblique showing left facets. (C) Oblique showing right facets.

and also connect the spinous processes. Therefore, on marked flexion occasionally a fracture of the spinous process might occur. This fracture is, of course, not so significant except that it shows that more severe damage may have occurred.

Hyperextension injuries do occur. However, these cause marked anatomic disruption which may not be apparent. First of all, many hyperextension injuries would cause injury in the first or second vertebrae, since most motion of this sort takes place at this area. However, we must consider injuries which may occur in the cervical spine from C-3 to C-7. With hyperextension, the ligamentum flavus is compressed and extends forward, decreasing the size of the neural canal. The cord is angulated sharply against this area and can be damaged.[13] In severe hyperextension injuries, the anterior ligaments can be ruptured and the spine opened up with stretching of the cord and injuries to the neural arch or ligaments of the spine. This injury is quite extensive and would involve a very strong force in severe hyperextension.[4] Barnes[1] feels that hyperextension injuries are more likely to occur in the older patient with an arthritic involvement which has caused loss of mobility of the spine. Under these circumstances, with no gradual stretching permitted, the force is applied until one area gives way.

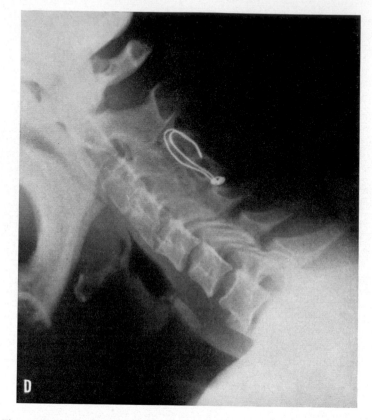

Fig. 5—(D) Lateral 6 years follow-up fusion extends beyond operative site.

The cervical spine can be fused by exposure of the spinous processes posteriorly while the head remains in traction. This can be done easily under local anesthesia. The area is exposed subperiosteally. Bone chips are turned down on spinous process and laminae; then grafts, autogenous or homogenous (from bank), are inserted. In addition to this, it is felt in this institution that wiring the spinous processes is usually worthwhile. Rodgers[11] advocates drilling holes through the base of the spinous process. However, the senior author states that these pull out readily. He advises looping wire through the neural arch, then catching the loop over spinous process, and finally tying the free ends down around a lower spinous process. This gives a force in both dorsal and ventral direction rather than just a posterior compressive effect (fig. 6).

After a reduction or replacement of cervical injury, there may be a recurrence of deformity, particularly in external fixation. This is one more good reason why internal fixation should be done. [5, 11]

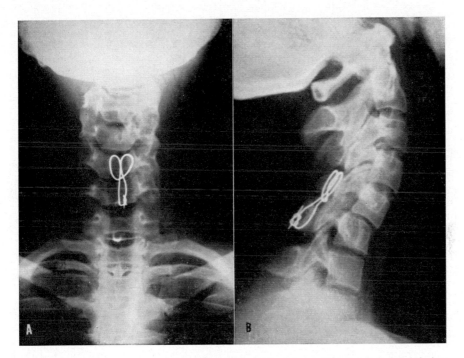

Fig. 6— A. B. Auto accident December 1951. Neck injury. Traction by head halter — 3 weeks; then neck brace. Slight weakness, left triceps muscle. December 1952, fusion done. Fishhook traction beneath zygomatic process; subsequent good recovery.

Fig. 6–(A) AP after wiring and fusion. (B) Lateral after wiring and fusion note persistent dislocation.

Cervical spine fractures are all potentially dangerous. Rodgers' [11] three cardinal points sumarize well the treatment of this problem:

1. The cord must be protected at all times.
2. Reduction must be complete or pain and recurrence may ensue.
3. Fixation must be adequate or recurrence will follow.

References

[1] BARNES: Paraplegia in cervical spine injuries. J. Bone & Joint Surg. *30 B*: 235—244, 1948.

[2] BARTON, L. G.: Reduction of fracture dislocation of cervical vertebrae by skeletal traction, Surg. Gynec. & Obst. *67*: 94, 1938.

[3] BLOCKEY and PURSER: Fractures of the odontoid process of the axis. J. Bone & Joint Surg. *38 B*: 794, 1956.

[4] BÖHLER: Treatment of Fractures. Translated by Hans Tretter et al. New York, Grune & Stratton, 1956, vol. 1, pp. 423—449.

⁵ CONE and TURNER: Treatment of fracture dislocation of cervical vertebrae by skeletal traction and fusion. J. Bone & Joint Surg. *19*: 584, 1937.

⁶ CRUTCHFIELD: Treatment of injuries of cervical spine. J. Bone & Joint Surg. *20*: 696, 1938.

⁷ DAVIS, A. G.: Injuries of the spinal column. From BLOUNT, W. P., Ed.: American Academy of Orthopedic Surgeons. Instructional course lecture, Ann. Arbor, Mich., J. W. Edwards Co., 1946, vol. VI, pp. 73—94.

⁸ DURBIN: Fracture dislocation of cervical spine. J. Bone & Joint Surg. *38 B*: 734, 1956.

⁹ GROGONO: Injuries of atlas and axis. J. Bone & Joint Surg. *36 B*: 397—410, 1954.

¹⁰ HOEN, T. I.: A method of skeletal traction for treatment of fracture dislocation of cervical vertebrae. Arch. Neurol. & Psychiat. *36*: 158, 1936.

¹¹ RODGERS, W. A.: Treatment of fracture dislocation of cervical spine. J. Bone & Joint Surg. *24*: 245, 1942.

¹² SCHNEIDER: Cervical traction. Internat. Abstr. Surg. 1957. *104*, 521—529 (June) 1951.

¹³ TAYLOR, A. R.: Mechanism of Injury to the spinal cord in the neck without damage to the vertebral column. J. Bone & Joint. Surg. *33 B:* (Nov.) 1951.

¹³a — and BLACKWOOD: Paraplegia in hyperextension cervical injuries with normal radiographic appearance. J. Bone & Joint Surg. *30 B*: 245—248, 1948.

¹⁴ WATSON-JONES, R. I.: Fractures and Joint Injuries. Fourth edition 1955. Fractures and dislocation of the spine, 946—985.

CHAPTER 24

FRACTURES OF THE DORSAL AND LUMBAR SPINE

H. Balensweig, M.D.

Man was designed to walk on hands and knees. This is particularly evident in the dorsal and lumbar spine. The spine consists of a series of oval building blocks with thin lateral and posterior struts connected by a series of inter-vertebral fibrocartilages. The thin struts consisting of transverse processes, ribs and posterior elements are strung together by ligaments and short muscles. There is a second type of supporting mechanism consisting of the long trunk muscles.

It has been estimated that in forward flexion as high as 2000 pounds per square inch pressure may be built up, applied over a small area of a lumbar vertebra, which approaches the physiologic limit of endurance of the vertebral body. This is caused by the upright posture with the added weight of the trunk, head and upper extremities above the apex of the fulcrum in flexion. Simple forward flexion in patients with osteoporosis may be sufficient to cause a compression fracture of a vertebra.

The common denominator in most traumatic vertebral body injuries is forward flexion either resulting from a fall with the patient landing on feet or buttocks, or with a force applied to the upper portion of the trunk with the body in a flexed position (figs. 1 and 2). Even a weight landing on the head of an erect person will result in an angular compression vector. The spine is poised to flex, and motion occurs anterior to the stable fixative apparatus of the spine such as the muscles and ligaments connecting the posterior and lateral elements.

E. A. Nicoll [1] has tabulated the relative frequency of fractures in a group of miners in England. In a series of 166 fractures of the spine excluding the cervical spine and sacrum, the following distribution was observed:

Dorsal 10 and above	7		Lumbar 1	49
Dorsal 11	12		Lumbar 2	27
Dorsal 12	34		Lumbar 3	17
			Lumbar 4	12
			Lumbar 5	8

He then called attention to the observation that 66 per cent occurred between D-12 and L-2. Most of these fractures were the result of a rock-fall from the roof of a coal seam possibly 2 feet or less in height, with the patient crouched in the tunnel. This mechanism produces sudden hyperflexion of the spine. The predilection for the dorsolumbar junction can easily be explained. The rib cage attached to the dorsal vertebrae acts as a firm supporting mechanism for the dorsal spine and allows the dorsal spine with the rib cage

321

as a unit to flex on the lumbar spine, transmitting the force as an angular force to the dorsolumbar junction. Falls from a height are the most frequent cause of fractured spines. According to various series, anywhere from 3 to

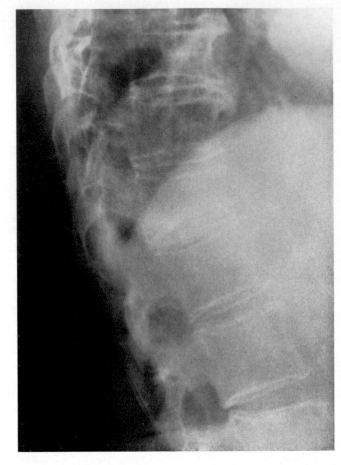

Fig. 1—Patient—I.G. Age 60. Somewhat overweight female who slipped on rug and landed on buttocks. She was seen the following day with some backache in dorso-lumbar region and mild abdominal distension. She was hospitalized 3 days later with 2 weeks of bed rest primarily for paralytic ileus. Ambulated with her usual corset and returned to work 3 weeks post injury.

12 per cent of patients with a fracture of the os calcis, have in addition a fracture of the spine.

Direct injuries to the spine, if relatively mild, may be transmitted into angular forces and again produce the same type of fracture as that from a fall. More severe forces applied to the fixed body produce fractures of the posterior elements if mild, or produce shearing fractures of the spine with disruption of the articular facet region and translocation of the upper segment on the lower, often resulting in paraplegia, if severe.

There is an intrinsic force which may produce fractures of the spinal column. Muscular contraction can produce fractures of the vertebrae or of the transverse or spinous processes. Fractures of the spinous processes are

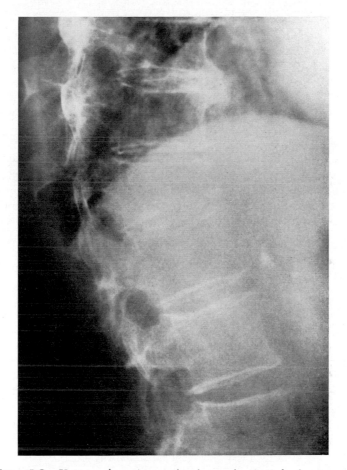

Fig. 2 Patient—I.G. X-ray taken 2 months later showing further compression of D-12 with patient asymptomatic except for some backache on arising in the morning. She was able to touch her toes and do housework as a housekeeper. It is interesting to note that the compression injury of D-12 occurred from below up. This is most often seen in pathological fractures but in this instance represented a usual compression injury in a slightly osteoporotic patient with a rigid dorsal spine secondary to arthritic changes.

most often noted at C-7 or D-1. These are called the clay shoveler's fracture because they are the result of sudden resistance to the powerful contraction of the trapezius muscles in the shoveling process. Such fracture can also occur from a glancing blow. An isolated fracture of the spinous process is extremely uncommon below the level of D-1 or D-2.

Fractures of transverse processes can occur from a direct blow in the lumbar area, but most commonly are the result of violent muscular contraction occurring while lifting or occurring in a fall in which the patient violently contracts his muscles as a form of involuntary protection. The transverse processes are pulled off by the quadratus lumborum and psoas muscles.

Another form of violent muscular contraction occurs in shock therapy and in epileptics. J. P. Kelly[2] reviewed the results of 37,000 electric shock treatments in 2,200 patients and identified 53 fractures with 21 occurring in the spine. D-4 and 5, 6 and 7 were most frequently fractured with a lesser number in D-8, 9 and 10. There were no fractures below D-10 except for 1 in L-2 and 1 in L-4. This, interestingly enough, is the direct opposite frequency from fractures occurring subsequent to a fall. It illustrates the results of a vertical compression force instead of an angular compression force.

Fractures of the spine are relatively frequent in the older age group and may even go unrecognized. These should be classified as pathologic fractures, based on softening of the bone. Trauma may be the precipitating cause, but osteoporosis is the underlying cause. In this type of fracture it is not uncommon to see multiple vertebrae involved, while in compression injuries subsequent to trauma in the younger age group, it is much more common to see single bodies involved. In addition, in the older age group, the type of fracture often differs, in that one will see a large impression caused by an expanding intervertebral disc breaking through the vertebral end plate (figs. 3 and 4). We then, of course, have the true pathologic fracture subsequent to a localized disease process in a vertebra or many vertebrae.

Diagnosis

Following an injury which may have involved the spine, the patient should be transported on a rigid support with a minimum of movement, leaving the patient in the position in which he has fallen if he is already prone or supine. If it is necessary to turn the patient, he should neither be flexed nor extended, but rolled as one piece. Transection of the cord has occurred on ill-advised attempts to move the patient. Following arrival in an emergency room, after attention to airway and shock, an evaluation of the patient as a whole is made without moving him. If there are any signs of partial paraplegia, a scout x-ray should be taken with the patient on the board or stretcher to evaluate whether or not the patient can be turned sufficiently to take adequate x-rays. Many new hospitals are now equipping themselves with radiolucent padded stretchers through which x-rays can be taken. In fact, these stretchers have detachable tops so that the patient can be moved on support to bed, operating room or x-ray room without physically shifting his position. Proper planning of an x-ray room requires a space at the bottom of the x-ray table large enough to introduce a stretcher with an overhead tube which can be moved over the stretcher to take diagnostic x-rays. Ingenious methods have been devised so that stretchers have legs without bars between them to allow the top of the stretcher to be placed directly on the x-ray table to utilize the bucky.

X-rays should be taken of the entire spine in anteroposterior and lateral views with particular attention to the dorsolumbar area, since this is the most

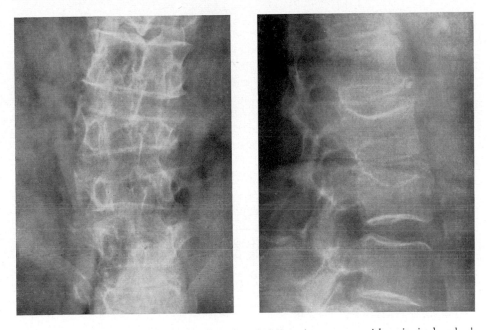

Figs. 3 and 4—Mrs. I. N. Age 74. Slipped and fell and was seen with pain in her back radiating down the right leg with inability to bend back. X-rays show compression of L-2 and 3 with marked expansion of intervertebral discs, and also reveals diffuse osteoporosis. One month after injury the patient had no complaint except difficulty getting out of bed. Over the next year and a half she had no back complaints except for 2 mild attacks of sciatica without back pain. X-rays typical of osteoporosis with compression and marked changes by x-ray without symptoms.

frequently involved. The x-rays must be of adequate detail to show the posterior elements and to allow a diagnosis of whether the fracture is stable or unstable. This is the prime consideration in deciding on future therapy.

Pitfalls in diagnosis do exist. Scheuermann's disease can imitate a fracture but usually can be differentiated by the ragged outline of the superior and inferior tables of the vertebrae and also since it usually involves more than one vertebra, usually in the mid-dorsal area. Occasionally, there can occur epiphysitis of the lumbar vertebra simulating a chip fracture. If films are of adequate detail, this so-called chip fracture will have smooth rounded edges.

Many people in the middle age, heavy laborer group with short trunks and prominent abdomen will have a wedging of D-11 or 12. Occasionally, this cannot be differentiated from a fresh fracture except by subsequent x-rays. Reparative process should be visualized within six to eight weeks if this is a fresh fracture.

Old fractures can be separated from new fractures by trying to account for the bone which has been compressed. If a simple wedging is found with an even texture to the entire body in detailed x-rays, the fracture is probably old. In fresh fractures of the impacted type, one will see an increase of density where the cancellous bone has been crushed into itself. In addition there will usually be a sharp step on the anterior margin. Another aid is that quite frequently old fractures show a tendency to bridging from the fractured vertebra to the one above. The disk space is often narrowed at this level.

A stable fracture is one in which the posterior elements are intact. The posterior longitudinal ligaments, the interspinous ligament, the ligamentum flavum and the posterior neural arch are intact. In this type of injury, motion will not cause further displacement of the fracture. These types are the chip type; the hyperextension chip type which is quite rare, the anterior wedging type and the lateral wedging type.

In an unstable fracture the posterior supports have been lost. They can at times simulate the stable wedging type on casual inspection of the x-ray, but on closer inspection one will find a horizontal fracture of a spinous process or a widening between spinous processes or a fracture of the neural arch. If one is in doubt, it is better to take flexion and extension x-rays, allowing the patient to flex and extend as much as he can tolerate. On moving himself a patient will not do further harm, but manipulation by an x-ray technician may.

Treatment

It is now generally accepted that fractures of the dorsal spine which are stable do not need reduction or immobilization. It has been shown by past experience that most fractures of the dorsal spine cannot be reduced by hyper-extension and if reduced are usually not maintained in the reduced position. If maintained for even as long as five or six months in the reduced position, follow-up x-rays over the next year will show gradual collapse to the original position. The difficulty of maintaining reduction is that one must include the neck and shoulders. Difficulty in reduction comes from the tendency for the rib cage to prevent reduction. The prime indication for not attempting reduction or immobilization is the far better results to be obtained from mobilization of the spine after a period of three to four weeks of bed rest. There is still a large field of debate in the severe compression injuries of D-12. A certain percentage of these can be successfully reduced and maintained. One group feels that anatomic reduction will prevent subsequent backache while the other group feels that the benefits to be obtained from anatomic reduction are outweighed by the benefit of early mobilization.

Watson-Jones, who formerly was a strong proponent of reduction and immobilization of fractures of the spine, in his fourth edition of *Fractures and Joint Injuries* [3] now believes that simple wedged compression fractures of a vertebral body which are stable are best treated by a short period of rest with exercises, followed by increasing periods of exercise therapy and ambulation in fractures occurring in the elderly people and in most simple compression fractures of the dorsal spine at all ages. He still feels that fractures in the dorsolumbar area in young people are best treated by reduction and immobilization in plaster (figs. 5—7).

E. A. Nicoll[1] on the other hand, feels that all stable fractures should be treated by so-called functional treatment. In his review of fractures of the dorsolumbar spine in a large series of miners with a two to five year follow-up, he came to certain conclusions: No patient with surgical fusion of the

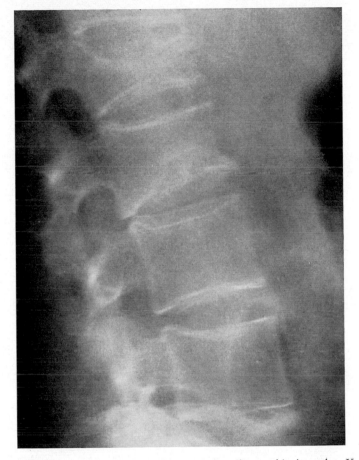

Fig. 5—Mr. L. K. 54 year old salesman landed heavily on his buttocks. X-rays show 50 per cent compression of L-1 and 20 per cent compression of L-2 with severe pain.

spine returned to the coal face; 55 per cent of patients treated by functional methods returned to heavy work, while 27 per cent returned to work if treated by the plaster technique.

He also attempted to evaluate the relationship of back deformity to work capacity. Of patients with an anterior wedge injury who recovered without deformity, 37 per cent returned to heavy work. Of those with residual deformity, 38 per cent returned to heavy work.

E. A. Nicoll also described a type of fracture which he calls the lateral wedge fracture, not well described in the literature but not extremely uncommon. This consists of an injury sustained with both flexion and side bending, resulting in a wedging deformity seen best in the anterior posterior view. Among his series there was an anterior wedge in 58 per cent, a lateral wedge in 14 per cent, a fracture-dislocation in 19 per cent and fracture of the neural arch in 9 per cent.

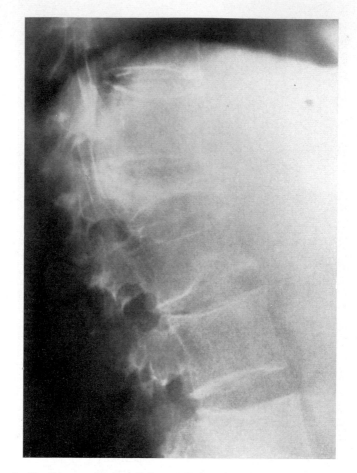

Fig. 6—Mr. L. K. $1^{1}/_{2}$ months post injury. Further compression of L-1 almost complete with gibbus and severe pain.

The prognosis in patients with a lateral wedge fracture was poorer than in those with an anterior wedge fracture. Of those with anterior compression 40 per cent achieved complete function, while only 21 per cent with a lateral wedge achieved complete function. Two patients with a lateral wedge fracture, otherwise stable, developed paraplegia. Local pain was a fairly common finding, occurring in 93 per cent of patients with a lateral wedge fracture.

His routine was three to four weeks of bedrest with extension exercises for

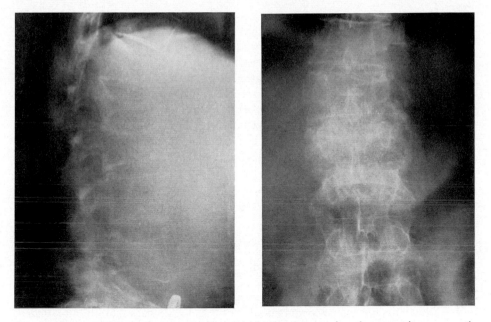

Fig. 7–Mr. L. K. 3 months post injury with further progressive change and osteoporosis in lumbar spine. Also spontaneous early compression of L-4. Subsequent films showed compression also of L-5. Patient had severe traumatic compression of L-1 and 2 following relatively minor injury and subsequently spontaneous compressions of 2 further lumbar vertebrae. The only abnormality found is polycythemia. Malignancy was ruled out.

the trunk and legs. Following this, during the fourth to eighth week, there were group exercises, gradually increasing in severity, followed by hardening for work between the eighth and twelfth week with the patient actually going into a practice coal mine.

Reduction of a stable fracture of the wedge variety depends on an intact anterior longitudinal ligament. Reduction is a desirable treatment in selected fractures in young adults. The technic outlined by Watson-Jones [3] uses 2 tables, one higher than the other, and separated by the space between the shoulders and knees of the patient, with the patient lying face down resting the knees on the lower table and the arms on the upper table. In this position with the patient awake, gravity will reduce the fracture, assuming that the anterior longitudinal ligament is intact. This technic is the safest and simplest. In addition it keeps the entire trunk free of any apparatus so that plaster can easily be applied in the corrected position. The plaster should extend from the symphysis pubis to the clavicle and should be well moulded. After the plaster is hard, the patient is started on extension exercises for the trunk. An aid to performing this with the patient comfortable is to inject a small amount of Novocain about the spinous process of the involved vertebra. There almost always is some stretching and tearing of the interspinous ligaments, and Novocain in this area will relieve most of the pain which occurs during reduction of this fracture.

If there is only mild wedging or if the patient is physiologically in the middle to old age group, the functional treatment is the treatment of choice. A loosely fitted plaster or a brace does not treat the fracture but simply immobilizes the patient's trunk and prolongs the time necessary for recovery of the musculature. In the older age group with weak abdominal muscles and generalized muscle weaknesses, some form of flexible external support may be of benefit primarily to support the abdominal muscles. The aim in this older age group is not to obtain a very flexible trunk but to obtain relief of pain with moderate mobility of the trunk. A simple, wide elastic abdominal support is more comfortable and serves the same function as a formal back brace in the older age group. In females with osteoporosis and compression injuries, a firm corset is usually of benefit but exercises should be stressed. One must be a realist and accept the weak abdominal musculature in the older age group.

Unstable Fractures

It is in the unstable or potentially unstable fracture that serious problems occur.

On admission to the hospital patients with paraplegia have two main medical problems. One is the problem of nursing, since they should be turned about every 2 hours to avoid pressure sores and kidney stones. The other problem is whether or not exploration is indicated. One school of thought feels that exploration is not indicated because of the infrequency with which decompression does any material good. The other school of thought is that even if one out of one hundred is relieved of cord or nerve root pressure by decompression, it is a significant gain. In either case the decision of whether or not to explore should be made within a few hours after admission since nerve root and cord compression of over 6 to 12 hours may cause irreversible damage.

The other problem is that of being able to nurse the patient. If the fracture is grossly unstable and the trunk shifts through the site of fracture on turning the patient, open reduction and fixation by two plates is indicated whether or not the paraplegia is complete. This fixation can greatly simplify the nursing problem and there will be spontaneous anterior fusion before the plates loosen up. Holdsworth and Hardy [4] in reviewing their experiences in 68 cases of paraplegia from fracture in the dorsolumbar area, stated that 16 cases were treated by plaster. They developed pressure sores and "our experience of external fixation by prolonged immobilization in plaster has been quite disastrous."

Some fracture-dislocations are stable in the dislocated position and can be left in this position. They will heal spontaneously to provide a firm anterior fusion. It is at times amazing how much one body can be shifted on another without producing paraplegia. Reduction if desired can sometimes be obtained by traction. Attempts at hyperextension are ill advised except with an open procedure, because potentially unstable fractures on hyperextension will have angulation occurring posteriorly with further cord and root compression.

At the operating table, it is wise to place the patient prone over a kidney rest. With the spine exposed, one can guide it back into proper position by using local traction on spinous processes and it often is of aid to flex the spine to unlock the facets. At times it is necessary to nibble away locked facets.

The late aftercare depends on the amount of damage. All paraplegics who have sustained damage in the dorsolumbar region can be taught to walk again with braces and crutches. Those with some root escape having control of hip musculature are the best candidates for ambulation. The others will be best off in a wheelchair but should be provided with braces and taught to ambulate for occasional use.

Indications for Operation

As outlined previously, an unstable displaced fracture with or without complete paraplegia often will benefit from open reduction and internal fixation with metal plates in order to facilitate nursing care.

Pathologic compression fractures with paraplegia or evidence of cord or nerve root pressure should have a decompression. The surgery permits one to do an open biopsy and at the same time relieve cord pressure. Hemangioma of a vertebral body and Paget disease are prime offenders among the benign group, causing pathologic fractures with nerve root or cord pressure. Hemangioma is more common in the young to middle age group while Paget's disease is more common in the older age group. A recently seen patient, 10 years ago at the age of 50 developed weakness of arms with staggering gait and progressive weakness of legs. He had a decompressive laminectomy in the upper dorsal area for Paget's disease and presently has no neurologic findings except for some wasting of the interosseous muscles of the hands.

Metastatic disease of the spine can cause cord compression by either direct expansion of the lesion itself or secondarily by collapse of a vertebral body. It is far better to relieve the cord pressure and have a patient who can ambulate and be comfortable for the rest of his life rather than have a hopeless paraplegic.

Decompressive surgery with x-ray radiation is indicated. The response is excellent when the pressure is secondary to collapse of a vertebral body, while it is less sure when the cord pressure is caused by infiltration of tumor. At times the tumor causes cord damage by involvement of the blood supply locally and decompression will not cause any material change.

Traumatic spondylolisthesis of L-4—L-5 or L-5—S-1, should be operatively fused. They have a tendency for late slipping even though maintained in plaster for a prolonged time.

Potentially unstable fractures with x-ray evidence of widening between the spinous processes indicating tearing of the posterior soft tissues probably will be maintained by local spine fusion limited to the involved body and the one above. They may also recover with plaster therapy but are more prone to have prolonged backache. Fusion will at times shorten the period of disability.

Comminuted fractures, particularly in the midlumbar area and lowlumbar area, are often associated with ripping of posterior elements. While these will solidify with time and prolonged immobilization in corrective plaster, they tend to have a very prolonged disability and spine fusion again will tend to shorten the period of disability. It also will actually shorten the period of plaster immobilization. Spine fusion should be limited to the affected body and the one above with occasionally the inclusion of the one below if there is evidence of intervertebral disc damage at this level also.

We have reported only one case of proven intervertebral disc herniation in the lumbar region associated with a fracture of the spine. This would suggest that an intact intervertebral disc is stronger than the adjacent bone.

In conclusion we recommend the functional or exercise treatments for fractures of the spine as advocated by G. Perkins[5] unless there are specific reasons why another method should be pursued. Loosely fitting plasters which do not reduce a compression injury and braces which almost never reduce a compression injury serve no purpose other than to remind the patient that he is sick and has a broken spine. When the external support is removed, the patient continues to walk around as if in a firm cage. He is now well muscle-bound. When reduction and immobilization are indicated, exercise is still an essential part of treatment. It would be a shame to forget the excellent results obtained during the last World War in rehabilitation centers where the efficacy of group exercises and intensive active physiotherapy was proven.

References

[1] NICOLL, E. A.: Fractures of the dorso-lumbar spine. J. Bone & Joint Surg. *31 B:* 376—394, (Aug. 3) 1949.

[2] KELLY, J. P.: Fractures complicating electro convulsive therapy and chronic epilepsy. J. Bone & Joint Surg. *36 B:* 70—79, (Feb.) 1954.

[3] WATSON-JONES, R.: Fractures and Joint Injuries, ed. 4. Baltimore, Williams and Wilkins Co., 1955.

[4] HOLDSWORTH, F. W. and HARDY, A.: Early treatment of paraplegia from fractures of the thoraco-lumbar spine. J. Bone & Joint Surg. *35 B:* 540—550, (Nov.) 1953.

[5] PERKINS, G.: Rest and movement. J. Bone & Joint Surg. *35 B:* 521—539, (Nov.) 1953.

CHAPTER 25

INJURIES TO THE SPINAL CORD

Herbert Parsons, M.D.

Injuries to the spinal cord are among the most tragic seen. In an instant, a vigorous, healthy individual may be rendered suddenly paraplegic or, still worse, if the injury is in the cervical region, tetraplegic. High cervical cord injuries of any magnitude result in sudden death due to respiratory paralysis.

Etiology

In time of war injuries to the spinal cord are frequent, resulting most commonly from high velocity missiles, gunshot wounds, or shell, bomb or mine fragments. Fortunately, similar injuries occur only rarely in peace time.

By far the greatest number of civilian patients with cord injuries have been involved in automobile accidents. Some have been hit directly, such as pedestrians. Others have been riding in, or driving, a car which has been in a collision. There may be a resultant whiplash type of cervical injury with a fracture dislocation of the cervical spine, or there may be direct compression and fracture of the spinous process and laminae of a vertebra with secondary cord compression.

Industrial accidents account for a number of such injuries, with heavy objects striking the back directly or sometimes falling on the shoulders, resulting in a compression or jackknifing of the spine with compressed portions of the vertebral bodies projecting posteriorly into the spinal canal, impinging on, or transiently squashing, the cord.

Some accidents have occurred as the result of falls, such as down stairs, down elevator shafts or out of windows.

All too frequently people dive without looking, either into an empty swimming pool or into shallow water, with the disastrous result of injuring the cervical spine and cord.

It is surprising how, on occasion, the blade of a knife or dagger can be so forcibly driven through the heavy coverings of bone, muscle and ligaments of the back as to reach the spinal cord.

Pathology

In most instances of severe injury the spinal cord damage results from sudden changes in the bony confines of the spinal canal, but in a few the damage is due to herniation of the intervertebral disk, particularly in the cervical or lumbar region.

The actual damage to the cord itself may vary anywhere from a brief concussion of the cord to contusion with edema and hemorrhage, to hematomyelia, to compression by bone, disk or hemorrhage, and infrequently from laceration or severance of a segment of the cord.

Anatomic Factors

The spinal canal varies considerably in its diameter. It is narrowest in the thoracic region, and relatively wider in the cervical and lumbar portions. The cord itself is larger in the cervical and thoracolumbar segments. It then splays out into the cauda equina at the conus, situated at the level of the first and second lumbar vertebrae. The lower spinal canal in the lumbar region contains no cord substance but only the nerve roots making up the cauda equina. There is, therefore, a relatively larger space occupied by spinal fluid in the lumbar region and a relatively smaller space occupied by nerve tissue in this region. The same is true, to a lesser degree, in the cervical portion of the canal. This anatomic variation has definite practical implications and accounts for the fact that there can be considerably more bone displacement in the lumbar and upper cervical regions without associated neural damage than is possible in the narrower confines of the thoracic area.

In certain abnormal conditions, such as in achondroplastic dwarfs, the spinal canal is flatter and smaller in diameter owing to the fact that the pedicles making up the arch of the spinal canal are shorter than normal. Injuries to the bony or disk portions of the spine are much more apt to result in cord or nerve damage in such individuals. There are similar, but less marked, variations in normal persons. Other congenital defects of the bony spine may also increase the susceptibility of the spinal cord to injury. Diseases of the spine, such as extensive demineralization of vertebrae, Paget's Disease, and the presence of tumors — metastatic or primary — may be pre-existing factors which can result in cord damage from relatively mild injuries. A spine made rigid by arthritis is apt to fracture when sudden force is applied to it.

Symptoms and Signs

Patients sustaining injuries to the spinal cord, unless there is an associated head injury or unless intoxicated, are usually immediately aware of sudden paralysis and loss of sensation of the involved extremities and trunk. They may actually collapse or fall if in the standing position when the injury occurs. They can often describe the mechanism of the injury and whether there has been acute flexion or acute extension of the spine at the time, or whether there has been a direct blow to the back or neck.

Pain at the site of injury or cord compression may be of varying degrees, at times mild and at times severe. Pain may be particularly severe in injuries involving the cauda equina. Patients with injuries involving the atlas or axis usually will not be able to turn the head voluntarily from side to side. If the injury involves the low cervical spine, there will be pain on attempted flexion of the neck, or the head and neck will be tilted or held in flexion. There may be acute tenderness over the site of injury and a kyphotic swelling or ecchymosis visible at this level of the spine. Missile wounds of entrance are frequently found a considerable distance from the spine itself. Stab wounds are usually situated to one side of the spine. The spinous processes often prevent stabs directly over the midline from reaching the cord. Partial cord lesions are more common as a result of stabbings than complete transections.

Complete cord injuries in the lower cervical and upper thoracic region result in diaphragmatic or paradoxic respirations caused by paralysis of the intercostal and accessory muscles of respiration. Such patients soon fill up with pulmonary secretions because they are unable to cough them up. If breathing is entirely diaphragmatic, respirations may become exhausted in the course of a few days' time. Patients with complete cervical cord lesions, who survive, may run a high fever because of loss of control of the sympathetic sweating mechanism over much of the body and extremities. Other signs of sympathetic nerve involvement may be evident, such as a Horner's syndrome. The arms may be completely or only partially paralyzed, depending on the level of the lesion in the cervical spine. If the traumatic myelitis is at the C-6 level, there may be weak voluntary flexion of the elbows but no voluntary extension, and the biceps reflex will be absent. When the lesion in the cervical cord is a segment lower, the paralysis will involve chiefly finger movements and the biceps reflex will be preserved, though the triceps reflex will be absent. At the eighth cervical and first thoracic level, sensation is lost along the ulnar aspect of the fingers, hands and forearms. Lesions involving the thoracic cord are best localized by the segment level of sensory loss.

Immediately following a complete injury to the cord, there is not only a flaccid paralysis and sensory loss below the level of the lesion but there is complete absence of all reflex activity, both deep and superficial, below the level of the lesion, with the exception that there may be a slow vermicular flexion response to plantar stimulation.

Urinary retention occurs no matter what the level of injury, but may frequently be overlooked, particularly if there happens to be some overflow incontinence. It is common even with partial cord lesions. In spite of anal sphincter relaxation and fecal incontinence, considerable abdominal distention is commonly present with injuries of the spine, cord and cauda equina.

When the period of spinal shock, or flaccidity and areflexia, is past, an interval varying from days to weeks to months, spontaneous contractions of the lower extremities begin to appear and may be precipitated by almost any stimulus on the feet and legs. A mass reflex consisting of dorsiflexion of the toes and feet, and flexion of the knees and hips appears. Spasticity, strongly active deep reflexes and clonus become apparent. Flaccidity persists indefinitely with lesions of the cauda equina unless normal function is regained.

A unilateral partial cord lesion produces the familiar Brown-Sequard syndrome, or variations of it. In this there are motor paralysis and pyramidal tract signs on the side of the lesion, sometimes with posterior column signs such as position or vibratory sensory loss, but impaired or absent sensation for pain and temperature on the side opposite the lesion. Hematomyelia should be suspected when there is a dissociation between the area of loss of sensation to pain and the area of loss of touch.

Certain spine injuries, notably laterally situated disk herniations, produce primarily root signs. As these occur most commonly in the lower lumbar and low cervical regions, there is either pain radiating down the legs in a sciatic nerve root distribution to the ankle or foot, with associated paresthesiae in the toes, or there is pain radiating into the shoulder and down the arm, with associated paresthesiae in the fingers.

Lesions of the sixth cervical nerve root, between the fifth and sixth cervical vertebrae, usually produce paresthesiae in the radial fingers, including the thumb. The biceps reflex is often diminished in such cases and there may be weakness of flexion of the elbow. Lesions of the seventh cervical nerve root, between the sixth and seventh cervical vertebrae, usually produce paresthesiae, predominantly in the index and middle fingers, but not including the thumb. With such lesions the triceps reflex will usually be diminished and there may be weakness of extension of the elbow. Lesions of the eighth cervical nerve root usually produce paresthesiae in the ulnar aspect of the fingers, hand and forearm.

The fifth lumbar nerve root is the one usually compressed by disk herniations at the interspace between the fourth and fifth lumbar vertebrae. The paresthesiae will most commonly involve the medial aspect of the foot and toes.

The first sacral nerve root is the one usually compressed by disk herniations at the lumbosacral interspace and the resulting paresthesiae usually involve the lateral aspect of the foot and toes.

A diminished or absent ankle jerk suggests that the nerve root compression is at the lumbosacral interspace (although it may also be at L-4-5), whereas a diminished knee jerk suggests that it is at L-4-5, or higher.

Neck movements, forward or lateral flexion, and extension, commonly aggravate the pain when a herniated disk is compressing one of the cervical nerve roots, and bending or straight leg raising almost invariably aggravates the root pain due to compression by a herniated disk in one of the lower lumbar interspaces. When the patient with lumbar root compression is standing, a list of the trunk is usually away from the side of the pain when the disk herniation is laterally situated in relation to the root, but may be toward the side of the pain when the herniation is medially situated in relation to the root.

Atrophy of lower leg muscles and weakness of dorsi or plantar flexion of the feet and toes, especially the great toe, may be found with root compression in the lower lumbar region. Weakness of plantar flexion is best tested by having the patient rise up on the foot and toes in the standing position so that he has to raise the full weight of the body.

Sensory changes on the toes, foot and lateral aspect of the lower leg may be present but are not as dependable as the reflex and motor signs. Isolated sensory loss in the saddle region indicates involvement of the sacral roots of the cauda equina and usually is accompanied by urinary retention.

X-Rays

X-rays of the spine of patients with cord damage may be helpful in evaluating the extent of the associated bony injury, or presence of foreign bodies, but should be obtained with a minimum of moving the patient. Stereoscopic views may give more information than single views. Oblique views of the spine may at times be necessary, but good anteroposterior and lateral views are usually of most value. X-rays frequently fail to reveal the full extent of the bony injury.

In patients with signs of root compression in the cervical region, x-rays will usually reveal flattening or reversal of the cervical lordosis due to associated muscle spasm, and in the lumbar region flattening of the lumbar lordosis. Narrowing of an intervertebral disk space indicates degeneration of an intervertebral disk and may be suggestive of a disk herniation at that level but is not a reliable aid in localization, particularly in the lumbar region. Multiple, narrowed intervertebral disk spaces are frequently seen in association with hypertrophic arthritic changes of the spine and merely indicate disk degeneration as part of the degenerative process without there being any protrusion or herniation of the disk into the spinal canal or intervertebral foramina.

In patients who have had several episodes of root compression, the narrowed interspace is particularly unreliable for localization as it may have resulted from one of the previous attacks and the herniated disk producing the most recent episode may be found at a different level.

Lumbar Puncture

Lumbar puncture for manometric evidence of a spinal fluid block, complete or partial, on bilateral jugular compression, or for evidence of an elevated spinal fluid protein due to block, may well help to sway ones decision for or against operation.

Myelograms

Myelograms are performed whenever it is felt that they would contribute information of value in the operative management of a case, but are not done routinely. They are most helpful in determining the exact level of an intraspinal block found on lumbar puncture, when the clinical and x-ray evidence is not conclusive. They are also helpful in demonstrating the presence, and full extent, of an intraspinal mass, particularly when there are unilateral or bilateral cord signs, or bilateral cauda equina signs. They occasionally help to establish the diagnosis of avulsion of the roots of the brachial plexus by demonstrating a leak of Pantopaque out from the spinal canal at the site of a tear in the dura.

The indiscriminate use of myelograms in every case is probably unwise. After performing a myelogram it is sometimes difficult to aspirate the Pantopaque completely and relatively large amounts may have to be left behind. In some instances there may be considerable meningeal reaction to the myelogram, though fortunately this is usually only transient. At other times the residual Pantopaque may be blamed, probably in many instances unjustly, for the persistence of back and root pains, or for headaches when droplets are seen inside the skull. Myelographic artifacts are sometimes misleading. Laterally situated disk herniations may not be visible in the myelogram.

In most cases, patients with good signs of root compression have sufficient clinical evidence of localization and sufficient indication for operative intervention to make myelography unnecessary.

Treatment

The proper management of patients with acute injuries of the spinal cord has been the subject of much discussion. The handling of these patients immediately after the injury has occurred is most important so that further damage to the already injured cord will not occur.

They should not be moved from the scene of the accident until plans are formulated to transport them to a hospital where adequate care can be given. A firm stretcher or flat surface, such as a door, should be used, and with plenty of helping hands and with the head supported by gentle traction in the case of cervical injuries, the patient can be slid or rolled onto the stretcher. Patients with injuries to the cervical spine are best transported in the supine position as this requires less turning of the head and neck, and allows for greater ease in breathing in a patient whose respiration may already be embarrassed. The head should be immobilized with laterally placed sandbags, shoes or a blanket roll.

Patients with injuries to the thoracic and lumbar spine can be transported in the prone position, particularly when it is suspected that there may be fractures of the laminae resulting from a direct blow to the back. When the injury has resulted from compression of the lumbar spine without likelihood of fracture of the spines and laminae, or when it may have resulted from hyperextension of the lumbar or thoracic spine, the supine position may be used.

When the cervical spine is injured, it is unwise to attempt reduction of a fracture dislocation at the scene of the accident any more than is accomplished by gentle, direct traction on the head.

When the patient arrives at the hospital, x-rays can be obtained while he is still on the stretcher, before being moved to a bed. Moving should be kept at a minimum. Portable x-rays can be used when necessary, although frequently they are inadequate when the thicker areas of the trunk are being examined. It is safest for a doctor to be present while the films are being obtained, to prevent undue moving of the patient by the technician.

After bringing the patient to his room, if there is a considerable area of sensory loss, he should be placed in bed on an air or foam rubber mattress, an alternating air mattress or a Stryker frame.

Any degree of urinary retention, a distended bladder, should be relieved by an indwelling Foley catheter which can be connected either to a tidal drainage apparatus or intermittent drainage. It is wise to keep the urinary tract sterile with an antibiotic, such as Gantrisin, or other antimicrobial agent, when the catheter has to remain in place for a long time.

Abdominal distention may be relieved with a rectal tube and other appropriate measures.

After due evaluation of the physical and neurologic status of the patient, and after correcting any degree of respiratory obstruction and surgical shock that may be present, attention will be directed to further surgical management of the case.

Open or compounded injuries will of necessity require operative débridement, inspection of the injury to the cord and careful primary closure of the wound in order to prevent leakage of spinal fluid. If the wound is left open and a fluid leak results, meningitis will follow.

It is generally agreed that extensive injuries to the cauda equina, which are unusually painful, (even if not open), are best treated by operation with decompression, removal of any indriven fragments of bone and, where it seems reasonably feasible, reapproximation of torn nerve roots much as one would treat peripheral nerves. It is not altogether clear why much of the pain should be relieved after simple toilet of the injured area, even when torn nerve roots cannot be reapproximated. Partial cauda equina lesions, in which pain is not severe and which are not showing evidence of progression often do well without operation.

It is agreed that any spinal cord injury in which the lesion seems to be getting worse under observation warrants exploration and decompression.

Injuries to the cervical spine and cord are usually first treated with traction. Skeletal traction with Crutchfield tongs, or with the Raney modification of Crutchfield tongs which has a flange on the tong, applied under local anesthesia with the patient in bed, is the simplest and preferred method. If tongs are not available, wires may be passed extradurally between bur holes in the skull and traction applied to the wires. Another method of merit, when the scalp is badly damaged or infected, consists of placing hooks around the zygomatic arch on each side and applying traction to the hooks. A spreader is used to keep the traction from pressing against the side of the head. At first only a 10 pound weight is tried, but if this is not adequate to reduce a fracture dislocation, greater weights up to 35 pounds can be added for short periods and the weight cut down as soon as the dislocation is reduced. The head of the bed is placed on shock blocks for counter traction. If there is no improvement after a reasonable period of observation, open reduction may be resorted to. The vigorous manipulations of cervical spine injuries formerly used may be hazardous.

Unfortunately, it is not possible to differentiate by clinical means whether a cord lesion is complete due to anatomic disruption or merely because of physiologic loss of function though anatomically intact. It is in the realm of complete cord lesions that there is the greatest divergence of opinion. Some believe that all cord injuries should be explored and decompressed, and others believe that no complete cord lesion should be operated on. Others take an intermediate point of view and operate only on those in whom there is x-ray evidence of compression of the spinal canal by bone fragments or in whom a spinal fluid block can be demonstrated by lumbar puncture.

It must be acknowledged that very few patients, probably less than 5—10 per cent, in whom evidence of a complete cord lesion is found on neurologic examination soon after injury, whether physiologic or other, will ever regain much useful motor function. An improvement in function, dropping of the level several segments, occurs commonly, both in patients who have been operated on and in those who have not. Exploration may at times be helpful in determining the prognosis when extensive damage to the cord is found, but one is frequently disappointed when, at operation, the cord appears grossly normal and yet never regains any significant motor function. Both patients and their families are rarely satisfied that everything possible has been done unless the cord has been visualized at operation.

Partial cord lesions, on the other hand, may show gradual improvement for periods as long as two years after the injury has occurred.

Although operation has rarely been felt to be indicated for partial cord lesions unless there is an associated open wound, Schneider has emphasized the value of operation in what he calls the syndrome of acute anterior spinal cord injury. In this there is impaired motor function with pyramidal tract signs and evidence of spinothalamic tract involvement (impaired or absent sensation for pain and temperature) but with sparing of the posterior columns and some preservation of position and vibratory sensation. Under such circumstances he feels that division of the attachments of the dentate ligaments, which hold the cord anteriorly in the spinal canal, is helpful in allowing greater return of cord function. Occasionally midline disk herniations have been found and removed in such cases. Certainly, whenever a herniated disk is suspected as contributing to cord compression, operative intervention is justified. Also when abundant callus formation around a fracture site seems to be either embarrassing a return of cord function or making the patient's condition worse, decompression may be worthwhile.

Any patient with a disk herniation in whom there is a serious neurologic defect, such as impending paraplegia. Brown-Sequard signs, urinary retention or foot drop, deserve prompt operative intervention.

On the other hand, many patients, in whom a laterally herniated disk has produced signs of compression of only a single root, will recover spontaneously and operation may be deferred unless pain and disability persists or becomes worse. Once the root pain has been relieved, recovery will usually follow even though atrophy and some motor weakness, corresponding to the muscles supplied by that particular root, are evident. For this reason a preliminary period of bed rest, with or without traction, is usually advisable.

Most cervical spine fracture dislocations which have been satisfactorily reduced by skeletal traction are maintained in traction for a period of about 6 weeks until sufficient healing has taken place to keep them from slipping. They are then placed in a cervical neck brace or collar. The type of open collar with pads under the chin and occiput and over the upper chest and shoulders, separated by turnbuckle bars, is much cooler than the completely padded leather variety and more easily adjusted. This is worn for a period of three to six months, at first continuously and later during waking hours only. Neurologic findings are evaluated repeatedly. The position of the vertebrae is checked with frequent x-rays and if there is a tendency for the dislocation to recur, fusion may occasionally be necessary.

Dislocations between the atlas and the axis producing cervical cord injuries are first reduced with traction and then fused. Rib grafts may be used or the type of clothespin graft suggested by Gallie. The laminae of the atlas and the axis are wired to the graft, and the laminae of the atlas are also wired to the spinous process of the axis. Heavy silk sutures may be used rather than wire.

When decompressions or exploratory laminectomies have been performed lower in the cervical spine, fusion is rarely necessary unless there is evidence of recurrent dislocation.

Compression fractures and dislocations in the lumbar region which are closed may be reduced by hyperextension in bed by placing a roll of blankets beneath the appropriate area of the mattress or by placing the patient in reverse, with the head at the foot of a hospital bed, and raising the knee lift. Another method consists of hyperextension on a strap in the prone position. After reduction has been accomplished, they may be immobilized, either with a brace or plaster. When there is considerable associated neurologic impairment, decompression and open reduction may be necessary, particularly if simple hyperextension does not result in prompt reduction. If there is a tendency for the dislocation to recur, fusion will have to be done.

Fracture dislocations in the thoracic region are usually produced by considerable force because this part of the spine is heavily buttressed. They are difficult to reduce by any method. Operative decompression is usually necessary. Because of the relatively small caliber of the spinal canal in this region, there is almost invariably marked associated cord damage in such injuries.

When patients with compression fractures or fracture dislocations of the thoracic or lumbar spine are first permitted to get up after a period of bed rest, a supporting brace or corset should be used. Plaster body casts may also be used if sensation is intact but should never be applied over an extensive area of diminished or absent pain sensation, as they will almost always produce pressure sores.

Laminectomies for exploration of cord injuries can be done either under local or general anesthesia, but in the event of cervical spine or cord injury, if an endotracheal tube is inserted it should be done without manipulation of the neck. If there are bilateral cord or cauda equina signs, a total laminectomy of the involved area should be done. If there are only unilateral cord signs or only unilateral root signs, a hemilaminectomy will usually be adequate. With spine injuries, exposure of the spines and laminae should be done under direct vision and the muscles not dissected blindly from the spines and laminae, as is done in the usual laminectomy, for fear of plunging the elevator through a fracture in the laminae and further injuring the cord.

Tales are told of the cord, in severe injuries, squeezing out like toothpaste when the dura is opened, but this is rarely the case if the dura is first opened well above and below the site of injury. A blunt, short nerve hook can then be inserted between the dura and arachnoid and the dura rapidly split longitudinally over the site of injury with a single sweep of the instrument allowing any swollen cord and overlying arachnoid to bulge out over a wide opening in the dura. The dentate ligament attachments may be cut on either side. Any indriven bone fragments or spicules should be removed and search made for a herniated disk. This can be removed either transdurally or extradurally, whichever seems most appropriate. Midline disk herniations usually have to be removed transdurally. Lateral disk herniations may be removed either transdurally or extradurally. Occasionally, when there are marked root signs in the cervical region, laterally herniated disk material may not be encountered until the intervertebral foramen is unroofed and the nerve root well exposed. If there is any considerable swelling of the cord, the dura should be left open for purposes of decompression. Otherwise it may be closed again.

The long-term care of paraplegic patients is a subject which has received much attention and shown great progress during and after World War II and the Korean conflict, and it will be touched on only briefly. It properly requires the combined efforts of a medical, neurosurgical, plastic surgical and urologic team.

Great effort should be made to prevent infection in the genitourinary tract with appropriate drainage of the bladder and the prompt treatment of urologic complications such as epididymitis, pyelonephritis, abscesses and stones, as they arise. The goal is to establish an automatic bladder which empties itself at intervals with minimal effort, whenever this can be accomplished.

The care of the skin in the area of analgesia is also most important. Much can be done in the prevention of decubiti by frequent changing of position at regular intervals, the use of air mattresses which distribute weight over much of the body rather than on bony prominences, and by keeping the bedclothes smooth and dry. The worst decubiti are prone to develop over the bony prominences of the iliac crests, greater trochanters, ischial tuberosities and sacrum, but also are frequently seen on the knees and heels. If they do develop over the iliac crests, trochanters and ischial tuberosities they should be excised, the underlying bone removed and soft tissue flaps used to cover the defects. Decubiti over the sacrum, knees and heels will usually clear up spontaneously if care is taken to keep further pressure off these points. Amputations and hip disarticulations have, at times, been resorted to but have not been very satisfactory, the patients finding it difficult to maintain balance under these circumstances.

The problem of pain and painful spasms of the extremities was formerly greater than at present and resulted in the use of chordotomies, anterior rhizotomies and intrathecal injections of alcohol or phenol to control them. With better management of urinary infections and decubiti, these pains and spasms have become less frequent and, as time goes on, regress.

Nutrition is difficult to maintain in these patients, but with the use of nourishing high vitamin and high protein diets, and getting the patients into an upright position as soon as it is safe to do so, nutrition can usually be fairly well maintained.

Bowel control can be managed first by enemas every other day and later by establishing regular daily bowel habits.

The first effort at rehabilitation is directed at strengthening the muscles of the arms or, at least, those that are left, then in training the patient to take care of his own daily needs and, when possible, to get in and out of bed to and from his wheelchair by himself.

Considerable effort was at one time expended in trying to get these patients ambulatory with the use of braces. Although this is possible in many cases, the excessive effort required in a person already finding it difficult to breathe has resulted in many returning to a wheelchair.

Probably the most important thing of all in the management of the paraplegic is to give him something to do which he is interested in, and to help him find an occupation in which he can become financially independent. Once this has been accomplished, he can be considered to be fully rehabilitated and many of his other problems become relatively insignificant.

Prognosis and Summary

The outlook for patients with injuries to the spinal cord is quite variable. In those in whom there is neurologic evidence of a complete cord lesion the chance of recovery of significant motor function is not good. The higher the lesion in the spinal cord, the worse the prognosis. The mortality for patients with complete lesions of the cervical cord is still high, no matter how they have been treated. Most patients with thoracic or lumbar injuries to the cord or cauda equina will survive unless there are other serious associated complicating injuries. Patients with partial cord injuries will often show slow but gradual improvement over long periods of time. The outlook for patients with injuries to the cauda equina is distinctly better than for those with injury to the cord itself.

Most patients with herniated intervertebral disks compressing a single nerve root, whether in the lumbar or cervical regions, will usually do well, either recovering spontaneously with rest or following removal of the herniated disk when necessary. But when there is cord compression by a midline disk herniation in the cervical region, the outlook is much less favorable and depends on the extent of damage to the cord.

Modern methods of rehabilitation have done much, not only in prolonging the lives of paraplegics but also in giving them back their independence and returning them to useful occupations in society.

References

[1] BRADFORD, F. K. and SPURLING, R. G.: The Intervertebral Disc. Springfield, Ill., Charles C Thomas, 1945.

[2] CAMPBELL, E. and MEIROWSKY, A.: Penetrating Wound of the Spinal Cord. In BOWERS, W. F.: Surgery of Trauma. Philadelphia, J. B. Lippincott Co., 1953.

[3] COMARR, A. E. and KAUFMAN, A. A.: A survey of the neurological results of 858 spinal cord injuries. J. Neurosurg. 13: 95—106, 1956.

[4] COVALT, D. A., COOPER, I. S., HOEN, T. I. and RUSK, H. A.: Early management of patients with spinal cord injuries. J. A. M. A. 151: 89—94, 1953.

[5] DAVIS, L.: The Principles of Neurological Surgery. Philadelphia, Lea & Febiger, 1953.

[6] —: Treatment of spinal cord injuries. Arch. Surg. 69: 488—495, 1954.

[7] FREEMAN, L. W.: Treatment of paraplegia resulting from trauma to the spinal cord. J. A. M. A. 140: 949—958; 1015—1022, 1949.

[8] —: Injuries of the spinal cord. Surg. Clin. N. A. 34: 1131—1146, 1954.

[9] GRINKER, R. R., BUCY, P. C., and SAHS, A. L.: Trauma to the central nervous system. In Neurology. Springfield, Ill., Charles C Thomas, 1960, chap. 15: pp. 914—986.

[10] MARTIN, J.: The treatment of injuries of the spinal cord. Collective review Internat. Abstr. Surg. 84: 403—416, 1947.

[11] MATSON, D. D.: The Treatment of Acute Compound Injuries of the Spinal Cord. Am. Lect. Series. DeBakey, M. E., Spurling, R. G. and Woodhall, B., Eds. Springfield, Ill., Charles C Thomas, 1948.

[12] MUNRO, D.: The Treatment of Injuries to the Nervous System. Philadelphia, W. B. Saunders Co., 1952.

[13] POOL, J. L.: The Neurosurgical Treatment of Traumatic Paraplegia. Am. Lect. Series. De Bakey, M. E., Spurling, R. G. and Woodhall, B., Eds. Springfield, Ill., Charles C Thomas, 1951.

[14] PRATHER, G. C. and MAYFIELD, F. H.: Injuries of the Spinal Cord. Springfield, Ill., Charles C Thomas, 1953.

[15] SCHNEIDER, R. C., CHERRY, G. and PANTEK, H.: The syndrome of acute central cervical spinal cord injury with special reference to mechanisms involved in hyperextension injuries of cervical spine. J. Neurosurg. 11: 546—577, 1954.

[16] SCHNEIDER, R. C.: The syndrome of acute anterior spinal cord injury. J. Neurosurg. 12: 95—122, 1955.

[17] SPURLING, R. G.: Lesions of the Cervical Intervertebral Disc. Am. Lect. Series. De Bakey, M. E., Spurling, R. G. and Woodhall, B., Eds. Springfield, Ill., Charles C Thomas, 1956.

[18] WANNAMAKER, G. T.: Spinal cord injuries. J. Neurosurg. 11: 517—524, 1954.

[19] WHITHE, J. C.: Injuries to the spinal Cord and cauda equina. In CARE, E. F., Ed.: Fractures and Other Injuries. Chicago, Ill., Year Book Publishers, Inc., 1958, Chap. 15, pp. 177—202.

CHAPTER 26

ACUTE BACKACHE

PETER-CYRUS RIZZO, M.D.

Discussions of back injuries must include information of the structures and tissues involved. The most common area of injury is the lower back.

The lumbar fascia is a most important structure since it surrounds the muscles of the back and acts to protect and support them. It is the first vulnerable tissue and is described as a continuation of the tendons of three muscles rather than a true fascial investment. These muscles are the latissimus dorsi, serratus posterior inferior and internal oblique. This tissue is anchored to the vertebral column in three layers: an outer or posterior, a middle and an inner layer.

The outer layer extends from the tip of the spinous processes of the lumbar and sacral vertebra. The upper attachment is to the last rib and the lower to the outer lip of the iliac crest and the iliolumbar ligament. The middle layer is from the free ends of the lateral transverse processes of the lumbar vertebrae. The inner layer arises from the bases of the same transverse processes. The outer and inner layers of this fascia extend laterally to unite at the outer edge of the erector spinae muscle. This muscle fills the interval between these layers. As this conjoined fascia extends laterally, it is joined by the inner fascial layer, and the interval between these layers is occupied by the quadratus lumborum muscle. Superiorly, these layers blend to form the lumbocostal ligament; inferiorly they form the iliolumbar ligament.

Knowledge of the anatomic arrangement of the fascia readily localizes the areas of strength and weakness of the back. The most common sites of pain are the lumbosacral area and the lumbodorsal costal junction, where the fascia is thinnest and weakest and where mobility is greatest. The transverse process attachments are so strong that injury to this region is associated with a fracture of the bony process.

The bony structure in this area comprises the five lumbar vertebrae, the sacrum and the innommate bones. Of all the joints formed by these structure, the lumbosacral joint is the most vulnerable. It is the junction of the freely mobile spine with relatively fixed spine. The torso weight is borne by the opposing surfaces of the first sacral segment and the fifth lumbar vertebra, which is separated by the intervertrebral disc and also the apophyseal joints.

Further sources of increased vulnerability may be the many congenital variations which may contribute to structural weakness. One of these variations is incomplete developmental fusions of the lamina, resulting in a spondylolysis or some degree of slipping or spondylolisthesis. Other variations which are considered factors making for weakness are asymmetry of the

345

lumbar facets, increased lumbosacral lordosis or partial sacralization of the lumbosacral joint.

Tissues that surround these bones are subject to injury with resultant derangement. These ligaments and joint components include the intervertebral fibrocartilage which contains the nucleus pulposus, the anterior longitudinal ligament, the posterior longitudinal ligament, capsule of the apophyseal joints, the ligamentum flavum, interspinus ligament, supraspinus ligament, lumbosacral and iliolumbar ligaments.

The paraspinal muscles pad these bones and joints. Transverse muscle nestles closest to the laminae and spinous processes. These are the rotators, multifidus and semispinalis. The longitudinal muscles are the sacrospinalis, erector spinalis and quadratus lumborum which are contained in the previously mentioned lumbar fascia.

The lumbar plexus of nerves passes through bony canals at the junctions of the vertebrae. The canals through which the anterior divisions of the fourth and fifth lumbar nerves emerge are long. Accompanying the nerves is a venous plexus. Engorgement or overdevelopment of this plexus, especially if associated with injury, may compress and irritate the nerve roots, thus accounting for symptoms of nerve root irritation and radiating pains.

Injury, whether traumatic or chemical, causes inflammation locally. The consequence of such inflammation is congestion and edema, caused by a slowing up of local circulation which, in turn, causes a local engorgement of the smaller vessels and slowing of circulation. To relieve this engorgement there is an osmotic interchange of fluid. The excess fluid is deposited in the interstitial tissue, resulting in edema which causes pressure on nerve ends and accounts for the pain and swelling. The degree of inflammation is proportional to the extent of the local injury. The degree and resolution of this local inflammation is also influenced by the degree of inflammatory reaction.

The repair or resolution process may be best illustrated by the burn injury. As we know, burns are classified by many as to degree, depending on penetration and tissues involved. The deeper the burn, the more severe the scars of resolution. Interpolating this scarring to trauma, we can also estimate to some degree the residual scarring, limitation of function and symptoms expected. The more severe the injury, the more extensive the residual cicatrix.

The examination includes a careful history. It should elicit the patients age and occupation, the mode and manner of onset of the trauma as well as history of previous back injuries or similar episodes. A history of bending over and inability to straighten up or the sensation of a snapping or tearing is most often due to a facet or small joint slipping and would call for treatment different from that for trauma associated with a blow or straining episode. Previous medical or surgical conditions or injuries may have some bearing on the symptoms.

An accurate description of the character of the pain — duration, localization or radiation, recurrent or constant — is important. Causes for aggravation, such as posture changes, or activity and manners of relief should be recorded.

The examination of the patient should begin with observation from the time he sits at the doctor's desk until he has disrobed. Formal examination of the patient when stripped is, in fact, an observation of conscious motions of various phases of his unconscious acts of standing, sitting, walking and attitude changes.

As the patient walks look for limp or foot drop, and if possible identify the cause of limp, whether due to pathology involving the joints of the extremity or muscular paralysis.

As he stands note the spinal posture. Are the shoulders and pelvis level? Is there a scoliosis, tilt of the trunk, increase or decrease of normal physiologic curves?

Mobility of the head, neck and upper extremities is measured, and associated or referred complaints noted. In litigation cases, inspection of the hands for callus is important. In a manual worker, callus will soften and disappear after three months of inactivity.

Motions of the spine are noted in the planes of flexion, extension, lateral bending, rotation and hyperextension. Points to recognize are whether there is reversal of the lumbar spine, muscular spasm, voluntary rigidity or deviation of the trunk from the midline with flexion. Is there rigidity of the spine as associated with arthritis? Hyperextension limitation in an otherwise flexible spine may indicate a myositis or nerve root pressure. Motions which are accomplished with jerkiness and which are not rhythmic suggest a subjective limitation.

With the patient in a sitting position, the spine is normally relaxed and legs dangle easily. Variations may indicate nerve root pressure fracture, myositis or some other underlying pathology. The ankle and knee reflexes are tested. The knees are extended. Tilting of the pelvis backward with pulling in the hamstring muscle bilaterally is associated with contracture of the hamstrings, which may indicate a possible developmental condition, but may also be a sign of sprain. Unilateral tilting and limitation of knee extension with pain radiation to the lumbar area can be a manifestation of nerve root pressure. This extension of the knee test is the equivalent of the Lasègue test in the supine position.

With the patient supine, the leg lengths are measured and the circumferences of the calves and thighs noted. Variations of leg lengths are not uncommon and may account for backache due to postural strain. The shorter leg may measure slightly more in circumference at the thigh or calf. There is often a difference in circumferential measurements in lesions due to a disc protrusion. This is also associated with some weakness of the dorsiflexors of the toes, and these muscles should be tested against resistance. Sensation to sharp and dull stimuli is tested. It is important to differentiate between a stocking type of hypoaesthesia or hyperaesthesia and one that follows a definite anatomic pattern. Although there may be some overlap of these sensory areas in a true disc lesion, it does not encompass the entire extremities.

Hip flexion is tested with the knees flexed. Restriction of motion is due to hip pathology. In the most severe backache, flexion can be accomplished to beyond 90 degrees. Straight leg raising (Lasègue) puts the hamstring muscles and sciatic nerve on tension and locks the pelvis. The range is recorded for either side and associated and referred symptoms are noted.

Limited rotation of the hip (Patrick) performed with the hips and knees flexed is due to hip pathology.

Stress on the sacroiliac joints is accomplished by placing the patient close to the table edge and hyperextending the straight leg.

With the patient in prone position, hyperextension of the hips and spine motion range are measured. The tone of the glutei and paraspinal muscles is palpated. Ranges of motion are diminished in osteoarthritis and with discogenic disease. In this position the spine is systematically tested for local tenderness.

Costovertebral angle tenderness is associated with sprains of the quadratus lumborum and erector spinae attachment. The lumbar fascia attachment is a vulnerable area and accounts for symptoms in the upper lumbar spine. Fortunately, acute symptoms are not prolonged, as in the lumbosarcal spine, but may be nagging. Fracture of transvere processes of L-1 is associated with very exquisite tenderness. Kidney tenderness is more diffuse and more lateral.

Spinous processes and interspinous ligaments are tender in vertebral body fractures, acute sprain and to a lesser degree strain due to poor posture.

The articular facets of L-5 to S-1 are symptomatic in sprains due to hyperextension or acute flexion injuries, strain or poor posture. Radiating pain to the legs and tenderness in this area with the spine slightly flexed indicate nerve root pressure.

Tenderness of the dorsum of the sacrum is found with exaggerated lordosis due to postural or muscular strain or due to protective spasm secondary to lumbosacral sprain.

Iliac crests, the origin of the iliolumbar muscles, are tender with sprains or myositis.

Transverse process, iliolumbar ligament and erector spinae tenderness is associated with fracture at the spinous process, strain of ligaments secondary to faulty posture and acute muscle and ligament sprains.

Tenderness of the posterior iliac crests and posterior superior spines of the ilium follows sprains and strains.

Spinous processes of L-5 and S-1, are tender in faulty posture and possibly in spinae bifida occulta.

The area between the posterior inferior and the posterior superior spine of the ilium is sensitive to sacroiliac lesions, especially strains or sprains.

At the sacrosciatic notch, tenderness is due to superior gluteal nerve sensitivity and may also be due to swelling of the sacroiliac joint.

Sacrococcygeal junction tenderness is found in sprain, strain or fracture.

Sciatic nerve trunk tenderness appears in nerve root pressure symptoms, especially in disc lesions.

The information in the preceding praragraphs is used as a basis to localize the injury and to formulate therapy.

Treatment is divided into four phases: (1) physical and assurance, (2) medical and therapeutic, (3) mechanical and (4) surgical.

All acute back injuries should be treated as soon as possible. This is best accomplished in a hospital where the patient is assured of complete rest and full nursing care. The temptation to get out of bed or the necessity to entertain guests and well wishers is avoided. While in bed, a pillow under the knees will relieve the affects of hamstring pull on the pelvis which causes tilting and stretching of the painful muscles or ligaments. A firm bed will relax the spinal muscles and a small pillow in the lumbar area often relieves pain. Pelvis traction may be provided. This is preferred to leg traction and avoids the complication of phlebitis which sometimes arises when the legs are bound. If a pelvic sling is not available, one can be improvised using a wide swath with ropes tied to either side.

Gentle spinal manipulation is of value, especially if the history is that of an acute catching pain of the back and inability to straighten up and there is a tilt of the trunk. Such a history implies that there is a subluxation of an apophyseal joint, usually at the lumbosacral junction. Considerable and often miraculous relief can be obtained by spinal manipulation. My method of choice is to have the patient supine with his knees flexed and thighs drawn tightly against the abdomen. This can be accomplished in the most acutely painful back and locks the pelvis. The patient uses both hands to hold the knee on the painless side. The other leg is gently extended, first in the midline, and then flexed again and rotated internally and externally while being extended. A snapping when felt or even heard indicates that the joint is free.

Complete rest and relaxation is essential, and to this purpose sedation is prescribed. Usually codeine $^1/_2$ to 1 grain with Empirin compound is sufficient every four hours. However, I do not hesitate to order Demerol or other narcotics. After the first 24 hours, barbiturates in any of many forms may be sufficient. The simplest is phenobarbital $^1/_2$ to 1 grain every four hours. Aspirin in a dosage of 10 grains every 3 to 4 hours may be sufficient after the acute seige, as it acts both as an analgesic and an anticongestant. Muscle relaxants are of some benefit, but do not give startling results. The principal drug is mephenesin in combinations with glutamic acid. Several such drugs are commonly used and prescribed in dosages up to 2 grams per 175 pounds of body weight. The tranquilizers are also being prescribed, essentially for their psychic relaxing properties. They have been of benefit in the tense individual. One of the most dramatic relaxants is curare, which should be given only under close supervision because of possible curarization, symptoms of which are heavy eye lids, diplopia or marked general relaxation. An antidote must always be quickly available in the form of neostigmine 0.5 to 1 cc. Tubocurarine in aqueous solution gives a very transient effect. In a peanut oil base, the curare is released in about 45 minutes and lasts 12 to 24 hours. The dosage is 1.25 cc. per 150 pounds. It has been our experience that 0.75 cc. given one to three times a day is often enough. Injections are made intramuscularly into the buttock. It is not to be rubbed in nor any local heat applied. Local injections of 1 per cent Novocain plain have proven very beneficial, especially when a point of local tenderness can be established.

Five to 10 cc. is injected into this trigger point, using a 22 gage needle $1^1/_2$ to 2 inches long. When the area of maximum pain is located, the fluid is injected in multiple points as one would in puncturing a shoulder bursa. This may be repeated on two to three occasions at two day intervals. If there is nothing more than very temporary relief after the third injection, the therapy should be discontinued as having no effect.

Mechanical treatment includes all modalities that affect local circulation favorably and relieve congestion. Hot moist packs for periods of 15 to 30 minutes at intervals of every three to four hours can be applied with simple turkish towels or with an elaborate hydrolator. Dry heat in the form of an electric pad, hot water bottle or infrared lamp is relieving and is best used at intervals, as with the moist heat. If pain increases after the use of heat, then cold packs may be used. There are many electrical and electronic machines which place the heat deeper in the tissues. This form of therapy is reserved for office treatment, as in unskilled hands severe injuries can occur. However, I have found that these modalities are often much abused and too many promises are made for their miraculous affects. When they are used, the period of therapy should not exceed several months, yet I have examined cases who receive such therapy two to three times a week for years. The effect of such long therapy is an increase of fibrosis. Effective and sometimes miraculous relief in short periods is accomplished by the various forms of diathermy and ultrasonic machines. Massage is relieving and is recommended both for home and office. Medications used during or after massage include gentle to concentrated rubifacients. Care to avoid blistering is important. Simple rubbing or muscle-kneading in its various forms is beneficial.

Prognosis

The prognosis in the 20 to 30 year groups is usually very good if there are no extreme congenital defects or evidences of arthritis. Recovery is usually complete within four to six weeks.

The age group of 30 to 40 may have a slightly more prolonged period of symptoms because of arthritis and soft tissue changes. This is especially true in the nonsedentary worker who, over a period of years, has developed some soft tissue scarring as a result of minimal sprains. The period may extend to 8 to 12 weeks.

As one approaches the older age group, one must consider the many soft tissue injuries, scarring and natural attritional changes of the structures. The period of symptomatology may be further prolonged so that it may extend to 6 to 9 months. However, other factors beside tissue wear enter into the picture.

Functional symptoms also become more pronounced. These are influenced by the urge to retirement. The job becomes too hard. The patient is discontented with his work, his associates or his financial status. Such factors are to be suspected especially if the injury described is not capable of producing tissue damage that would cause prolonged disability.

IV. CHEST AND ABDOMEN

CHAPTER 27

INJURIES TO THE CHEST

CRANSTON W. HOLMAN, M.D.

Severe thoracic injuries may involve not only extensive areas of the chest wall but, most important, usually cause serious damage to the intrathoracic viscera, including the lungs, heart, great vessels and diaphragm. In those who survive the initial injury, immediate treatment follows the general principles of therapy for trauma – namely, the control of bleeding, the correction of shock, the prevention of pain, the proper care of the wound and the prophylactic administration of antibiotics.

Since chest injuries almost always compromise ventilatory efficiency to some degree, other immediate measures should be taken to prevent or reduce anoxia. For instance, although a patient may be in shock, he should be placed slightly upright rather than in the head-down position so as to facilitate respiratory function. Also, it is wise immediately to give oxygen either by mask, nasal catheter or oxygen tent, whichever is most practical. It is surprising that patients, who soon after injury show no respiratory embarrassment, in a relatively short time become dyspneic and cyanotic, evidence of respiratory decompensation. Particularly for such patients, manipulation for examination and x-ray should be done rapidly and kept to a minimum.

A classification based on clinical and pathologic findings that applies to any individual case is difficult to set up, but in general injuries may be divided into nonpenetrating and penetrating. In the main, most of the serious complications such as pulmonary edema, hemothorax and pneumothorax are common to both, and as the following case histories will illustrate, their treatment is much the same irrespective of the type of injury in which they may occur.

Anoxia Secondary to Pulmonary Edema

The first case illustrates the effects of anoxia secondary to pulmonary edema in a patient with rather severe lung injury but with minimal involvement of the chest wall.

A 65 year old man, hit by an automobile, did not lose consciousness but had severe pain in the right chest. Since he had no other ill effects, he worked for eight hours, but at the end of that day his pain had increased, and because of difficulty in breathing he came to the hospital for examination and treatment. X-rays revealed fractures of the sixth and seventh ribs in the midaxillary line on the right side, but there was no evidence of shock, fluid in the chest or pneumothorax. Because of dyspnea and a suggestion of cyanosis he was hospitalized. Strapping was applied to the right chest, which made him reasonably comfortable, and he was given sedation. By the third day his temperature had risen to 40° C., and at this time he was somewhat dyspneic and slightly cyanotic in spite of the fact that he was in an oxygen tent (Graph 1). The most distressing feature, however, was his restlessness, incoherence and lack of co-operation. It was thought by those who saw him that the man possibly had a brain injury, but after negative neurologic, spinal fluid and skull x-ray examinations, some mental disturbance was suggested. A psychiatrist offered the tentative diagnosis of possible delirium tremens. These points are mentioned and emphasized because the patient presented typical symptoms and signs of chronic anoxia seen particularly in the older age group or in those with pulmonary fibrosis due to antecedent disease. During the next week of his admission, as his temperature gradually fell to normal, he became mentally alert and co-operative coincident with the improvement in his color and decrease in respiratory rate.

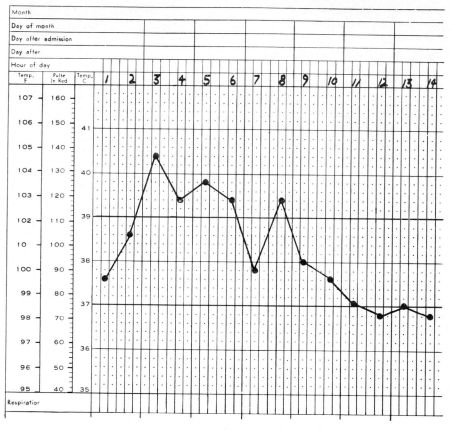

Graph 1.

The case illustrates the variable signs and symptoms that may result from acute and chronic anoxia. Needless to say, the excessive neurologic and psychiatric examinations with their attendant manipulations only contributed to his difficulty.

Hemothorax

The next patient illustrates the treatment of hemothorax, a common complication of either closed or open injuries, some degree of which is seen almost always in the perforating injury of the chest.

This patient was also struck by an automobile, was admitted to the hospital shortly after injury, and was found to have multiple lacerations, with several fractured ribs on the right in addition to fractures of both bones of the right forearm. He was in a mild degree of shock, was quite dyspneic, and already had developed considerable subcutaenous emphysema, the latter pathognomonic of lung perforation. The immediate treatment consisted of placing the patient in a slightly upright position; he was given oxygen (95 per cent oxygen and 5 per cent carbon dioxide) by mask, adequate sedation (demerol and sodium phenobarbital), prophylactic antibiotics, a transfusion of whole blood, and his chest was strapped. On this regimen his condition improved so that within a few hours x-rays could be obtained. These showed no evidence of fluid, but, by the third day (fig. 1), there was evidence of fluid in the right pleural cavity. This was aspirated on two successive days and a total of 900 cc. of blood was removed.

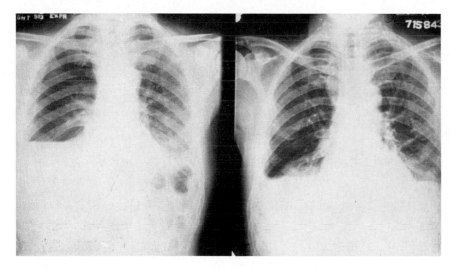

Fig. 1—Hemothorax — before and after aspiration.

Ideally, in the treatment of hemothorax, aspiration is delayed for 48 hours, with the hope that the blood may prevent continued bleeding by exerting tamponade on the lacerated lung. If, however, anoxia develops, fluid should be removed to improve ventilatory efficiency. When possible, only 500 cc. should be aspirated at one time since rapid evacuation of large amounts may only initiate further hemorrhage. After 48 to 72 hours, it is safe to begin gradual re-expansion of the lung by daily aspiration, limiting the amount to 500 cc. at any one time. Air replacement of the fluid aspirated should *not* be done. The relatively early removal of blood is important so that fibrothorax is prevented — a rare complication if this method of therapy is followed.

Tension Pneumothorax

Next illustrated is the treatment of tension pneumothorax — most commonly found in patients with perforating injuries, but in this instance a complication of chest wall contusion associated with fractured rib.

A 61 year old woman was admitted to the hospital shortly after she struck her side against the seat in a lurching bus. She was in considerable pain, quite dyspneic, but showed no evidence of shock. She was immediately placed in an oxygen tent and soon after an x-ray revealed minimal pneumothorax of the left chest. Twenty-four hours later the dyspnea and pain had increased, and another x-ray revealed increased pneumothorax with a shift of the mediastinum towards the opposite side. The pleural cavity was aspirated in the second intercostal space anteriorly and approximately 1000 cc. of air removed, with immediate improvement in the dyspnea. In addition, the

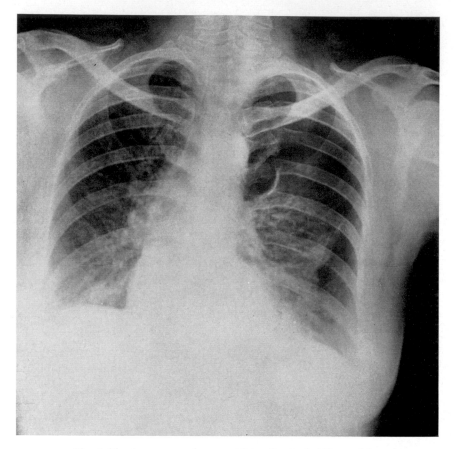

Fig. 2—Tension pneumothorax with mediastinal shift to right.

third to seventh intercostal nerves were blocked posteriorly just to the left of the vertebral column, with considerable relief of pain. However, in less than two hours' time, her dyspnea had again increased, she was cyanotic in spite of the fact that she was in an oxygen tent, and another x-ray (fig. 2) revealed an increase in pneumothorax and an increase in the shift of the mediastinum. With these findings, it was obvious that insertion of a catheter for constant decompression was indicated. Accordingly, under local anesthesia and without transporting the patient to the operating room, a 16 caliber French catheter was inserted in the pleural cavity through the second anterior intercostal space with immediate relief of symptoms. The catheter was connected to a tube placed under water, and 12 hours later moderate suction was started. Within 48 hours the lung was completely expanded (fig. 3) and the tube was removed four days after its introduction.

Needless to say, early recognition of tension pneumothorax is most important not only to re-expand the nonfunctioning injured lung, but also to prevent the serious complications of mediastinal shift — namely, compression of the ipsilateral lung and inadequate filling of the right heart because of compression and distortion of the vena cava. Although there is a dif-

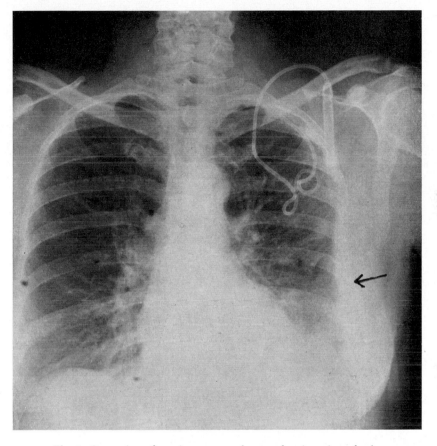

Fig. 3—Correction of tension pneumothorax after insertion of tube.

ference of opinion as to whether suction should be used immediately after the introduction of a tube into the pleural space, there is some virtue in gradual re-expansion to prevent reopening of the lung perforation.

Ruptured Diaphragm

The next patient illustrates the failure to establish an early diagnosis of a ruptured diaphragm, a possibility which should always be considered in the severely wounded patient.

This 67 year old woman was admitted shortly after being struck by an automobile and was found to have multiple fractures, including both legs, both arms and several ribs in the lower left chest — the latter causing relatively little pain and for this reason receiving no particular attention. During the first two and a half weeks, the lower extremities were operated on and her condition seemed to be progressing satisfactorily when one evening she complained of severe substernal pain radiating to the left shoulder and down the left arm. It was thought she probably had either coronary occlusion or an embolus, and x-rays of the chest disclosed a density in the left lower chest. The following day she complained of difficulty in swallowing, and a barium swallow revealed that the barium remained in the stomach, which was in an abnormally high position. The question arose

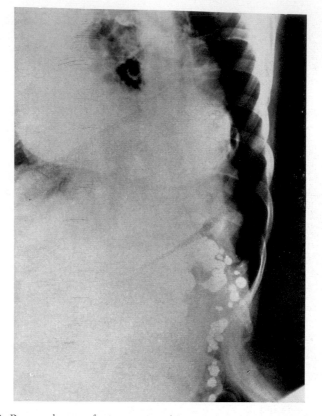

Fig. 4—Pneumothorax after pneumoperitoneum in rupture of diaphragm.

as to whether the patient had a pleural effusion with paralyzed diaphragm or whether the stomach had herniated through a rent in the diaphragm. 500 cc. of air was injected into the abdominal cavity and after placing the patient in an upright position, the x-ray (fig. 4) showed a large amount of air in the pleural cavity, thus establishing the presence of a diaphragmatic hernia. At operation a large rent was found in the diaphragm through which the stomach and a portion of the colon had herniated.

In patients with multiple injuries, the possibility of ruptured diaphragm is often overlooked and its diagnosis may be difficult. The use of a Levin tube, a small barium swallow and pneumoperitoneum are valuable diagnostic aids.

Traumatic Asphyxia

Traumatic asphyxia produces an immediate dramatic appearance of a violescent discoloration of the face, neck and upper extremities, the areas drained by the superior vena cava (*see* Frontispiece). Found only in patients following a sudden compression injury of the thoracic cage, it probably results from sudden increase in intrathoracic pressure which causes obstruction of the superior vena cava. The striking discoloration is due not to extravasation of blood but to thromboses of small venules and capillaries. Unfortunately, this same process may occur in the brain, and a patient whose progress seems to be satisfactory up to the fifth or sixth day may lapse into a coma and die. For this reason, prognosis must be guarded for a week. We have used no specific therapy in this condition, but in view of the venous and capillary thromboses, anticoagulant therapy might be of value in some cases.

Multiple Rib Fractures or "Stove-in" Chest

The next condition to be considered — namely, multiple rib fractures associated with paradoxical respiration, is always potentially dangerous. Often associated with multiple injuries that frequently command our immediate attention, its serious nature may not be recognized until the development of complications that defy all efforts in treatment. For this reason, after the emergency care of the associated injuries, the thoracic injury should be given first priority in treatment.

The most urgent problem, the maintenance of an unobstructed airway, is extremely difficult. Within hours after injury the traumatized lung becomes edematous and pours secretions into the tracheobronchial tree. Unable to cough with an effective expulsive force because of the unstable rib cage, the patient literally drowns in his own secretions. Immediate tracheostomy provides the only satisfactory means for maintaining an unobstructed tracheo-

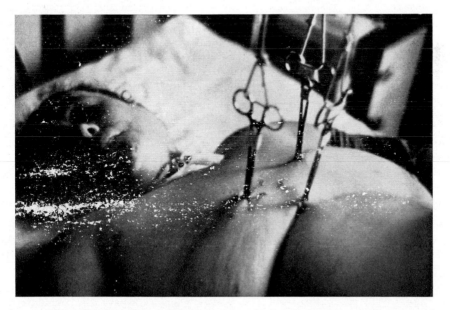

Fig. 5—Tracheostomy and traction on rib cage for "stove in" chest.

bronchial tree, and only when this is insured can definitive treatment of associated injuries be safely undertaken. During the first critical days, constant nursing care is essential to provide frequent and gentle aspiration of the voluminous secretions. The striking improvement that follows simple tracheostomy, since first suggested in 1951 by Carter and Guiseffi, [1] has been so impressive that it should be our first step to prevent the serious and sometimes fatal complications of chest wall injuries associated with paradoxical respiration.

Occasionally, additional stabilization of the chest wall may be indicated. This can best be done by applying traction on the rib cage by means of towel clips that have been placed around a rib on either side, connected to balanced suspension from an overhead fracture frame (fig. 5).

Open Sucking Wound

We now turn to a few of the problems encountered in penetrating wounds of the thorax, the most immediately serious of which is the open sucking wound. The open thorax results in complete collapse of the lung on the involved side, and the mediastinum, unless fixed, is dislocated toward the opposite side with consequent compression of that lung and further decrease in respiratory function. It is little wonder then that a fatal outcome is likely unless the wound is quickly closed with whatever type of compression bandage is available at the time. When proper facilities are available, the wound should be surgically closed — if it is the result of a knife wound, several through-and-through sutures will suffice; if it is grossly contaminated or severely traumatized, débridement followed by closure is indicated. In the latter case, a catheter for drainage should be placed in the most dependent part of the pleural cavity.

Packing of these wounds, rather than surgical closure, should never be done. The pack always leads to some degree of chest wall infection and too often results in an empyema.

Combined Thoracoabdominal Injury

Combined thoracoabdominal wounds require operation as soon as the patient's condition permits. The diagnosis is often difficult, and occasionally is only possible after a thorough exploration of all intra-abdominal and retroperitoneal organs. Any perforation of the left lower chest may be associated with a subdiaphragmatic injury to the spleen, kidney, splenic flexure of the colon, or stomach, and there are some who advise routine abdominal exploration irrespective of the clinical findings on abdominal examination. At the time of laparotomy, wounds of the diaphragm can be satisfactorily closed, and, if indicated, intrathoracic exploration can be carried out by extending the incision into the chest. In the presence of massive hemothorax, pneumothorax, mediastinal shift, or a laceration of the diaphragm, or if the chest has been opened, catheter drainage of the pleural cavity is indicated.

Cardiac Tamponade

Injuries to the heart and pericardium are rarely seen in connection with nonpenetrating trauma. In the "steering wheel" injury described by Beck,[2] cardiac contusion should always be considered a possibility and the patient carefully observed for signs and symptoms suggesting coronary disease.

Acute cardiac tamponade, characterized by dilatation of the neck veins, almost imperceptible pulse and blood pressure, inaudible heart sounds and a quiet heart on fluoroscopy may complicate stab wounds of the anterior chest. Such patients may be relatively free from symptoms for a short time, only to collapse as the pericardium becomes filled with blood. There are two schools of thought as to the best therapy — one favors aspiration and the other advises immediate surgical exploration. Because of the numerous satisfactory reports of aspiration, it would seem wise to aspirate the pericardium initially. Except in an extreme emergency, this should always be done in the operating room so that if improvement is not prompt, exploration can be done immediately. If exploration is carried out, it should be anticipated that on opening the pericardium, active and profuse hemorrhage may be encountered. In this event, the bleeding point is occluded by digital pressure until the area can be satisfactorily visualized and sutured. A communication between the pericardial and pleural spaces should be established and the latter drained with an indwelling catheter.

Summary

Initial treatment of thoracic injuries should follow the established principles of therapy for injuries of any part, but with emphasis on the early administration of oxygen. Pain that is not relieved by the usual amounts of sedation may be controlled by the paravertebral injection of procaine into the intercostal nerves. Open sucking wounds of the thorax demand our most urgent attention and should be closed immediately by whatever means available. Tension pneumothorax should be corrected immediately by aspiration. In the event of recurrence, constant suction should be instituted, best done by means of a catheter introduced through the anterior second intercostal space. Tracheostomy should be routinely employed in thoracic injuries associated with paradoxical respiration. Any injury to the lower chest cage should direct one's attention to possible injuries of the diaphragm and intra-abdominal viscera.

References

[1] CARTER, B. N., and GUISEFFI, J.: Tracheotomy, a useful procedure in thoracic surgery, with particular reference to its employment in crushing injuries of the thorax. J. Thoracic Surg. *21:* 495, 1951.
[2] BECK, C. S.: Contusions of the heart. J. A. M. A. *104:* 109, (Jan. 12) 1935.

CHAPTER 28

INJURIES TO THE ABDOMEN

S. W. MOORE, M.D.

The treatment of traumatic injuries to the abdomen involves anesthesia, fundamental principles of wound treatment, multiple injuries, shock, blood replacement, antibiotics, fractures of the pelvis and complicating injuries, kidneys, bladder, chest, blood vessels, x-rays and mass casualties. Though these subjects are all most important in connection with injuries to the abdomen, they will be treated only briefly here to provide space for additional points which will not be stressed elsewhere in this volume.

Abdominal injuries can be divided into (1) nonpenetrating or subcutaneous, where there is no break in the skin and (2) penetrating, which will also include the perforating. In the perforating, the "trauma" has passed through the abdominal wall, as with a bullet wound. Even the skin may deflect a "spent" missile, and often the bullet can be felt just beneath the skin after having gone through the entire body save the skin on the other side.

Associated Injuries: Some injuries to the abdomen will lead us to suspect an associated injury. Again, at times, the associated injury will cause us to overlook an abdominal injury.

Fractured ribs, spine or transverse processes frequently are seen with rupture of the spleen or liver.

X-rays are most important in considering injuries to the abdomen. Almost every injury, but especially severe ones, should have x-ray examination. When we wish to confirm or eliminate a diagnosis by x-ray, it is important to request examination for that particular condition. Never be satisfied with a negative x-ray report when the clinical examination points to an injury. There is no sign, symptom or indication on which we can make the complete diagnosis, but rather we must consider the total picture.

Symptoms: All abdominal trauma is potentially serious regardless of immediate symptoms. A delayed rupture usually means the original rupture was not diagnosed. One immediate symptom is shock, which is the result of trauma or hemorrhage or both. Immediate symptoms may be due to peritoneal irritation of a chemical nature, gastric juice, bile, intestinal contents or bleeding. Later symptoms may be due to delayed hemorrhage or peritonitis.

Pain usually occurs immediately following trauma, then subsides with rest and sedation. Pain together with tenderness is the best indication of the site of injury. As soiling of the peritoneum continues, pain increases. Pain in the shoulder or neck indicates irritation of the diaphragm.

Pulse goes up with bleeding, shock and soiling of the peritoneal cavity.

Temperature is of very little immediate help. Later it goes up.

Vomiting is variable and gives little indication of any specific injury. Vomiting of blood strongly suggests injury of the stomach or upper gastro-intestinal tract.

Blood in the urine is evidence of injury to the bladder or kidneys, while blood in the rectum is evidence of injury of the rectum or colon or, at times, central rupture of the liver.

An accurate history concerning the nature and details of trauma is most helpful in determining the nature of the injury.

Signs are variable. Tenderness and rigidity are most marked over the site of the injury; however, there can be marked damage with no physical signs at the time of first examination. For this reason, it is important to establish a baseline of initial physical findings: temperature, pulse, blood pressure, hematocrit and x-ray. Peristaltic sounds are usually absent if perforation has occurred.

X-ray may well show fractures. Air under the diaphragm means injury to a gas-containing viscus.

Laboratory: Urine and blood counts are mandatory. Although the latter are not completely dependable, the white blood count becomes elevated with hemorrhage or chemical peritonitis. The hemoglobin and hematocrit must be repeated at intervals when the patient is being watched for hemorrhage.

It is a mistake to think of abdominal exploration as a harmless procedure. In the presence of other serious injuries, the mortality is such that the greatest care should be exercised to reach an accurate diagnosis by some other means.

There is no substitute for an accurate and careful physical examination, and thorough x-rays and laboratory work.

Incisions: In most situations the right midrectus muscle splitting incision is best. In case the lesion is thought to be on the left, the approach should be on that side. These incisions can be extended up or down; they can be extended into the chest or across the abdomen. They do not get in the way of colostomies. A transverse incision is usually not good. The most difficult lesion to find is probably a perforation of the splenic flexure of the colon, but again, subcostal incisions have little place in treating traumatic wounds of the abdomen.

Preoperative Care: These patients should be started on antibiotics and have a tube passed into the stomach, preferably a double lumen Miller-Abbott tube. This can then be placed into the small intestine at operation. With trauma to the abdomen, blood is usually lost and whole blood, not plasma, serum or crystalloid solution, should be given as replacement. Of course, if blood is not available, the others must be used. An in-dwelling catheter is necessary in many cases and desirable in most.

Postoperative Care follows preoperative care. Mortality and complications are caused by missed lesions, blood loss and infection. We must be careful in the examination both before and at operation not to miss perforations or other trauma. After operation, as well as during operation, lost blood must be replaced, the gastrointestinal tract decompressed, and antibiotics used. Where there is cyanosis and difficulty in breathing, tracheotomies must be considered, particularly in associated chest lesions.

Thoraco-abdominal wounds should be mentioned. Here the thorax, abdomen, and diaphragm have all been injured at the same time by the same trauma. If the patient breathes well and is not bleeding, the chest injury usually is not as urgent as the abdominal injury because there is always the possibility of perforation of the gastrointestinal tract and peritonitis. In all of these cases, it is mandatory that the abdomen be explored. This can be done through the chest, through the abdomen, or by the combined thoracoabdominal approach where both body cavities and the diaphragm are all opened through the same incision. Despite fear of infection from entering the chest if the gut has been perforated, it may be better to enter the chest and clean out the material already leaked in from the abdomen. With perforating wounds, the path of a missile can usually be plotted very accurately. With penetrating wounds by bullets or shell fragments, an x-ray will help in locating the missile. When the right diaphragm is traversed, the liver is almost always damaged. The best approach to the bare area of the liver is through the chest.

Abdominal Wall: Hemorrhage into or beneath the rectus muscle may be caused by a blow or violent muscular effort. In the upper abdomen it may be confused with an acutely inflamed gallbladder, in the lower abdomen with acute appendicitis or an ovarian cyst. The hematoma results from rupture of the rectus muscle with consequent tearing of the artery and vein.

The hematoma does not pass the midline or lateral border of the rectus muscle. Exploration is usually necessary to establish the diagnosis. Removal of clot and ligation of vessels hastens healing.

Penetrating wounds demand care in the operating room. The entire abdomen should be prepared for a laparotomy, and the wound excised. Penetration of the peritoneum makes exploration of the abdominal cavity mandatory. At times the seriousness of the situation may lead one to incise the abdomen directly and to take care of the original wound later.

Remember that all wounds which cause visceral injuries do not always occur in the anterior abdominal wall. Sir Gordon Gordon-Taylor reports that in only 60 per cent of intra-abdominal injuries seen in England during World War II was the wound of entrance in the anterior abdominal wall; in 20 per cent it was in the back, while in the other 20 per cent the injury occurred in the buttock. Again this shows the importance of a complete and detailed examination under a good light.

Peritoneoscopy has been recommended in questionable cases of stab and gunshot wounds of the abdomen. As in all other procedures, a negative report is of no value.

Stomach: Because of its size and position, the stomach is most often injured and may be associated with other visceral lesions. Many of the injuries are extensive and difficult to repair, particularly near the esophagus, the fundus or high on the lesser curvature. Openings in the stomach are rarely single, and with an anterior perforation, the posterior perforation must be searched for, even if it is necessary to open the lesser peritoneal cavity. At times the posterior wound may be repaired through an enlarged opening in the anterior wall of the stomach. Gastric wounds tend to have considerable hemorrhage. Gastric ulcers may perforate during air raids. Acute dilation of the stomach is prone to occur after "blast" injuries, particularly those of the chest. The stomach appears better able to take care of a perforation than any other portion of the intestinal canal.

The primary aim of the surgeon is to save life. Simple suture of a stomach lesion, if possible, is the procedure of choice. Gastroenterostomy is rarely indicated save to restore continuity of the gastrointestinal tract. Total gastrectomy should be attempted only as a last resort.

With rupture of the stomach, duodenum or small intestine there may be hemorrhage, spreading peritoneal irritation and shock. The usual signs are abdominal tenderness and spasm, rising pulse and white count, nausea, vomiting and reduction in audible peristaltic signs. Vomiting is no more frequent in wounds of the stomach than in wounds of other abdominal viscera. X-ray may show free air under the diaphragm, or there may be absence of liver dullness and pain in the shoulder or neck due to irritation of the diaphragm. Blood in the vomitus is a good sign of gastric injury. In cases of abdominal injury, we must remember, "It is safer to look and see than to wait and see." In suspected wounds, pass a Levin tube. Restore blood loss and start antibiotics. There are only two signs diagnostic of gastric perforation: emission of undigested food from an abdominal wound; actual observation of a perforation or laceration in an eviscerated stomach.

In World War II, 9 out of 10 injuries to the stomach were complicated by wounds to other viscera. Forty per cent of all soldiers with gastric injuries died. When the stomach was injured alone, the mortality was 28 per cent. But when there were other associated injuries, it was 42 per cent.

Duodenum: Few wounds of the duodenum are reported, and recovery in these is exceptional. The duodenum is well protected from most trauma, but owing to its fixed position and the fact that it passes in front of the vertebral column, it is particularly vulnerable to compression injuries against the spine, as when it is caught between the spine with trauma applied to the abdominal wall. Usually the trauma is nonpenetrating. The symptoms at first may be minimal. However, with extravasation of duodenal contents and digestion of retroperitoneal tissue, there is most extensive pain, tenderness, and rigidity. Fever and leukocytosis increase. X-ray may show air. Radiopaque substances are introduced by some to show perforation.

At operation the duodenum is most unsatisfactory to explore. The presence of a retroperitoneal hematoma, or the finding of bile or a greenish-yellow discoloration of the peritoneum makes a careful examination mandatory. This can be done from the right by incising the peritoneum and mobilizing the duodenum; from the left by incising the peritoneum at the ligament of Tritz. If possible, suture the lesion. It may be necessary to excise the entire duodenum as for cancer of the head of the pancreas. These lesions are often associated with injury to the pancreas, fracture of the spine or hemorrhage due to damage to large blood vessels in this area. In World War II they were almost always associated with other injuries, and the mortality was 56 per cent. A good number of these injuries were missed early in the war. They must be thought of and sought or they will be overlooked and found only at autopsy.

Small Intestine: In the intestinal tract the number of bacteria increases as we go lower, and the impression is gained that injuries to the large bowel are more dangerous and carry a higher mortality than those to the small intestine. This is not borne out by figures from World War I.

The most important factor in the successful management of injuries of the small intestine is the finding and treatment of all openings. This requires a careful examination of the entire tract. Whether one starts at the cecum and goes up, or at the ligament of Tritz and comes down, is immaterial. The vital point is not to spend twenty minutes repairing a lesion, and then after exploring further find it necessary to resect this portion of the bowel. In 27 cases of fatal gunshot wounds in which autopsy was done, McGowan found that in 15, or over half, visceral lesions had been overlooked at the time of operation. When a perforation is found, mark it with a long black suture and go until the entire small gut is examined. Again, hemorrhage is the immediate cause of death and peritonitis the later.

Intestinal obstruction occurs due to trapping a loop of small bowel between injured bony structures. Beware of treating vomiting following trauma by a tube in the stomach until a definite diagnosis is made. Be on the alert for intestinal obstruction.

It is interesting that multiple wounds due to birdshot will heal and seal off. It may be best in these to pursue an expectant course of treatment.

The treatment must be completed by using plication if feasible, and resection when necessary. Do not bring the small intestine (ileostomy) outside save as a last resort.

Perforation is most common at the fixed points, such as the ileocecal valve or the ligament of Tritz. Perforation of the intestine in children is rare.

In World War II, mortality in injuries of the jejunum and ileum was 30 per cent. Always assess the total damage before starting a resection.

Large Bowel: As one would expect, injuries to the large intestine carry a high mortality. A large portion of this tract is retroperitoneal, making it difficult to find all perforations, and these openings give rise to a particularly virulent retroperitoneal cellulitis. Although the splenic and hepatic flexures are difficult to repair or even to examine, exploration should start at the ileocecal valve and include the entire large bowel. World War II injuries of the colon had a mortality of 35 per cent – 22 per cent when injured alone and 40 per cent in multivisceral injuries.

Perforations of the right colon, if small and if treated within eight hours, can be closed. If large, a large mushroom catheter may be sutured in the bowel and brought out. In more extensive injuries, exteriorization of the damaged bowel is preferred. In general, primary closure is the best treatment if the condition of the bowel permits. Again in this instance the Miller-Abbott tube is useful.

Satisfactory approach to the splenic flexure is often difficult, and as a rule, exteriorization is preferable to an attempt at suture. A thoraco-abdominal approach is indicated if the wound involves both the chest and the abdomen. The presence of blood behind the descending colon should always suggest a retroperitoneal injury.

The sigmoid colon as a rule lends itself readily to exteriorization. With a short mesentery or thick abdominal wall, it may be better to close the perforation and do a proximal colostomy.

Rectum: Wounds of the rectum are seldom mentioned when speaking of intra-abdominal injuries. They are difficult to diagnose when the general peritoneal cavity is opened. Large numbers of injuries to the rectum occur by way of the buttocks; the most important factor here is to think of the injury and to look for it. In case of doubt, open the peritoneal cavity. Exploration of the perineum with débridement is readily carried out. If necessary, the coccyx and a portion of the sacrum may be excised. Colostomies are mandatory. Remember the possibility of injury by the proctoscope and by the practical joker with the air hose to the seat of the pants. Both are lethal weapons. The presence of fresh blood in the rectum is presumptive evidence of injury to the rectum or colon. The perirectal tissue should be drained.

Foreign bodies in the rectum are always more difficult to remove than to introduce. At times this calls for an abdominal approach. If pressure from above is not sufficient, the rectum must be opened. When the rectum is opened without preoperative preparation, do a proximal colostomy.

When intestinal contents have been spilled into the abdominal cavity, it is important to remove all such material mechanically by suction and swabbing. An attempt to cleanse the abdomen by flushing with normal salt solution or other fluid often carries the fecal material to inaccessible recesses of the peritoneal cavity and does more harm than good.

Drainage: It has been shown long ago that effective, prolonged drainage of the general peritoneal cavity is not possible. A material introduced as a drain becomes walled off within a few hours. If there is persistent oozing of blood or question of bile drainage, a soft drain may be used for 24 hours.

When possible, bring drains and colostomies out of stab wounds.

Wound Closure: Before closing, remember that overlooked perforations are a major cause of death. Gauzes and pads are left more frequently after operations for traumatic conditions than after operations performed under ordinary conditions. These are the wounds most often infected and disrupted. Where haste is essential, through and through sutures of silver wire, silkworm gut, or silk are best. If time permits, a layer closure should be carried out in addition to through and through sutures.

In World War II, three out of four injuries to the colon and rectum were multiple injuries. The important points learned in this were (1) exteriorization of the wounded segment and (2) the proximal colostomy.

Liver: The liver is the largest organ in the abdomen and is frequently injured, largely by accidents occurring as a result of our rapid means of transportation. We have blast injuries of the liver together with penetrating wounds produced by knives and missiles. The many causes account for a great variation in the types of lesions found in the liver.

Nonpenetrating trauma may produce:

1. Rupture of capsule and liver parenchyma.

2. Subcapsular rupture or rupture of the parenchyma with an intact capsule.

3. Central rupture without injury to the capsule or the periphery of the parenchyma.

The immediate results of massive liver injury are exsanguinating hemorrhage and accompanying shock. Pain is often absent in the right upper quadrant as are signs of hemoperitoneum. Coexisting injuries of other intra-abdominal organs are often present.

Operation should be done after treatment for shock and hemorrhage has been instituted. There is no one way to treat all injuries of the liver. If possible, suture a laceration as if after a biopsy. Gelfoam, muscle or omentum sutured into a liver defect may at times control the hemorrhage. Detached or devitalized fragments of the liver should be removed. Packing of the liver wound and drainage of the area has been a most unsatisfactory means of treatment, but at times it must be done.

The removal of packing often is associated with severe hemorrhage or persistent drainage of bile abscesses and necrosis of liver tissue. Great caution must be exercised in removing the packing.

Foreign bodies, including bullets and bits of clothing, should be removed at the initial operation if the condition of the patient permits and if they are accessible. This can be done more easily at this time than later. If left, an external sinus that drains bile and infected material will result. If the unperitonealized portion of the liver is the site of the foreign body, it is probably better to approach this directly through the chest at a later operation than to transect undamaged liver tissue in an effort to remove it through the anterior approach.

Remember that high velocity bullets and jagged shell fragments as well as blunt forces often cause damage far beyond the grossly apparent injury. Cyanosis due to anoxia is common with thoracic injury. Jaundice is not apparent for several days. No liver function tests are of any help in the early management of these patients. Peritoneal aspiration to determine presence of blood is used by some, but I have never liked it.

It has been shown many times that antibiotics are particularly important in injuries of the liver.

Drainage should always be carried out in case there is leakage of bile. With gelfoam packing, bleeding may be controlled and the abdomen closed without drainage. A dry gauze pack to a bleeding liver while one is repairing another injury will usually stop the bleeding. Shock is the most common cause of death. In World War I expectant treatment was carried out with a mortality of 66 per cent. In World War II with operation, the mortality was 27 per cent.

Subcapsular or central rupture of the liver may give rise to bleeding into the biliary tract. Sandblom has called this "hemobilia." It may cause hematemesis and melena, biliary colic, biliary obstruction or gallbladder distention. It should be looked for in all cases of liver injuries with vague symptoms. Because of their location in the interior of the liver these injuries do not give rise to hemorrhage and bile leakage into the peritoneal cavity.

The right lobe of the liver is six times the size of the left and is injured five times as often.

Complications result chiefly from inadequate draining and include subphrenic abscess, bile empyema, and intrahepatic abscess.

Gallbladder and Bile Ducts: These are injured in many ways, including the aspiration needle. The mortality is high because they are not thought of, and because only minimal symptoms are associated with bile in the peritoneal cavity until late.

Injuries to the gallbladder are treated by closure of the perforation with drainage of the gallbladder. In all injuries of the gallbladder, drainage of this organ should be carried out. At times it is feasible to drain through the perforation if this is in the fundus. Injury to the cystic duct calls for a cholecystectomy. At times it may be necessary to ligate both ends of the cystic duct, drain the gallbladder and remove it later. However, the gallbladder should be removed at the first operation if possible. In case the distal cyst stump is not accurately identified, the common duct should be drained by T-tube.

Treatment of Injuries to Biliary Ducts: The ideal way to repair these injuries is end-to-end suture or repair over a T-tube. If these are impracticable, one will have to study the individual problem. Remember, it is always better to re-establish the continuity of the biliary tract. Lesions are frequently overlooked. It may be possible to implant the proximal end into the stomach or duodenum or to ligate the proximal end and anastomose the gallbladder to the stomach or duodenum. As a last resort, drain and hope for an external biliary fistula. But drain all these patients.

Spleen: This is the most common single entity requiring operation. The spleen may be injured by contusions, blasts, direct blows, knives, missiles, as well as at the operating table. There may be damage to blood supply, a complete tear of the spleen, or a subcapsular rupture and hematoma. These give rise at times to a delayed rupture or hemorrhage.

The most reliable sign of splenic injury is evidence of severe hemorrhage and hemoperitoneum, the presence of a mass, or dullness in the splenic area. History of injury in this area, presence of broken ribs, or external injury leads one to suspect it.

Rupture of the spleen may give rise to multiple peritoneal transplantation of splenic tissue.

Before operation, we must make provisions for adequate transfusion. Operation may dislodge clots and reactivate bleeding. Usually the spleen is normal in size and can be grasped quickly. The important thing is to stop bleeding. Clamp the splenic pedicle, ligate the splenic artery, or make pressure on this artery. After bleeding is controlled, remove the spleen. Remember, the stomach and tail of the pancreas are closely associated with the spleen. The spleen is much more readily mobilized if the posterior peritoneum is incised. It can then be brought into the wound. There is no really good incision, but probably the best is a high left rectus. This can be extended in any direction. The main difficulty with a subcostal incision is "your diagnosis may be wrong." Except for very minor wounds, suture of the spleen should not be attempted. The spleen should be completely removed. Firm fixation of the spleen limits shifting its position and adds to its susceptibility to injury by blunt forces. From the standpoint of splenic injury alone, there is no need for administration of antibiotic agents. In World War II, wounds of the spleen had a 25 per cent mortality, and 75 per cent had multivisceral injuries.

Pancreas: Individuals with wounds of the pancreas usually do not survive long enough to reach a hospital. In World War II the mortality was 57 per cent and 98 per cent of the cases had multivisceral wounds. It is a rare injury, and all persons with it are in shock when first seen. The injury is frequently missed. In no case would clinical findings arouse suspicion that the pancreas had been injured. The position renders it vulnerable to blows above the umbilicus which crush it against the vertebral column. The friability of the pancreas facilitates the escape of external secretions when it is traumatized. This leads to severe cellular reaction in the surrounding tissue.

At operation, devitalized portions of the pancreas are removed. Ducts should be sutured if possible, otherwise ligated. Blood serum amylase is of value in diagnosing pancreatic injury. It may be elevated considerably due to traumatic pancreatitis. Glycosuria and hyperglycemia may be present. Pack for bleeding and always drain.

Summary

1. If it is suspected that a penetrating wound involved the peritoneal cavity, it is mandatory to explore the abdomen with the least possible delay.

2. Localized tenderness and muscle spasm are valuable guides to the site of injury.

3. In stab and gunshot wounds of the abdomen, most deaths are due to overlooked perforations of the intestine.

4. There is no substitute for a careful history and physical examination.

5. Do not let an opening in the stomach or small intestine communicate with the outside through an abdominal incision. If possible, all openings and drains should be through stab wounds.

6. Complications following abdominal injury include: shock, peritonitis, abdominal distention, intestinal obstruction, infected wounds, wound dehiscence, gastrointestinal fistula, intraperitoneal abscess, anaerobic infection, secondary hemorrhage, thromboembolism and anuria.

7. The surgeon must realize that diagnostic aids are of importance only when they are positive. Careful repeated physical examination and thoughtful analysis of each case still afford the best opportunity for correct diagnosis.

References

[1] Early care of acute soft tissue injuries. Chicago, Illinois, Committee on Trauma, Am. Coll. Surg., 1954.

[2] Medical Department, United States Army, Surgery in World War II. Washington, D. C., General Surgery, Office of the Surgeon General, Department of the Army, 1955, vol. 2.

[3] MORTON, J. H., HINSHAW, J. R., and MORTON, J. J.: Blunt trauma to the abdomen. Ann. Surg. 145: 699—711, 1957.

[4] SANDBLOM, P.: Hemorrhage into the biliary tract following trauma — Traumatic hemobilia. Surgery 24: 571—586, 1948.

[5] WISE, W. D.: Multiple peritoneal transplantation of splenic tissue following traumatic rupture of the spleen. Surg. Gynec. & Obst. 96: 427—429, 1953.

[6] MIKAL, S. and PAPEN, G. W.: Morbidity and mortality in ruptured liver. Surgery 27: 520—525, 1950.

[7] COTTRELL, J. C.: Nonperforative trauma to abdomen. Arch. Surg. 68: 241—251, 1954.

[8] GLENN, F. and MOORE, S. W.: Traumatic wounds of the abdomen. Surg. Clin. N. A. 23: 556—574, (April) 1943.

CHAPTER 29

TRAUMA TO THE KIDNEY, URETERS AND BLADDER

Victor F. Marshall, M.D.

The physician caring for the victims of trauma must view the patient as a whole while simultaneously diagnosing and treating the individual injuries. Such possibly associated disorders as shock, hemorrhage, severe head injury, open thoracotomy and cardiac tamponade nearly always take *immediate* precedence over the damage to the genitourinary tract — for the reason that the former are likely to be more immediately life-threatening. On the other hand, the patient's genitourinary damages frequently do not receive proper attention largely because the associated injuries are more readily evident, more common or more generally publicized. Early and late disasters are not rare following injury to the urinary tract, but many can be avoided and nearly all mitigated. Patients have been dramatically saved from acutely near-fatal injury, only to become urinary cripples because damage in that out of the way tract was overlooked and the therapy there, too little and, especially, too late.

Renal Injuries

The simplest renal injury is a minor contusion, and complete recovery may be expected clinically (fig. 1). In fact, many subtle contusions go unnoticed. A little flank pain and some red cells temporarily in the urine are usually the only indications of a mild contusion, and pyelography is nearly always normal. It is important, however, to know that a previously abnormal kidney can be seriously damaged by forces otherwise considered quite minor. For example, significant gross hemorrhage or dangerously aggravated infection may follow a relatively light blow to a hydronephrotic kidney.

Major contusions, commonly with some slight rupture or laceration, nearly always present clinical evidence. Patients with a major renal contusion have flank pain, hematuria and at least a tendency to shock. A capsular tear may permit a small or moderate perirenal hematoma. Spasm and tenderness in the flank are usually found, but if these signs seem particularly notable anteriorly, the possibility of intraperitoneal damage must also be considered. In fact, renal injuries from violence such as occurs in war time have been associated with intraperitoneal lesions of significince so frequently as to demand consideration in every case. When the injury has been thoraco-abdominal, multiple sites of serious damage in addition to the renal lesion can nearly always be anticipated.

Renal ruptures and lacerations are prone to cause serious difficulties. When such a lesion extends into the collecting portion of the urinary tract as well as through the renal capsule, urinary extravasation is probable. However, the clinical evidences of extravasation are commonly delayed because renal function is often in abeyance at least temporarily, and during

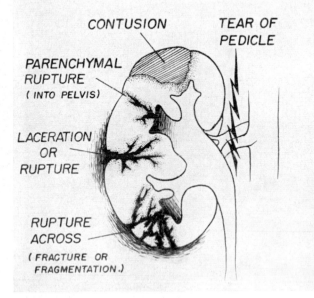

CONTUSION   TEAR OF PEDICLE

PARENCHYMAL RUPTURE (INTO PELVIS)

LACERATION OR RUPTURE

RUPTURE ACROSS (FRACTURE OR FRAGMENTATION.)

Fig. 1—Diagramatic representation of common traumatic renal lesions. From Textbook of Urology by V. F. Marshall, with permission of the publishers, Paul B. Hoeber, Inc.

this time considerable sealing by clot formation and inflammation may take place. Some time later infection may break down this seal, so that it is advisable to observe the patient, almost continuously for about two weeks and to use antibacterial drugs prophylactically. A clearly minor extravasation may be treated expectantly (fig. 2), but major extravasations are best drained surgically within a day or so (fig. 3). An intravenous pyelogram and careful following often suffice in the cases of lesser damage, but if all does not progress well or information is not adequate, retrograde pyelography may be indicated (figs. 4 and 5). It is valuable to realize that the damage is usually more extensive than the clinical and pyelographic findings portray.

Serious hemorrhage from the traumatized kidney is the most obvious immediate concern, although it is not the most common result of renal trauma. The signs of major and continuing bleeding are the clearest indications for immediate or very early operative intervention – increasing mass in the flank, increasing shock, etc. In these circumstances, it is of the utmost importance to have information about the opposite kidney because removal of the involved one is often the most direct way to avert the threat to life. A flat film of the abdomen may not only provide useful information concerning the traumatized side but may also reveal the size and position of the supposedly good kidney. Unless the blood pressure remains very

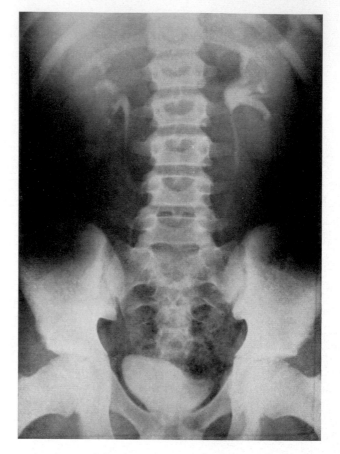

Fig. 2–Intravenous pyelogram following a blow to the right flank. Note slight extravasation of contrast downward from renal pelvis near kidney (this looks almost like a lower calyx) and filling defect in the renal pelvis probably caused by clot as well as some rupture. Note normal left kidney.

low or the emergency is extreme, an intravenous pyelogram is nearly always in order – even more to reveal the opposite kidney than to study the injured one (fig. 6). Such pyelography can be made in bed, using portable radiographic equipment. In some circumstances retrograde pyelography may be required to gain the necessary information. At operation, the supposedly good kidney can be palpated transperitoneally if necessity demands, but under no circumstances should a nephrectomy be done in the absence of reasonable information concerning the mate of the traumatized kidney

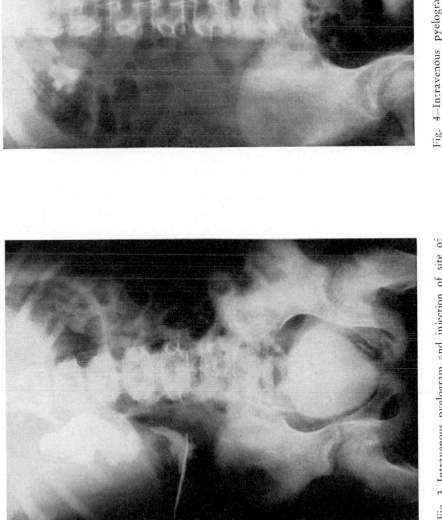

Fig. 4—Intravenous pyelogram after a fall in which the patient landed with the right flank across a concrete block. The upper calyces function but the lower part of kidney is not visualized. Note the normal left kidney.

Fig. 3—Intravenous pyelogram and injection of site of surgical drainage of an extravasation around right kidney. The right kidney was hydronephrotic before the trauma and ruptured through the lower calix. Note normal left kidney.

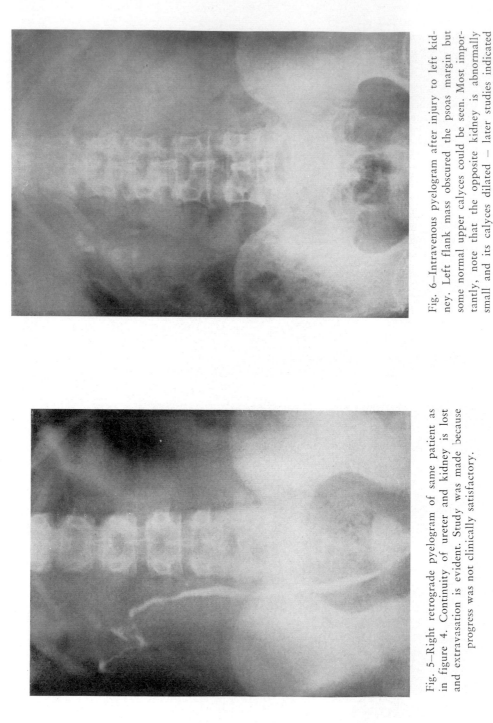

Fig. 6—Intravenous pyelogram after injury to left kidney. Left flank mass obscured the psoas margin but some normal upper calyces could be seen. Most importantly, note that the opposite kidney is abnormally small and its calyces dilated — later studies indicated a contracted pyelonephritic organ.

Fig. 5—Right retrograde pyelogram of same patient as in figure 4. Continuity of ureter and kidney is lost and extravasation is evident. Study was made because progress was not clinically satisfactory.

(fig. 7). If the patient has only one reliable kidney and operation is indicated, it is mandatory to perform repair only. On occasions, the blood loss may be from an open wound in the kidney or down the ureter. A tear across the renal pedicle is a rare event, but prompt surgical control has prevented some fatalities (many exanguinate before reaching a hospital).

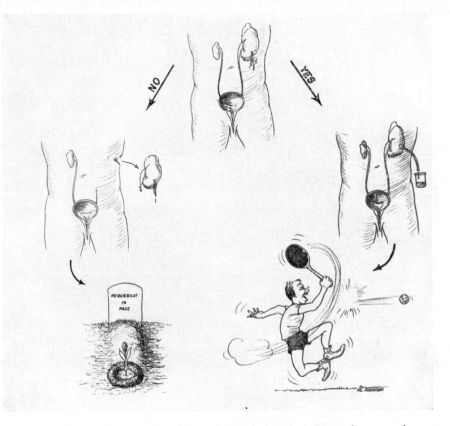

Fig. 7—To emphasize the necessity of knowing the opposite kidney when a nephrectomy is contemplated.

Ureteral Injuries

Ureteral injury from external violence is rare and likely to be associated with extensive damage in the area. Obviously the ureteral damage must be recognized and then controlled, or urinary infection and extravasation will add serious hazard both immediately and later. If there is good reason to believe that the continuity of the ureter has been interrupted by the external force, at the least, a simple surgical drainage is in order. Intravenous injection of indigo carmine at the start of operation may facilitate this diagnosis at exploration and aid in the localization of the injury. As with renal injuries, knowledge of the opposite side is of the greatest value.

Only rarely is nephrectomy permissible immediately following a ureteral injury. This holds even when the status of the opposite upper urinary tract is known to have been normal some time earlier, because patients thus greatly traumatized are likely to need all available renal function for convalescence. If a ureteral repair with external drainage is not feasible, transplantation of the ureter to the skin at any convenient level or nephrostomy above a ureteral ligation can be the method of choice. Prophylactic antimicrobial drug therapy is a great aid, though not the fundamental correction. Follow-up examinations, including intravenous pyelography and urinalysis, should be made at least a few months later and preferably for a year or two even if all appears highly satisfactory. Late hydronephrotic atrophy, infection, chronic uremia and hypertension are well known sequelae of renal or ureteral damage.

Injuries to the Bladder

Contusions, punctures, extraperitoneal and intraperitoneal ruptures may result from trauma to the urinary bladder. Contusion alone is not often recognized clinically, but can be the cause of red cells found transiently

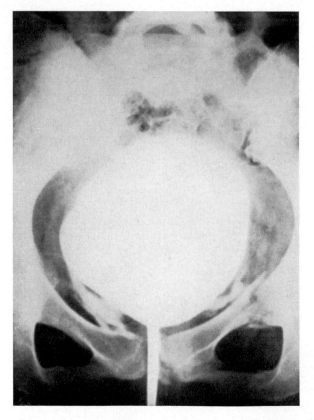

Fig. 8—Radio-opaque cystogram revealing extraperitoneal extravasation on both sides near the vesical base.

in the urine. Of course, hematuria of some degree accompanies all significant vesical injuries. Perforations via the abdominal wall call for the general measures advised in the care of external wounds (tetanus prophylaxis, etc.) and especially for measures to prevent urinary extravasations into the local

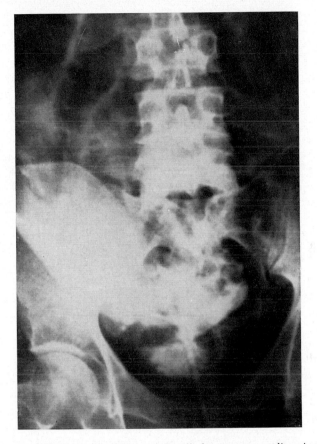

Fig. 9—Radio-opaque cystogram revealing nearly all the contrast medium inside the peritoneum (the blotchy contrast in the pelvis extending over the shadows of the sacrum and right iliac bone).

tissues or the peritoneum. The insertion of a cystostomy tube (occasionally through the wound itself) must always be favored as *drainage by cystostomy is the keystone to successful management* of major injuries to the bladder. A transurethral catheter also is useful, but it is pertinent to realize that this irritates and obstructs the urethra and prostate, and thus aggravates infection, which a cystostomy tube does not. In addition, because of its larger caliber a cystostomy catheter often functions better, particularly if clots and debris are present. Foreign bodies within the bladder should be removed at some convenient early time because they maintain infection and sooner or later tend to become incrusted into calculi. The bladder rarely ruptures unless it is distended at the time of the accident, and most are intraperitoneal in direction. It is important to know that a patient with a ruptured bladder may be able to pass some urine. A tendency to shock and signs of lower peritoneal irritation appear promptly with large ruptures but may develop slowly if the leakage is not free. When rupture is suspected, gentle clean catheterization provides information concerning possible urethral damage and particularly permits a cystogram with one of the contrast media used for intravenous pyelography (figs. 8 and 9). The entrance of the contrast medium into torn veins is quite common and accordingly only media tolerated intravenously are advisable. Injection of air is conducive to embolism. Instillation of a certain quantity and measurement of the return constitutes a test so unreliable and often misleading as to make it, at least, useless. (For example, a rupture without free leakage will give a falsely favorable test yet an intact organ with clots may provide an unfavorable test.) If there is a good suspicion of vesical rupture, cystostomy is indicated. The rent in the bladder should be simply sutured if at all feasible, but a large caliber cystostomy tube is the essential element in management. The incidence of additional intraperitoneal injuries is so great that at least a brief inspection there is nearly always advisable at the same time. Concerning cystostomies, it is better to do a few too many than a few too few — and promptness excels procrastination! Of course, general supportive measures and antimicrobial drugs are valuable in the program. Extraperitoneal ruptures, while less common than the intraperitoneal, provide similar indications except that the physical findings tend to be more localized to the pelvic area. Sometimes extravasation can be felt by rectal examination (and evidences of other damage, such as urethral rupture, may come as a surprise). The extra-peritoneal ruptures call for drainage, cystostomy and general supportive measures. Injuries at surgery and from irradiation have been considered as outside the scope of this chapter.

The following general program should provide sufficient specific diagnosis of urologic injury to permit logical therapy. The history taking and physical examination may be done simultaneously in true emergencies, but concentration on first one and then the other is more conducive to accuracy. A history of previous genitourinary disorders may be of major importance, yet questions in this direction are too often forgotten in the rush. Included in the physical examination are the characteristics of the pulse, the blood pressure, and other observations relative to possibly developing shock; and the patient should be carefully observed from time to time in this regard as well as concerning the likelihood of possibly associated injuries. The patient should be asked to void and the specimen saved for urinalysis. Watching the patient void may provide useful information. For example, a prompt, large caliber, forceful, continuous stream of grossly clear urine militates strongly against major urethral damage and partly against vesical rupture. A flat film of the abdomen is usually helpful and gentle catheterization is often indicated to test the urethra, obtain urine and permit cystography. Intra-venous pyelography can hardly be overemphasized as a diagnostic tool.

Cystoscopy and retrograde pyelography are reserved for specific indications – especially the indication that clearly needed information has not been obtained by the simpler and safer steps of the preliminary portion of the program. Developments may call for a change in plan of management at any time.

References

1 CLARKE, B. G., and LEADBETTER, W. F.: Management of wounds and injuries of the genito-urinary tract: A review of reported experiences in World War II. J. Urol. *67:* 719—739, 1952.

2 CULP, O. S.: Treatment of ruptured bladder and urethra: Analysis of 86 cases of urinary extravasation. J. Urol. *48:* 266—286, 1942.

3 LEWIS, L. G.: Treatment of wounds of the bladder and urethra: Surg. Clin. N. A. *24:* 1402—1409, 1944.

4 LYNCH, K. M., Jr.: Traumatic urinary injuries: Pitfalls in their diagnosis and treatment. J. Urol. *77:* 90—95, 1957.

5 ORKIN, I. A.: Management of trauma to the kidney. Internat. Abstr. Surg. *89:* 313—334, (Oct.) 1949.

6 SARGENT, S. C., and MORQUARDT, C. R.: Renal injuries. J. Urol. *63:* 1—8, 1950.

CHAPTER 30

INJURIES TO THE URETHRA AND GENITALIA

John W. Draper, M.D.

Injuries to the male urethra from external or internal trauma may cause contusion, laceration or rupture. The characteristic complications and sequelae of serious injury depend on the location of the trauma. The triangular ligament is the dividing fascial plane between the anterior and posterior urethra. Figures 1 and 2 illustrate the different pathways for extravasation of blood and urine in patients having rupture of the urethra anterior or posterior to the triangular ligament. If, however, the ligament itself is torn, extravasation may proceed in either direction from either side of the ligament.

The diagnosis of avulsion of the posterior urethra may be made from a history of severe injury often associated with fracture of the pelvis, bleeding from the urethra, pain in the lower abdomen and inability to void. Examination may reveal swelling of the lower abdomen with pain on gentle pressure. Usually, rectal examination reveals the prostate to be dislodged

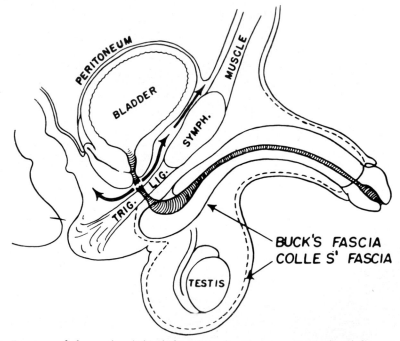

Fig. 1—Rupture of the urethra behind the triangular ligament. (Reproduced from the Textbook of Urology by V. F. Marshall through the courtesy of the publishers, Paul Hoeber, Inc.)

upwards in the pelvis and surrounded by boggy tissues infiltrated with fluid. It may be impossible to pass a catheter into the bladder. Injection of diluted intravenous contrast agent will demonstrate extravasation at the site of injury. Associated fractures of the bony pelvis are usually demonstrated on these films.

The management of this injury calls for prompt treatment of associated shock and re-establishment of continuity of the urethra. The retropubic approach to the urethra with end-to-end anastomosis over a catheter is the ideal treatment. However, because of technical difficulties, this is rarely accomplished. Therefore, the usual procedure is to identify the severed ends of the urethra by means of a retropubic exposure; pass a 24 French Foley catheter through the anterior urethra, guide it across the defect in the membranous urethra and inflate it in the bladder. Gentle traction applied to this catheter will appose the severed ends of the urethra. This approximation my be helped by passing mattress sutures on long straight needles from within the bladder out through the perineum and fastening them over rolled gauze to provide traction. Cystostomy drainage is always advisable because of the frequent failure of urethral catheter drainage. Loose particles of bone should be removed, and the extravasated blood and urine evacuated. Adequate drainage of the retropubic area is important.

Injury to the posterior urethra from internal violence is usually the result of instrumentation or electrosurgical procedures on the prostate. A physician

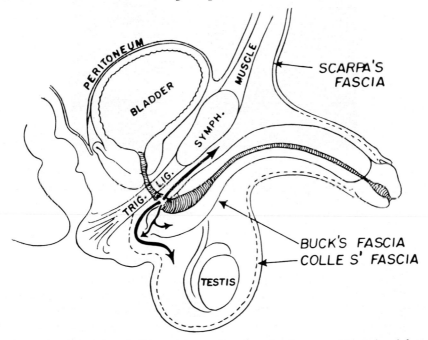

Fig. 2—Rupture of urethra (bulb) anterior to the triangular ligament. (Reproduced from the Textbook of Urology by V. F. Marshall through the courtesy of the publishers, Paul Hoeber, Inc.)

usually causes these injuries and he should diagnose and treat them as soon as they occur.

Laceration of the posterior urethra without loss of continuity is treated by drainage and urethral catheter.

Simple contusion of the urethra may produce edema and so require a catheter.

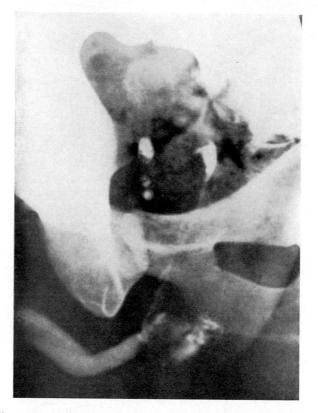

Fig. 3–Incomplete rupture of the urethra from straddle injury.

Injury to the urethra distal or anterior to the triangular ligament often results from internal or external violence. Internal injury in this part of the urethra is also usually caused by instrumentation. External trauma to the perineum as the result of straddle injuries compresses the bulb of the urethra against the symphysis pubis. If the injury is slight, the diagnosis is made from the history of injury and the presence of bleeding, which may be independent of urination or may be washed out with the urine. A soft catheter may be passed to the bladder if the continuity of the urethra is intact. The urethrogram is a diagnostic procedure. Toxic local anesthetics should not be injected into the traumatized urethra because of the danger of absorption. Death has followed the injection of procaine and similar agents into the injured urethra.

Figure 2 illustrates the various pathways of extravasating urine and blood in the more serious straddle type of injury. The perineum, scrotum and penis may become infiltrated with blood and urine. The diagnosis is made from the history of injury, bleeding from the urethra and swelling in the perineum, scrotum or shaft of the penis. The swelling may increase with voiding as urine follows along the fascial planes.

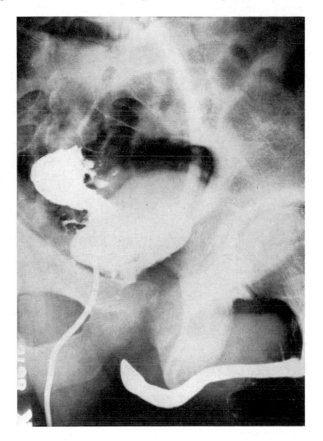

Figure 4.

Figure 3 is a urethrogram of a patient who had incomplete rupture of the urethra from a straddle injury. The point of injury is seen in the bulb, with extravasated media in the perineal tissues and a thin trickle of contrast media following the partially severed urethra to the bladder.

Figure 4 is a combined cystogram, urethrogram and proctogram. The film was made three months after the soldier stepped on a mine which exploded and tore away part of the rectum and urethra. Colostomy and cystostomy were done as emergency procedures, and when the patient's condition permitted, he was sent to a base hospital for further definitive treatment. He had had no erection since his injury, three months before he was admitted over the sacrum. Sensory examination was negative. The coccyx was nontender and the radiogram revealed a transverse, undisplaced fracture of the midsacrum as outlined by the arrows. Treatment consisted of bed rest only, no other therapy being necessary. Figure 3 is a roentgenogram of a 4 year old boy who fell against a corner of his bed and suffered

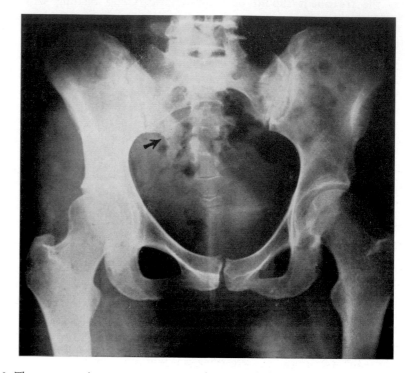

Fig. 2—The arrow points out a transverse fracture of the sacrum. There is seldom any serious associated neurological deficit with this injury.

pain in his back. He had pain on walking. There was tenderness over the sacrum and tenderness of the coccyx on bidigital rectal examination. X-rays revealed anterior displacement of the last coccygeal segment due to the pull of the anococcygeal muscles. He was placed at bed rest for two weeks until he was comfortable, and he was asymptomatic six weeks after injury. Again these fractures require nothing more than symptomatic therapy. Closed replacement can be attempted. This procedure, however, is usually doomed to failure, as the muscle pull will cause recurrence of the displacement. The patient should be warned that the period of healing can be prolonged, owing to the muscle forces continually in play. If severe disability due to pain persists after heat and bed rest, the patient need not necessarily be labelled an hysteric or a psychoneurotic. Watson-Jones [1] strongly states that coccygectomy should be considered in those patients who have severe disability following coccygeal fracture.

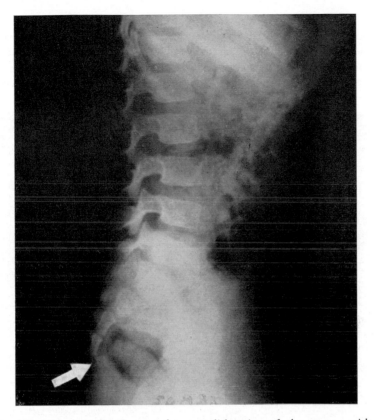

Fig. 3—In this child there has been a fracture dislocation of the coccyx with anterior displacement being maintained by the pull of the ischiococcygeal ligaments and surrounding anococcygeal muscles.

Fractures of the Pubis

These are the most frequent fractures of the pelvis and usually extend through one of the two major rings of the pelvis. The first ring is the brim of the pelvis separating the false and true pelvis. The second or vertical ring is that formed by the sacrum and ilium continuing down to the acetabulum. It has been demonstrated that the pelvis is an extremely well constructed structure. The pelvis remains intact under large degrees of force until one portion of the structural arches (rings) fails. Once one portion of the arch fails, however, the remainder of the arch rapidly disintegrates, and therefore one must always look for a second fracture of the pelvis when the first is demonstrated. For example, if the superior and inferior rami of the pubis are fractured, the sacroiliac joint should be carefully examination to see whether it is intact or whether some type of dislocation has taken place. Usually, the diagnosis of pelvic fracture can be easily confirmed by x-ray deformity. There is usually pain on motion of the lower extremities, tensing of the abdominal muscles or on sitting.

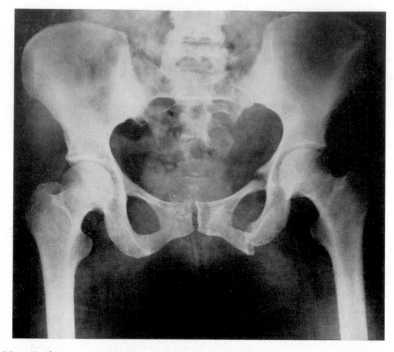

Fig. 6—Here is demonstrated definite left sacro-iliac dislocation with the classical upward (and posterior) displacement of the ilium.

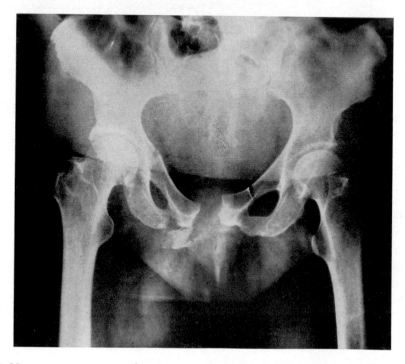

Fig. 7—Here are present several serious anterior pelvic injuries. The soft tissue damage associated with the bony deformities are the cause of great morbidity and mortality.

pared to the opposite side. After supportive therapy is carried out, reduction by manipulation can be attempted and then spica casting can be applied. Traction is another method of treatment using adductor tubercle traction with a Steinman pin and up to 30 pounds of weight. The usual complication associated with sacroiliac dislocations is that the reduction cannot be adequately accomplished or maintained. Traumatic arthritis of the sacroiliac joint is a frequent sequel, and if pain and disability become marked, Smith-Petersen sacroiliac fusion may be necessary.

Figure 6 is an x-ray of a 43 year old woman who was hit by a truck. She suffered open fracture of the olecranon, fractured ribs and fractured transverse processes of the lumbar spine. There was a fracture of the pubic and ischial rami and dislocation of the right sacroiliac joint. This picture shows that the ilium is displaced superiorly on the sacrum and that it rides some 2 to 3 cm. higher than the contralateral iliac crest. This patient

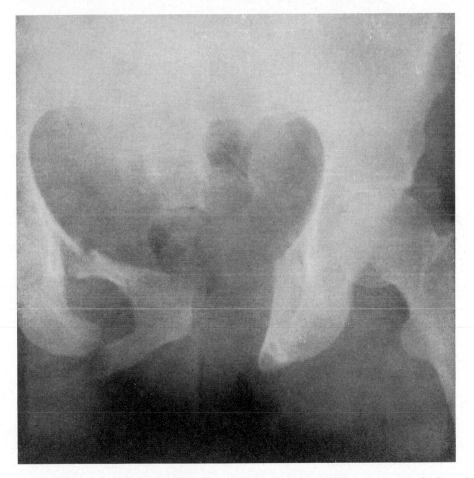

Fig. 8—(A) In these bilateral pubic and ischial fractures the left pubic and ischial rami have been displaced and rotated 90 degrees anteriorly.

was treated on a Bradford frame with bed rest for six weeks and had no sequelae.

Figure 7 demonstrates multiple injuries to the pelvis in a patient who had been hit by a truck. There are fractures of both pubic and ischial rami, and there is suggestion of a dislocation of the right sacroiliac joint. This injury is almost akin to a crushed pelvis.

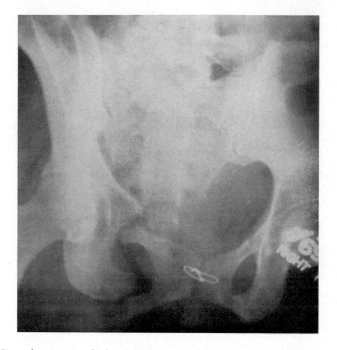

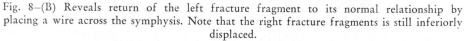

Fig. 8—(B) Reveals return of the left fracture fragment to its normal relationship by placing a wire across the symphysis. Note that the right fracture fragments is still inferiorly displaced.

Occasional severe pubic or ischial fractures are amenable to direct surgical intervention. Marked displacement of a pubic fracture may be corrected by an anterior surgical approach with replacement of the fracture and fixation by wire. Such an injury and the corrective procedure are demonstrated in figure 8.

Crushed Pelvis

The so-called "crushed pelvis" is a very severe injury; it rarely comes to treatment because it is associated with an extremely high rate of immediate or rapid fatality. Multiple arterial and visceral injuries almost always accompany the crushed pelvis. There can be any variation of fracture or combination of fractures as can be seen in figures 7 and 8. Treatment is aimed at support and at care of soft tissue injuries.

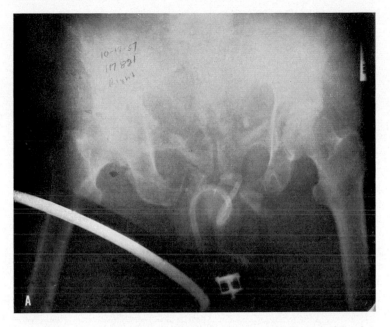

Fig. 9–(A) The multiple comminuted fractures in this partially "crushed" pelvis are well demonstrated. Note the urethral catheter which could not be passed into the bladder prior to cystotomy and laparotomy.

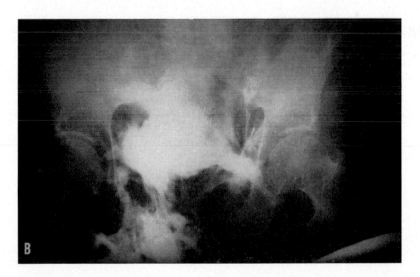

Fig. 9–(B) Here is well demonstrated a urethral rupture. The contrast medium injected by catheter has extravasated into the soft tissues.

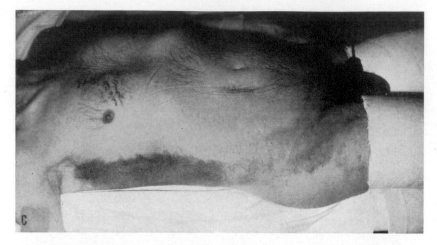

Fig. 9—(C) This is a clear demonstration of the large amounts of blood which collect in the retroperitoneal and dependent spaces following serious pelvic injury.

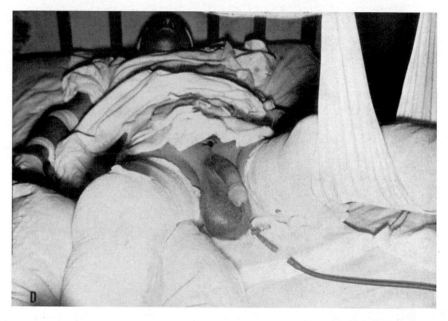

Fig. 9—(D) The large scrotum hemorrhage associated with urethral transection is well demonstrated here.

Urologic injury and retroperitoneal hemorrhage are frequently encountered in the "crushed pelvis." Aggressive diagnostic and therapeutic measures must be employed to save a patient sustaining such an injury. Figure 9 demonstrates several of the findings noted in this syndrome. This middle-aged man was crushed by the rear wheels of a pick-up truck while working

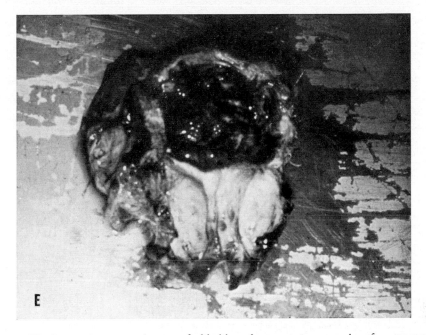

Fig. 9–(E) Post-mortem specimens of bladder demonstrates necrosis of postprostatic urethra and marked hemorrhagic cystitis.

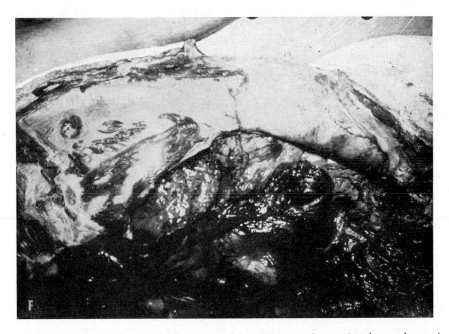

Fig. 9–(F) An autopsy view of the peritoneal cavity reveals massive hemorrhages into the leaves of the mesenteries of the large and small bowel and hematoma collects in the extraperitoneal tissues.

on a construction project. He sustained multiple fractures of the extremities and "crushed pelvis" (fig. 9 A). Cystography (fig. 9 B) revealed a ruptured urethra. The extent of hemorrhage associated with the pelvic fracture is well illustrated in figure 9 C. Here there is marked ecchymosis of the right flank and posterior thorax. Figure 9 D demonstrates the scrotal hemorrhage associated with urethral rupture (distal to the pelvic diaphragm). Figure 9 E illustrates the necrotic ruptured urethra, and figure 9 F illustrates marked peripelvic hemorrhage (autopsy specimens).

Diagnosis

Main points in diagnosis and treatment:

1. Bed rest is required for the various fractures, and it almost always leads to relief of symptoms.

2. Specimens of the urine should be checked immediately, and if necessary there should be cystography and catheterization. Abdominal examination should be carried out immediately and should be repeated frequently to see if there is any progression of signs or symptoms. Despite the patient's pain it is wise to withhold any large amount of analgesia which may mask abdominal findings. Immediate care of shock is, of course, important, and is carried out as it is in any other type of hemorrhagic shock. The incidence of ileus is relatively high owing to the retroperitoneal hemorrhage which so frequently accompanies pelvic fractures. The usual method of treatment for this is nasogastric suction, denial of oral intake, and administration of intravenous fluids. Prostigmine or urecholine can be used to hasten return of peristalsis. However, we seldom use parasympathomimetic drugs for this purpose at The New York Hospital. After six to eight weeks the patient has usually returned to full motion except in cases of complicated fractures which enter the sacroiliac joint or the acetabulum.

Complications of Pelvic Fractures

1. The most frequent complication and soft tissue injury accompanying pelvic fractures is urologic injury.

2. Rectal injury is rare. Diverting colostomy with repair of any rectal or rectosigmoid laceration can be carried out if the defect is above the peritoneal reflection. If the defect is below the peritoneal reflection, simple diverting colostomy is the procedure of choice. Proctoscopy is rarely necessary since rectal injuries with these fractures are extremely uncommon.

3. Sacral root injuries are also rare. There may be saddle anesthesia or incontinence, and here the treatment is purely symptomatic.

4. Retroperitoneal hemorrhage is a frequent finding at autopsy in multiple injuries. The lumbar veins are frequently torn, and since these vessels are fairly large, such injury can lead to a serious exsanguinating hemorrhage. Supportive therapy by the use of blood or blood substitutes is the only treatment possible. Exploration in the hope of stopping the bleeding is seldom of any avail.

5. One of the main reasons for fearing pelvic fracture in a girl is the possibility that there may be cephalopelvic disproportion when the patient grows up and bears children. Over the last five years at The New York Hospital, 26,000 pregnancies have been carried out to term. Among these women, 15 had a previous history of pelvic fractures. Of these, one underwent elective cesarean section because of cephalopelvic disproportion; three required forceps delivery, one as a prophylactic measure and two because of lack of progress; one aborted; the other ten underwent normal, full-term spontaneous deliveries. It was believed that 3 of the 15 patients who suffered previous fractures had some element of dystocia due to the injury. Accordingly we believe that at the time of confinement all patients with a history of pelvic fracture should be given a pelvic x-ray series to rule out cephalopelvic disproportion. This should be carried out even if the intrapelvic measurements are normal.

6. With the use of safety devices in automobiles, there has been the feeling that a "seat belt syndrome" may come into being. The seat belt, of course, exerts its main snubbing and restraining forces across the pelvis and upper femora, and many people interested in this problem have considered the possibility that the belts may cause an increase in pelvic fractures in automobile accidents. In 1,000 cases of injuries sustained while seat belts were in use, there was no increase in the incidence of abdominal or pelvic injuries. This is not yet statistically significant, and further data are still forthcoming.

Summary

Barring entrance into the sacroiliac joint or acetabulum, pelvic fractures of themselves seldom require definitive therapy to the bony injury. However, associated soft tissue injury and retroperitoneal hemorrhage are the main problems which must be dealt with efficiently, thoroughly, and immediately. Immediate urinalysis, catheterization to determine integrity of the urethra and bladder, and cystography are most important in treating possible urologic complications. Soft tissue injuries to other than the genitourinary tract are rare, except for massive retroperitoneal hemorrhage which must be treated by the usual method of treating hemorrhagic shock; symptomatic treatment of the osseus lesions by bed rest is usually all that is required.

V. THE EXTREMITIES

CHAPTER 32

FRACTURE DISLOCATIONS OF THE SHOULDER GIRDLE

Philip D. Wilson, Jr., M.D.

Anatomic And Functional Considerations

The shoulder girdle is a structure comprised of three bones – the clavicle, the scapula and the upper end of the humerus – and three articulations – the sternoclavicular, the acromioclavicular and the glenohumeral joints. This relatively complex mechanism functions as a unit to allow free movement of the arm in all planes, so that the hand, which is so distinctive to man, may perform all of its vital functions.

The *sternoclavicular joint* is doubly compartmented by an intra-articular fibrocartilaginous disc and has strong supporting ligaments. It allows forward protrusion and backward retraction of the clavicle and a certain amount of rotation and angulation. The *clavicle* when viewed from above presents an S curve, the leading curve of the S being in the medial one-half and the backward curve in the outer portion. Its medial articulation has already been described. Its *lateral articulation* is with the acromial process of the scapula to which it is bound by the acromioclavicular ligaments. It also, occasionally, has an intervening incomplete fibrocartilaginous disc. The strong coracoclavicular ligaments extend from the outer or backward portion of the S curve to the coracoid process of the scapula. They are relatively inelastic and prevent free angulation of the scapula on the distal end of the clavicle. The *scapula* is a broad, thin bone providing an articular surface for the head of the humerus, and a broad surface for muscular attachments. It is free to move on the chest wall by means of a large subscapular potential space or bursa. The clavicle and scapula together form a bony strut which supports the arm and which, at the same time, is capable of extending the range of all movements performed in the glenohumeral joint. As the result of angulation in the sternoclavicular joint and rotation of the clavicle on its longitudinal axis, the scapula can be rotated about 60 degrees, and this movement accounts for about one-third of elevation of the arm from the side.

The glenoid itself is much smaller than the humeral head and is enlarged by a cartilaginous lip or labrum glenoidale. The articular capsule (including its three glenohumeral ligaments) is rather lax, allowing the humeral head great freedom of movement. Under the acromion and the coraco-acromial ligament lies a large bursa, which extends out under the deltoid. The floor of the subacromial or subdeltoid bursa is formed by the musculotendinous cuff, a conjoint structure made up of the subscapularis in front, the supraspinatus on top, and the infraspinatus and teres minor behind. It is interrupted only at the point where the biceps tendon emerges from its intracapsular position on its way to the intertubercular sulcus. The cuff muscles are not only the prime movers in rotation, but are absolutely essential to the movement of abduction. With the deltoid alone, abduction cannot be accomplished. A force couple action is necessary in which the rotator muscles stabilize the upper end of the humerus against the glenoid while the deltoid levers the humeral shaft upwards. In elevating the arm from the side, scapular rotation and glenohumeral abduction operate concomitantly to provide a smooth motion, aptly termed "scapulohumeral rhythm" by Codman.

Closely adjacent to the shoulder girdle lie the vital structures of the axilla and base of the neck, the subclavian vessels and brachial plexus. They are sometimes involved in injuries of the clavicle or shoulder joint. The axillary nerve deserves special emphasis since it passes from the posterior cord of the brachial plexus under the neck of the humerus and is not infrequently injured by dislocation of the shoulder. It supplies the teres minor and deltoid muscles, and sends a cutaneous branch to the skin overlying the tip of the acromial process. By examining the cutaneous sensation in this region, an injury of the nerve often can be diagnosed when the shoulder is too painful to move.

Sternoclavicular Joint

Dislocations of the sternoclavicular joint are rare. Only four cases, have been well enough documented to make evaluation worth while. One case resulted from a specific injury. Closed reduction was attempted, but it did not appear that much was accomplished. The inner end of the clavicle remained prominent, but there was no pain or interference with function. The three other cases were more in the nature of recurrent subluxations. One subsided with protection alone, but another was repaired by means of a fascial sling. In each instance, prominence remained, but again function was unimpaired and there was no pain. X-ray diagnosis is difficult in these cases but is facilitated by laminography.

Clavicle

Fractures of the clavicle are relatively common and usually result from a blow against the shoulder. Displacement is usually caused by the weight of the upper extremity, which drags the outer fragment downwards, and in the absence of end-to-end apposition, there is overriding.

In children, the fracture is often of the greenstick variety and usually occurs in the middle third. Considerable angulation can be accepted, especially in young children, since growth will tend to overcome the deformity. End-to-end apposition is desirable in order to provide some stability, but is not absolutely necessary. Open reduction is seldom if ever indicated and immobilization is best secured and length maintained by a figure of 8 dressing, either made from a strap, which is kept tight by daily adjustment, or of plaster combined with sling support of the arm.

After completion of growth, fractures of the clavicle are usually complete and are most common in the middle third or at the outer end close to the acromioclavicular joint. Accurate reduction is advisable to prevent ugly prominence in middle third fractures, though sometimes this is caused by exuberant callus. Function is not disturbed unless there is gross angulation or displacement. Manipulative reduction can often be achieved after local anesthesia under suitable sterile precautions, and sometimes is facilitated by the use of towel clips placed on the bone through the skin. If marked displacement cannot be overcome by conservative measures, open reduction with metallic fixation is usually advisable. A square clavicular pin has been found most useful, but the surgeon should be quite certain that it is strong enough and adequately placed since there is a strong tendency toward recurrence of the deformity. The S-shaped curve of the clavicle makes intramedullary insertion of the pin difficult and usually it will have to be passed through the cortex of at least one fragment. This is best done by passing it retrogade into the distal fragment, then reducing the fracture and tapping the pin back into the proximal fragment. The end should be buried just underneath the skin, since this will allow early mobilization, which is the great advantage of skeletal fixation. After open reduction and intramedullary fixation, bony union is often delayed, but nonunion must be very rare since it has not been encountered in the 26 cases studied.

Fractures of the outer portion of the clavicle sometimes involve the acromioclavicular joint, and when they do are best treated by resection of the outer end. In performing this operation, one should be careful to preserve the coraco-acromial ligaments. Otherwise, the outer end of the remaining fragment tends to become unduly prominent as the rest of the shoulder girdle drops away from it. For undisplaced fractures, treatment should be the same as for those in the middle third.

Acromioclavicular Joint

Acromioclavicular separation can be classified into two general types; first, those with minimal displacement, in which the coracoclavicular ligaments are not ruptured and second, those with gross displacement, where the ligament is badly torn. The best way to demonstrate the severity of injury is by taking an AP x-ray of both shoulders with the patient holding a 5 pound weight in the hands.

When separation is slight, some form of immobilization is all that is necessary, and an elastic traction strapping maintained by an interconnecting rubber link with pressure over the clavicle on the top and with pressure underneath the olecranon below will usually be sufficient. The forearm is best left unsupported so that its weight applied over the fulcrum provided by pressure against the under surface of the olecranon will tend to raise the shoulder and thus overcome the downward displacement of the acromion. Careful nursing attention is necessary in order to prevent undue discomfort or pressure sores.

In the presence of gross displacement, it is almost impossible to maintain reduction by this means. Open reduction is better for these cases since it minimizes the period of immobilization and favors a better result. Fixation is best maintained by means of Steinmann pins or fairly heavy Kirschner wires across the acromioclavicular joint into the clavicle. (When internal fixation is used, the patient should be prepared for its removal at the end of six weeks.) At the same time, the coracoclavicular ligaments should always be explored and repaired. In older cases, or in the presence of severe damage, a fascial sling passed from coracoid to clavicle will be helpful. If there is associated fracture of the outer end of the clavicle, removal of this section of the bone is advisable. Functional results are usually pretty satisfactory. In a heavy-muscled individual, residual mild displacement will not be apparent, whereas, in a thin person, the undue prominence may be ugly and make the patient unhappy. There may sometimes be pain, but this is rarely disabling.

Scapula

Fracture of the scapula is not a particularly common injury. It is usually caused by a direct violence, and the fractures are frequently comminuted. Associated injury of the ribs should be looked for. Radical or open therapy has not been necessary in our cases, despite involvement of the glenoid in several instances. Unless trauma has been extensive, usually only immobilization with a sling and early pendulum exercises are necessary. When there is a fracture across the base of the acromial process, it is usually slow to heal and sometimes persists as a fibrous union. Operative interference is required only when the incomplete union is painful, since function is usually quickly regained.

Shoulder (Glenohumeral) Joint

Anterior dislocations of the glenohumeral joint are relatively common, and next in frequency to fractures of the clavicle. Displacement is usually to the subcoracoid position but sometimes is subglenoid. The large majority of our cases have occured in the age group of 40 and over. Only a few have been epileptics, but one should always question the patient for a history of convulsions.

Reduction is usually easily secured in cases seen soon after injury and often is affected by simple traction, without anesthesia. There are many methods of reduction, and almost everyone has his favorite. The least traumatic is done with the patient in the face prone position, with the arm hanging over the edge of a table or stretcher. The patient can hold a weight in the hand to add to the traction, or this can be produced by the surgeon. Patience and gradual steady traction are the keys to success. The arm should be gently externally rotated if traction alone does not accomplish reduction. This method, or any that uses steady traction, is usually successful. If reduction is difficult to secure, or if the case is more than a few hours old, anesthesia is helpful.

Subsequent to reduction, the arm should be retained in a sling for a period of a week, then circumduction exercises begun. It is important to emphasize, however, that this plan of postreduction, therapy is indicated only in the older age group. A review of our cases of recurrent dislocations indicates that they all developed from injuries occurring in young people, most of them in the age group of 10 to 30. Though it is an open question whether the length of the period of immobilization has much to do with the tendency toward recurrence, immobilization should be maintained for at least three weeks in young people. Nicola[3] has actually recommended eight weeks, and since stiffness is less to be feared in this age group, it is probably better to err on the conservative side. X-rays of the original injury rarely indicate the cause of recurrence. A view of the arm in internal rotation will frequently show a compression fracture of the posterior portion of the head of the humerus, but this often does not appear until after there have been several recurrences. A "Bankhart lesion"[4-6] of the antero-inferior portion of the labrum glenoidale has been the most frequent finding in our operative cases.

Posterior dislocations, though rare, do occur. When recurrent, they are not necessarily the result of any specific injury since they may be due to a congenital laxity of the joint. These cases occur among young adolescents who are continually coaxed by their fellow students to demonstrate the trick of popping the shoulder in and out. If the child can be taught to refrain from this activity, very often the shoulder will tighten up spontaneously with passage of time. True traumatic posterior dislocations are recognizable from the internally rotated position of the arm. This is readily seen in the x-ray though one may be fooled if one does not look carefully. An axillary view, or at least an AP view in three separate rotations, is helpful in making accurate diagnosis. Though reduction may not be difficult, retention of the reduced position often is. It has been pointed out by Wilson and McKeever[7] that the temporary use of a Kirschner wire passed through the acromion into the humeral head provides sufficient stability to preserve reduction. Open reduction with repair of the posterior capsule was used successfully in one of our cases where closed reduction had been found most unstable.

Complicated Dislocations: Out of 50 anterior dislocations, fracture of the greater tuberosity occurred 13 times. There was no correlation to the extent or nature of injury. Usually, reduction is no more difficult than in simple dislocations and in the large majority of cases, reduction of the dislocation will at the same time accomplish anatomic reposition of the fractured tuberosity. However, healing time is definitely prolonged and circumduction exercises should be started early, in most cases, about two weeks after injury in order to prevent later stiffness. If there is a persistent displacement of all or a portion of the greater tuberosity, (and this occurs more frequently in the presence of comminution), one must assume that there has been a rather extensive tear in the musculotendinous cuff and open reduction is indicated. Suture of the torn portion of the cuff is necessary in order to maintain reduction, and if carried out early will prevent permanent disability.

Injuries can occur to the brachial plexus or axillary nerve and one should always examine for the circulatory status as well as for nerve function. In the only case of axillary nerve paralysis due to dislocation explored by the author, the nerve was found in continuity, and neurolysis sometime after the injury had occurred did not seem to help in this case. However, treatment of the nerve injury should be carried out with the same principles in mind as will be discussed in the section on peripheral nerve injuries.

Delayed unreduced dislocations are unfortunately still anything but rare. It is often difficult to secure a stable, closed reduction four weeks or more after injury, and open operation may be indicated in these cases. At operation, the glenoid cavity will have to be enlarged by removal of scar tissue and the musculotendinous cuff will usually have to be incised in order to complete reduction. The results in these cases will, of course, not be as satisfactory as in one in which a closed reduction was performed shortly after dislocation. However, some degree of function without pain will often result.

The remainder of complicated dislocations of the shoulder comprise a group of injuries most difficult to treat. Fortunately, they are not common. They are better called fracture dislocations, since the dislocation is only a small part of the injury and is often missed at the time of initial treatment. The fractures may involve the surgical neck, the tuberosities, or the humeral head itself, or all three together, and are often markedly comminuted. No generalizations can be made about this group, and anyone who has had any experience with them knows that they are frequently complicated problems to handle. Closed reduction is all but impossible to obtain and open reduction, though advisable, is at best difficult. When operating, be careful to avoid injury to the axillary artery, since this sometimes is compressed by the humeral head and can easily be lacerated. Aseptic necrosis of the humeral head often presents itself as a delayed and disastrous complication. Where injury is too extensive to enable satisfactory closed or open reduction, removal of the head of the humerus with the substitution of a Neer prosthesis [8] is justified. When this prosthesis is used, the surgeon should be careful to get as good a repair of the musculotendinous cuff as possible. Simple resection of the humeral head usually leads to a flail shoulder, whereas the use of the metallic prosthesis has resulted in a modicum of function with less pain.

In fractures of the surgical neck of the humerus, one will often note that the humeral head lies low in the glenoid though it is actually not dislocated. Sometimes an erroneous diagnosis of dislocation will be made. The cause of this relaxation of the shoulder is not known. It may be due to a pain reflex or to soft tissue injury. In any case, no specific treatment of the subluxation is indicated. With healing of the fracture and protection of the shoulder, the subluxation is overcome, and exercise usually does not have to be delayed. [9]

In dealing with injuries of the shoulder girdle, always remember that its prime function is to mobilize the hand. Do not forget the hand while treating the shoulder. Remember that edema will cause stiffness of the fingers and a stiff hand is much worse than a stiff shoulder. It is necessary, therefore to remind the patient to move his fingers from the start. Begin pendulum exercises of the shoulder as soon as possible, even with the arm still in a sling.

References

1 INMAN, SAUNDERS and ABBOTT: Observations on the function of the shoulder joint. J. Bone & Joint Surg. *26:* 3, 1944.

2 CODMAN, E. A.: The Shoulder. Boston, Thomas Todd Co., 1934.

3 NICOLA, T.: Acute anterior dislocation of the shoulder. J. Bone & Joint Surg. *31 A:* 153, 1949.

4 BANKHART, A. S. B.: An operation for recurrent dislocation (subluxation of sterno-clavicular joint). Brit. J. Surg. *26:* 320, 1938.

5 —: Pathology and treatment of recurrent dislocation of the shoulder joint. Brit. J. Surg. *26:* 23, 1938.

6 —: Recurrent or habitual dislocation of the shoulder joint. Brit. M. J. *2:* 1132, 1923.

7 WILSON, J. C. and McKEEVER, F. M.: Traumatic posterior (retroglenoid) dislocation of the humerus. J. Bone & Joint Surg. *31 A:* 160, 1949.

8 NEER, C. S. H.: Articular replacement for the humeral head. J. Bone & Joint Surg. *37 A:* 215, 1955.

9 THOMPSON, F. R., and WINANT, E. M.: Unusual fracture-subluxations of the shoulder joint. J. Bone & Joint Surg. *32 A:* 575, 1950.

CHAPTER 33

FRACTURE OF THE HUMERUS

WILLIAM COOPER, M.D.

This chapter is concerned with simple fractures of the humeral shaft exclusive of the elbow and shoulder regions, which are dealt with elsewhere. These are fractures which, for the most part, are easily treated by a variety of methods; good results may be expected in most cases. They usually unite readily, often despite careless and even inadequate treatment. Unlike fractures in other long bones, shortening is not a serious problem unless marked, and angular deformities within limits are obscured by the overlying muscles, or compensated for in the extensive range of motion in both elbow and shoulder. Paradoxically, the complications of fractures of the humerus though infrequent, constitute some of the most difficult of all fracture problems.

The form which a fracture of the humerus takes is quite variable. It may be transverse at any level, spiral, or comminuted to any degree. The origin and mechanism of injury generally explains the nature of the fracture. These range from tests of strength which may produce the historic spiral fracture to the shattering effects of crushing injuries and transmitted stresses from falls on the outstretched hand. For the most part, the configuration of the fracture is no reliable guide to difficulty in management or speed of repair. The fracture which is simplest in appearance may actually prove most reluctant to unite.

Muscle stresses do tend to displace the fragments but rarely to an important degree. Anatomically, one expects abduction of the proximal fragment when a fracture is below the insertion of the supraspinatus but above the pectoralis major. When the fracture is between the insertions of the pectoralis and deltoid, the proximal fragment tends to adduct. Distal to the deltoid insertion, the proximal fragment again is often found abducted. Actually, malposition results less from muscle pull than it does from the force of injury, the lack of support for the arm, and from injudicious manipulation.

Most uncomplicated fractures of the humeral shaft may be satisfactorily treated by sugar-tong splints of plaster of Paris, perhaps bandaging the splinted arm to the trunk, and maintaining the forearm in a collar and cuff sling. This is especially true for spiral fractures and high fractures which are only slightly angulated. The splint should begin in the axilla, fit closely around the elbow and be carried upward as far as the acromion. It is bandaged in position before hardening. Elbow and axilla must be well padded to avoid friction and pressure. This simple immobilization limits further angulation of the fragments, maintains relative alignment and prevents or discourages distraction. It has the advantage of simplicity, and provides most patients with fair comfort even during the initial period of fracture healing. The sugar-tong splint, bandage and sling may be considered the first line of defense in the treatment of most fractures of the humeral shaft. In fractures high in the shaft when the deformity is slight and the fragments impacted, the sugar-tong splint may be omitted, because the sling alone is sufficient.

The hanging cast has achieved great but perhaps undeserved popularity in the treatment of humeral fractures. Its use has oversimplified the management of this injury at the expense of sound principles of fracture care. In most instances the traction which the cast produces is not required, and in no instance is separation of the fracture fragments desirable. If traction were required, the hanging cast would be rendered ineffective when the patient was recumbent. Its widespread use has probably contributed to a greater incidence of non-union than would otherwise be encountered with this rapidly healing fracture. The hanging cast should be used only with caution and with a clear recognition of the dangers and penalties. A light hanging cast does have occasional value in the management of certain comminuted fractures where there is shortening or over-riding of the fragments.

Certain humeral shaft fractures require special handling if prompt union in satisfactory position is to be obtained. These include (1) high fractures in which the angular deformity is great, (2) transverse fractures with wide displacement or poor stability, (3) fractures with interposition of soft parts between the fragments preventing reduction and (4) fractures presenting neurologic or vascular complications.

Marked angular deformity, especially with adduction of a short proximal fragment, should be reduced if satisfactory alignment and range of motion are to be restored. This is generally accomplished by manipulation under anesthesia. Local anesthesia is likely to prove insufficient and general anesthesia is preferable. Following reduction, maintainance in an abduction shoulder spica with the arm abducted may be required to retain alignment. This should be employed for approximately six weeks and followed by a sling and the gradual institution of active motion. These measures usually suffice to allow healing.

Some transverse fractures with displacement require manual reduction under anesthesia. If satisfactory reduction is accomplished, it is followed by the application of a sugar-tong splint, bandage and sling. If interposition of soft parts interferes, or if reduction is unstable, open reduction and fixation is justified. The anterolateral approach to the humeral shaft described by Henry assures adequate visualization of most fracture sites. If there are signs of radial nerve palsy, a posterolateral approach is recommended to allow exposure of the nerve.

Intramedullary pin fixation of humeral shaft fractures is not justified as a routine procedure. When, however, adequate reduction is difficult to attain, Rush pins provide a satisfactory means of controlling position of the fragments. The fracture is reduced through a short incision followed by placement of a curved intramedullary pin extending through the greater tuberosity to the external condyle. If further stability is required, a supplemental pin may be driven proximally through the medial epicondyle. Other entrance sites can be employed. Blind passage of the nail requires special reduction equipment, flouroscopy technic, and often a measure of pure luck for success. It cannot be recommended for routine use. The most suitable fractures for intramedullary fixation are transverse fractures in the middle and lower thirds of the shaft and spiral fractures in the middle and upper thirds. In certain instances it is also useful in high unimpacted fractures. It is important that a nail of adequate size and length be employed. If the diameter of the nail is too small, rotation of the fragments will occur, and if the nail is too short, the fixation in cancellous bone will be inadequate.

Following intramedullary fixation, a plaster cast is not usually required and early exercise of the shoulder and elbow may be instituted, even on the third or fourth postoperative day. It should again be emphasized that internal fixation of fresh humeral shaft fractures is not usually indicated and should never be employed as a routine measure. Intramedullary fixation of patho- logic fractures, on the other hand, is of specific advantage in their management.

Other methods of internal fixation may be of value in selected cases in which a stable reduction cannot be secured. Multiple screw fixation is often well suited to long oblique and spiral fractures. A bone plate and screws are occasionally advisable for transverse fractures.

If motion can be demonstrated at the fracture site after five to six weeks of immobilization in a sugar-tong splint, delayed union should be suspected and the fixation should be considered inadequate. Application of a spica is advisable at this point to provide more secure fixation of the fracture fragments. If union should fail to occur after an additional twelve to sixteen weeks, open operation and bone-grafting would be advisable to hasten consolidation.

Most fractures of the humerus will develop sufficient union in five to six weeks to permit removal of the sugar-tong splint and bandage. If there is no motion on clinical examination, and x-rays demonstrate early callous forma- tion at the fracture site, active exercise for both the shoulder and elbow may be initiated. The arm is kept supported in a sling, but at least twice daily it may be removed for pendulum exercises of the shoulder. In addition, the shoulder should be carried gently through a full range of motion. Passive assistance to the shoulder is permitted, provided that it is painless. On the other hand, passive manipulation of the elbow is never justified. Active elbow exercises are, however, instituted at the same time that shoulder motion is started. Persistent shoulder stiffness may be a problem following fracture of the humerus, especially in the elderly patient, while serious limitation of elbow function is unusual unless forcible manipulation has been employed. Active motion of the fingers, hand and wrist should, of course, be encouraged from the very onset.

The complications of delayed union, radial nerve palsy and brachial artery damage are dealt with elsewhere. Fortunately, they are uncommon, as is residual disability following humeral shaft fractures. Indeed in fractures of the humerus, after four to six weeks immobilization and a few further weeks of exercise to regain shoulder and elbow motion, most patients should be able to resume their previous activities.

References

[1] ALTMAN, H.: Metallic fixation for pathologic fracture and impending fracture of long bones in patients with osseous metastases. J. Internat. Coll. Surgeons *19:* 612, 1953.

[2] BLOUNT, W.: Fractures in Children. Williams and Wilkins, Baltimore, 1955.

[3] BÖHLER, L.: Treatment of Fractures. Grune and Stratton, New York, 1957.

[4] BREMMER, R. A., and JELLIFFE, A. M.: Management of pathological fractures of the major long bones from metastatic cancer. J. Bone & Joint Surg. *40 B:* 652—659, Nov., 1958.

[5] BURGESS, E. M. and ROMANO, R. L.: Fractures in the aged. Clin. orthop. *11:* 28—29, 1958.

[6] CAVE, E. F. et al.: Fractures and Other Injuries. Yearbook Publishers, Chicago, 1958.

[7] DAVIS, C. B., Jr., Fractures of the humerus. J.A.M.A. *146:* 430, (June 2) 1951.

[8] HADJISTAMOFF, B.: New method of portable skeletal traction for compound fracture of humerus. J. Internat. Coll. Surgeons *12:* 875—882, (Nov.) 1949.

[9] JONES, L.: Fracture of upper end and shaft of humerus; simple conservative method of treatment. Surg., Gynec. & Obst. *83:* 126—128, July, 1946.

[10] LA FERTE, A. D., and NUTTER, P. D.: Hanging cast. Ann. Surg. *114:* 919, 1941.

[11] MASSIE, W. K., and ECKER, A.: Internal fixation of bone and neurorrhaphy; combined lesions of radial nerve and fracture. J. Bone & Joint Surg. *29:* 977—989, (Oct.) 1947.

[12] RUSH, L. V., and RUSH, H. L.: Intramedullary fixation of fractures of humerus by longitudinal pin. Surgery *27:* 268—275, (Feb.) 1950.

[13] SEDDON, H. J.: Nerve lesions complicating closed bone injuries. J.A.M.A. *135:* 691—694.

[14] STEWART, M. J. and HUNDLEY, J. M.: Fractures of the humerus. A comparative study in methods of treatment. J. Bone & Joint Surg. *37 A:* 681—692, (July) 1955.

[15] STREET, D. M., HANSON, H. H., and BREWER, B. J.: Medullary nail; presentation of new type and report of case of fracture of humerus. Arch. Surg. 55—423, 1947.

[16] WATSON-JONES, R.: Fractures and Joint Injuries. Williams and Wilkins, Baltimore, 1955.

CHAPTER 34

INJURIES TO THE ELBOW

PRESTON A. WADE, M.D.

Fractures and dislocations of the elbow joint are very common in both adults and children and many of them are exceedingly difficult to treat so as to achieve a satisfactory result. Particularly in children, these fractures are perhaps the most challenging with which the surgeon has to deal.

The hinge joint of the elbow and the rotary motion of the forearm are essential for the proper function of the prehensile quality of the hand. Any serious interference with elbow joint motions may make the hand and arm useless. It is therefore essential that the integrity of the elbow joint be meticulously preserved. Although it is possible to accept marked anatomic displacements in other joints, such as the shoulder, the fragments of fractures in the elbow must be replaced accurately so as to allow free motion of the tightly held joint. Although it is possible to excise the upper end of the radius above the bicipital tuberosity and still achieve good function (if there is no injury to the distal radial-ulnar joint), it is essential that the articulation between the humerus and the ulna be carefully preserved.

The elbow joint is also the most frequent site of two serious complications: one seen early, Volkman's ischemic paralysis; and the other, occuring as a late complication, myositis ossificans. Fortunately neither of these complications is common.

Volkman's Ischemic Paralysis

Because the anterior cubital space is tightly confined within the lacertus fibrosis fascia, injuries in this region often result in tremendous swellings when displacement, edema and hemorrhage beneath the fascia cause serious interference with circulation to the forearm. After an injury to the elbow joint, excessive swelling may result in pain, pallor and paralysis of the muscles of the forearm, indicating impending Volkman's ischemic paralysis. If the condition is not recognized quickly and treated adequately, the tragic permanent disability of flexion contracture of the hand may result. The most important considerations are prompt reduction of the fracture and elevation of the limb. It is also essential that no constricting circumferential bandaging be applied so as not to add to the constriction of the contents of the ante-cubital space. In many instances flexion of the joint may be the proper position for maintaining reduction of the fracture, but extension may be necessary to allow return of the radial pulse. Maintenance of circulation is much more important than maintenance of the position of fracture fragments. If reduction, plaster immobilization and elevation of the limb do not afford return of circulation, it then may be necessary to apply skeletal traction through the upper end of the ulna just below the olecranon (fig. 6 C and D) for suspension and elevation. If circulation does not return to the hand within a few hours, it is then necessary to operate on the antecubital space and incise the lacertus fibrosis fascia, thus decompressing the area. Usually this will suffice to correct the situation, but if there has been an injury to the brachial artery, it may be necessary to resect and graft this vessel.

Myositis Ossificans

This condition is an ossification of subperiosteal hematoma and calcification within the fibers of the brachialis anticus muscle with eventual ossification of its fibers (fig. 1 B). It occurs frequently enough in this area to make it

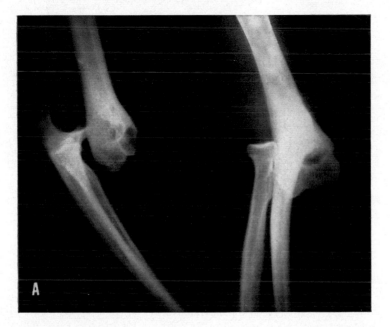

Fig. 1—(A) Dislocation of elbow without fracture in adult of 35.

necessary for a surgeon to always consider its possibility. There is no known cause for the deposit of calcium in this area, and one can never predict whether or not myositis ossificans may occur. It is probably the result of stripping up of the periosteum due to marked displacement of the fracture fragments and should therefore be considered as a possibility in severely displaced fractures with marked swelling. There is no specific treatment for this condition, but it is known to occur more frequently in those cases in which manipulation has been excessive. The possibility of the formation of calcium should be considered in all fractures about the elbow, and frequent x-ray examination will pick up the beginning signs of calcium deposit in the stiffened elbow. There is only one essential treatment, and that is to discontinue passive joint stretching which often is responsible for the condition. The elbow joint should never be passively stretched after injury under any circumstances. The pernicious habit of urging children to carry pails of sand to stretch the stiffened elbow and the continued passive stretching of the masseuse are most certain to cause the stiffening to become more severe and permanent. Sir Reginald Watson-Jones has advocated that the stiffened elbow never be referred to a physical therapy technician so that there be no

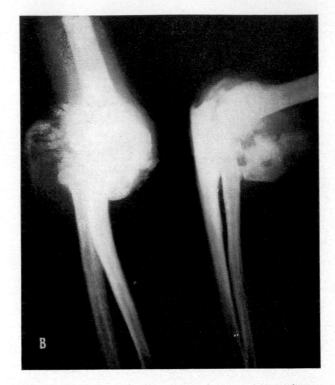

Fig. 1—(B) Six months later. Extensive myositis ossificans.

temptation to stretch the limb. The elbow joint will regain normal motion if the patient is allowed to use the arm and to move it actively within the limits of pain. It takes considerable patience on the part of the doctor, the parent and the patient himself to allow nature to take its proper course and to refrain from attempting to hasten recovery by means of stretching. Passive stretching of the joint causes tearing of muscles, further hemorrhage and formation of granulation tissue and scar, which further increases the loss of motion. It is well to keep in mind the admonitions of Böhler and the aphorisms illustrated in Chapter 15 (figs. 1 and 2).

Fractures in the Lower end of the Humerus — Supracondylar Fractures

Supracondylar fractures occur most frequently in children. Transcondylar, dicondylar and intercondylar fractures (T-fractures) occur most frequently in adults.

The supracondylar fracture is usually sustained by a fall on the extended arm. Most commonly the fracture is short and oblique from the front of the bone upward and backward, and the distal fragment is usually displaced posteriorly and angulated anteriorly (fig. 2). On rare occasions, when the

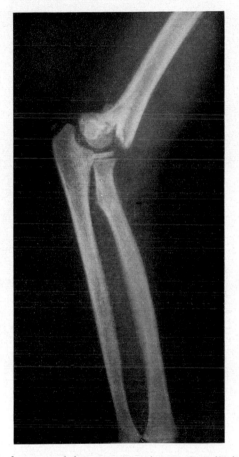

Fig. 2—Supracondylar fracture of humerus. Usual posterior displacement with anterior angulation.

fracture results from a fall on the flexed elbow, the displacement of the distal fragment is anterior (fig. 3). The posterior displacement of the distal fragment and the subsequent angulation is often one cause of interference of circulation in the forearm, and prompt replacement of the fractured fragment will often result in return of normal circulation. For this reason, delay in the treatment of fractures about the elbow is not justifiable.

In the usual supracondylar fracture (fig. 2), reduction is best accomplished by manipulation. The patient should be given a general anesthetic, and traction applied to the long axis of the limb. After traction has corrected the overriding, the fragment is pulled forward and held by means of flexion of the forearm. At the same time, lateral displacements are corrected, the lower fragment being pushed inward if it is displaced outward, and pushed outward if it is displaced inward. Portable x-rays should be taken after

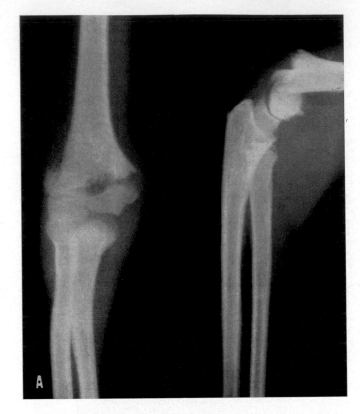

Fig. 3—(A) Supracondylar fracture of humerus with anterior displacement and posterior angulation. This is unusual displacement.

reduction has been accomplished, and if it is not perfect, the limb should be gently manipulated again until proper reduction has been effected.

Flexion of the forearm causes the triceps to act as a splint posteriorly and usually all that is necessary to hold the fragments in place. The flexion can be maintained by a posterior molded plaster splint. Care must be taken that flexion does not obliterate the radial pulse. If there has been so much swelling that the mere flexion of the forearm causes the obliteration of the radial pulse, then a compromise must be made, and the arm extended to a point where the radial pulse returns. Even if one must accept some recurrence of displacement, it is necessary to accept this displacement to protect the circulation. In some instances it is necessary to elevate the limb with skeletal traction in order to maintain reduction and circulation at the same time. Dunlop's traction has been advocated for treatment of these fractures, particularly where there is considerable swelling and where circulation may be impaired, but we prefer skeletal traction through the proximal ulna.

The lateral x-ray of the supracondylar fracture may show a so-called "fishtail" deformity (fig. 4) which indicates a rotation of the distal fragment

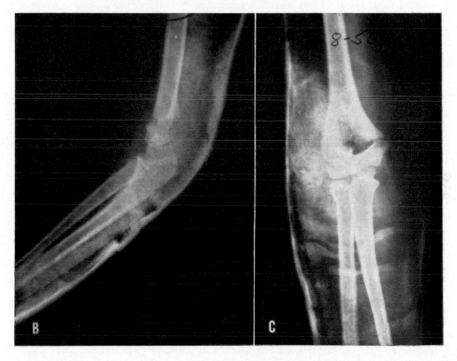

Fig. 3—(B and C) After reduction and immobilization in extension by means of posterior plaster splint.

showing an anteroposterior view of the proximal fragment and a lateral view of the distal fragment. This can be corrected by proper rotation with the arm in supination after reduction has been accomplished.

If the fracture is of the less common type where the distal fragment is displaced forward (fig. 3 A), the reduction is accomplished by traction in the line of the long axis of the arm and the reduction is maintained by extension (fig. 3 B and C).

Immobilization of the flexed elbow is accomplished by means of a posterior plaster slab and careful application of circumferential bandaging, the arm being held in a sling applied to the elbow and wrist.

The immobilization of the anteriorly displaced fragment is accomplished by means of a posterior slab with the arm in full extension. This is one of the few exceptions in which immobilization of the elbow in extension is permissible (fig. 3).

After three weeks the fracture is usually stable enough to allow removal of the plaster and extension of the elbow to a right angle. The elbow immobilized in extension may be flexed to a right angle after three weeks.

Supracondylar fractures of the humerus in children occasionally require use of internal fixation by means of transfixion with Kirschner wires. The Kirschner wires should be inserted under x-ray control, and they should be removed after a period of three weeks.

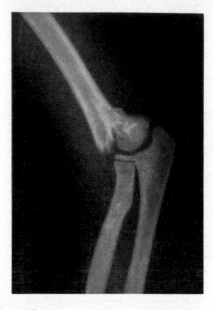

Fig. 4—"Fishtail" appearance of supracondylar fracture. The shaft is seen in anteroposterior view while the rotated condylar fragment is seen in lateral projection. To reduce this fracture the condylar fragment must be rotated into position.

After-Care of Supracondylar Fractures in Children

These fractures usually heal enough to be removed from their immobilization after three weeks and immobilization should rarely be necessary after a period of four weeks. Active elbow motion should be instituted immediately, and it is the responsibility of the surgeon to insist that the active exercises be done properly and frequently enough to be useful. After the fourth or fifth week, the patient's arm should be removed from the sling and he should be allowed to use it normally. Under no circumstances should forced manipulations be attempted. Massage and diathermy are contraindicated. It takes considerable patience on the part of the doctor, the surgeon and the parent to await return of full function.

Forward Displacement of the Lower Humeral Epiphysis in Children

Occasionally, a fall on the flexed elbow will cause a detachment of the whole of the cartilage of the lower end of the humerus including the epiphysis, the capitellum, trochlea and medial condyle. This anterior displacement is often overlooked because it is not recognized that the normal forward tilting of the epiphysis is exaggerated. If unrecognized, the extension of the elbow may be permanently limited.

The reduction of the displacement is accomplished by manipulation and the elbow immobilized in extension.

Intercondylar Fractures (T-Fractures) and Comminuted Fractures of the Elbow

The intercondylar fracture may be sustained in adults by a direct fall on the point of the elbow. The comminuted fractures occur in adults as a result of severe falls on the elbow or are sustained when an automobile strikes the exposed elbow of the driver of a passing car. This is the so-called "baby-car fracture" described in English literature.

The intercondylar fracture may be treated by manipulation and immobilization in plaster, but often the reduction cannot be accomplished or maintained without operative intervention and internal fixation of the displaced fragments. This internal fixation may be accomplished by screws or transfixion by means of threaded Kirschner wires (fig. 5).

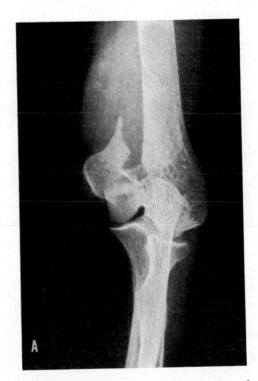

Fig. 5—(A) Intercondylar fracture with medial displacement of medial fragment.

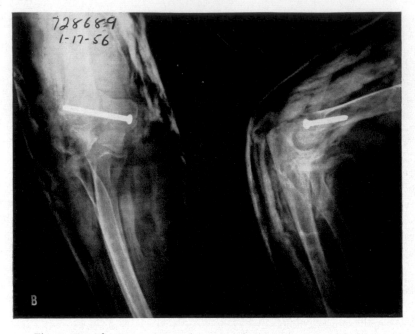

Fig. 5–(B) After operation and internal fixation by means of screw.

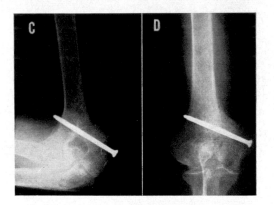

Fig. 5–(C and D) Six months follow-up. Function good.

In many instances the comminution of fragments of the lower humerus as well as the olecranon may be so great as to make it impossible to fit them together. In these instances, elevation with skeletal traction through the upper end of the ulna is the most effective means of treatment (fig. 6). It is amazing how well the fragments fall into position when the arm is elevated with a wire through the olecranon, and in this position motion in the elbow may be begun very early so as to prevent late stiffening.

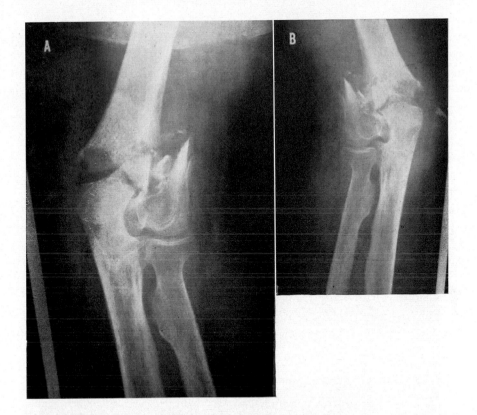

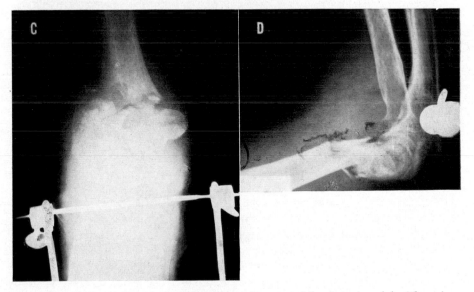

Fig. 6—(A and B) Comminuted supracondylar fracture of humerus in adult. There is an intercondylar as well as supracondylar fracture with marked comminution. Operative reduction and internal fixation is very difficult in this case. (C and D) After traction by means of wire through upper end of ulna. Note satisfactory reduction of fragments by molding of fragments.

Fractures of the Lateral Condyle

This injury usually occurs between the ages of 5 and 15. The separated fragment of the lateral condyle includes the epiphysis of the capitellum and sometimes the adjacent part of the trochlea (fig. 7). If there is no displacement of the condyle, immobilization is all that is necessary. If, however, there is

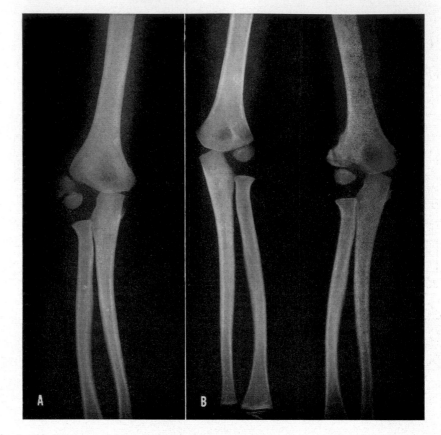

Fig. 7—(A) Fracture of lateral condyle of humerus in child of 6. This must be reduced and fixed by means of suture or metal to prevent nonunion or malunion. (B) Three months after operative replacement and fixation by means of catgut suture. There is apparent deformity of condyle but position of capitellar epiphysis is good.

marked displacement and rotation of the fragment caused by the pull of the extensor muscle of the forearm, it is necessary to operate on the lesion and to replace the fragment accurately in position. If this is not done, there may be a failure of proper growth of the capitellum with resulting increased carrying angle and awkward deformity (fig. 8). The fragment may be fixed in position by means of simple catgut suture, but may be more securely fixed by means of transfixion with threaded Kirschner wires which can be removed in a period of about three weeks.

Fractures of the Medial Epicondyle

Avulsion of the epiphysis of the medial epicondyle caused by traction of the flexor muscles of the forearm is a common injury to the elbow in children. If there is very little displacement, immobilization is all that is necessary. If the displacement is marked, or, if as is commonly the case, the epiphysis

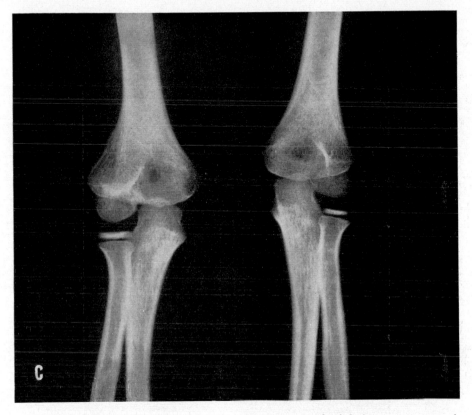

Fig. 7—(C) Three year follow-up. The affected condyle on the left is normal except for slight enlargement.

has been displaced within the elbow joint (fig. 9), it is necessary to operate on the elbow, taking care to protect the ulnar nerve and to remove the fragment from the joint and fasten it to its normal position on the medial condyle by means of catgut or silk. It is also proper to fix the condyle by means of removable Kirschner wires. Some surgeons prefer to excise the fragment and attach the tendon to the condyle.

Fracture of the Capitellum of the Humerus in Adults

This fracture is unusual, but it is important because it must be recognized and properly treated in order to establish good function of the elbow joint.

The fracture usually involves the articular surface of the lateral condyle (fig. 10 A), and it is displaced anteriorly and rotated superiorly. Because of the fact that the fracture is intra-articular and has no soft part attachments to preserve the blood supply, avascular necrosis of the loose fragment may result, leading to a painful elbow. These fractures should always be operated on and

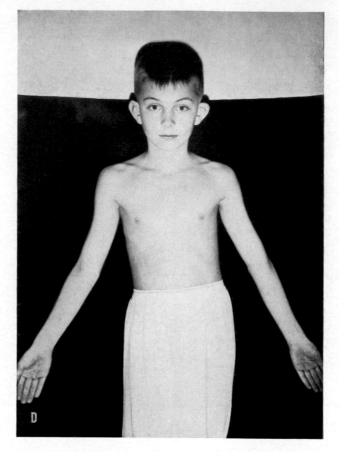

Fig. 7—(D) Five year follow up. Normal carrying angle of affected (right) elbow.

the fragment either removed (fig. 10 A and B) or replaced and fixed in position by means of removable transfixion wires (fig. 10 C). Removal of the fragment does not result in a severe loss of function, but it is preferable to attempt replacement of the fragment.

The elbow should be immobilized in neutral position so that any minor loss of motion will not be serious.

The Fracture of the Radial Neck in Children

The injury sustained to the upper end of a child's radius is usually a fracture through the neck with varying degrees of displacement of the head.

If the fracture is incomplete or if there is a slight displacement of the radial head, no reduction is necessary and immobilization for a short period of time is the extent of the treatment.

If there is a displacement greater than 45 degrees (fig. 11), then reduction is necessary. With the elbow in extension, the head of the radius may often be corrected by firm pressure over the displaced radial head while the forearm is being adducted. It is surprising how often a markedly displaced radial head in a child may be replaced by manual manipulations.

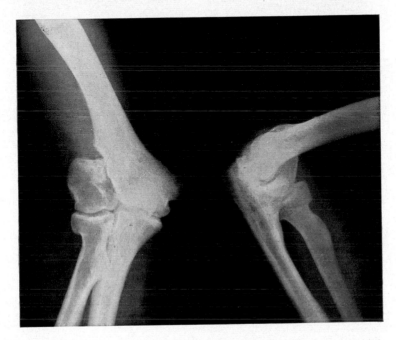

Fig. 8—(A) Male of 34 who sustained this fracture at age of 6. The lateral condyle was not reduced and deformity resulted.

If the displacement of the radial head is not greater than 45 degrees, nature will correct the displacement by reshaping the upper end of the shaft of the radius so that the x-ray presents a "double exposure" appearance (fig. 12).

If the displacement is great so that the head is completely displaced from the shaft or if manual manipulation does not give satisfactory reduction, then operative reduction is necessary (Chapter 17, fig. 1).

The head of the radius should never be removed in a growing child. When the displaced fragment is exposed, it is replaced in its proper position and sutured in position by means of catgut or silk.

If a suture does not hold the fragment in place, a Kirschner wire may be driven through the lateral condyle of the humerus into the center of the radial head and on into the intramedullary canal of the radius. This wire may be removed after a period of ten days when the head is stuck in position.

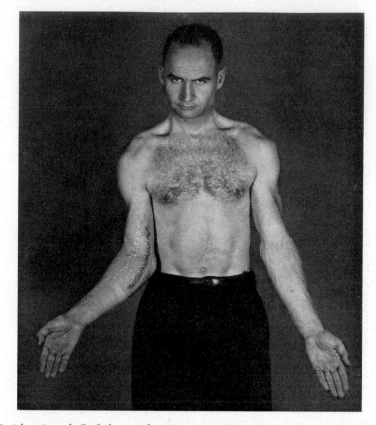

Fig. 8—B (above) and C (below) After 28 years ulnar developed as result of abnormal stretching of ulnar nerve caused by marked increased carrying angle. Photograph after transplantation of ulnar nerve.

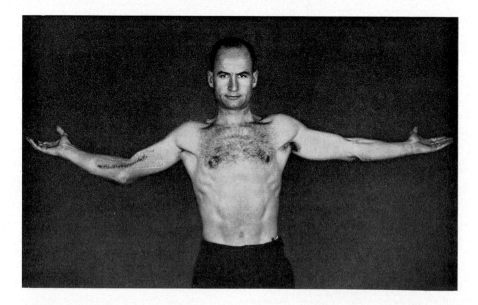

The transfixion of the epiphysis by the wire does not cause any growth disturbance.

Because the epiphysis may be injured in spite of replacement of the fragment, growth disturbances may occur and occasionally a nonunion will result (Chapter 17, fig. 1).

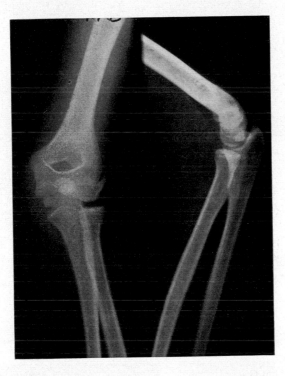

Fig. 9 Fracture of medial epicondyle with displacement of fragment into the joint. This must be removed from joint by operation. It may be sutured in position or removed.

Fracture of the Head of the Radius in Adults

This fracture occurs as the result of a fall on the extended hand and often the displacement is very slight. Even if the fracture involves a large area of the articular surface of the radius, if there is no displacement, no manipulation is necessary. The elbow is immobilized in flexion for a period of a week or ten days and then active motion is instituted, and the results should be excellent. Occasionally, even with minimal displacement there will be a minor degree of limitation of supination and a few degrees of loss of extension. This, however, does not interfere with function of the joint (fig. 13).

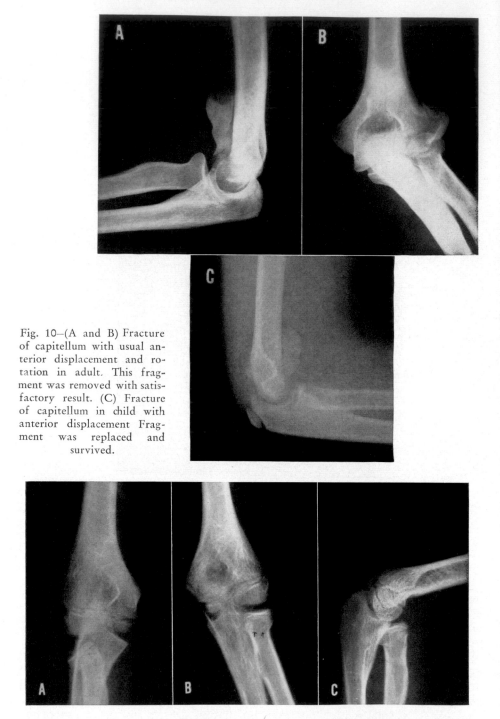

Fig. 10—(A and B) Fracture of capitellum with usual anterior displacement and rotation in adult. This fragment was removed with satisfactory result. (C) Fracture of capitellum in child with anterior displacement Fragment was replaced and survived.

Fig. 11—(A) Fracture of neck of radius in child of 8. There is angulation of more than 45 degrees and reduction is necessary. (B) After manual manipulation and satisfactory (C) Two months post reduction. Function normal.

If there is a displacement of the entire head or a fragment of the head of the radius (fig. 13 A), it is essential that the fragment or the entire head be removed in order to preserve the full pronation and supination of the forearm (fig. 13 C).

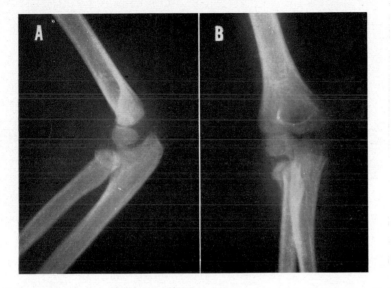

Fig. 12—(A and B) Fracture of radical neck with displacement of head less than 45 degrees.

The operation is accomplished through a lateral incision, care being taken not to injure the posterior interosseous branch of the radial nerve. The common extensor tendon is divided, and the radial head is exposed. The head and a portion of the neck of the bone are removed immediately above the orbicular ligament. If it is possible, the periosteum should be replaced over the end of the bone in order to prevent calcification in the hematoma which may follow. The elbow is then immobilized at a right angle with the arm in the neutral position, and after a period of ten days to two weeks, motion may be instituted.

In most instances the removal of the head of the radius results in perfect function of the elbow, but on occasion, particularly where there has been an injury to the distal radial-ulnar joint, a shifting of the radius occurs, giving symptoms at the wrist. It is therefore unwise to remove the head of the radius unless there is proper indication. If there is a single small fragment, this can be removed leaving the remainder of the head and neck to preserve the length of the radius.

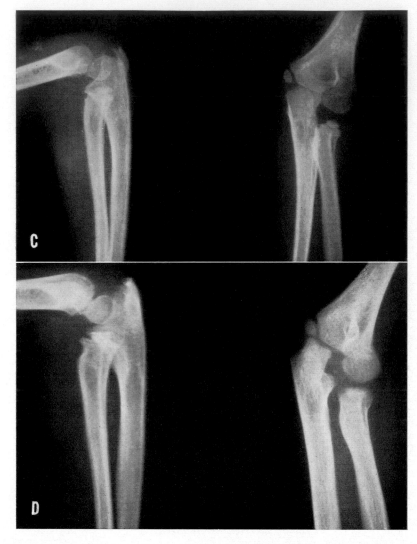

Fig. 12—(C) One month later. Note new shaft being formed. (D) One year later. Upper end of radial shaft reformed, giving "double exposure" appearance in x-ray. Function normal.

Optimum Time for Operation

The optimum time for operation on the head of the radius is within the first 48 hours after the accident has occurred, because there is then less possibility of the development of myositis ossificans. If operation is delayed for three or four weeks after the injury, there is much more likelihood of a deposit of calcium with the resulting limitation of motion. If the patient is not seen until late, operation is better delayed for six or eight weeks following the accident.

Fractures of the Olecranon

Fractures of the olecranon in adults occur very commonly as a result of a fall on the elbow, but they are quite rare in children. Fractures of the olecranon are comparable to those of the patella where there is a combination of muscle pull and leverage over the flexed joint. The olecranon process may

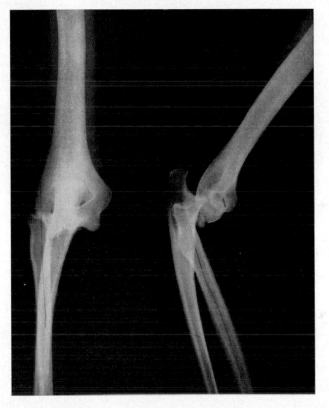

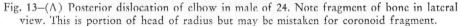

Fig. 13—(A) Posterior dislocation of elbow in male of 24. Note fragment of bone in lateral view. This is portion of head of radius but may be mistaken for coronoid fragment.

be pulled proximally by the triceps muscle. If the integrity of the extensor mechanism of the elbow is intact and there is no displacement of the fractured fragment of the olecranon, then no reduction is necessary, and the patient may be immobilized in extension for a period of ten days and gradual motion restored.

If there is displacement of the proximal fragment of the olecranon (fig. 14 A), operation is mandatory, and the fragment must be replaced and fixed in position. The fracture is exposed and reduced and may be fixed by one of several methods.

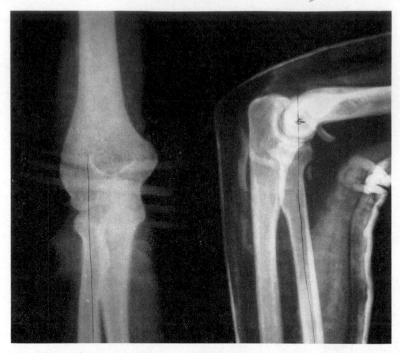

Fig. 13–(B) After reduction of dislocation. The loose fragment is anterior to joint and is obviously lozenge shaped fragment of head of radius. It must be removed.

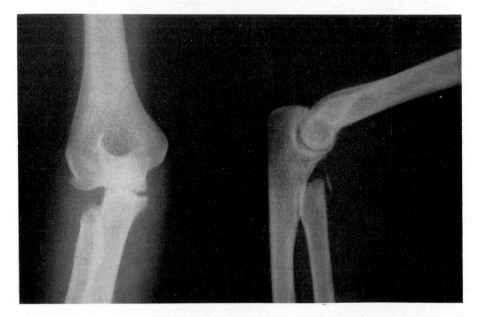

Fig. 13–(C) After operative removal of fragment and radial head and portion of neck. The remaining small bone chip should have been removed at operation. It might be a nidus for development of myositis ossificans.

The fragment may be fixed by means of stainless steel wire sutures (fig. 14 B), the drill holes being driven through the fragments transversely so that the wire will avoid articular surfaces and so that the wire and knot will not be subcutaneous and will be buried in soft tissue. The wire must be of sufficient strength to hold the fragments in position because the tremendous

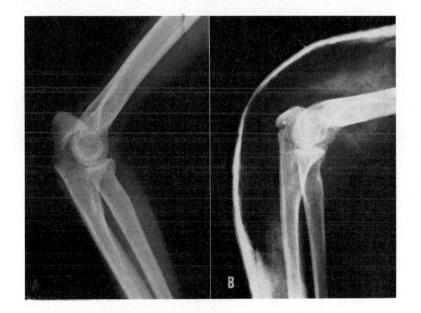

Fig. 14–(A) Typical fracture of olecranon process of ulna with displacement. Operation is necessary. (B) After fixation by means of circumferential figure-of-eight stainless steel wire. As is often seen with this method, displacement of minimal degree recurred.

leverage at the elbow joint will cause separation and rotation of the fragments if fixation is not secure.

If the fragment is small, it may be excised, and the triceps muscle sutured to the olecranon by silk or wire (fig. 15).

Fixation by means of the intramedullary screw (fig. 16) is a very satisfactory method, but of necessity, the screw must be long enough to firmly engage the intramedullary canal of the ulna so that it will not pull out. If a shorter screw is used, it must not only transfix the proximal ulnar fragment, but also the cortex of the shaft of the distal fragment of the ulna.

After operation, the elbow is immobilized by means of a plaster slab for a period of about ten days, after which protected active motion may be instituted. The fixation must be firm, since the healing of the olecranon is slow and imperfect immobilization will allow separation or rotation of the proximal fragment.

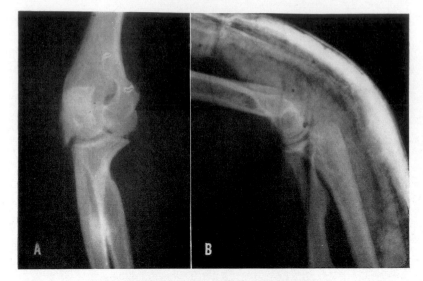

Fig. 15–(A) Fracture of olecranon with displacement. (B) Postoperative x-ray after excision of fragment and suture of triceps to ulna.

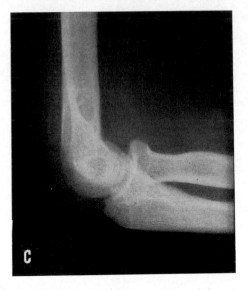

Fig. 15–(C) One year follow-up. Normal function.

Dislocation of the Elbow Joint

Dislocation of the elbow joint (fig. 17 A) may occur at any age, and particularly in children, it may be confused with the supracondylar fracture. An x-ray examination is necessary to confirm the diagnosis.

If there is no associated fracture, reduction of the dislocation is easily accomplished by means of traction. There is no need for hyperextension, as the reduction is usually easily accomplished by means of simple traction alone.

The elbow is then immobilized in partial flexion for a period of about ten days, and if there has been no associated fracture, active motion may be carefully instituted. After a period of three weeks, all immobilizing apparatus should be removed and motion encouraged.

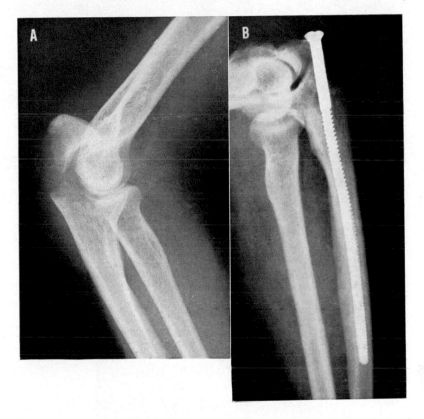

Fig. 16—(A) Fracture of olecranon process with marked displacement. (B) After reduction and immobilization by means of long malleable vitallium screw. Note the screw follows curve of ulnar intramedullary canal. This form of fixation is the strongest to prevent angulation and separation. Early motion is possible.

Since the dislocation of the elbow is often associated with considerable stripping up of the periosteum and hematoma formation, it is essential that one remember the admonitions mentioned previously in this chapter that the elbow joint should never be passively manipulated and that active motion be the only form of physiotherapy used. Frequent x-ray examination will reveal the calcification of a beginning myositis ossificans. In dislocation of the elbow, the prognosis should always be guarded because of the complications which may result (fig. 1 and fig. 17 B).

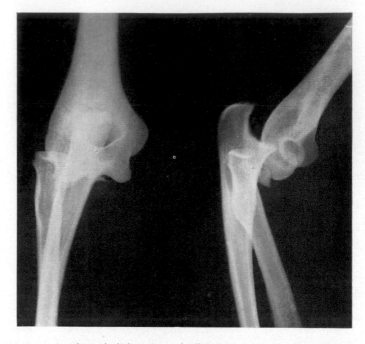

Fig. 17—(A) Posterior lateral dislocation of elbow joint. Easily reduced by traction and flexion. Note loose fragment of bone. This should have been removed.

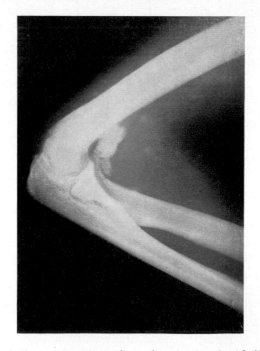

Fig. 17—(B) Six months later. Myositis ossificans has developed with limitation of motion.

Fracture-Dislocation of the Elbow

Dislocation of the elbow is often associated with a fracture of the head of the radius (fig. 13 A) or a fracture of the coronoid process. It is often difficult to recognize the site from which a fragment has been separated, but after reduction of the dislocation, the diagnosis can usually be made

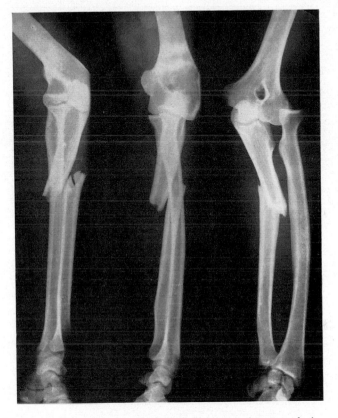

Fig. 18—(A) Monteggia fracture (extension type). There is a fracture of ulna at junction of upper and middle thirds of ulna with displacement. There is anterior and lateral dislocation of radial head.

(fig. 13 B). A displaced fragment of the head of the radius is often mistaken for a fracture of the coronoid process.

After the reduction of the fracture, if the fragments of the head of the radius or the entire head of the radius remains displaced, it is then necessary to excise the radial head (fig. 13 C). After the operation, the elbow is immobilized in a plaster splint in the neutral position, and immobilization maintained for at least two weeks. Motion is begun gradually, and great care should be taken to see that the elbow is not manipulated.

Monteggia Fracture

The Monteggia fracture is a serious type of injury which occurs in adults and in children in which there is a fracture of the upper end of the ulna or the shaft of the ulna with an anterior or posterior displacement of the head of the radius. If the fracture of the ulna is angulated anteriorly and the head

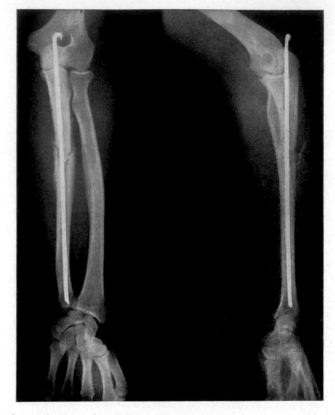

Fig. 18–(B) After reduction of radial head (operative reduction was necessary to remove interposed ligament) and reduction and internal fixation of ulnar fracture by means of Rush nail.

of the radius is displaced anteriorly, it is called the extension type of fracture (fig. 18). If the ulna angulates posteriorly and there is a posterior dislocation of the head of the radius, it is termed the flexion type of Monteggia fracture (fig. 19).

In the child the fracture of the ulna can often be reduced and the dislocation of the head of the radius reduced perfectly. After three weeks of immobilization, early active motion is encouraged and the result is usually good.

In the adult, reduction and maintenance of reduction may be impossible to achieve without internal fixation, and it is our practice to operate on all of

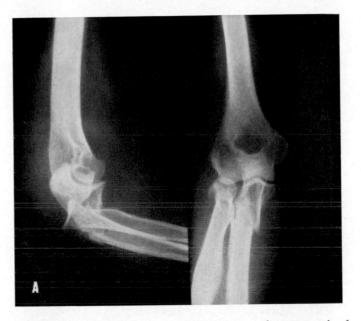

Fig. 19–(A) Monteggia fracture (flexion type). Fracture of upper end of ulna with posterior angulation and posterior dislocation of radial head.

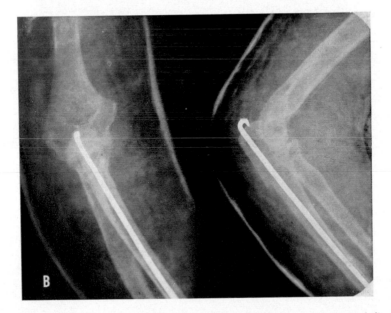

Fig. 19–(B) After reduction of radial head (closed) and reduction and internal fixation of ulnar fracture by means of Rush nail.

these fractures if perfect reduction is not easily accomplished by manual manipulation and if the reduction cannot be perfectly maintained in plaster.

In most instances, it is necessary to expose the fracture site of the ulna and fix it internally by means of an intramedullary rod (fig. 19 B). The use of a plate to fix the ulna is not satisfactory since nonunion is apt to result and

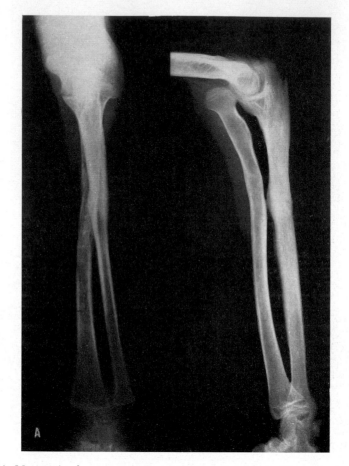

Fig. 20—(A) Monteggia fracture unreduced. The radial head dislocation has not been reduced and the ulnar fracture has healed.

the angulation of the ulna may recur as a result of loosening of the plate. After the fracture of the ulna is perfectly reduced, the radius may fall into position if the ligament is not displaced within the joint. However, in most instances it is necessary to expose the head of the radius and to replace it within the orbicular ligament. If the head of the radius is at all unstable, it may be fixed in position by means of a Kirschner wire transfixing the lower end of the humerus and driven through the head of the radius into the intramedullary canal of the radius. This wire can be removed after three weeks, and the radius may be expected to remain in position.

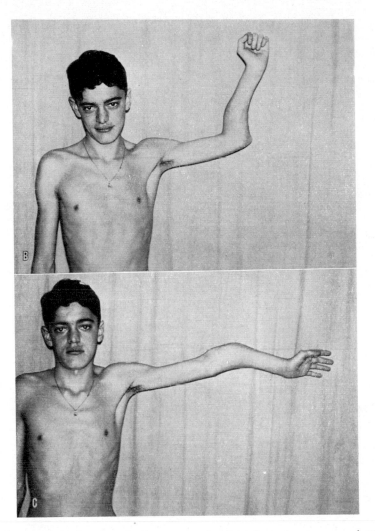

Fig. 20–(B and C) Deformity of elbow as result of ineffectual treatment of Monteggia fracture.

The head of the radius should never be excised in a Monteggia fracture because the radius is apt to shorten on the ulna causing troublesome symptoms at the wrist.

If the Monteggia fracture is not recognized and the dislocated head of radius reduced, a serious deformity and disability results. In these cases late excision of the head of the radius may achieve some slight improvement in motion but the deformity persists (fig. 20).

References

¹ BLOUNT, W. P.: Fractures in Children. Baltimore, Williams & Wilkins Co., 1954.

² BÖHLER, L.: The Treatment of Fractures, ed. 4. Translated by E. W. Hey Groves. Baltimore, W. Wood, 1935 (ed. 8 in German. Wien: Maudrich, 1942).

³ CAMPBELL, W. C.: Operative Orthopedics. St. Louis, C. V. Mosby Co., 1949.

⁴ HENRY, A. K.: Extensile Esposure. Baltimore, William & Wilkins Co., 1945.

⁵ KEY, J. A., and CONWELL, H. E.: The Management of Fractures, Dislocations, and Sprains. St. Louis, C. V. Mosby Co., 1951.

⁶ SMITH, F. M.: Surgery of the Elbow. Springfield, Ill. Charles C Thomas, 1954.

⁷ WATSON-JONES, R.: Fractures and Other Bone and Joint Injuries, ed. 4. Baltimore, Williams & Wilkins Co., 1955.

CHAPTER 35

FRACTURES OF THE FOREARM

PAUL W. BRAUNSTEIN, M.D.

This Chapter is limited to a discussion of those fractures of both bones of the forearm which do not involve the elbow joint and which are not distal enough to be considered in that group of fractures named "Colles' fractures." In other words, we will consider those fractures of one or both bones of the middle two quarters of the forearm. We shall try to describe the method of treatment employed at our institution rather than attempt to cover all others presently available and the different opinions of various authorities as to the best of these.

Fractures of Both Bones of the Forearm in Children

As has been mentioned elsewhere in this book, we feel very strongly that no operative intervention should be carried out in fractures of the forearm in children who still have some bone growth remaining. Closed reduction under general or local anesthesia is perfectly acceptable and almost never is there indication for open reduction. Angulation and displacement will correct themselves with time. It must be made clear that we do not advocate that children's fractures should not be treated. Rather we feel that adequate treatment should be carried out and no other treatment resorted to in the form of operative reduction of shaft fractures of the forearm.

Following closed reduction, the child's arm is immobilized in a long-arm plaster with the hand in pronation, supination or midposition, the position which gives the most adequate alignment of the fractured bones being selected.

The arm is immobilized until solid callus has bridged the defects. In a recent series studied at The New York Hospital, several children refractured the forearm between the eighth and twelfth week following the first injury. To prevent this type of refracture, we have encouraged immobilization through the twelfth week. It should be mentioned that such refractures have occurred only in the forearm and not in other long bones such as the tibia, femur or humerus.

Fractures in Adults

Closed reduction of the shaft of both bones of the forearm may be attempted, but if an adequate and accurate reduction is not obtained and maintained, internal fixation is necessary. Closed reduction should always be performed under general anesthesia, and at the time of casting of the extremity it is most important to remember the muscle pulls which operate along the shaft of the forearm. In proximal radial fractures the proximal

447

fragment is supinated by the supinator group of muscles while the distal fragment is pulled into pronation by the pronator teres and pronator quadratus (fig. 1). Fractures in the midshaft usually lie in more supination of the proximal fragment or equal amounts of supination and pronation of the proximal fragments but marked pronation of the distal fragment due to the pull of the pronator quadratus. According to the muscle pulls placed on a single radial fracture, it is then necessary to place the hand in supination

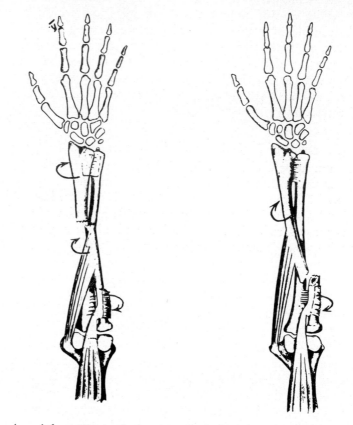

Fig. 1—As adapted from Watson-Jones, a proximal third fracture of the radius will result in marked supination of the proximal fragment owing to the pull of the biceps and supinator, while the distal fragment will be thrown into marked pronation by the pronator teres and quadratus. On the right it will be noted that a mid-third fracture, if below the insertion of the pronator teres, will result in mid-position of the proximal fragment and pronation of the distal fragment due to the pull of the pronator quadratus.

or pronation depending on the level at which the fracture occurs. A proximal radial fracture would require the hand to be placed in supination while a distal radial fracture would require the hand to be placed in either mid-position or slight supination according to the main pull on the proximal fragment as determined by x-ray.

Single Bone Fractures of the Forearm

Most single bone fractures are extremely difficult to treat because the unfractured bone acts as a splint to hold the fractured fragments apart. For example, a radial fracture will have separation at the fracture site because of the splinting action of the intact ulna. Most single bone fractures are caused by direct trauma on the site of fracture rather than by transmitted force through the hand or wrist (i.e. "nightstick" fracture of midshaft of ulna.)

If the single bone fracture is undisplaced, simple external plaster immobilization is sufficient for treatment. However, even in the undisplaced fracture the period of immobilization will be annoyingly long (i.e. four to eight months or longer) owing to the aforementioned splinting action of the opposite intact bone.

Fractures of the Radius: Fractures of the distal third of the radius are difficult to treat. These fractures have a relatively high incidence of non-union and mal-union. Recently Hughston [3] has brought out very dramatically the number of distorting forces playing on a solitary distal third radial fracture. The weight of the hand, the pull of the brachioradialis insertion, the pronating tendency of the pronator quadratus, and the force of the thumb abductors and extensors lead to a high degree of failure in closed reduction in this type of fracture. He reported 92 per cent failure of closed reduction.

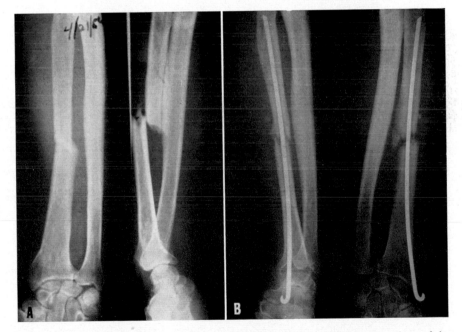

Fig. 2—(A) A midshaft solitary radial fracture is present with complete loss of bony continuity (day of injury). (B) Here, fracture fragment alignment has been re-established by Rush pin fixation introduced distally. Despite the use of bone chips, note the relative distraction due to the splinting action of the intact ulna.

He stressed the use of rigid fixation. In fractures of the middle two quarters of the shaft of the radius we have favored intramedullary fixation by exposing the fracture site and placing moderate amounts of bone chips into it. Figure 2 A reveals a solitary midshaft radial fracture, note the distraction of the oblique fracture with complete loss of contact of the fracture fragments. This patient was treated with intramedullary fixation with a round Rush

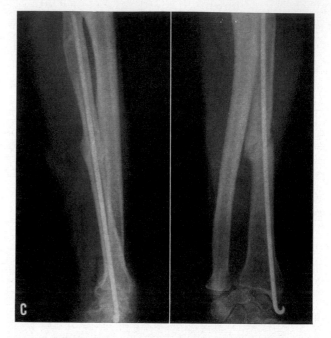

Fig. 2—(C)Twenty-one months later, there is complete healing and bony continuity across the fracture site. It is believed that this long period of healing is required due to of absorption at the fracture site and distraction of these fracture fragments by the opposite intact bone.

pin introduced through the radial styloid process and a fair amount of bone chips was placed about the fracture site (fig. 2 B). In this patient there was delayed union as might be expected with the intact ulna. However, figure 2 C shows the healed radius 21 months after injury.

Fractures of the Shaft of the Ulna Alone: Fractures of the shaft of the ulna also tend to lead to distraction of the fracture fragments by absorption at the fracture site and splinting action of the intact radius. In those fractures where there is no displacement of the ulnar fragments, we have tended to leave them in place and treat them by simple plaster immobilization. However, in those with displacement we have leaned toward open reduction and insertion of a round Rush pin. Figure 3 A demonstrates such a fracture in the distal third of the ulna. Note that there is some displacement, and with the rather poor healing qualities of the distal ulna, even this slight displacement tends to lead to delayed union. Figure 3 B demonstrates the insertion of an

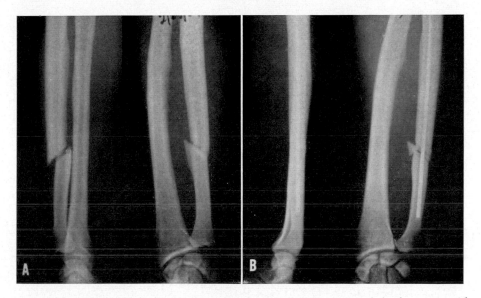

Fig. 3.—(A) This fracture has approximately 50 per cent displacement of the fragments with an intact radius. Note definite relative distraction of the fragments even with rather minor displacement. (B) Following insertion of an intramedullary rod there is exact anatomical alignment except for minimal interosseous comminution.

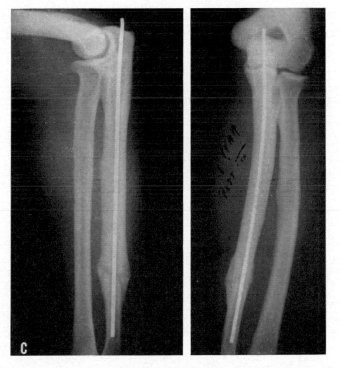

Fig. 3.—(C) One year following operation complete healing and bony bridging have occurred. Again the long healing period is due to the splinting action of the opposite intact bone.

intramedullary rod down the ulna with adequate reduction of the fracture fragments. Figure 3 C shows healing at the end of one year postoperatively with good callus formation, good bony crossover at the fracture site and adequate maintenance of position at the fracture site.

There is frequently delayed or nonunion in solitary forearm bone fractures. Therefore rigid internal fixation is utilized to overcome relative distraction of the opposite bone. Plates lead to rigid fixation with slight distraction which may possibly be overcome by muscle pull in intramedullary type of fixation. It is our opinion that plaster immobilization is required for shorter periods of time if the patient has internal fixation, though healing is not accelerated by this means. It is possible, however to have the patient begin active motion before healing has been recognized and this favors more complete rehabilitation.

Fractures of Both Bones of the Forearm

Frequently fractures of both bones of the forearm are attacked by closed reduction. We feel that it is imperative to obtain and to maintain accurate reduction, and it is in solving this problem that most difficulties arise. In recent years we have come to operate on these fractures more frequently. We have no proof that this either delays or hastens healing, but we do believe that it leads to more rapid mobilization of the upper extremity and hence to more rapid rehabilitation. In the distal or midthird fractures of

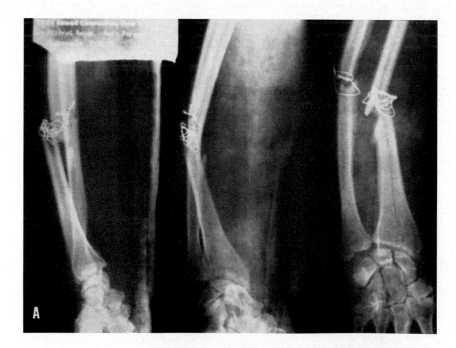

Fig. 4—(A) Here inadequate wiring of the mid-shaft fractures of both bones has led to angulation and distraction and would probably have gone on to nonunion.

both bones of the forearm, we have been using Rush pins. We have not had any experience with the diamond shaped pins which, it is said, tend to decrease rotary displacement of the fracture fragments after internal fixation. In certain instances of fractures of both bones it has been found sufficient simply to fix one of the two bones to maintain stabilization. However, in most cases, unless it proves technically too difficult, both bones have been

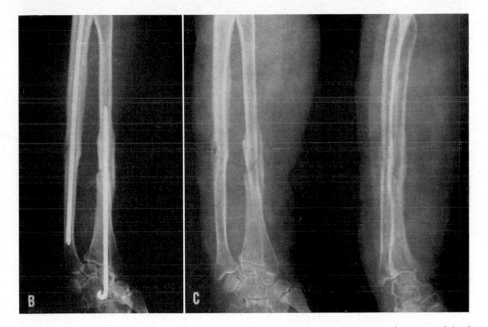

Fig. 4—(B) Adequate alignment has been accomplished by intramedullary fixation of both bones. Note introduction of the radial Rush pin through Lister's tubercle has led to inability to completely insert the pin, therefore necessitating removal at a later date. (C) Here, following removal of the pins, adequate healing has taken place. It should be noted that in this patient, autogenous bone grafts have probably aided rapid healing.

fixed by the intramedullary pinning method. Lane plates or other types of rigid plate fixation have been abandoned because of the impression that with the relative distraction of the fragments due to bone absorption at the fracture site, healing is prevented or delayed. Figure 4 A demonstrates a patient in whom internal fixation with wires did not prevent both displacement and angulation at the fracture site. Though fixation was not completely adequate, Rush pins were placed proximally from the ulna and distally from the radius. It will be noted that the radial pin was not placed in far enough owing to "hanging up" of the Rush pin in the shaft of the radius proximal to the fracture site (fig. 4 B). One year postoperatively it will be noted that the internal fixation appliances have been removed and there was solid bone healing at the fracture sites (fig. 4 C).

Introduction of a distal Rush pin through the radial styloid is a technically difficult procedure. Figure 5 A demonstrates the beginning of the introduction of a thin Rush pin through the radial styloid. Note that the direction of the pin is towards the interosseous cortex of the radius. Very frequently the pin will penetrate this cortex and hang up in the soft tissue in the extra-

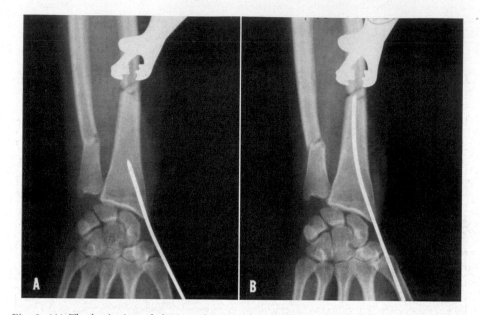

Fig. 5—(A) The beginning of the introduction of a thin Rush pin through the radial styloid. Note that the direction of the pin is towards the interosseous cortex of the radius. Very frequently this pin will penetrate this cortex and hang up in the soft tissue in the extra-cortical portion of the forearm. (B) Note the extreme bend that must occur in the introduced portion of the Rush pin so that it can reach the fracture site while still in the intra-medullary canal. Our attempts at closed blind nailing have been extremely unsuccessful and we have resorted to small incisions at the fracture site to facilitate reduction and fixation.

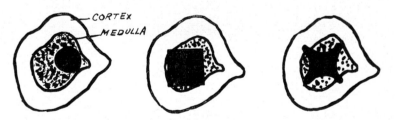

Fig. 6— This diagram illustrates the theoretical benefits of square or self-broaching pins over the round Rush pins. Here the square and self-broaching pins impinge upon the cortex and so prevent rotational movement at the fracture sites.

cortical portion of the forearm. Figure 5 B is a picture taken slightly after figure 5 A. Note the extreme bend that must occur in the introduced portion of the Rush pin so that it can reach the fracture site while still in the intra-medullary canal. Our attempts at closed blind nailing have been unsuccessful and we have resorted to small incisions at the fracture site to facilitate reduction and fixation.

Recently there have been innovations in intramedullary fixation of the forearm. These have consisted of square or "self-broaching" pins to replace the round Rush pins. The principle on which these designs has been based is that a square or self-broaching pin will impinge on the thick cortical bone

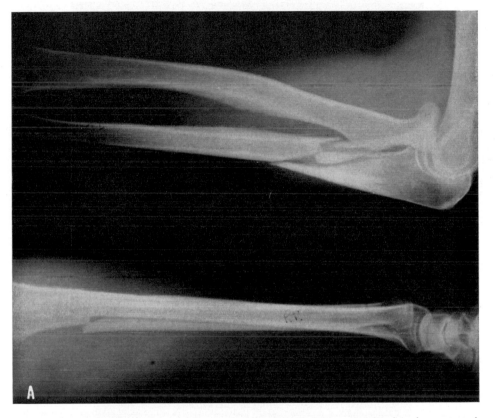

Fig. 7—(A) Monteggia fracture with anterior dislocation of the radial head is demonstrated here. While occasionally successful closed reduction does not assure maintenance of reduction of the radial dislocation owing to re-displacement of the previously reduced ulnar fracture.

and thereby help prevent rotation. With these self-broaching or square pins, it is believed that external plaster fixation can be discontinued at an earlier date without rotation stress and strain contributing to delayed union or nonunion.

In fractures of the forearm treated by open reduction, autogenous cancellous bone chips are inserted at both fracture sites following reduction and fixation. However, the amount of chips must not be excessive, as there have been rare reported instances of cross-union when too many chips are employed.

bones of the forearm is accompanied by infection, usually following an open
fracture or an open reduction of a closed fracture, the infection must first be
controlled, then the wounds must be closed and finally on-lay bone grafting
must be performed at a later date when the wound has become supple and
all evidence of infection has disappeared. Figure 8 A shows the consequence
of an infection in an open fracture of both bones of the forearm. Note the

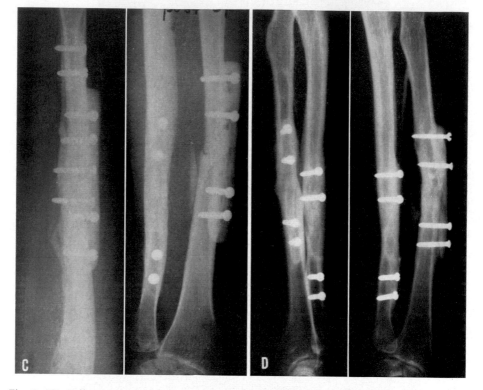

Fig. 8–(C) Following removal of plaster six months after operation, healing has begun but
is not complete. (D) Several years later, complete healing of the grafts and bones has
occurred.

absorption of the bone ends and the complete lack of continuity in the
forearm. Here on-lay bone grafts were placed and held by screw fixation.
Figure 8 B, taken several years later, shows complete healing of the bones
with acceptance of the on-lay bone grafts. Figure 8 C is a follow-up picture
9 years later showing complete healing at the site of nonunion.

Summary

We have considered a very small and special group of fractures, namely
those of one or both bones of the forearm not in its distal or proximal
quarter. We have tended more and more toward open reduction with rigid
internal fixation as the procedure of choice. Closed reduction can be

attempted, and if adequate reduction can be maintained, it is, of course, desirable. We feel that closed reduction often fails, and hence we have resorted very frequently to open reduction. Single bone fractures of the radius or ulna are difficult to handle. The intact bone tends to act as a splint to keep the fractured fragments apart. Here, internal fixation, though it has not accelerated healing, has certainly led to more rapid mobilization of the injured extremity. Both bone fractures have been treated by round Rush pin internal fixation, fixing either one or both of the bones. At the time of internal fixation it is wise to first attack the fracture that is more difficult to reduce, and then to handle the fracture that is more easily reduced. We believe that the use of bone chips in small amounts (not enough to encourage cross-union) has proved helpful in obtaining healing in a large percentage of cases. We have given up plate fixation of forearm fractures, as the plates tend to lead to relative distraction at the fracture site. Monteggia fractures have been treated by reduction of the radial head dislocation and open reduction and internal fixation by Rush pin, and screw fixation of the ulna if necessary. In open fractures we have occasionally used internal fixation at the time of original débridement, but we feel it is safer to postpone this procedure until the primary wounds of débridement have healed.

References

[1] BRADFORD, C. H. et al.: Fractures of both bones of forearm in adults, Surg. Gynec. & Obst. *96*: 240—244, (Feb.) 1953.

[2] HALL, R. H. et al.: Intramedullary fixation of fractures of forearm. South M. J. *45*: 814—818, (Sept.) 1952.

[3] HUGHSTON, Jack C. Fracture of the distal radial shaft. J. Bone & Joint Surg. *39-A*: 249—260, (April) 1957.

[4] ROBERTSON, R. C.: Intramedullary fixation; evaluation of 20 successive unselected cases. Am. J. Surg. *85*: 496—502, (April) 1953.

[5] THOMPSON, J. et al.: Kuntscher nailing in problem cases. Am. J. Surg. *85*: 486—495, (April) 1953.

[6] WATSON-JONES, B.: Fractures and Joint Injuries, ed. 4. Baltimore, Williams & Wilkins.

CHAPTER 36

COLLES' FRACTURE

ROLLA D. CAMPBELL, JR., M.D.

Injury, Pathology and Deformity

This fracture of the distal radius gains its name from original description in the literature of 1814 by Abraham Colles of Dublin, writing in the Edinburgh Medical and Surgical Journal.[14] It is usually due to a fall on the outstretched hand, and results in posterior and outward displacement of the small distal fragment of the radius with an associated supination type of rotary displacement of the distal fragment. The ulnar styloid may or may not be fractured and displaced. The radial fracture frequently is comminuted and may extend into the wrist joint.

If the deformity is left unreduced the patient will have a so-called silver fork deformity with a posterior bump at the fracture site where the distal segment remains posteriorly displaced, including the wrist and hand. In addition, there will be shortening of the radius with prominence of the ulna. If the dorsal tilt is not corrected there may be a significant percentage of loss of flexion. However, it is remarkable what good function can be retained in asymptomatic wrists in spite of considerable components of all three of the deformities mentioned above (fig. 1).

Treatment

Although there are many surgeons who say, "Anyone can treat a Colles' fracture," the pathologic anatomy presents very difficult problems in maintaining reduction and in regaining full function.

Traction

It is agreed that reduction is usually easy to obtain. Merely to exert traction on the wrist and maintain it for a few minutes, especially applied to the thumb and index finger, will achieve correction of the radial shortening, dorsal tilt and radial deviation (figs. 2 and 3). However, to maintain reduction requires art; to obtain both normal anatomy and excellent function requires much more knowledge and ability than is usually accorded patients with these injuries.

Manipulation and Splinting

The secret of holding a good reduction includes not only obtaining it by sufficient traction but by placing the wrist in full pronation and as much ulnar deviation and traction as are tolerated. These three principles are rated in importance as just stated: Pronation, ulnar deviation, and flexion, the

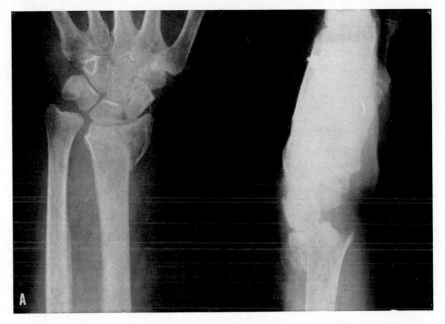

Fig. 1–(A) Original injury demonstration in a 60 year old school teacher.

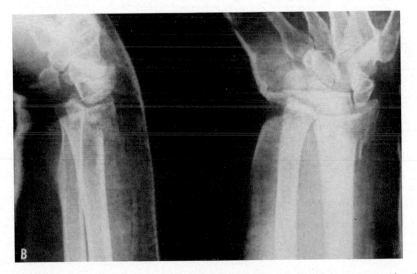

Fig. 1–(B) Reduction was attempted by index digital and thumb traction under local anesthesia. A long arm circular cast was applied. The patient would not agree to hospital admission for general anesthesia. These post-reduction x-rays show that the elements of radial shortening and dorsal angulation persist.

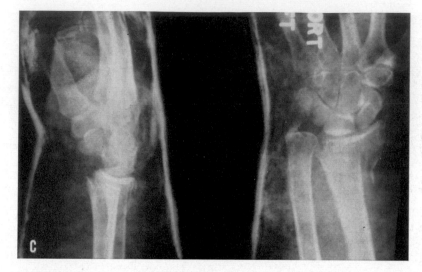

Fig. 1–(C) Four days later, the patient still refusing general anesthesia, local anesthesia was again employed for change of cast and attempted re-reduction with thumb and index finger traction as shown in Fig. 1–(D).

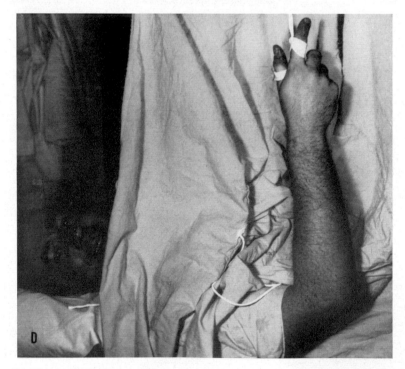

Fig. 1–(D) This method of gauze loops around the thumb and index finger, holding the arm suspended against gravity, plus additional weights tied to the brachium, is frequently useful to prevent loss of reduction at early change of cast. However, unless supplemented by general anesthesia, it does not usually allow the relaxation needed for full reduction. The congestion of the distal portion of the looped digits often prevents the surgeon from applying sufficient traction both in amount and duration.

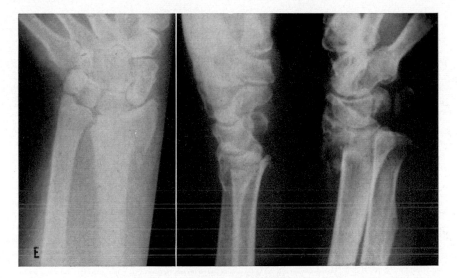

Fig. 1—(E) These x-rays were taken on the eighth day after injury at a third attempt at reduction under local anesthesia with the wrist in traction as described in Fig. 1—(D) (above). No improvement was obtained. The patient still refused general anesthesia and stated agreement to accept the deformities of radial shortening and some dorsal angulation.

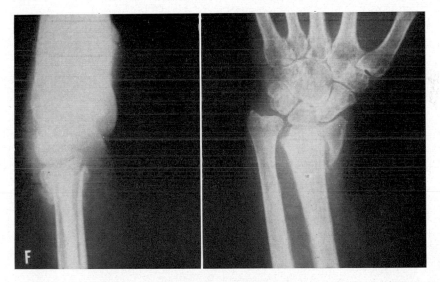

Fig. 1—(F) Result at ten weeks after injury. Because of known malunion to be expected, early emphasis was placed on regaining motion. The cast was cut below the elbow at ten days. Besides having full normal shoulder and hand motion in the injured arm, the patient had the following range of motion in her wrists: Pronation/supination normal; flexion 60 degrees; extension 70 degrees. She has had no complaints of pain or weakness in the injured wrist. The cast was discarded at six weeks.

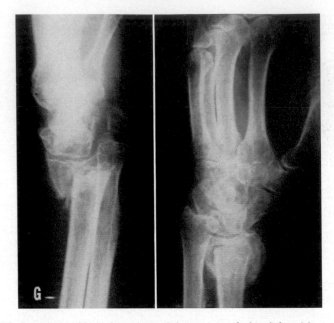

Fig. 1–(G) These oblique films show better the extent of the deformities remaining. The patient was advised that she might need excision of the distal ulna eventually, but for the last year she has been asymptomatic.

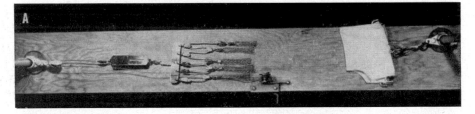

Fig. 2–(A) An ingenious wrist traction device inspired at The Roosevelt Hospital and set up by Dr. Walter Wichern and Dr. Robert Bacon (J. A. M. A., Vol. 146, 1951). The board is radiolucent to allow fluoroscopic control during reduction. The gauge permitted exact knowledge of the amount of traction winched up to the multiple wire mesh finger and thumb grippers.

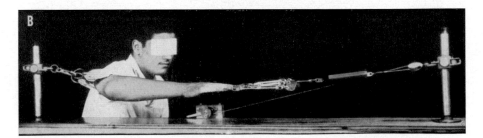

Fig. 2–(B) The elbow is held in flexion by the brachium sling. The posts hold the arm elevated in traction to permit casting in pronation and supination.

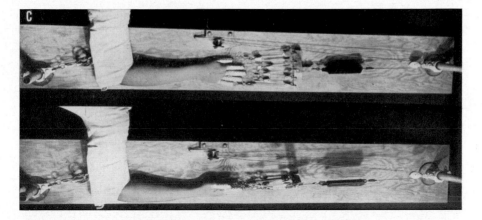

Fig. 2--(C) The authors quoted experience in 75 cases, in all of whom reduction was obtained under local anesthesia in this traction machine without any ill effects on the fingers. This method offers much better control, and the fingers and thumb, protected by adhesive taping under wire mesh grippers, tolerate traction better than the single gauze loop technique demonstrated in Fig. 1--(D). The only disadvantage of having such a useful device as the Wichern-Bacon winch board in the fracture room is that residents find it too easy to use and do not learn other methods.

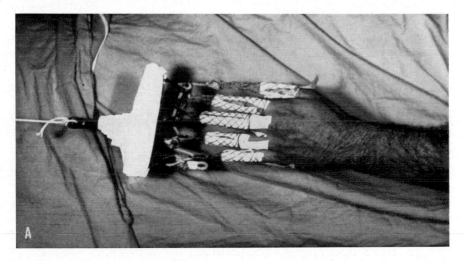

Fig. 3--(A) At first traction is applied to all five digits for ten minutes, or less if reduction is noted sooner.

most important of which is pronation (fig. 4). Bad late results are more often due to radial displacement of the distal fragments and wrist than to dorsal tilt deformity, which is the reason why ulnar deviation is stressed more in maintaining reduction than is flexion. An additional consideration in this regard is that it is very difficult to maintain action of finger flexion in the full flexed position of the wrist. One should not forget, however, that as much flexion as is well tolerated will aid in maintaining reduction of the Colles' fracture. Especially not to be forgotten is the fact that these fractures are supination injuries and that pronation is the most important key in gaining and maintaining reduction. Sugar-tong splints are especially useful in holding these three elements of reduction and offer the advantage that this compression can be loosened or increased, according to the tolerance of the soft tissues (figs. 5—7).

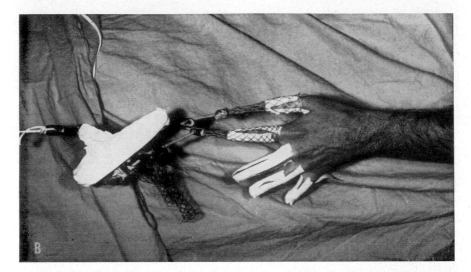

Fig. 3–(B) For the last few minutes (usually five) traction is concentrated on the thumb and index finger. This may be confined to the thumb alone for application of plaster.

Casting

Long arm volar and dorsal plaster splints held by circumferential ace bandaging may be used instead of sugar-tongs previously described. The elbow is usually maintained at 90 degrees or slightly more flexion so that the hand will be somewhat elevated when the arm is hanging at the side. The ace bandages offer some advantage of continuing proper pressure if they are loosened or rewrapped more securely as needed. After the initial swelling has subsided, the plaster slabs may be wrapped in with circular plaster bandages. This technic may be applied also to the sugar-tong splints.

Instability of the Colles' Fracture: Many individuals cannot tolerate the position necessary to hold reduction (fig. 8). In these problem cases it is important to realize that one is treating soft tissues first, and x-ray representation of bone alignment second. Because of the element of comminution of the dorsal architectural surface of the distal radius or of the cortex of the proximal fragment, which makes the fracture unstable if not held in some pronation, ulnar deviation and flexion, the surgeon has either to accept the inevitable malunion by letting the wrist out of the optimum position of stability for the fracture, or else to add internal fixation.

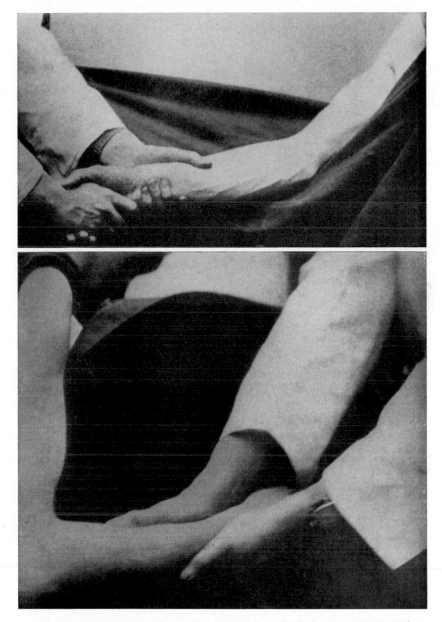

Fig. 4—(A) These illustrations from the excellent textbook by Dr. P. D. Wilson and Dr. W. A. Cochran: Fractures and Dislocations, Philadelphia, T. B. Lippincott Co., 1928, show the incorrect method (above) and correct manipulation (below) for controlled reduction of a Colles' fracture. One has only to try the latter technique to appreciate how effective it can be, especially if some traction is applied at the same time to the thumb and index finger while the thenar eminence of the operator's hands gives reduction by pronation-flexion force on the fracture site. Furthermore, this method of thenar eminence pronation reduction force on the soft tissues over the fracture site is less traumatic than direct thumb pressure over the dorsal prominence of the displaced distal fragment.

Internal Fixation

Internal fixation can be of several types:

1. Transfixion of the distal radial fragment to the proximal ulna. The disadvantage of this method is that pronation/supination are impossible until removal of the transfixion metal, with the possible permanent loss of forearm rotation (figs. 9 and 10).

2. Transfixion of the distal radial fragment to the proximal radius by Kirschner wires or Roger-Anderson apparatus. This is often impossible because of lack of sufficient body in the distal fragment to support internal fixation.

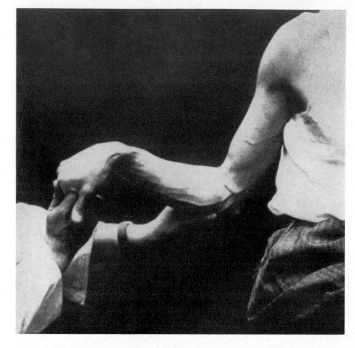

Fig. 4–(B) When this position of reduction is achieved, as shown in Wilson-Cochran, the Colles' fracture is stable and will not slip while plaster is being applied. If the patient can tolerate this position for a period of three, four, or five weeks, a good anatomical result will be achieved. Unfortunately, relatively few patients will be able to maintain hand function in this position, especially with the soft tissue trauma already present from the fracture.

3. Distal proximal transfixion either by:

a. Roger-Anderson apparatus to the proximal radius and distal first metacarpal (fig. 11).

b. Transfixion Kirschner wires to the proximal olecranon and metacarpus.

c. Traction on the thumb by transfixion wire through the proximal phalanx to a long-arm cast in which the countertraction is the flexed elbow, or transfixion wire through the olecranon and incorporated into the cast.

Of these last three, the Roger-Anderson apparatus to the proximal radius and distal first metacarpal is the most sound, both mechanically and physiologically, because it allows early pronation/supination, often without need for cast.

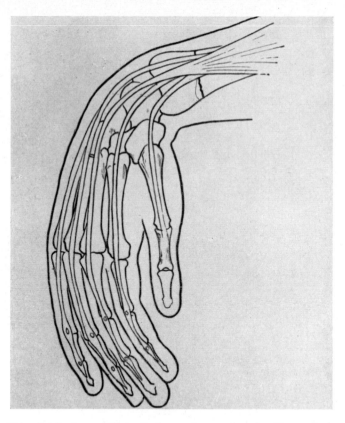

Fig. 4 (C) This sketch from Wilson-Cochran shows why the Cotton-Loder position of pronation, ulnar deviation and flexion is effective in holding reduction. The extensor tendons of the digits are thus drawn tightly over the distal fragment to hold it in place. Very occasionally, one sees adhesions of these tendons in tenodesis to the fracture site of a late complication demanding release. This complication may simulate a partial radial nerve palsy.

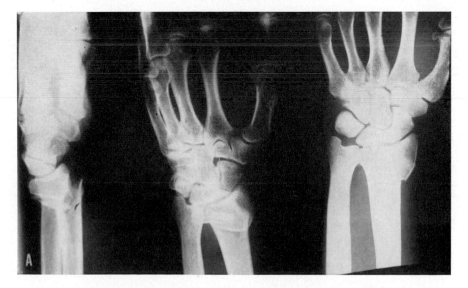

Fig. 5—(A) This patient is a surgeon, aged thirty.

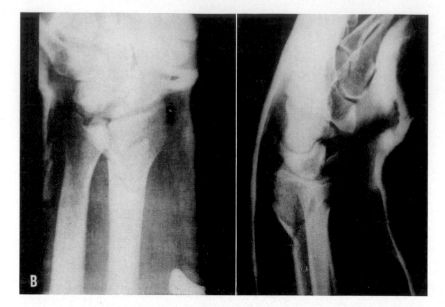

Fig. 5—(B) Reduction in the traction machine under local anesthesia was placed in the Cotton-Loder position in sugar-tong splints. These were loosened or tightened daily as needed to keep firm but not occlusive pressure. After the first five days, the patient was seen only two or three times each week. This position was maintained for six weeks. (This reduction was achieved by a resident surgeon on the Trauma Service at the Roosevelt Hospital.)

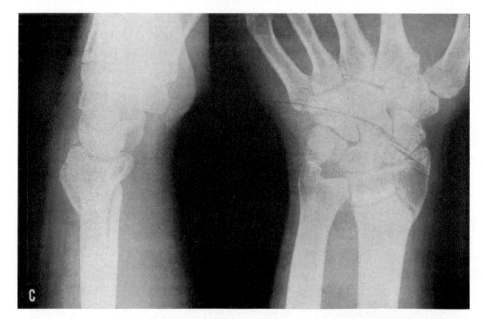

Fig. 5—(C) An excellent anatomical result was obtained. Of most importance is the fact that this man has full return of motion and strength in the wrist and hand and is asymptomatic. His youth, plus close observation and care of the splints, permitted mainte-nance of the Cotton-Loder position of stability of reduction.

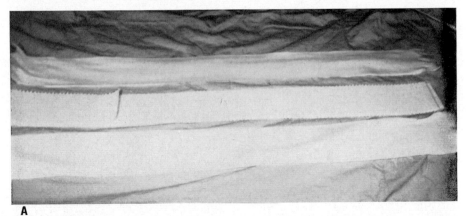

A

Fig. 6—(A) Technic in making comfortable sugar tong splints for the forearm and wrist includes Curity gauze on either side of plaster slab, which is four or five layers thick and six inches wide, on both sides of the plaster permits easy rewrapping as is frequently required in the use of this method.

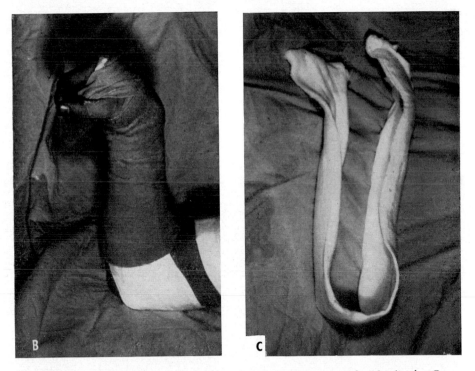

B   **C**

Fig. 6—(B) This shows the splints holding the elbow, forearm and wrist in the Cotton-Loder position. Full finger flexion must be maintained to touch the palm, and wrist flexion is reduced if necessary to allow this motion. Strong finger flexion is, of course, not possible in this position, but the range must be maintained.

Fig. 6—(C) The sugar tong splint manufactured from materials seen in Fig. 6—(A) and on the patient in Fig. 6—(B). It is light and effective in most individuals. Some elderly or very obese patients cannot tolerate even light constriction. Ace bandage, and less extensive splinting may have to be substituted.

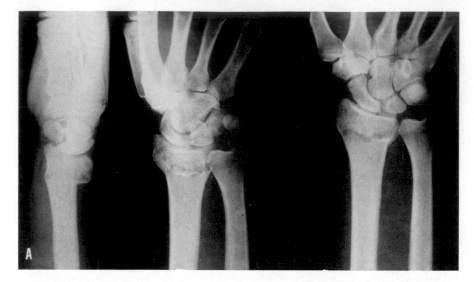

Fig. 7–(A) A Colles' fracture in a young housewife.

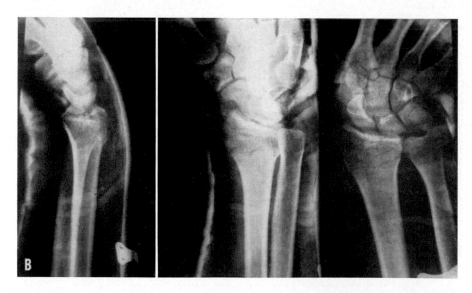

Fig. 7–(B) Excellent reduction was gained in the traction machine under local anesthesia and held in the Cotton-Loder position by sugar tong splints and Ace bandage. The patient was seen frequently (several times each week) and the bandage kept snug for six weeks, when a short arm circular cast was applied in neutral position. The splinting was well tolerated.

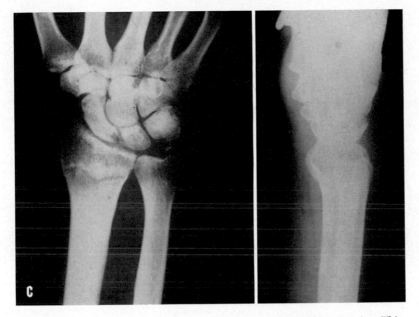

Fig. 7—(C) At ten weeks, x-rays show excellent position at the fracture site. This patient went on to regain full normal wrist and hand motion and strength. (This case is presented through the courtesy of Dr. Tom Dring.)

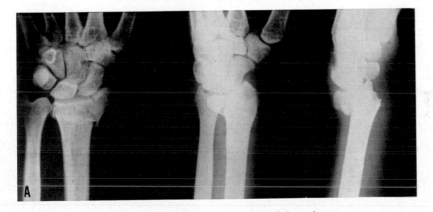

Fig. 8—(A) A Colles' fracture in a young adult male accountant.

At a meeting of the American College of Surgeons Committee on Trauma with associated committees of Eastern Canada, New England and New York-Brooklyn, this method was described as it was used at Peter Bent Brigham Hospital in 1956, where it had given excellent results in approximately 50 cases.

A transfixion loop of Kirschner wire through the first metacarpal was employed, attached to a Steinmann pin, with the Roger-Anderson pins holding the proximal radius. Illustrations are shown of a modification of this technic

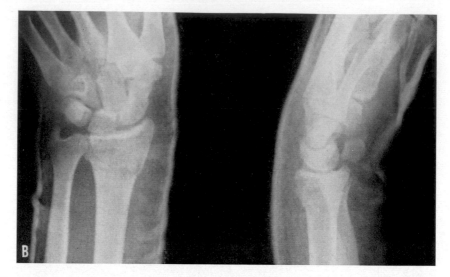

Fig. 8–(B) A good reduction was obtained in the traction machine and the patient put up in sugar tong splints to hold the Cotton-Loder position.

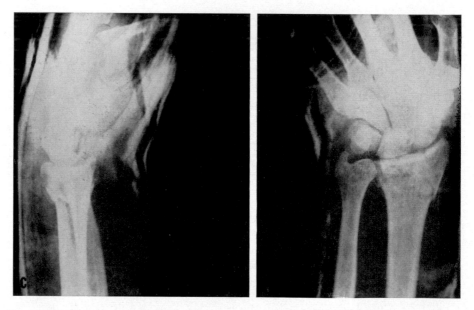

Fig. 8–(C) The patient could not tolerate the full Cotton-Loder position in spite of loosening the sugar tong splints repeatedly. Therefore, at ten days, a circular long arm cast was applied with less severe ulnar deviation, flexion and pronation. Index finger and thumb traction were maintained during change of cast but, as can be noted in the above x-rays, some radial shortening and dorsal angulation recurred.

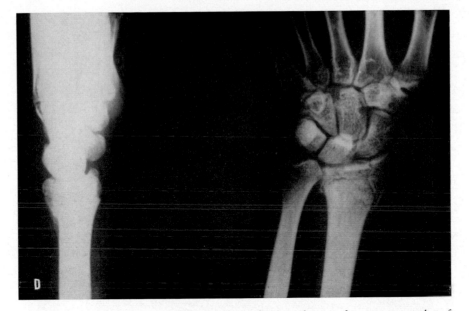

Fig. 8–(D) Position of final result is noted to be less than perfect at ten weeks after injury. The patient had been in a short arm cast for the previous month. In spite of interim exercises, the patient still has only about 75 per cent strength at the end of one year and only 75 per cent full motion in all directions. This cases typifies the small amount of slippage of reduction which is so difficult to prevent.

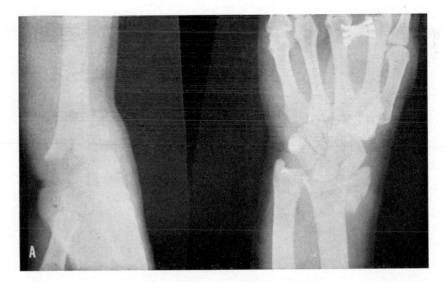

Fig. 9–(A) A Colles' fracture with considerable radial comminution and shortening in a housewife aged 44. An early treatment, of course, was removal of the ring!

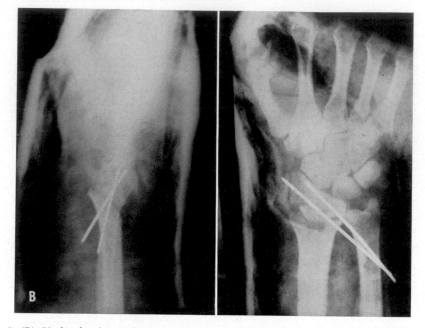

Fig. 9–(B) Under local anesthesia and thumb and index finger traction, length could be regained but tended to be lost as soon as traction was released, even after application of a long arm cast in the Cotton-Loder position. Therefore, transfixion wires were applied from the ulnar direction through the distal ulna and radius while the patient's hand was still in traction. The wires were cut off beneath the skin and a long arm cast applied with the wrist in neutral position.

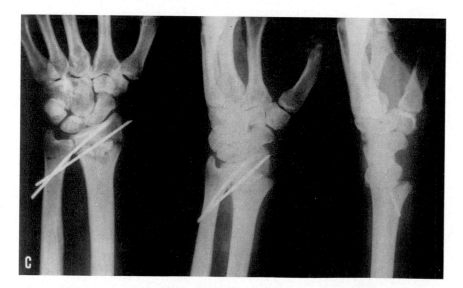

Fig. 9–(C) These wires were left in for eight weeks, after which a short arm cast was applied and strenuous active efforts made to regain pronation/supination.

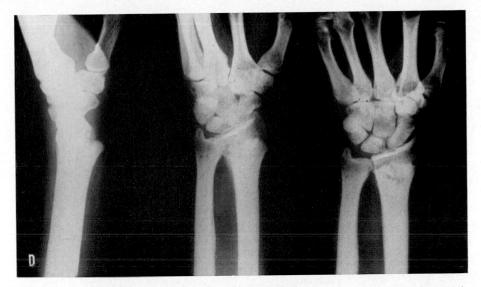

Fig. 9—(D) An excellent anatomical and full normal functional result was achieved. The patient had no median nerve irritation or flexor tendon symptoms from the residually prominent anterior radial beak at the fracture site.

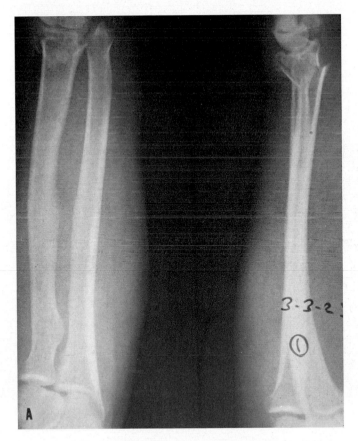

Fig. 10—(A) A Colles' fracture in a 28 year old electrician.

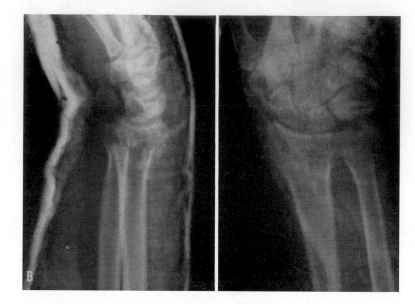

Fig. 10–(B) Under local anesthesia, a fairly satisfactory reduction was obtained in the traction machine.

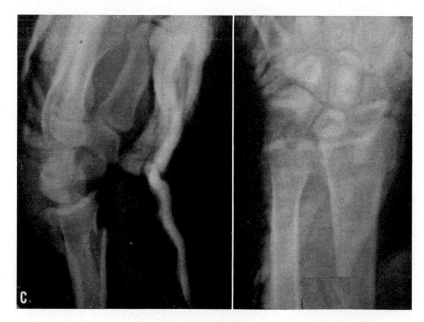

Fig. 10–(C) Reduction was not maintained, however, even in a long arm cast in considerable Cotton-Loder position. These views are at five days after injury.

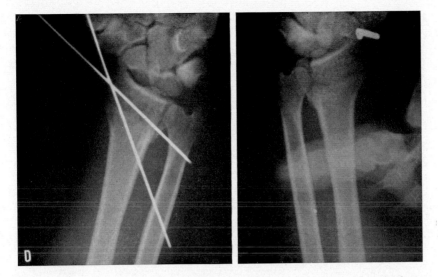

Fig. 10–(D) The upper right film shows closed reduction under general anesthesia with the patient's wrist being held in the Cotton-Loder position os shown earlier in Fig. 4–(B). The marker at the far right was placed on the skin as a guide for the surgeon in applying wires from the radial sides which were placed in transfixion to the ulna. This operation was performed at six days after injury.

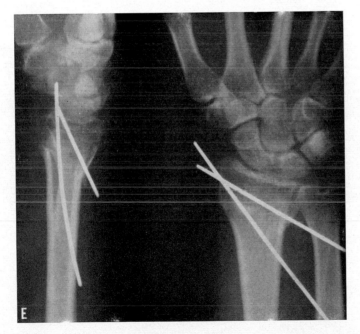

Fig. 10–(E) These x-rays show excellent position and advanced healing at six weeks when the wires were removed. The patient had been in a long arm cast with the wrist in neutral position until this date, when a short arm cast was applied and strenuous active efforts made to regain pronation and supination.

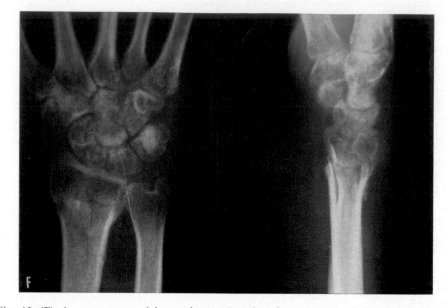

Fig. 10—(F) Appearance at eight weeks, two weeks after removal of the wires. A short arm cast was maintained two more weeks, but was split on the ulna side so that the patient could slip it off for gentle active exercises in warm water twice daily. He had full normal motion and strength, and his injured wrist was asymptomatic at one year when seen in recent follow-up.

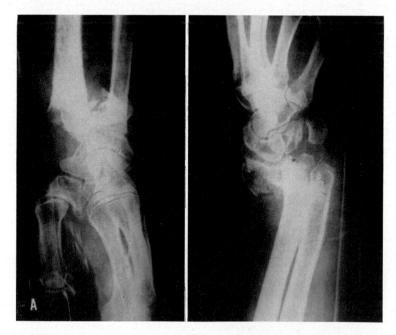

Fig. 11—(A) This was a severely comminuted, open, badly displaced Colles' fracture, complicated by dirty wounds at the wrist which required frequent dressing, in an elderly lady.

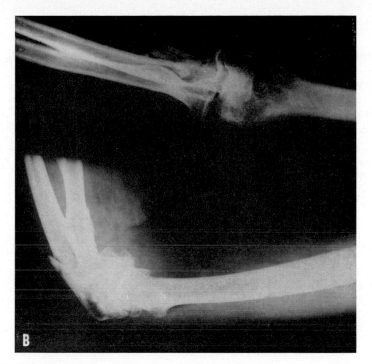

Fig. 11–(B) In addition, there was a Monteggia fracture dislocation of the ipsolateral elbow with the fracture of the proximal ulnar shaft and of the radial head.

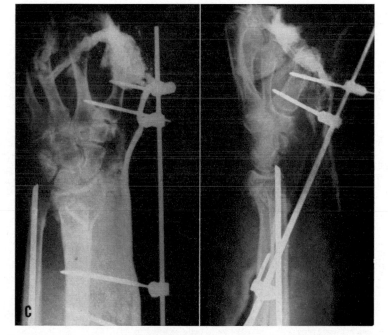

Fig. 11–(C) Roger-Anderson type transfixion splinting of the first metacarpal bone and proximal radial shaft stabilized the wrist after reduction under general anesthesia. Also the radial head was removed and the ulnar shaft held in reduction by an intramedullary Rush pin. A plaster slab was applied to the forearm for only a few days.

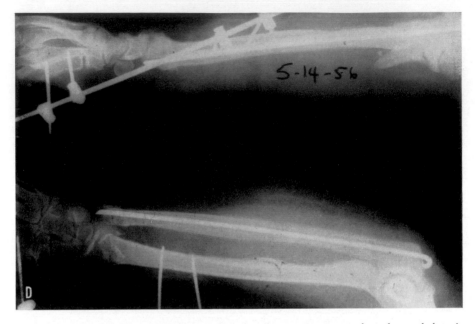

Fig. 11–(D) On the fifth postoperative day the plaster was removed, and guarded active use of the hand and wrist and elbow encouraged.

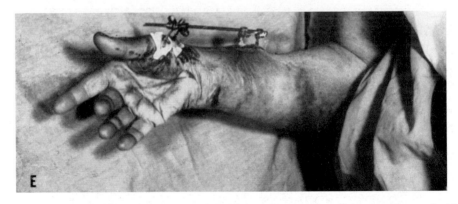

Fig. 11–(E) The apparatus holds the thumb in a position of partial opposition and aids hand function. The wound over the ulnar area of the wrist is seen in this photograph.

(fig. 11) in which two transfixion pins were used for the distal first metacarpal and the proximal radius attached to a Steinmann pin external support. This method of external support is of great advantage in open fractures of the distal radius and ulna where a wound requires frequent dressing.

Maintaining Function

If the position of maintenance of reduction of the wrist described above cannot be held due to soft tissue intolerance, and if the surgeon elects not to

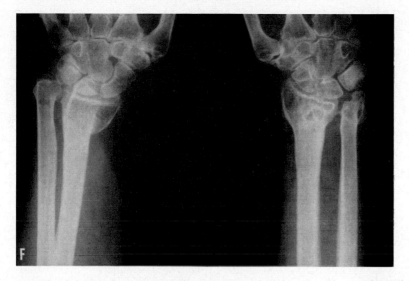

Fig. 11—(F) The final result is seen in the AP view of both wrists above. The right had received the transfixion pin treatment; the left had been injured several years previously and had received cast splinting for an ill-remembered interval "elsewhere."

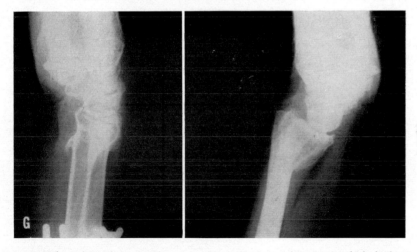

Fig. 11—(G) These lateral views show the final result in the wrist, which had received transfixion on the left above and in the opposite wrist, which had received conventional treatment elsewhere as seen on the right above.

use internal or external fixation adjuvants, a certain amount of loss of reduction will occur in any or all of the original components of deformity because of the lack of cortical support in the dorsal and radial aspects of the fracture site. This problem can be accepted temporarily while soft tissue swelling is allowed to subside, with the patient hospitalized and the wrist constantly elevated, in which case secondary reduction under general anesthesia may be

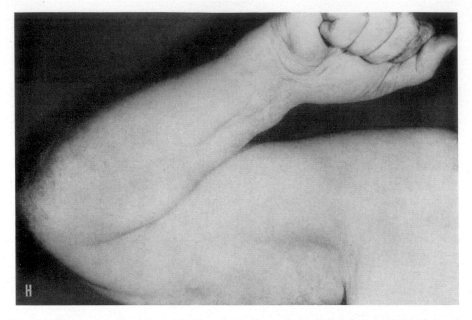

Fig. 11—(H) An excellent functional result in the wrist and hand was obtained by the transfixion pins and Steinmann pin splint. Also, a good result was achieved in the elbow. Full normal elbow, wrist and hand range of motion and strength were regained. The patient has been asymptomatic.

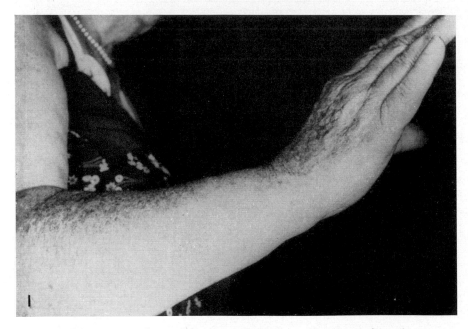

Fig. 11—(I) There was no infection from the wounds of compounding or from the pin tracts. The transfixion pins were removed at ten weeks and the patient was last seen one year after injury and is still doing well.

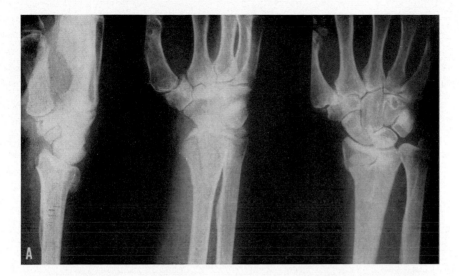

Fig. 12–(A) A small amount of dorsal angulation, dorsal displacement and radial shortening is seen in the wrist of this obese, middle-aged typist.

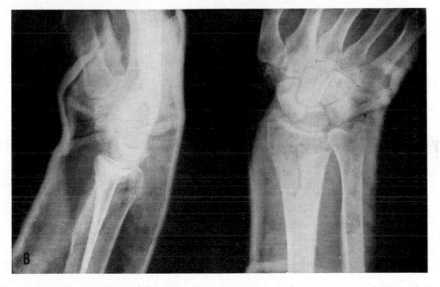

Fig. 12–(B) An excellent reduction was obtained by the traction machine and local
anesthesia. A long arm cast was applied in much less than the full Cotton-Loder position
because of considerable soft tissue swelling.

carried out with the position of maintenance of reduction tolerated. If this
second attempt is not successful in obtaining or maintaining reduction, it is
very important that the x-rays be ignored in an effort to regain early
pronation/supination and relatively early recovery of total full motion of
the wrist flexion, extension and radial and ulnar deviation (fig. 12). These

may be realized by cutting the cast down below the elbow in the first month
after injury to permit pronation/supination (fig. 13), and univalving the cast
on the ulnar side at the end of six weeks and spreading it so that it can be
removed several times daily for gentle active efforts to gain full wrist
function in all directions. If there are late problems of ulnar prominence at

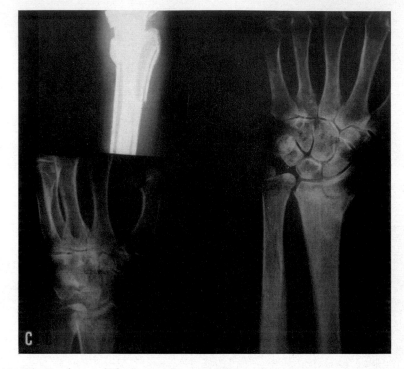

Fig. 12–(C) Further radial shortening occurred in spite of frequent recasting by the
thumb-index finger traction method. However, an excellent functional result was obtained.
The x-rays are at ten weeks after injury, when plaster was discontinued. A long arm cast
had been employed for the first three weeks and then a short arm cast substituted to allow
early pronation/supination efforts. The patient finds no difficulty from 80 per cent normal
wrist motion in all directions.

the wrist or distal radial ulnar arthritic symptoms, a Darrach procedure [1, 7]
of excision of the distal ulna should be performed (fig. 14).

   Reverse Colles' Fracture (Smith's Fracture): This fracture represents results
from a reversal of the elements of traumatic forces applied to the wrist from
those described above. The distal radial fragment is comminuted on the
anterior portion of the distal radius, and displaced and tilted anteriorly.
Like the Colles' fracture, it may involve a certain amount of radial shortening
and radial deviation, and may be associated with a fracture of the ulnar
styloid. It may also involve comminution into the wrist joint.

   The reduction is again largely dependent on adequate traction, usually to
the thumb and index finger, with the important difference that the rotary

element of displacement of the distal fragment of pronation is corrected and maintained in reduction by a position of full supination. Also, of course, a certain amount of dorsiflexion must be used, if tolerated, in some ulnar deviation (fig. 15). All of the criteria otherwise described for the Colles' fracture pertain in treating the reverse Colles' fracture or so-called Smith's fracture (fig. 16).

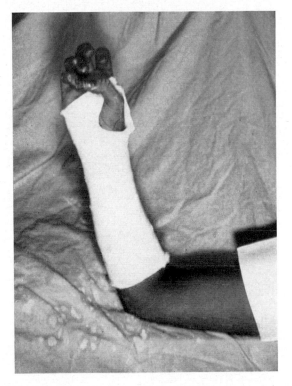

Fig. 13—This short arm cast required only one roll of three-inch plaster bandage. The patient has enough thumb room to reach the fifth finger in opposition as shown here. The distal flexion area of the palm is left exposed to permit full metacarpal phalangeal flexion.

Associated Injuries and Complications of Colles' Fracture: Any person who falls on the outstretched hand may have other injuries besides the Colles' fracture anywhere in the line of force. Infrequently, fractures of the metacarpus are seen; more frequently, but still rarely, are noted carpal injuries which may include total midcarpal row dislocations, or isolated carpal injuries such as dislocation of the lunate anteriorly or fracture of the navicular.

Occasionally, associated trauma to the elbow may be noted, as in one case of Monteggia fracture seen in the illustrations, which is indeed rare. The possibility of associated radial head fractures must be remembered and looked for. At times a dislocation of the elbow may occur with the Colles' fracture.

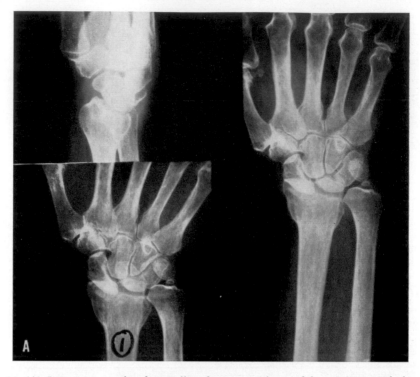

Fig. 14—(A) Late poor result of a Colles' fracture with painful prominence of the ulna from radial shortening. There was also dorsal angulation of distal radius.

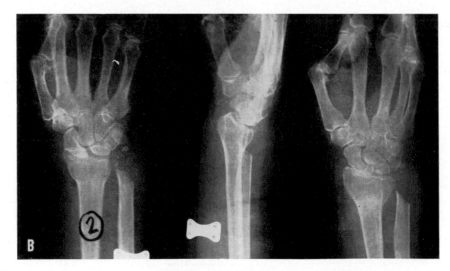

Fig. 14—(B) Painless wrist function returned after Darrach procedure of excision of the distal ulna.

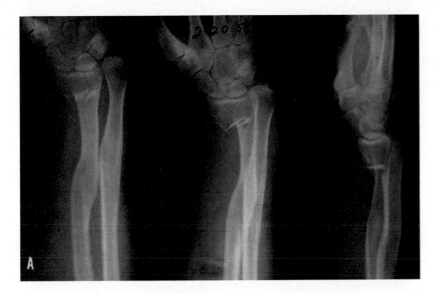

Fig. 15–(A) A Smith's, or reversed Colles' fracture in a middle-aged male with volar displacement of the distal radius, radial shortening and radial deviation. These are rare fractures caused by a fall on the back of a volary flexed wrist. This patient had had fractures of both bones of the forearm previously.

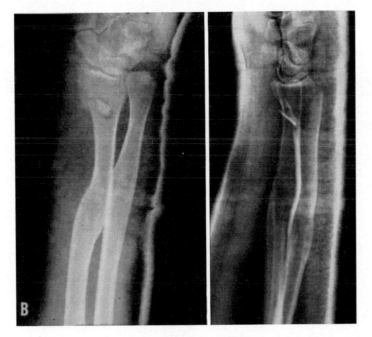

Fig. 15–(B) After reduction in the traction machine under local anesthesia. Note that the wrist is not flexed.

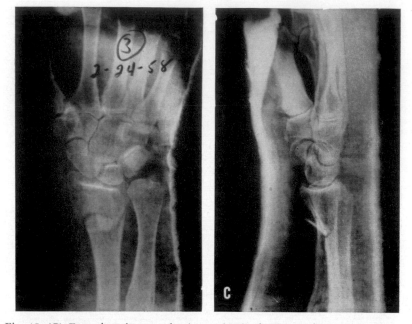

Fig. 15–(C) Four days later; reduction maintained. Note volar comminution.

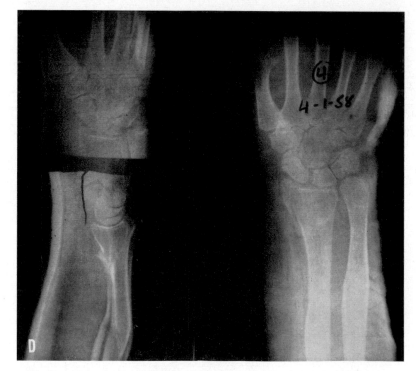

Fig. 15–(D) Six weeks later; angulation reduction has been maintained, but some radial shortening has occurred.

One should always test shoulder motion, because the line of force could include a subcapital fracture of the upper humerus, cuff tear, or anterior dislocation of the shoulder.

Late complications of Colles' fracture may include attrition rupture of extensor tendons from the chronic trauma of motion over dorsally displaced

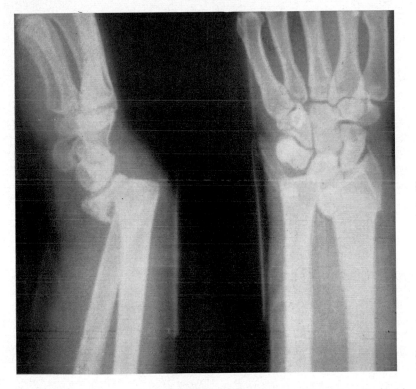

Fig. 16—(A) This severe Smith's type fracture in a twenty-three year old female was incurred in an automobile accident.

sharp radial fragments. This problem is most frequently demonstrated in late rupture of the extensor longus of the thumb.[5] Occasionally, late rupture of flexor tendons may occur.[3]

Not infrequently a severely displaced Colles' fracture will be associated with median nerve palsy. This problem will present the surgeon with a challenge of decision as to whether or not it is imperative to explore the median nerve or wait to see if return of function will occur as swelling subsides. Certainly if median nerve palsy, partial or complete, exists, any extreme position of maintenance of reduction should be decreased to more neutral alignment of the hand with the forearm, cutting constricting bandages or plaster splint down to skin even if this will mean loss of some of the position of reduction. The author would rather explore a median nerve

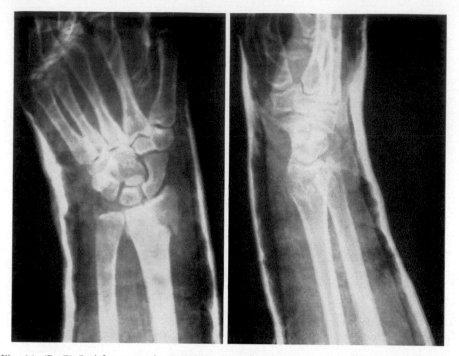

Fig. 16–(B, C) Satisfactory reduction was achieved by manipulation of traction, supination, ulnar deviation, and dorsiflexion under general anesthesia. A long arm cast was used with the elbow at 90 degrees.

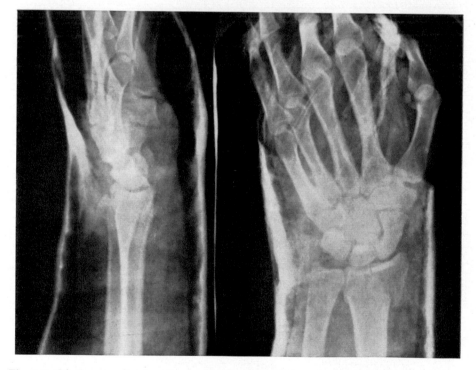

Fig. 16–(D) Some radial length was lost by the mistake of cutting the cast away from the first metacarpal at ten days to allow more thumb action. However, no further loss of reduction occurred.

needlessly than wait without reward in hopes that return of function will occur without surgery through conservative means, but the consensus of his associates has been to favor the nonsurgical procedures described above.

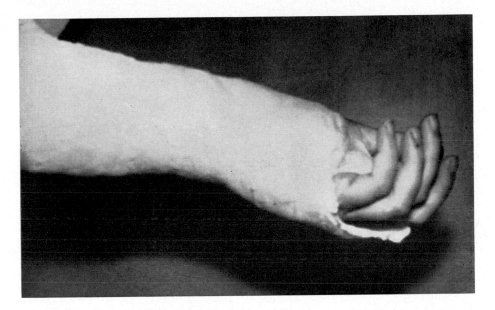

Fig. 16 (E) The cast is shown holding this Smith's type distal radial and ulnar fracture in full supination and some dorsiflexion and ulnar deviation.

Basic Principles

In treating fractures of the Colles' or Smith's type it is most important to remember that the wrist serves only to aid in function of the hand. At all costs, complete hand function must be retained. This means that if the cast holding a beautiful reduction is too tight, it must be loosened without hesitation, even at the cost of loss of reduction of the fracture, in order to relieve swelling of the hand. If median nerve pressure has resulted in palsy and this is not relieved by loosening the cast, serious consideration must be given to early exploration of the median nerve or the use of internal or external transfixion, which will maintain reduction of otherwise seriously displaced fractures causing palsy. The surgeon should always believe the patient when he complains of pain of a persistent or increasing type in the wrist or hand, even in the absence of swelling, and not hesitate to open a cast or release constricting bandages. If possible, it is very important to hospitalize all patients who have considerable primary swelling or whose fractures are so extensive that they threaten soft tissue health even after reduction. Every patient should be seen within a few hours after reduction, with repeat visit on a daily basis or more often if needed for symptoms of pain or signs of swelling, numbness or weakness of the hand.

Maintenance of a cast or fixation which limits pronation/supination in the elderly beyond three weeks is a serious threat to recovery of rotation of the forearm.

It is also very important to remember that the wrist is attached to the elbow and the shoulder. Not only should every cast be cut back in the palm proximal to the distal flexion crease and away from the thenar eminence of the thumb so that full metacarpal-phalangeal flexion and opposition are permitted, but also, when the cast is cut below the elbow, it should be sufficiently low to permit full flexion so that the patient can reach the mouth and the back of the head. Every patient, regardless of the length of cast on his arm, should be encouraged from the beginning to practice shoulder motion several times daily to maintain full abduction and rotation. Otherwise, good wrist anatomy may be associated with a frozen shoulder.

The basic philosophy in treating Colles' and Smith's fractures comes from the realization that although it is often impossible to maintain normal anatomy at the fracture site, there is no excuse for final residual significant limitation of hand, wrist, elbow or shoulder motion. [2, 4]

References

[1] APFELBACH, G.: Ulnar resection for malunited Colles and Smith fractures. Quart. Bull. Northwestern Univ. M. School 27: 1—5, 1953.

[2] BACORN, R. W.: Colles fracture, 2000 cases from New York State Workmen's Compensation Board. J. Bone & Joint Surg. 35 A: 643, (July) 1953.

[3] BRODER, H.: Rupture of flexor tendons associated with malunited Colles fracture. J. Bone & Joint Surg. 36 A: 404, (April) 1954.

[4] CASSEBAUM, W. A.: Colles fracture. J.A.M.A. 143: 963, (July) 1950.

[5] CHRISTOPHE, K.: Rupture extensor pollicis longus following Colles fracture. J. Bone & Joint Surg. 35 A: 1303, 1953.

[6] DePALMA, A. F.: Comminuted fractures of the distal end of the radius treated by ulnar pinning. J. Bone & Joint Surg. 34 A: 651—662, (July) 1952.

[7] DINGMAN, P.: Darrach procedure. J. Bone & Joint Surg., 34 A: 893, (Oct.) 1952.

[8] GECKLER, E. O.: Treatment of comminuted Colles fracture. J. Internat. Coll. Surgeons. 20: 596—601, 1953.

[9] KEY, J. A.: Compression and extension fractures at wrist (Colles fracture). Geriatrics 10: 17—25, 1955.

[10] KNAPP, M. E.: Treatment of some complications of Colles fracture. J.A.M.A. 148: 825 (March) 1952.

[11] LOVELL, E. S.: New aid in management of Colles fracture. Am. J. Surg. 84: 375, (Sept.) 1952.

[12] MASON, H. L.: Colles fracture; survey and results. Brit. J. Surg. 40: 340, 1953.

[13] MASON, M. L.: Management of Colles fracture. Med. Illus. 8: 837, 1954.

[14] PELTIER, L. F.: Abraham Colles and Colles fracture. Surgery 35: 322 (Feb.) 1954.

[15] SALLAM, A. M.: Artificial wrist (intentional pseudarthrosis in Colles fracture). Brit. M. J. 2: 1463, (Dec.) 1954.

[16] SHIPP, F. L. and SPENCER, F. A.: Colles fracture — surgical pitfall. Surg. Clin. N. A. 32: 727, (June) 1952.

[17] STRONG, J. M.: Treatment of Colles fracture. Surg., Gynec. & Obst. 101: 107, (July) 1955.

[18] WICHERN, W. and BACON, R.: Traction Device for Fractures of the Forearm. J.A.M.A. 146: (July) 1951.

[19] WILSON, P. D. and COCHRANE, W. A.: Management of Fractures and Dislocations. Philadelphia, J. P. Lippincott Co. 1928, pp. 656—657.

CHAPTER 37

FRACTURES AND DISLOCATIONS OF CARPAL BONES

Howard D. Balensweig, M.D., and Irvin Balensweig, M.D.

Injuries to the wrist are the most common injuries seen by the fracture surgeon. Nothing is as disabling as the loss of use of the hand. We eat with our hands, we dress with our hands, we work with our hands and we even think with our hands. In a large series of all injuries to the wrist, approximately 14 percent were injuries to the carpus. Among these, 70.8 percent were injuries to the navicular bone, 5.6 percent were injuries to the lunate and 14.3 percent were injuries to the triangular bone. The remainder made up approximately 9 percent.

Anatomy of the Wrist

The radius is the main bone of the wrist, with the cup-shaped articular surface being tilted about 20 degrees ulnarward and 15 degrees palmarward. In some people the radial styloid is long and in others it is short. It articulates with the distal ulna as a separate relatively extrinsic joint of the wrist, and the radio-ulnar joint is the one that is primarily concerned with rotation. The radial styloid lies approximately one-half inch distal to the ulnar styloid in the normal wrist.

The proximal carpal row consists of the scaphoid, lunate, triquetrum and pisiform. The pisiform is actually an accessory bone and does not play any real part in the function of the wrist except as a portion of the buttress on the ulnar side for the transverse carpal ligament. It is primarily a sesamoid bone in the flexor carpi ulnaris.

The distal carpal row consists of the distal half of the scaphoid, the lesser multangular, the capitate and the hamate. The greater multangular is usually considered in the distal carpal row, but is primarily the articulating bone for the thumb.

Functional Anatomy

When one considers the wrist as a connection between the forearm and the hand, one main unit is the third metacarpal, which is firmly attached to the capitate, connecting the hand to the distal carpal row. The capitate is the keystone bone in the distal carpal row, which moves on a cup-shaped joint formed by the proximal pole of the scaphoid and the entire lunate bone. The proximal pole of the scaphoid and lunate as one unit moves on the distal end of the radius. This arrangement is the stable connection between the radius and the hand. Dorsiflexion and palmar flexion occur at the radial carpal joint and the joint between the proximal and distal carpal rows. The greater portion of the dorsiflexion occurs between the lunate and the radius, approximately two-thirds occuring here and one-third between the capitate and the lunate. In palmar flexion, the reverse is true.

Ulnar and radial deviation occur primarily through the radiocarpal joint, and in this motion the distal ulna enters into the wrist as a functional unit since it carries the ulnar collateral ligament, and on radial deviation the lunate swings over and articulates with the triangular ligament arising from the ulnar styloid and attaching to the ulnar side of the distal radius.

The thumb is an independent unit separate from the hand and articulating with the wrist through the greater multangular and the distal portion of the scaphoid and lesser multangular.

The wrist also serves as a protective mechanism for the soft tissues running from the forearm into the palm. There is a definite, fan-shaped channel running into the palm, on the ulnar side formed by the hook of the hamate and the pisiform bone and a portion of the triquetrum. On the radial side it is formed by the tubercle of the scaphoid and the greater multangular.

In the front of wrist, the carpal tunnel contains the flexor tendons and the median nerve, the nerve lying immediately beneath the transverse carpal ligament and on top of the flexor tendons to the fingers. Compression of the median nerve has recently been recognized secondary to injuries of the wrist joint.

Examination of the Wrist

Examination of the wrist should take cognizance of all available information. The history, including, if possible, the mechanism of injury; the present complaints in detail including questioning as to paresthesias; local examination as to deformity of the wrist, points of tenderness, circulation, neurologic status and ranges of motion. We recently saw a 15 year old boy who had a hyperextension injury of the wrist. The initial x-rays were negative. The examination revealed hypesthesia in the distribution of the median nerve, and over the next few days this went on to complete anesthesia. Eventually, x-rays revealed a greenstick type fracture of the distal radius. In this case, he probably had a stretching of the median nerve associated with a hematoma about it. If he had been older, the most likely diagnosis would have been a dislocation of the lunate with spontaneous reduction.

The most important part of the examination is the taking of x-rays of both wrists in identical position in multiple views. They should not be read wet. If the x-rays prove negative and patient has pain over the snuffbox area, a light plaster cast should be applied and repeat x-rays taken in two to three weeks. If patient has symptoms and the x-rays are again negative, they should be repeated two weeks later. Fractures of the navicular may take up to four weeks to show themselves. Ligamentous injuries associated with circulatory changes to the lunate may take four to eight weeks to demonstrate themselves by x-ray. When there is still doubt, magnified x-rays can be taken by a special technic using a pin hole in a lead plate in front of the tube and placing the wrist about 6 to 8 inches away from the plate. This will produce magnification and at times demonstrates fractures not otherwise visualized.

Although fractures of the distal radius are rarely associated with injuries to the carpus, they can occur. Anywhere between one-half of 1 per cent and

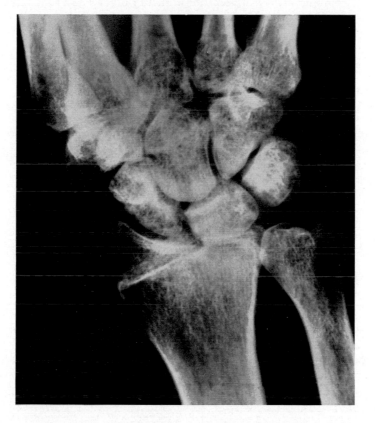

Fig. 1—Anteroposterior view of wrist showing healed fracture of radial styloid process, with disruption of the relationships between the lunate and scaphoid or navicular, secondary to this type of injury.

2 per cent of fractures of the radius have associated fractures of the carpus. Two types of fracture may be associated with fracture of the wrist—the type which runs transversely through the base of the radial styloid, or that which runs obliquely into the wrist joint from below up, entering in the region between the lunate and scaphoid. These may be associated with fractures of the waist of the scaphoid or associated with subluxation of the lunate and circulatory changes. A further type of injury to the distal radius resulting in a lesion of the carpus is that of the longitudinal type of fracture of the distal radius which opens up and allows the carpus to slide in between the fragments; in addition there is the type or injury in which the anterior

or the posterior half slips. Associated with this longitudinal fracture the carpus may be dislocated either anteriorly or posteriorly. These injuries are very difficult to handle. The problem is more properly taken up in a discussion about Colles' type fractures, but we would suggest that in the younger age group where this type of fracture cannot be reduced closed, one is warranted in doing an open procedure. In the older age group, there is too much comminution to hope to maintain satisfactory reduction.

Lunate and Perilunar Dislocations

A fall on the outstretched hand with forced dorsiflexion of the wrist most often results in a Colles' type fracture. On occasion we have a dislocation of one or more of the carpal bones with or without associated fracture. In the young adult, the radius may be sufficiently strong so that the injury occurs in the carpus. Hyperextension applied through the carpus may attack either the anterior ligamentous structures in the capitate lunate joint, the lunate radial joint or both. The most common injury is that of anterior dislocation of the lunate. In this we have two degrees of dislocation. The milder degree of dislocation of the lunate results from rupture of the anterior structures betweeen the capitate and lunate and rupture of the posterior attachments of the lunate to the radius. The lunate then rotates 45 to 90 degrees on its anterior connection to the distal radius. In the second degree of dislocation, all attachments of the lunate to the radius and carpus are ruptured and the lunate may rotate as much as 180 degrees, lying completely anterior to the wrist joint.

When the lunate is more firmly fixed to the radius than the capitate, we may have a perilunar dislocation, usually backward. All possible varieties of perilunar dislocation exist. The lunate may be the only bone fixed to the radius while the remainder of the carpus dislocates posteriorly. The lunate and proximal half of the scaphoid may remain attached and the rest of the carpus go posteriorly. The lunate and entire scaphoid may remain in place with the remainder of the carpus going posteriorly. Many of these cases are more complex and we get various chip fractures of the remainder of the carpal bones associated with the basic type of dislocation. One of the commonest types of perilunar dislocation is associated with the fracture through the waist of the scaphoid, since the intercarpal joint runs through the scaphoid itself if one considers the capitate articulating with the lunate and scaphoid as one joint. Only the proximal portion of the scaphoid enters into this joint.

By far the commonest mistake among inexperienced people is to miss the diagnosis of a dislocation of the lunate or perilunar dislocation. It is most important to take the opposite wrist for comparison. Generally, one will see either overlapping of bones in a perilunar dislocation in the anterior posterior view along with malalignment of the axis of the capitate to the lunate, or a change in the shape of the lunate in lunate dislocations from square to triangular.

Fresh dislocations of the lunate and perilunar dislocation should be reduced as an emergency procedure under general anesthesia. The safest technic of reduction is to apply longitudinal traction with an assistant holding onto the flexed elbow and applying countertraction. One will feel a click and find that the dislocation has reduced itself. Repeated forceful manipulations will produce so much edema and trauma that one may end up with a median nerve palsy, swollen wrist and useless hand. If traction for 10 minutes with maximum force has not succeeded in reducing the dislocation, one is permitted to go through various maneuvers to attempt reduction. In anterior dislocations of the lunate, the next procedure is strong traction with the wrist dorsiflexed and gentle pressure applied to the anteriorly dislocated lunate from proximal distalward, since the lunate always rotates toward the upper arm. If these maneuvers are not successful, and they may not be in occasional severe dislocations of the lunate with ripping of all attachments, open reduction is then preferable to further manipulations of a traumatic nature. One should probably use a combined approach both anteriorly and posteriorly, although often the anterior approach alone is sufficient. If it is necessary to use a skid and bone hook, etc., to push the lunate back into a space not large enough to accept it from the anterior approach, it is preferable to open up posteriorly as well and use more gentle measures. If the dislocation still cannot be reduced, excision of the lunate is preferable to destroying the cartilage of the lunate in an attempt to replace it. Fresh injuries will almost never require excision of the lunate.

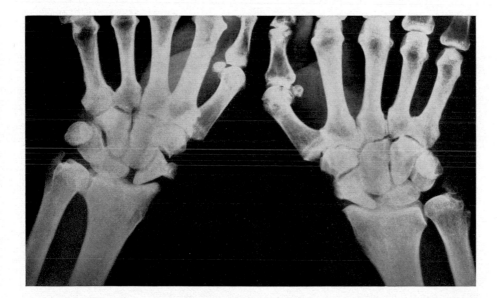

Fig. 2—Anteroposterior view, both wrists, in a heavy worker showing osteoarthritic lippings off the distal end of the navicular bilaterally, and definite separation between the lunate and scaphoid bones.

In reductions of the lunate delayed up to about three weeks, one is warranted again in attempting closed reduction and, if necessary, open reduction. Beyond three weeks, it is preferable to remove the lunate rather than to replace an almost surely avascular bone. If the patient engages in work that requires a strong but not a very flexible wrist, fusion of the wrist as a primary procedure following prolonged dislocation of the lunate is probably preferable to simple excision of the lunate.

C. J. Wagner[1] reviewed 78 carpal injuries in which there were various degrees of loss of the normal relationship between the lunate and capitate bones. He felt that cases of perilunar dislocation associated with fracture of the navicular, unless they could be perfectly reduced, should have a primary wrist fusion. Also, cases of perilunar dislocation associated with aseptic necrosis of the proximal pole of the navicular should have wrist fusion. In uncomplicated fractures of the navicular, immobilization until the fracture is healed will give a good functional wrist. This is because there is little intra-articular damage. When this same fracture is associated with a perilunar dislocation, one has massive damage to the ligamentous structures of the wrist with probably a moderate amount of damage to the cartilaginous covering of the bones. Immobilization for a prolonged period in the face of this type of damage will leave residual limitations of motion and often pain.

A type of injury not described in the literature but observed by us and akin to perilunar dislocation is that of disruption of the connection between the scaphoid and lunate bones. This may be the only injury detectable by x-ray or may be associated with a fracture of the navicular. It probably represents a form of complete perilunar dislocation which spontaneously reduced with some rotation of the scaphoid. In our experience this widening of the space between the scaphoid and lunate as seen in figure 2 leaves some permanent disability.

Fractures of the Lunate

Fractures of the lunate are very uncommon. Most often the lunate dislocates rather than fractures. Occasionally, we have chip fractures of the lunate often associated with perilunar dislocation or associated with spontaneously reduced perilunar dislocations. There occasionally is a horizontal form of fracture through the lunate caused by a twisting injury. We have also seen fractures of the lunate secondary to long standing Kienböck's disease of the lunate with a new injury (fig. 3). Treatment for fractures of the lunate consist of a few weeks of immobilization followed by active exercises if there is only a chip fracture. With a fracture through the body of the lunate six to eight weeks of immobilization are usually required.

Fractures and Dislocations of the Lesser Carpal Bones

Fractures of the carpal bones, aside from the lunate and scaphoid, are quite rare, as are dislocations. In crushing injuries to the hand, one may find linear fractures of the capitate, since it is the largest carpal bone. In other injuries to the wrist, one may find chip fractures, often of the triquetrum or back of the capitate. Usually these fractures require a short period of immobilization followed by active exercises. Occasionally, chip fractures on the dorsum of the wrist may be painful and require excision. Dislocations

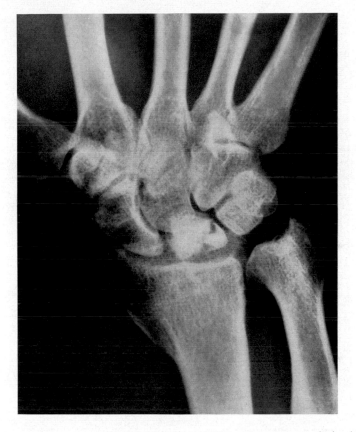

Fig. 3—Anteroposterior view of wrist, showing old Kienböck disease of the lunate bone with a fresh fracture through it. One can see a deformity of the distal radius and ulna, suggesting that he had had a fracture of the wrist in the past, probably productive of the Kienböck disease.

are extremely rare, and when they do occur should be promptly reduced, if necessary, by operation.

Fractures of the Navicular and their Sequelae

These fractures are overlooked quite often when accompanied by a Colles' fracture. The treating physician focuses his attention upon the fracture of the radius and ignores the navicular.

There are three main levels of injury of the carpal navicular, the most frequent occurring through the waist of the bone. The prognosis is about two-thirds for rapid healing and one-third for delayed healing or nonunion, depending on the amount of damage to the blood supply. The second most frequent level is through the distal third of the navicular, and healing in this region occurs in most of the cases, occasioned by the fact that the blood supply has not been materially damaged and the texture of the bone is

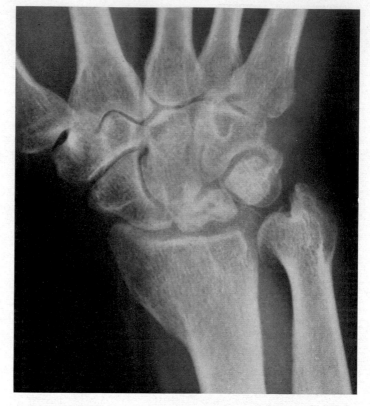

Fig. 4—Anteroposterior view of wrist, following old fracture of distal radius which extended into the wrist joint at the level of the lunate bone, and with resultant Kienböck disease of the lunate bone.

excellent. Fractures occurring through the proximal pole of the navicular are least frequent and union least apt to occur (fig. 5).

Aseptic necrosis is easily recognized in a wrist because the lesser fragment remains dense whereas the major fragment shows decalcification. If a fracture of the proximal pole of the navicular shows evidence of aseptic necrosis within three to six weeks from the time of trauma, it is safer to remove the loose fragment in order to obtain a satisfactory result rather than to wait for the possibility of union by prolonged immobilization.

We recently examined a patient who had fractured the carpal navicular and who failed to respond to the usual prolonged period of immobilization. The line of fracture was through the waist of the navicular and there was no accompanying aseptic necrosis. Because of persistence of pain it was decided to operate on this patient and remove the proximal fragment. The operative report specifically mentions the purpose of the operation and what was done, but we did not witness the operation. Instead of removing the proximal fragment, however, the distal one was removed. This patient obtained a most satisfactory result (fig. 7).

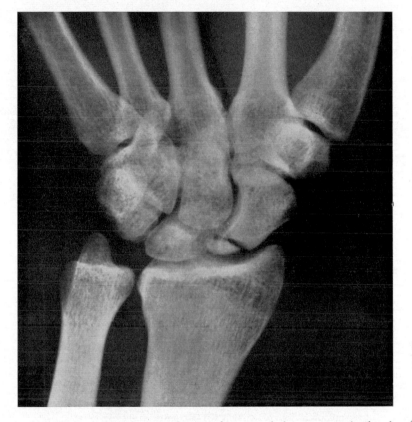

Fig. 5—Anteroposterior view of wrist, showing fracture of the very proximal pole of the navicular bone, about 8 weeks old. There is early aseptic necrosis of the proximal pole and rounding off of the fracture ends, indicating that this will probably go on to non-union.

In the presence of extensive arthritic changes, we believe that there is but one choice, and that is fusion of the wrist or, if the patient elects, surgical neglect. It is surprising how well people do if left to their own resourcefulness. There are many patients with ununited fractures of the carpal navicular with secondary arthritic changes who had been told that they suffered sprained wrists and still did remarkably well. Most of these were seen for other injuries and during the routine examination it was noted that they had injuries of the wrist and were x-rayed. We do not advocate neglect of proper treatment. Prompt immobilization maintained until healing takes place

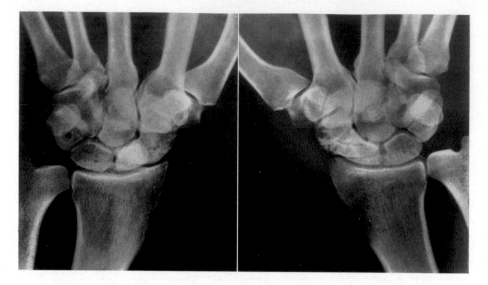

Fig. 6—Anteroposterior view both wrists, demonstrating old injuries to both wrists, resulting on one side in a fracture of the navicular, with aseptic necrosis of the proximal third; and on the other side a vascular change, not actual aseptic necrosis following an injury to the navicular bone.

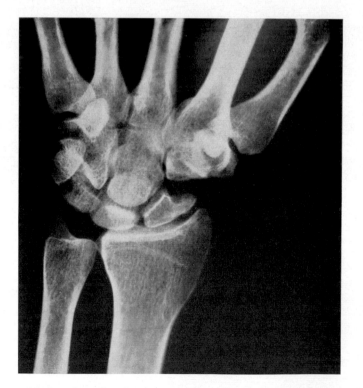

Fig. 7—Anteroposterior view of wrist, post-operative, showing accidental removal of distal half of navicular bone for non-union, with excellent clinical end result.

is the method of choice. However, it is wise to make certain reservations, depending on the situation as it is met with. It has been wisely stated that it is sometimes better to have nine carpal bones with comparatively mild discomfort rather than seven or eight carpal bones with a great deal of discomfort and deformity.

This subject was studied by J. S. Barr et al. [2] It was their feeling that treatment of nonunion was not particularly satisfactory. Out of fourteen men with nonunion, nine were treated conservatively without improvement, five were operated on, and of these, two obtained union with satisfactory results. Functional impairment was present in every case, although earning power was impaired in only 42 per cent of the cases. Of the fourteen wrists with nonunion, one showed a normal work capacity.

References

[1] WAGNER, C. J.: Perilunar dislocation. J. Bone & Joint Surg. *38*: 1198—1207, (Dec.) 1956.

[2] BARR, J. S., ELLISTON, W. A., MUSNICK, H., DeLORME, E. L., HANFLINN, J. and THIBODEAU, A. A.: Fracture of the carpal navicular bone and end result study in military personnel. J. Bone & Joint Surg. *35* A: 609—625, (July) 1953.

CHAPTER 38

FRACTURES IN THE HAND

LEE RAMSAY STRAUB, M.D.

Principles of Therapy in Fractures of the Hand

The aim of treatment of finger and palmar fractures is the early restoration of complete grasp and normal pinch. These objectives may not be obtainable in comminuted crushing injuries, but perfection, insofar as possible, should be the constant goal. Restoration of grasp and pinch with dexterity and strength requires (1) alignment, (2) mobility and (3) stability.

Alignment

Preservation of the longitudinal and transverse arcs of the hand is essential. The transverse arc of the palm is formed by the closely fixed relationship of the second, third, fourth and fifth metacarpals. The arch thus formed can be increased by flexion and rotation of the fourth and fifth metacarpals. The second and third metacarpals are relatively fixed. The first metacarpal opposes each of the other metacarpals and has been called the "hub of the wheel" by Littler. Full flexion of the second to fifth metacarpophalangeal joints with the proximal interphalangeal joints flexed and the distal interphalangeal joints extended brings each respective finger tip to very nearly the same point on the thenar eminence overlying the tuber of the scaphoid bone. This relationship is essential to normal pinch with all fingers. Proper rotary alignment of fractures of the metacarpals, the proximal phalanges, and to a lesser degree, the middle phalanges is required for proper grasp and opposition.

Longitudinal concavity in the hand makes for better grasp. It is formed by the natural curve in the volar shape of metacarpals and phalanges, by the attitude of all finger joints while in the resting position and by the prominence of the transverse carpal ligament with attached thenar musculature. The continuity of this arc is greatly disturbed by fractures with displacement into volar angulation, usually of the middle or proximal phalanges.

Immobilization of the thumb: Whether fixation of the thumb is done by splint or traction it should be placed in a position of wide opposition. If placed on a flat board in adduction and extension, a very resistant web space contracture may result.

Mobility

Preservation of motion in the interphalangeal and especially in the metacarpophalangeal joints requires a minimum of total immobilization, and this in an anatomically acceptable position. Interphalangeal joints should be held in the position of function (the position of rest; see Hand Injuries, fig. 5).

The collateral ligaments of the metacarpophalangeal joints are relaxed in extension, tight in flexion. If a metacarpophalangeal joint is splinted at 180 degrees, the collateral ligaments will shorten, thus producing a fixed extension contracture. The metacarpophalangeal joints of the second, third and fourth fingers should therefore be fixed in considerable flexion. In isolated noncrushing fractures, splinting should include only the finger requiring it — no others. Various methods of internal fixation provide, as their chief advantage, a means of early mobilization.

Stability

Osseous and articular stability are needed for strength and mobility in pinch and grasp. Finger strength and motion will be reduced by an ununited metacarpal fracture. Pinch will be weak at best, with an unstable interphalangeal joint. It would be better to have an arthrodesed joint in a functional position.

External Splinting of Hand and Fingers

Only the finger or fingers affected should be immobilized, whether the fixation is by plaster or by metallic splint. The splint should include the total ray involved, with tip showing and should extend above the wrist to provide better support. Whatever method of fixation is used, the finger should be in a position of function (rest position). This is a position of moderate flexion which can be determined readily as the position fingers assume when the entire hand is put at rest with the palm upward. Fingers should never be immobilized in the straight extended position by any means, nor should the hand be immobilized on a palmar basswood splint. A Universal splint (see Hand Injuries, fig. 4) may be used for limited periods. Finger traction of a number of types can be employed, but traction will seldom provide reduction. It is merely another means of immobilization once reduction has been obtained. Skin traction is almost useless and may be dangerous. It is unsafe to leave circular dressings of this type on a finger for any period, and the use of the oriental finger trap for prolonged traction is to be condemned because of its obvious compressive dangers. Finger pulp traction is widely employed, but because of skin sloughs is not as good as pin traction through bone. Skeletal traction can be done through the proximal half of the distal phalanx or through almost any portion of the middle phalanx of the lesser fingers (fig. 1). It can be done in either of the phalanges of the thumb. Due regard to the position of the lateral bands is necessary in placing a pin in a finger. Use of pins requires operating room care and technic. Traction is best accomplished over a curved volar splint as a rule, and the plaster portion of the splint must extend above the wrist for adequate anchorage. Elastic bands may be employed for tension, which may be increased by a Spanish windless. The banjo splint, holding all the fingers in full extension, has no place in treatment of fractures of the hand.

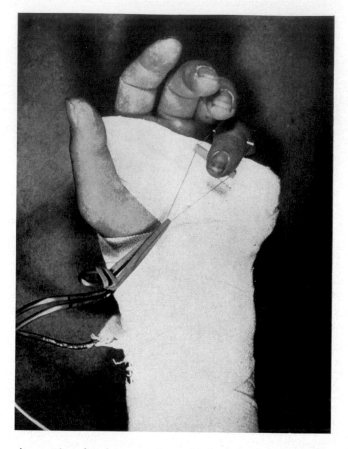

Fig. 1—Wire pin traction for fracture of proximal phalanx. Pin through mid-phalanx. Note the direction of the pull. (Courtesy Dr. Rolla D. Campbell Jr.)

Compound Wounds

Wounds compounded from within or without are an operating room problem. The same rules of exploration, cleansing and débridement apply here as in fractures elsewhere. The method of fixation must be determined by the degree of contamination in the period following the compounding. In general, internal fixation in a truly compound fracture is risky.

Period of Fracture Immobilization

Generally speaking, finger joints can be immobilized completely for only three to four weeks. Since four to six weeks may be required for fracture healing, consideration must often be given to the use of internal fixation. If prolonged external support is necessary, in most instances it should be removable so that gentle underwater exercises can be done.

Crush Injuries with Fracture

In this condition the fractures must usually be regarded as secondary. If there is any break in the skin, the fractures must be regarded as compound. The dangers of ischemia are present, and the soft tissue injury must be considered first. If the forearm has been involved, there may be a Volkmann's ischemia, and operative release of vessels and/or nerves may be a primary necessity. The hand may be molded over a Universal splint with a well padded compressive dressing. When desirable, internal fixation of fractures can be accomplished after edema subsides.

Crushing Injuries of the Distal Tuft

These injuries are very common in car door and industrial accidents. They are frequently compounded and may include injury to the nail or nail bed. It is of primary importance here, as in other compound conditions, to obtain a clean wound. Attention is therefore directed to the nail and the soft tissues more than to the fracture itself. Appropriate cleansing and gentle débridement of surely devitalized tissue is all that is done. The nail, if partially avulsed, may be removed. If merely lacerated, the nail should be retained for added support. Gentle dressings which will serve as immobilization are employed. It is best to disregard the fracture fragments as they give rise to little difficulty in the late result. Wounds should not be closed if there is any question of vitality of the skin margins. If the skin of the tip of the finger has been totally avulsed, it is well to resect a little phalanx to free enough good volar skin for closure. This will save many weeks of disability as compared to a free or pedicle skin graft.

The simple, noncompounded crush of the distal phalanx is best treated by a simple aluminum splint to protect against undue painful pressure.

Fractures of the Phalanges

The common types of transverse fractures of the phalanges are illustrated in figure 2. These result from direct blow. There may be injury of associated soft tissue, particularly of the flexor tendon mechanism. Careful evaluation of each fracture is important.

Treatment: Accurate reduction is imperative to good function. External fixation requires the use of traction over a curved splint. The splint should extend up the forearm. Traction with an outrigger and elastic band is done either with pin fixation in the distal phalanx or, if good reduction is obtained, with gentle traction to the tip of the finger nail. Here, traction serves as a means of fixation only; reduction must be obtained manually. The use of gauze rolls should be avoided, as they are, at best, a poor substitute for good immobilization. In applying traction or in immobilizing these fingers it must be remembered that in flexion the fingers all tend to meet and point toward the thenar eminence, or more specifically, the tubercle of the scaphoid. This direction of immobilization is essential to avoid rotary defects and malunion. Traction should be continued for three weeks. Splint immobilization in the

duction and fixation with buried transverse fine Kirschner wires which can be removed later, and then plaster fixation of the thumb as described for transverse fractures of the metacarpal base. (2) If there is comminution, however, this type of fixation will prove unstable and skeletal traction is desired (fig. 7). The pin can be passed transversely through the base of the distal phalanx or through the distal one-quarter of the proximal phalanx. Elastic band fixation should be then directed to an outrigger incorporated in the plaster cast. The position again should be one of abduction and opposition. The traction should be continued for four weeks, when fixation should be changed to a removable splint to be used in association with underwater exercises for two more weeks.

Bennett's fracture-dislocation probably presents more troubles in obtaining and retaining perfect reduction than any other fracture in the hand. Its treatment should not be undertaken lightly.

Dislocations and Fracture-Dislocations

Dislocations of the interphalangeal joints are by no means uncommon. When seen in the first hour or two, reduction without anesthesia is possible and, in fact, is usually done by the patient before he seeks medical advice. Radiographs should be obtained at once, whether or not the dislocation has been reduced prior to the patient's appearance so that any condylar fracture may be recognized. When reduction is delayed, general anesthesia is preferred. Steady manual traction in a straight line is preferred and will usually cause reduction with restoration of alignment. A splint is applied in the position of flexion. Reduction will be stable if there is no associated avulsion fracture. The presence of such a fracture with displacement suggests the necessity of open fixation of the fragment.

If the dislocation does not reduce by closed means with a reasonable firmness, but without added trauma, open reduction should be done at once. The patient should understand the possibility of this outcome before the administration of anesthesia. The condyles of the dislocated phalanx, usually the base of the middle phalanx, on passing volar to the distal portion of the proximal phalanx, have torn through the capsule or the volar plate and locked in this constricting band. This may be irreducible except by open means. Approach is made through a midlateral incision. The capsule is further opened and reduction accomplished.

Irreducible dislocation occurs most frequently at the metacarpophalangeal joint of the thumb (fig. 8). The phalanx is displaced dorsally on the metacarpal which passes through a rent in the capsule between the two heads of insertion of the flexor pollicis brevis. The flexor pollicis longus then passes beneath the dislocated condyles of the metacarpal rendering reduction by traction virtually impossible. Reduction is accomplished through a radiolateral incision. It is wise to identify and isolate the radiodigital nerve to the thumb, as this may be in close association to the flexor pollicis longus tendon as it passes round the metacarpal. A fine silk suture or two in the rent between the heads of the short flexor may be well placed.

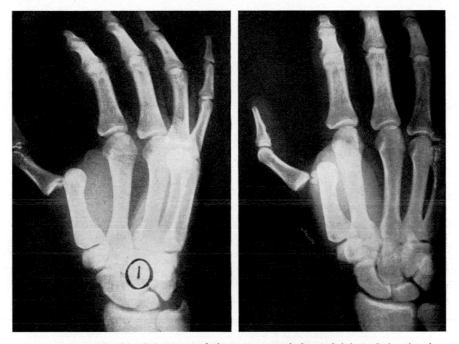

Fig. 8—(A) Irreducible dislocation of the metacarpophalangeal joint of the thumb.

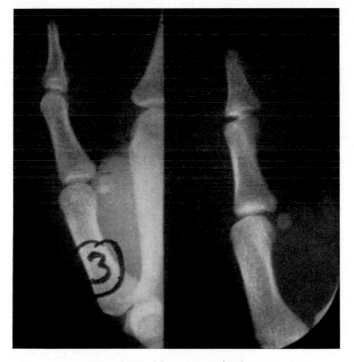

Fig. 8—(B) After open reduction.

Immobilizations in Fracture-Dislocations

The basic rules of hand immobilization apply here as elsewhere. The periods of immobilization must be kept to a minimum compatible with stability and maintenance of reduction. Position of immobilization is even more important in injuries to these joints than in those to the shaft of the phalanges or metacarpals. The so-called position of function is the acceptable position with rare exception. If a condylar oblique fracture complicates a dislocation, use of internal means of fixation may allow for earlier mobility and thus improve eventual function. Swelling will persist for at least six months and possibly a year, at a finger joint that has been dislocated, and these joints will remain sensitive to pressure for an equally long period. Patients must be reassured on this point.

Bibliography

ANDREIMI, G.: Avulsion fracture of the distal phalanges of the hand in relation to the insertion of the extensor tendons. Internat. Abstr. Surg. *103*: 72, 1956.

BELL, J. L., MASON, M. L., and ALLEN, H. S.: Management of acute crushing injuries of hand and forearm over 5 year period. Am. J. Surg. *87*: 370, (Mar.) 1954.

BRUNER, J. M.: Problem of postoperative position and motion. J. Bone & Joint Surg. *35 A*: 355, 1953.

BUNNELL, S.: Surgery of the Hand. Ed. 3. Philadelphia, J. B. Lippincott, 1956.

CLIFFORD, R. H.: Intramedullary wire fixation. Plastic & Reconstr. Surg. *11*: 366, (May) 1953.

GRAHAM, W. C.: Transplantation of joints to replace damaged articulation in hands. Am. J. Surg. *88*: 136, 1954.

LITTLER, W.: Textbook of Orthopaedic Surgery by M. B. Howorth, Philadelphia, W. B. Saunders Co., 1952.

MEMETHI, C. E.: Phalangeal fractures treated by open reduction and Kirschner wire fixation. Indust. Med. *23*: 148, (April) 1954.

PIGAUD, A. J.: Suggestion for surgical treatment of spiral fracture of the metacarpal bone with two or three fragments. Int. Abstr. Surg. *103*: 71, 1956.

VOM SAAL, F. H.: Intramedullary fixation in fractures of hand and fingers. J. Bone & Joint Surg. *35 A*: 516, 1953.

ZELENOCK, M. N., LARSEN, R. D., and POSCH, J. L.: Treatment of fractures of the hand. Arch. Surg. *75*: 320—338, (Sept.) 1957.

CHAPTER 39

INJURIES TO THE HAND

LEE RAMSAY STRAUB, M.D.

Prevention of Hand Injuries and Infections

Most hand injuries are preventable. Many are caused by carelessness or by devices which are mechanically unsound. Education of the householder and of the industrialist forms the heart of a preventive program. The elimination of dangerous practices in the home and of faulty tools can be encouraged by instructional programs in clubs, schools, the press and television. The enforcement of building codes has been effective in eliminating dangerous fittings such as the porcelain faucet handle. Care in the design of such utensils as can openers and vegetable peelers and the insulation of pot handles may considerably reduce the incidence of home hand accidents. Provision of high individual racks for the storage of sharp knives, and modern arrangements of hot surfaces for the protection of children's hands is proving worthwhile.

In industry there should be safety committees in all shops and installations. All machines must be provided with adequate safety guards. A nursing and first-aid staff should be on hand for the treatment of all hand injuries even the most minor, and a constant educational program should be conducted so that the injured worker will seek immediate treatment and thus possibly avoid prolonged disability. Operators who repeatedly injure themselves should be moved to other jobs and locations. Any wound that requires more than one dressing should be referred to the staff physician. Clinics handling injuries should classify the source of all injuries, both home and industrial, so that adequate studies will eliminate unnecessary hazards in the future.

Emergency Treatment

The initial definitive care must be correct, or irreparable damage may be done to the injured hand.

Open Injuries of the Hand

When the skin of the hand is opened by injury, clean wound-healing is the prime objective of emergency treatment. All other factors are secondary to this basic need.

The type and severity of the injury may vary greatly. The degree of contamination is never the same. The wound may be a razor cut or a jagged tear with loss of skin. It is here that fine surgical judgment must be exercised as to the means at hand to provide a noninfected hand with an intact skin coverage. If this basic fact is always borne in mind in the initial therapy after an injury, the problems of definitive hand surgery will be lessened. We can speak here only in general terms.

Emergency Treatment

Only the most superficial, open, nonpenetrating lacerations should be treated in an emergency room or office and then only when facilities are adequate for irrigation to the depths of the wound. The hand must be cleansed with soap and water for a 10 minute period, the depths of the wound thoroughly irrigated with normal saline and carefully inspected by an unhurried, gloved and masked examiner with good light. If involvement of tendon or nerve is found, dressing should be applied, and the patient transferred to the operating room for definitive care. If no deep structure involvement is present, skin closure is obtained with as few dermalon sutures as possible. No subcutaneous suture is used. Most often these procedures can be done without anesthesia. Occasionally, a local or regional block may be desirable. Finger tourniquet should not be used, as this may do permanent damage to vessels or nerves. Grossly contaminated wounds, more than six hours old, should not be closed, but only thoroughly cleansed and dressed. Clean wounds more than eight hours old should not be closed. Antibiotics should be given for any deep wound open more than two hours, and for all grossly contaminated wounds.

A tetanus toxoid booster should be administered for those patients who have received toxoid inoculations before. Others with deep, contaminated or puncture wounds should receive tetanus antitoxin.

General Anatomic Considerations

Figure 1 indicates the arrangement of the synovial sheaths. It will be noted that the infections of the sheath in the thumb and fifth finger may ascend into the forearm, whereas infections of the other three synovial sheaths will remain distalwards. Deep to these synovial sheaths, the palmar space is divided into three specific spaces. The hypothenar is enclosed by the thin fascia covering the hypothenar musculature. The thenar space is bounded by the fascia covering the thenar musculature and the midpalmar space. This latter space is of greatest importance. Its roof is formed by the fascia beneath the flexor tendons of the index, long, ring and fifth fingers. Its floor is formed by the fascia covering the third and fourth interosseous muscles, and the fascia covering the abductor muscles of the thumb. The medial border is ill defined. The fascial layer here makes for poor protection. The fascia arises from the third metacarpal shaft and extends radially to the region of the first lumbrical. Infection penetrates readily in that direction. On the ulnar border the midpalmar space is bounded by the fascia arising from the fifth metacarpal and extending over the hypothenar muscles. Distally, this space extends into the lumbrical canals of the ring and middle fingers; proximally, the space passes under the transverse carpal ligament and may extend into the forearm. Infections of the thenar and hypothenar space are generally less destructive than those of the midpalmar space or those of the synovial sheaths. Infections of the midpalmar space will direct backwards, because of the firm nature of the volar structures in front of them (fig. 2).

Palmar Incisions: Figure 3 shows the diagram of palmar incisions and incisions about the hand. Finger incisions should be midlateral and are indicated by the points of the volar creases. The neurovascular bundle will lie in front of this incision. Incisions in the palm should generally be curved and should not be vertical across flexion planes. They may parallel the

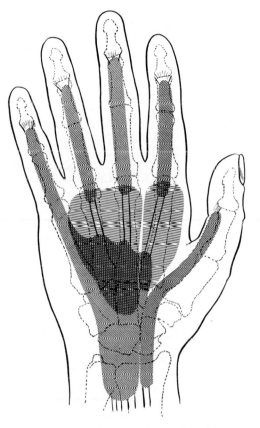

Fig. 1—The synovial sheaths (including the radial and ulnar bursae) are shown in diagonal lines. The mid palmar and thenar spaces are shown with horizontal lines.

palmar creases, but should not be directly in them; usually an 1/8 inch away will provide better healing. When incisions must cross the palmar or wrist creases, they should do so at an angle approximating 60 degrees. Incisions crossing the dorsal creases should also be placed at an angle approximating 60 degrees. Transverse incisions in the folds of the base of the fingers or the thumb are permissible. The proximity of the neurovascular bundle must be recognized and this area respected. Incisions into the length of the thumb should be midlateral, as in fingers. Incisions for whatever cause to the tactile ends of fingers or thumbs should be of the "alligator mouth" type as indicated.

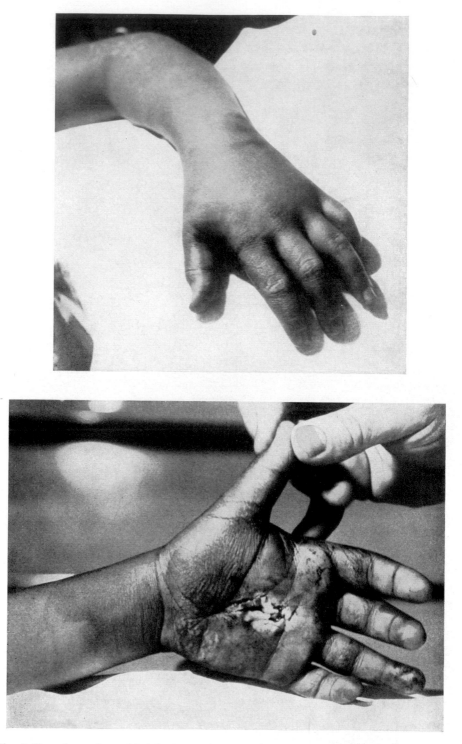

Fig. 2—Deep laceration with infection and loss of flexor tendons to the ring finger. Note
the dorsal edema caused by midpalmar space infection.

Tourniquet: Open surgery on the hand should be done under tourniquet. The automatic pneumatic tourniquets are satisfactory, but a simple blood pressure cuff elevated to a pressure of 275 to 300 mm. Hg. with both hoses and then occluded with a rubber-shod clamp is a satisfactory device. A flannel

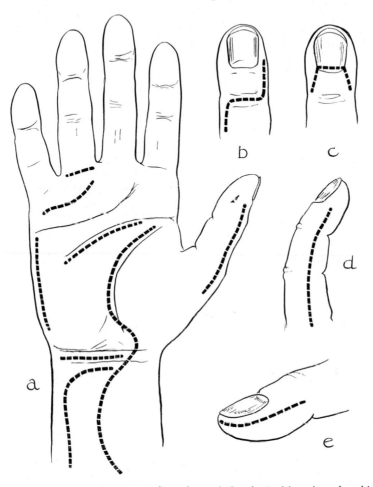

Fig. 3—Incisions in the hand. (A) For the palm and thumb. Incisions in volar skin of palm are best curved; may be parallel but not in the palmar creases: cross creases at 45—60 degree andgle. (B) For mallet finger — vertical extensions are midlateral. (C) For drainage of paronychia. (D) Exact midlateral for all finger surgery. (E) "Alligator Mouth" for pulp infections (felon).

bandage may be laid over the cuff to hold it neatly in place and to avoid rolling and undue local pressure. Before inflation of the cuff, blood should be occluded from the hand and arm by use of a sterile Esmarch bandage. The time limitation under tourniquet is 1½ hours. If the procedure must continue beyond that point, the tourniquet should be released for 15 minutes and then reapplied if needed. The use of finger tourniquets of any variety is to be avoided as there is a very real chance of injury to the neurovascular bundles. Cleansing and "débridement" of open wounds to the hand should be done initially without tourniquet, but definitive repair will require a bloodless view.

Cleansing or "Débridement" of Wounds

The term débridement is used with caution, since its mention conjures up many different interpretations. The actual excision of wounds is not desirable or feasible in the treatment of hand injuries, so the term wound-cleansing or wound lavage is better employed. Of the specialized tissues in the hand, the palmar skin is the most difficult to replace. This is thick skin with sub-cutaneous fat placed in fibrous cells, unique to this area and to the sole of the foot. Every effort should be made to preserve this skin. The deeper layers of the wound are débrided only of tissue that is obviously unviable. More important is the careful cleansing of the depths of the wound through the removal of all foreign substances by direct approach and by copious saline lavage. In wounds where deeper structures of tendons or nerves are involved, such a procedure should be carried out under anesthesia.

Anesthesia

General anesthesia is preferred for most hand surgery. However, in the treatment of hand trauma general anesthesia may not be possible because of recent ingestion of food. Local anesthesia is not practical and so in these instances regional anesthesia or brachial block may be required. When possible, regional anesthesia at the wrist is more favorable than brachial block, as the areas of anesthesia with the latter may be somewhat uncertain. It is possible to use an upper arm tourniquet with regional block anesthesia at the wrist.

The Diagnosis in Hand Injury

The examiner must, by careful examination, anticipate the aims of his surgical management. In any injury, be it open or closed, he must determine the status of the following:

1. The skeletal structures (bone, joint, ligament, muscle and tendon).
2. Nerve function (motor and sensory).
3. The circulatory status of the affected part.

Therefore, on initial examination he must test sensation and motor function and determine the nature of the injury. If there is reason to suspect infection, he must acquaint himself with the limits of the infection. If a laceration is present, he may inspect it superficially in the emergency room or in the office dispensary. If the wound obviously goes to a depth and there is sufficient nerve or tendon injury, further evaluation is an operating room procedure under anesthesia.

Radiography of the Hand and Wrist

X-ray studies of the hand are indicated in lacerations, just as they are in a crush injury. X-rays of the wrist should always be in four views, as standard anteroposterior and lateral projections may not reveal linear fractures in the scaphoid particularly, but also in other carpal bones. For the hand, anteroposterior and obliques are usually sufficient. Their value in trauma is not only to evaluate fracture and dislocation, but also to indicate a foreign body, such as glass or china, which may lie deep in the wound. Wood, unless painted, seldom appears in a radiograph.

Materials in Hand Surgery

The outlook for definitive secondary surgery is often spoiled by over-enthusiasm in the use of coarse materials and rough technics in the primary repair. It should be the aim of every surgeon working on the hand to use as little material below the surface of the skin as possible, and this material should be carefully selected. Absorbable materials cause too much reaction in the deep layers and around tendons and should be avoided. When silk is used, it should be the finest material compatible with the demands upon it. Where possible, and especially in the region of tendon sheaths, pull out wire technics are desirable as they leave no foreign material to cause later fibrosis and adhesion. If tourniquets are removed before final skin closure and adequate compression applied to the wound, only major vessels will require ligation. Here, 4 or 5–0 silk or cotton should be adequate. Skin should be closed with no. 34 to no. 38 stainless steel wire or 5–0 dermalon. Finally, adequate antibiotic and chemotherapeutic measures have greatly enhanced the opportunities of obtaining clean primary healing.

Splints

Splinting of the hand is a most important aspect of treatment in hand fractures and injury. The Universal splint (see fig. 4) is generally useful for emergency work, but more specialized splints are usually required in definitive care. The principles that apply to hand splinting are as follows:

1. Splinting of the metacarpophalangeal joint in extension for longer than three weeks will result in contracture of the lateral ligaments and loss in flexibility of the metacarpophalangeal joints. This may be permanent.

2. The preservation of the arch relationship of the first metacarpal to the remaining four metacarpals must be kept in mind in all molded splinting. Splinting of the hand in the flat position eliminates this arch, and through fibrosis may produce permanent deformity and loss of function.

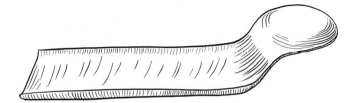

Fig. 4—The Universal splint. This allows the fingers to rest in the "functional position."

3. When possible, fingers and hands should be placed in the position of function (the position the hand assumes at rest; see fig. 5). This applies particularly to the immobilization of finger joints that have been damaged and may become stiffened because of infection, injury or fibrosis. In hand injuries, immobilization cannot be continued as long as it can in other joints, because of the dangers of fixation and fibrosis. Basswood splints and splints that hold the hand straight are to be avoided at all times. Bandage rolls for finger splints are inadequate in both shape and stability. Where possible, the

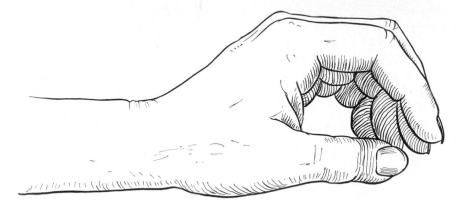

Fig. 5–Position of "function."

thumb should be immobilized in the position of opposition to the hand. Most times hand-splinting requires fixation of the wrist as well, in order to limit the excursion of long tendons. The position of fixation of the wrist will be varied according to the specific need of the immobilization.

Tendon Injuries

Lacerations (fig. 6): Lacerations can be divided into two groups: clean, and contused or dirty. The status of the wound and the time since injury will determine the course of treatment to some degree. With certain exceptions clean lacerations may be repaired when operated on within six hours after the time of injury. Contused lacerations may be repaired within four hours of injury, again with certain exceptions. In the latter group, a good deal of surgical judgement will have to apply as to the amount of contamination and/or crushing present. The area of tendon repair in the digits is best divided into three zones, as indicated. Zone I, or the profundus region. extends from the distal margin of the midphalanx pulley distally to the point of insertion of the profundus to the distal phalanx. Since this is beyond the pulley, a laceration here may be repaired in the time intervals indicated above. Better still, the tendon may be advanced to a new insertion up to a distance of 1½ cm. The profundus tendon may not retract because of its fixation by the lumbricales and vinculae. The tendon should be attached to a bed of bone in the distal phalanx. The Bunnell pull-out wire technic is preferred. Zone II. Lacerations in this area, clean or contused, are best cleansed and deferred for later free tendon-grafting. If the sublimis tendon alone is divided in this region, it is best sacrificed, leaving finger flexion entirely to the flexor digitorum profundus. If the profundus alone is divided and the sublimis remains functional, it is better to leave this situation unchanged than

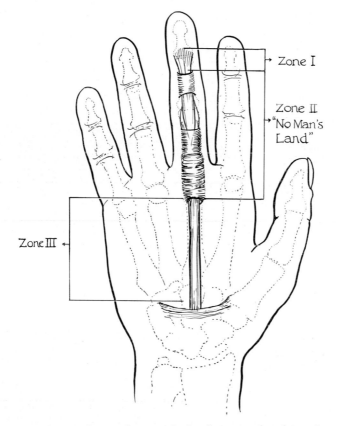

Fig. 6–Zones for tendon repair in flexor tendon laceration.

to do a free tendon graft to restore the profundus. Instability in flexion at the distal interphalangeal joint is seldom a serious disability. If it is, arthrodesis of this joint in a position of slight flexion is suggested. There is a transitional zone at the base of zone II, where the status may vary according to the position of the fingers at the time of injury. If a laceration occurs at the level of the metacarpal head with the fingers in flexion, a suture line of repair will pass beneath the metacarpal pulley on extension with resultant fixation. Such a lesion must therefore be considered to be in "No Man's Land." If the laceration occurs at this same level with the fingers extended, repair is possible, as the laceration will not pass underneath the pulley on extension. It is possible to remove a small portion of the proximal margin of this pulley in order to be certain that adherence to the pulley at the suture line will not occur.

Zone III represents the palmar area. In this zone, repair of one or both tendons is possible within the time limits specified. This situation holds true for tendon lacerations at and above the wrist as well. In lacerations around the region of the transverse carpal ligament, excision of the transverse carpal ligament is to be recommended.

Lacerations of the Flexor Pollicis Longus

The situation following laceration of the long thumb flexor is very similar to that in the fingers. The portion of the tendon in zone I, not beneath the pulley, can be advanced and repaired again, to the phalanx. Section in the region of the pulleys leads to more serious prognosis for primary repair, and while opinion varies here, it is probable that delayed free tendon-graft will assure the best result. Lesions above the pulley area and into the forearm can be treated by direct suture within the time allowances.

Extensor Tendon Lacerations

In clean wounds, direct repair of extensor tendon lacerations is readily undertaken. Because of the loose nature of the surrounding tissue and the lack of pulleys, the danger of adhesion, ever present in flexor tendons, is not a serious problem on the dorsum of the wrist and hand except at joints. Lacerations in the lower forearm to the level of the metacarpal heads can be repaired with nonabsorbable suture material or a pull-out wire suture technic. If the repair is secondary, and there has been retraction of the tendon and muscle belly, either a side anastomosis to an adjoining common extensor or a free tendon graft may be done. In lacerations of the extensor digitorum communis, the former method is the simplest and is effective. Total immobilization is continued for three weeks. Thereafter, a removable splint is applied. The wrist and metacarpophalangeal joints are held in nearly full extension.

A special type of extensor laceration occurs as a result of barehanded fisticuffs. Lacerations of the extensor tendon overlying the metacarpal head, by the opponent's teeth, produce a dangerous wound which penetrates to the metacarpophalangeal joint. The joint should be opened widely with an incision parallel to the extensor tendon, drained and immobilized in a position of function. There should be no attempt at primary closure.

Nerve Laceration

The same basic principles that governed tendon repair apply to the lacerations of the nerves. The time element in relation to an injury may be of vital importance. When the laceration is "clean," primary repair is desirable. While there are many ways of holding nerve ends approximated, perineural sutures of 7–0 eye silk are most frequently employed. The use of a jeweler's loop may facilitate the accurate approximation of small digital nerves and make possible the placement of 3 or 4 small sutures in these fine structures. Prognosis for recovery in digital nerve injuries is excellent. It is fair in medial nerve injury and less good in ulnar nerve injury as a rule. If the wound is contused and past the time limits, mere approximation of the nerve by a single suture is satisfactory. A final repair should then be done when the wound is soft and pliable and there is assurance that there is no potential of infection.

Rupture of the Extensor Pollicis Longus

Delayed rupture of the extensor pollicis longus following Colles' fracture is well known and has received wide attention in the literature both here and abroad. The tendon rupture at Lister's tubercle on the dorsum of the radius, is frequently not present initially, but is found after bone healing has taken place and function returned to the wrist.

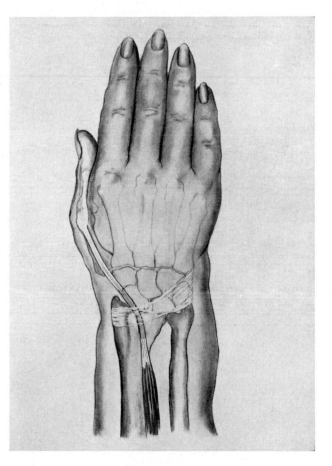

Fig. 7–Zone of rupture of extensor pollicis longus at Lister's tubercle. (Figs. 7 and 8 reproduced with permission of J. Bone and Joint Surgery, *38 A*: 1208—1217, (Dec.) 1956.)

Treatment: It is seldom possible to obtain an end-to-end anastomosis (fig. 7) of the extensor pollicis longus tendon following attritional rupture. The extensor indicis proprius may be used as a motor and the repair made away from Lister's tubercle so as to avoid adhesion.

Spontaneous Rupture of Extensor Tendons

Spontaneous rupture of the extensor digitorum communis tendons (fig. 8) may follow injuries or arthritis of the distal radio-ulnar joint, rheumatoid synovitis. Dorsal subluxation of the distal ulna increases pressure on these tendons as they pass beneath the dorsal carpal ligament. The tendons at this level are surrounded by a synovial sheath. The synovitis that results reduces the nutritional supply of the tendon. Fraying and eventual rupture follow.

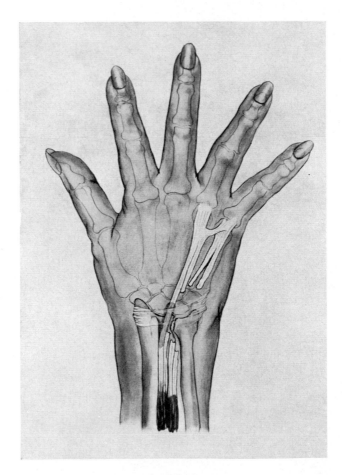

Fig. 8.–Spontaneous rupture of the extensor digitorum communis and the extensor digiti quinti over prominence of distal ulna.

Treatment: The recognition of synovitis at the dorsum of the wrist and its failure to respond to conservative measures indicates the need of synovectomy; the most effective prophylactic measure. The dorsal carpal ligament is left open. If the distal ulna is dorsal in its relationship, its distal 1½ inches are resected. When ruptured, tendons may be repaired by free graft or preferably, by side-to-side anastomosis with persisting intact tendons.

Mallet Finger

Rupture of the tendon (fig. 9) of insertion of the extensor mechanism from the dorsal distal phalanx results from sudden blows on the tip of the

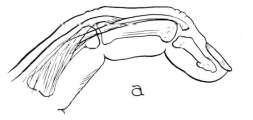

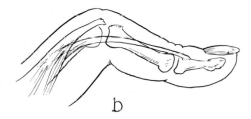

Fig. 9—(A) Mallet finger. (B) Boutonniere deformity.

slightly flexed finger. It is a frequent baseball accident and is sometimes called "baseball finger." A small fragment of distal phalanx may be avulsed with this tendon. In a complete lesion there is inability to extend the distal phalanx. A similar lesion may result from direct laceration over the extensor mechanism at the distal joint.

Treatment: Many methods of treatment have been advocated for mallet finger. The conservative measure most commonly employed is the application of a plaster splint to hold the finger with the distal joint hyperextended, the proximal joint flexed at 60 degrees, which allows relaxation of the lateral band and about 2 mm. slack on the extensor mechanism. This treatment will not be effective if the lesion is more than two weeks old. In recent years some operators have maintained this same position by using wire splinting, which longitudinally fixes the three phalanges. Others have used a shorter wire fixing only the distal phalanx on the midphalanx in moderate hyperextension. In any of these methods, the amount of hyperextension at the distal joint must be controlled by the appearance of the skin at the dorsum of this joint, as excessive hyperextension may lead to avascularity and necrosis of the skin. Bunnell has described an open operative procedure for repair of the tendon ruptures that come to treatment later than two weeks after injury. The tendon is approached through an L-shaped incision just proximal to the level of the distal joint. A no. 35 stainless steel pull-out wire is passed through the dorsal edge of the phalanx and out subcutaneously above the nail matrix. It is then passed through a drill hole at the tip of the nail. Splinting is continued for four weeks, but the wire is removed at three weeks.

It is probable that this lesion is largely overtreated. Since the extensor slip is not within synovial sheath and is surrounded by paratenon, the retracted tendon grows distalward in an attempt at repair which usually succeeds. A great majority of these deformities will disappear without treatment in from one to two years. The loss of extensor power will rarely persist beyond this, regardless of the treatment.

Recommended therapy, therefore, is as follows: Radiographs should be made on all patients. For the acute noncompound lesion, without avulsion of bone, the conservative method of plaster splinting with the dorsum of the splint left open for observation of the skin at the distal joint, is the treatment of choice. The splint is left in place for three weeks, when gently increasing activities are started. If a fragment of bone is avulsed from the dorsal distal phalanx with the tendon, the open pull-out wire method is used. In this instance the wire is passed through drill holes through the phalanx and brought out through the pulp where it is tied over a bolster. The wire is left in place for three weeks. The finger is splinted for four weeks. For open acute wounds primary closure with pull-out wire is advocated.

Delayed Treatment: If the lesion is over two weeks old and there is no avulsion of bone, the patient is reassured and no treatment advised. With displacement of a bony fragment, the open pull-out wire method described above is employed, as it is felt that these will have little chance of anatomical repair and the small bony fragment may be a source of mechanical irritation at the joint.

Bountonniere Deformity (see fig. 9)

This deformity results from a relative lengthening of the central slip of the extensor mechanism of a finger at the proximal interphalangeal joint. It may result from traumatic avulsion or open laceration of the tendon or joint capsule with tendon. The lateral bands tend to glide too far forward on the distal condyles of the proximal phalanx.

Treatment: Lacerations may be repaired, if within time limits, if they are reasonably clean, and if they are not the result of human bite. A fine pull-out wire technic to the dorsal base of the midphalanx may be used.

If a bony fragment is pulled from the base of the midphalanx, a similar type of repair is done.

If seen after recent injury, a closed avulsion without fracture of the midphalanx, treatment by operative repair may be considered. One should remember, however, that most of these deformities will correct themselves in from 9 months to 1 year without treatment. Should deformity persist after that time, lengthening of the lateral bands (Fowler) or release of the dorsal hood at the metacarpophalangeal joint (Littler) may restore balance in extensor function and overcome deformity.

Infections

Infections in the hand will require very careful evaluation as to the source and the direction of spread. Palpation for fluctuation is difficult in the palm. The appearance of edema at the dorsum of the hand, however, in all probability indicates a deep palmar space. The appearance of small superficial pustules in the palm at the web space or in the dorsum of the hand may not indicate the true nature of the lesion, as these may represent a so-called "collar button" abscess with a large, deep space infection pointing to a very small lesion subcutaneously.

Felons

A felon is an abscess in the tactile pulp of the finger. These may arise from contusion or from penetrating wounds such as those caused by needles. The vertical fibers supporting the tactile fat will tend to direct the spread of infection dorsally, sometimes to the paronychial area, or proximally to the tendon sheath, and rarely to the joint. Avascular necrosis of the bony tuft of the distal phalanx may occur. Treatment consists of adequate drainage through an alligator mouth incision and antibiotics. Initially, warm saline soaks may be effective in "gathering" the infection. Early recognition is important so that treatment will prevent the spread of infection proximally.

Paronychia

Infections involving the soft tissues peripheral to the nail are relatively common. These may be serious if not carefully checked. When fluctuation is present, open drainage is indicated. The proximal portion of the lunula of the nail may be removed. Incisions are then directed as shown in figure 3 to provide adequate drainage in this area. Antibiotics may be essential to the treatment and may modify the course of the disease.

Deep Space Infection

Infections of the thenar and hypothenar eminences are usually more readily controlled than those of the midpalmar space. Here the spread may be distally through the lumbricales canals and through the canal provided for the neurovascular bundle into the finger, or proximally beneath the transverse carpal ligament into the forearm. Infections may spread radially very readily because of the thin, loose structure of the fascia protecting and demarcating this side of the midpalmar space. Infections do spread dorsally and provide the all-important sign of dorsal edema. If all symptoms do not respond promptly to soaks and antimicrobial therapy, and if the abscess is localizing, adequate incision and drainage are essential to avoid severe disability in the hand. Constant observation and early treatment in the hospital are the watchwords in infections of the palm and synovial sheaths.

Finger Tuft Amputations

The loss of a distal finger tuft is a frequent injury resulting from machine tool accidents, slicers and the ordinary car door injury. If the lesion is transverse or dorsal with loss of a portion of the nail and some of the distal phalanx as well as the distal tip of the finger, the removal of enough of the distal phalanx to allow for dorsal closure of the volar skin will provide the quickest and surest method of healing. This will get the working man back on the job in the shortest possible time. If the remaining proximal portion of the nail is jagged and torn, it is best removed, but if it is intact in its bed, it can be left undisturbed and may actually function as a local splint. If the volar tactile surface of the flexor pad has been sliced off and is not available immediately for replacement as a skin graft, a graft from another area is desirable. A free thin, full thickness graft may be employed from the forearm or the arm. A pedicle graft may be raised from the volar base of the thenar eminence and attached to the flexed finger tip, or a pedicle may be raised from the dorsum of a neighboring finger and transferred to the affected fingertip. The donor site in the last two instances is replaced by a split-thickness graft. Moberg has transferred skin on a neural stalk to preserve sensation in the tactile area.

Closed Wounds of the Hand

Compression or crushing injuries: Crush injuries of the hand may produce severe permanent damage through fibrosis of the intrinsic structures of the hand following internal hemorrhage and ischemia. When seen, a very careful examination should be carried out at once with evaluation of circulation, motor function and sensation. The skin should be very carefully inspected for any compounding or puncture wounds. Radiographs are indicated to rule out fracture.

Treatment: Crushing injuries may be associated with shock, and generalized treatment of the patient in this regard is essential. For even moderately severe injuries, hospital admission is recommended. After thorough cleansing of the injured hand, a gently compressive dressing is applied to the hand and fingers, leaving only fingertips exposed with the fingers in the "position of function." The hand is kept elevated above the level of the heart and is cooled with an ice collar. Early active and assisted motion is recommended, optimum timing depending on the severity of the injury. The compressive dressing should be well padded and should extend up to the elbow even though the forearm is not involved. The fingertips should be evaluated hourly and the dressing changed frequently.

Subungual hematoma: This common condition results from the injudicious use of hammers. The hemorrhage beneath the nail, through pressure, may cause extreme pain.

Treatment: To relieve the pressure of the hematoma, the finger is thoroughly cleansed with soap and water and prepared with Merthiolate or other antiseptic. A sterile needle, or paper clip heated in a flame, is then passed, hot, through the nail. The hole through the nail can be made as well with a no. 11 Bard Parker blade which is rotated, drill-like, to make a hole, or a fine dental drill may also be employed. The hot needle has the advantage of causing very little pressure during the procedure. If this release is done within six hours of the accident, some of the hematoma can be expressed with resulting relief. If it runs over twelve hours, success is less likely. The nail is generally lost but regrows.

Bibliography

PULVERSTAFT, R. G.: Tendon grafts for flexor tendon injuries in fingers and thumb. J. Bone & Joint Surg. *38 B*: 175, 1956.

LITTLER, J. W.: Principles of reconstructive surgery of the hand. Am. J. Surg. *92*: 88, 1956.

PEACOCK, E. E.: Reconstructive surgery of the hand with injured central metacarpophalangeal joints. J. Bone & Joint Surg. *38 A*: 291, 1956.

PLEWES, L. W.: Sudeck's atrophy of hand. J. Bone & Surg. *38 B*: 195, 1956.

DICK, W.: Repair of tendons of hand. Internat. Abstr. Surg. *103*: 594, 1956.

BARCLAY, T. L.: Late results of finger tip injuries. Internat. Abstr. Surg. *102*: 200, 1956.

TENERY, JOHN H., and KOFFOOT, R. R.: Snake bite of hand; a case of observation of early and late treatment. Internat. Abstr. Surg. *102*: 303, 1956.

GOLDEN, L.: Reconstructive surgery of the hand in cerebral palsy and spastic paralysis resulting from injury to spinal cord. J. Bone & Joint Surg. *37 A*: 114, 1955.

TUBIANA, J.: Prognosis and treatment of Dupuytren's contracture. J. Bone & Joint Surg. *37 A*: 1155, 1955.

BOYES, J. H.: Evaluation of the results of digital flexor tendon grafts. Am. J. Surg. *89*: 1166, 1955.

CLARKSON, P.: Care of open injuries of the hand and fingers with special reference to the treatment of traumatic amputations. J. Bone & Joint Surg. *37 A*: 521, 1955.

LACROT, F.: Radiodermatitis of surgeon's hands; generalities and surgical treatment. Internat. Abstr. Surg. *102*: 305, 1955.

WATSON, A. B.: Some remarks on repair of flexor tendons in the hand with particular reference to technique. Brit. J. Surg. *43*: 35, 1955.

BOYES, J. H.: Repair of motor branch of the ulnar nerve in the palm. J. Bone & Joint Surg. *37 A*: 920, 1955.

GODFREY, J. D.: Early management injured hand. J.A.M.A. *155*: 1484, Aug. 21, 1954.

EDGERTON, M. J.: Immediate reconstruction of injured hand. Surgery *36*: 329, 1954.

FUSCO, E. M.: Fingertip reconstruction with palmar flaps. Am. J. Surg. *87*: 608, 1954.

MAXIM, E. S., WEBSTER, F. S., and WILLANDER, D. A.: Cornpicker hand. J. Bone & Joint Surg. *36 A*: 21, 1954.

UPCHURCH, S. E.: Management of common injuries. Ann. Surg. *139*: 650, 1954.

POSCH, L.: Mangle and severe wringer injuries of children. J. Bone & Joint Surg. *36 A*: 57, (Jan.) 1954.

KYLE, J. B., and EYREBROOK, A. L.: Surgical treatment of flexor tendon injuries; results obtained in consecutive series of 57 cases. Brit. J. Surg. *41*: 502, (Mar.) 1954.

MARBLE, H. C., and BURBANK, C. B.: Nerve grafts into hands. Am. J. Surg. *85*: 319, (Mar.) 1953.

WALDEN, R. H., and RUBIN, L. R.: Problem of repair of burned hands. Bull. Hosp. Joint Dis. *13*: 259, (Oct.) 1952.

FLYNN, J. E.: Problems with trauma. J. Bone & Joint Surg. *35 A*: 132, (Jan.) 1953.

ROBINS, R. H. C.: Use of post auricular skin grafts in treatment of traumatic amputation through terminal compartment of finger. Brit. J. Surg. *41*: 515, (Mar.) 1954.

MOBERG, ERIK: Personal communication.

CHAPTER 40

FRACTURES OF THE ACETABULUM AND DISLOCATION OF THE HIP

PRESTON A. WADE, M.D.

Fractures of the acetabulum and dislocations of the hip are now fairly common because of the increased number of injuries sustained in automobile accidents. Dislocation of the hip is most apt to occur in the young, healthy adult since the same force applied to a child's limb causes a fracture of the shaft of the femur, and in the adolescent a separation of the femoral epiphysis, while in the elderly person the break occurs at the weakest point, the neck.

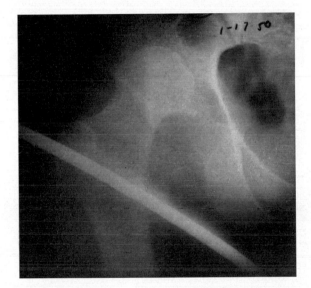

Fig. 1—Posterior dislocation of hip without fracture.

The weakest area in the hip joint is posteriorly and dislocation most commonly takes place when the patient sits in a car with his knees crossed, so that at the time of impact the knee closest to the dashboard receives the force of the blow which is transmitted posteriorly to the flexed adducted hip allowing posterior dislocation (fig. 1). With the limb in the neutral position, there is more apt to be a fracture of the lip of the acetabulum (fig. 2), or if the hip is slightly more abducted, a large section of the posterior portion of the acetabulum will be fractured and displaced outside the joint (fig. 3). If the limb is markedly abducted at the time of the accident, an anterior dislocation may result. If a severe force is applied to the abducted limb, a central

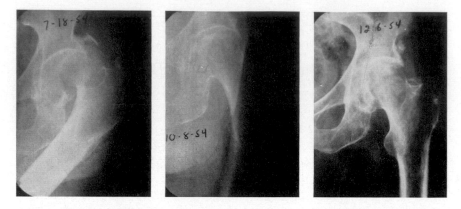

Fig. 2—(left) Posterior dislocation of hip with small fragment. (middle) Three months after reduction. (right) Five months after reduction.

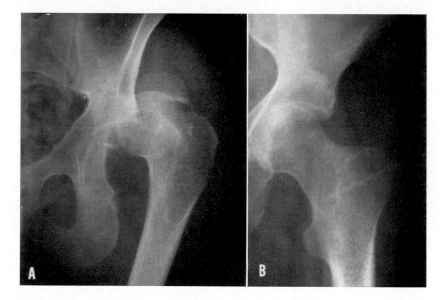

Fig. 3—(A) Posterior dislocation with large posterior lip fragment. Sciatic nerve involvement. (B) After reduction and fixation of fragment.

dislocation (fig. 5) may occur in which the head of the femur is driven through the roof of the acetabulum and may indeed actually rest in the intrapelvic position.

Since the force required to dislocate the hip is great, there are usually other severe concomitant injuries, and these may be so obvious and severe as to divert the attention of the examiner from the injured hip. In a review of hip injuries as a result of automobile accidents at The New York Hospital, we have found that other injuries to the same extremities, such as fractures of the patella, tibia and shaft of the femur on the same side may so dominate

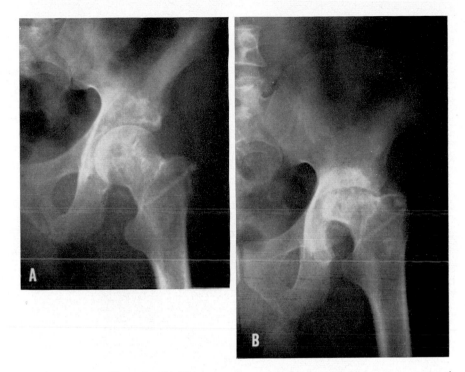

Fig. 4—Same case as figure 3. (A) Three months post operation. (B) One year postoperative. Avascular necrosis of head.

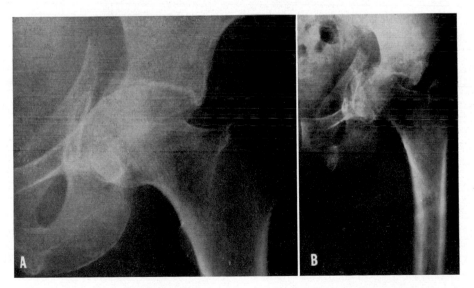

Fig. 5—(A) Central dislocation of femoral head with displacement of acetabulum — in traction. (B) After removal of traction. Central displacement of head has recurred.

the clinical picture as to make dislocation of the hip go unnoticed. We have had a number of cases in which the patient was properly treated for other injuries, but in which a disability of the hip was found after other injuries had healed. The late treatment of a dislocation of the hip or a fracture dislocation of the hip may present serious difficulties and will almost invariably result in a disability. It is therefore essential that one include a

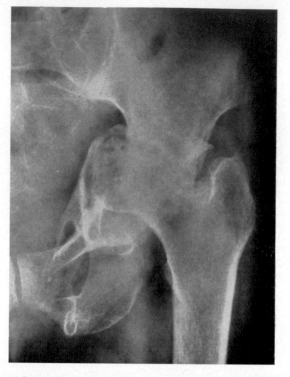

Fig. 6—Same case as figure 5. Avascular necrosis of head. Pain and limitation of motion necessitating fusion.

careful clinical and x-ray examination of the hip in evaluating the multiple injuries sustained in a severe accident. Fractures of the dorsal or lumbar spine are also often associated with dislocation of the hip, and the surgeon should be aware of the possibility of these injuries when evaluating the condition of the patient with a dislocated hip.

Treatment of Posterior Dislocation of the Hip

A patient with a posterior dislocation of the hip joint presents a typical deformity caused by shortening of the limb, marked adduction and internal rotation of the femur. The hip is painful, there is marked limitation of motion, and the head of the femur may be palpated posteriorly. Often there is little displacement obvious on examination if there is a subluxation of the head with a fracture of the posterior lip of the acetabulum so that the displacement of the head of the femur is not obvious except in the x-ray. Occasionally, the x-ray may be misleading, and although the head may seem to be in proper position, it may lie posteriorly in such a way as to make the usual antero-posterior view deceptive. It is important to obtain a good lateral view of the hip joint if there is any doubt in making the diagnosis.

The patient is placed supine on a padding on the floor of the operating room, and a general anesthesia administered. The operator flexes the hip and knee and applies traction in the neutral position in the long axis of the shaft of the femur as an assistant puts countertraction on the pelvis. Slow gentle traction in this position will usually suffice to reduce any dislocated hip whether it be an anterior or a posterior dislocation. It is usually unnecessary to use great force or to attempt to lever the head into position.

Postoperative Care

There is considerable difference of opinion as to the postreduction care of a patient with a dislocated hip. Many have advocated prolonged immobilization in plaster for a period of six weeks and ambulation without weight-bearing for an additional period of six months to a year. It is our feeling that in the pure dislocation of the hip joint, it is unnecessary to apply any form of external immobilization by either plaster or traction. We keep the patient in bed for a short time and then allow him to be ambulatory if there are no other serious conmitant injuries. We allow full weight-bearing within a period of three or four weeks.

Avascular necrosis of the femoral head (figs. 4 and 6) is one of the expected complications following a dislocation of the hip. There is considerable difference of opinion concerning the incidence of this complication, but it is recognized that it occurs in at least 20 to 25 per cent of the cases. It is our feeling that the fate of the femoral head is decided at the time of the orginal injury and that weight-bearing does not have any effect on the occurrence of subsequent avascular necrosis. We feel it is unnecessary to prolong the morbidity without some evidence that limiting weight-bearing is helpful.

It is said that dislocation of the hip is apt to recur if immobilization is not applied for six weeks. We have not seen a redislocation in any of our cases, and all have been treated by early ambulation and early weight-bearing.

If late aseptic necrosis and traumatic osteoarthritis occur in a patient with a dislocation, the condition may then be treated by arthroplasty, preferably using the Vitallium cup. If the head is considerably disintegrated, a metal prosthetic replacement may be inserted (fig. 7).

Traumatic ossification or myositis ossificans may occur about the joint, particularly if there be marked subperiosteal hematoma. It has been suggested that early ambulation causes an increase in the ossification. We have not found this to be true in our cases.

We have found, even in the presence of considerable myositis ossificans, that motion is only slightly limited (fig. 20 B). As in every other joint, passive motion, particularly by forceful manipulation, should be avoided.

Injury to the sciatic nerve is rare in a pure dislocation of the hip joint. If signs of sciatic nerve involvement are discovered, the nerve need not necessarily be explored primarily because it is rarely severely injured except in those cases where there is a fracture of the posterior lip of the acetabulum, in which case immediate operative reduction is essential.

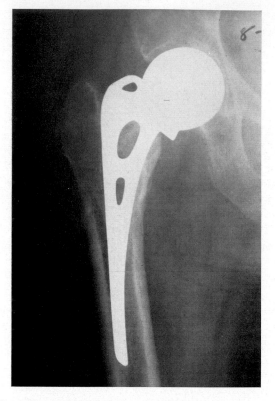

Fig. 7—Austin-Moore replacement for avascular necrosis.

Fracture Dislocations of the Joints

When a posterior dislocation of the hip is associated with a small marginal fracture of the posterior rim of the acetabulum which replaces itself after reduction of the dislocation (fig. 2) operative intervention is not necessary. If, on the other hand, there has been any evidence of sciatic nerve involvement with even a minor fracture of the acetabulum, operation and exploration of the nerve are mandatory.

When larger fragments of the posterior rim of the acetabulum (figs. 8 and 9) are displaced, it is necessary to operate immediately even if there is no obvious injury to the sciatic nerve. We use the posterior approach, and the fragment is replaced and fixed in position by one or two screws (figs. 8–10). On occasion it is difficult to fix the comminuted fracture of the acetabulum by

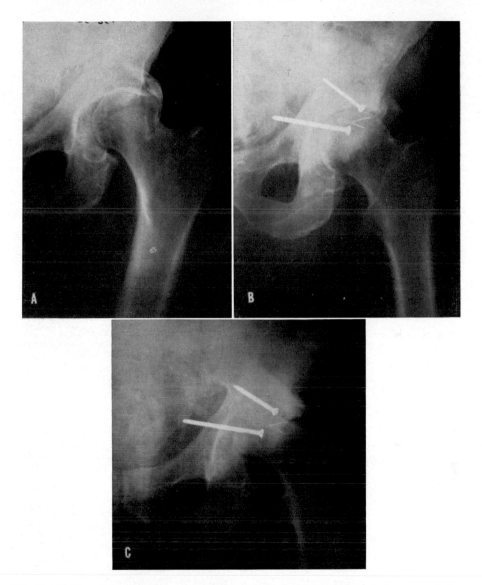

Fig. 8—(A) Posterior dislocation with posterior lip fragment displaced from acetabulum. (B) After replacement of fragment by means of 2 screws and wire sutures. (C) One year postoperative. Note avascular necrosis of head.

means of screws alone, and occasionally it is necessary to use a wire suture (fig. 11).

The sciatic nerve should be exposed and inspected in every operative case and appropriate treatment instituted. In the usual case there is only a contusion of the nerve, and freeing of the nerve from impingement of fragments of the acetabulum is all that is necessary.

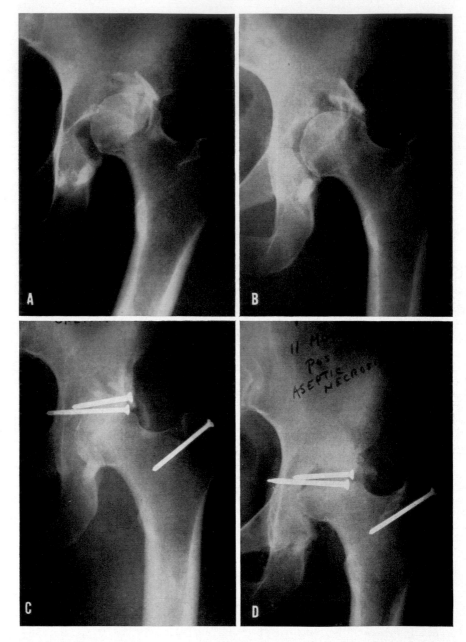

Fig. 9—(A) Posterior displacement with posterior lip fragment. (B) After two weeks in traction. (C) After operative replacement of fragment. Screw in greater trochanter is for replacement of fragment displaced in Gibson approach. (D) Eleven months postoperative. Avascular necrosis of head with disability.

Postoperative Treatment of Fracture Dislocations of the Hip

After a fracture dislocation of the hip joint has been repaired by operative means, it is essential that the joint be immobilized if there is any instability of the fragments of the acetabulum. The immobilization should be complete by means of a plaster spica. If the fragment of the acetabulum is quite stable, it may only be necessary to apply suspension in a Böhler frame or Thomas splint for two or three weeks.

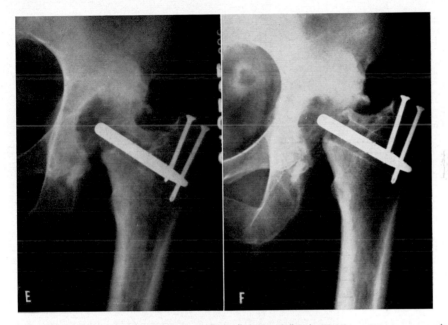

Fig. 9–(E) After Judet prosthesis replacement of femoral head. (F) One year postoperative.

Weight-bearing is allowed early if the fragment of the acetabulum is small, and if the hip joint is stable. If, on the other hand, there is a large fragment or if the stability of the acetabulum is questionable, it is then necessary to prevent weight-bearing for a period of many weeks.

Dislocation of the Hip with Fracture of the Femoral Head

As the head of the femur is displaced form the acetabulum, a fragment of the head may be fractured and displaced within the joint (fig. 12), the head fragment being sheared off by the edge of the acetabulum. Occasionally, the fractured fragment of the head is replaced in its proper position by mere reduction of the dislocation, and in such an instance, the fragment may be allowed to remain in place. In most cases, however, the small fragment undergoes avascular necrosis, and it is probably wiser to remove the fragment. If the fragment is displaced or if it remains within the acetabulum, it must be excised (fig. 13). If a fairly large segment of head and neck remains intact,

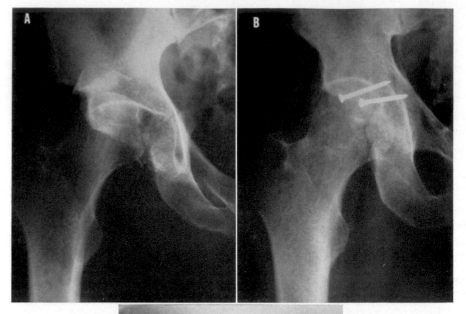

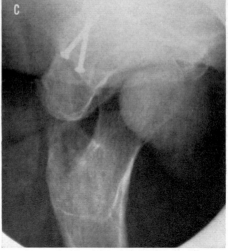

Fig. 10— (A) Posterior displacement with large fragment fractured from posterior margin of acetabulum. (B and C) After replacement by 2 screws.

one may expect that it will retain the function of the hip joint and allow full weight-bearing. In these cases, it is essential that full weight-bearing be restricted for a period of at least six months. It is obvious that in these cases aseptic necrosis and late osteoarthritis of the hip joint are more apt to result then if no injury to the head occurs. If the head of the femur is badly shattered (fig. 14) it is necessary to excise the remaining head portion of the neck and insert a metal prosthesis as a primary procedure.

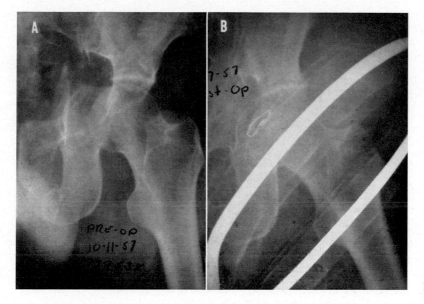

Fig. 11— (A) Posterior dislocation with large fragment posteriorly. The dislocation of femoral head is not always recognized. (B) After replacement of fragment by means of wire suture.

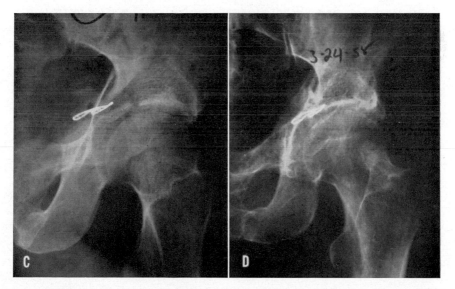

Fig. 11—(C) One month postoperative. (D) Six months postoperative. Note changes in acetabulum.

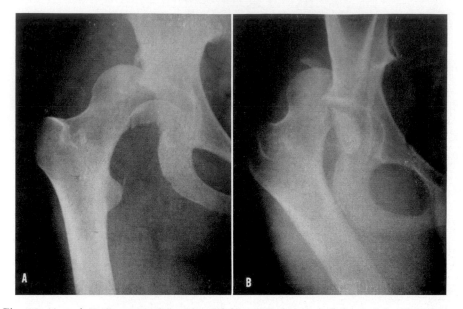

Fig. 12–(A and B) Posterior dislocation of hip with fracture of femoral head. Fragment of head remains in acetabulum.

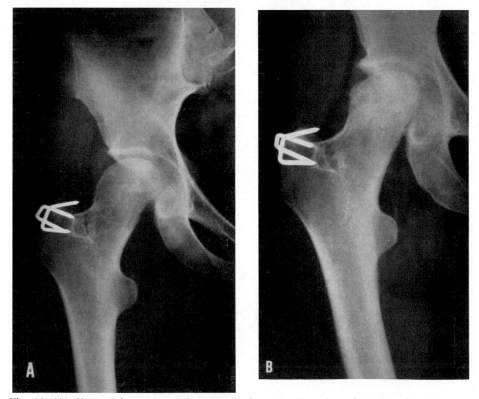

Fig. 13–(A) Six months postoperative. Weight bearing allowed at this time. (B) One year postoperative after removal of head fragment. No symptoms. Femoral head remains viable. (Courtesy of Dr. James Mithoefer, Cooperstown, N. Y.)

Central Dislocation of the Femoral Head

If a violent force is applied to the extremity with the hip in marked abduction, the head of the bone may be driven through the floor of the acetabulum and on occasion may lie within the pelvis (fig. 15 A and B). This is called an intrapelvic dislocation of the hip.

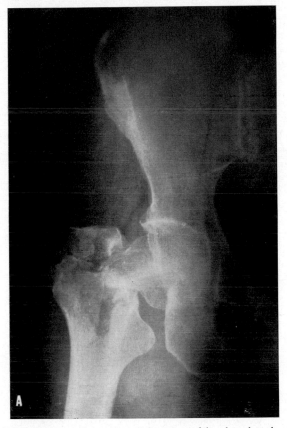

Fig. 14—(A) Comminuted fracture dislocation of head and neck of femur.

In this condition, skeletal traction in the line of the long axis of the femur should be applied with considerable weight. In the less severe cases, the dislocation may be properly reduced. It has also been advised that one apply lateral traction by means of skeletal traction applied to the greater trochanter in addition to the traction in the long axis of the femur (fig. 16). In severe cases, even strong traction on the greater trochanter is usually ineffective in reducing the dislocations, and considerable damage may be done by the wire or nail-pulling out of the greater trochanter. It is therefore preferable to perform open reduction in these severe cases rather than to try to depend on traction alone. Even in those cases in which perfect reduction of the dislocation is achieved and maintained, the resulting damage to the floor of the acetabulum and the head of the bone may result in avascular necrosis of the femoral head and an usually severe osteoarthritis which may progress quite rapidly and produce a severe disability of the hip joint.

In these cases we recommend immediate operation and the insertion of a Vitallium cup (fig. 17). If the cup chosen is somewhat oversized, it will form

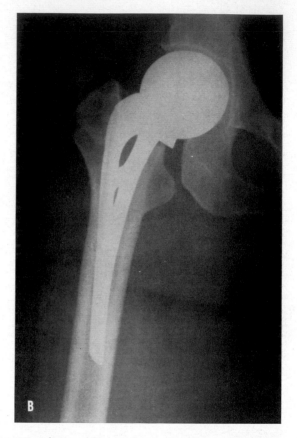

Fig. 14—(B) After replacement by Austin-Moore Vitallium prothisis.

a new roof for the acetabulum and will serve a dual purpose of immediate treatment of the dislocation and of the anticipated complication of osteoarthritis. It does not, of course, have any effect on the avascular necrosis and eventual disintegration of the head, but it is a form of treatment which nay delay symptoms as a result of this complication.

Dislocation of the Hip Joint Associated with Ipsolateral Fracture of the Shaft of the Femur

A rare combination of injuries is sometimes seen in dislocation of the hip and fracture of the shaft of the femur. Such a case is illustrated in figure 18.

Figure 18 A shows that the dislocation of the hip causes a marked separation of the fragments of the femoral shaft. Such a distraction in a fracture of the

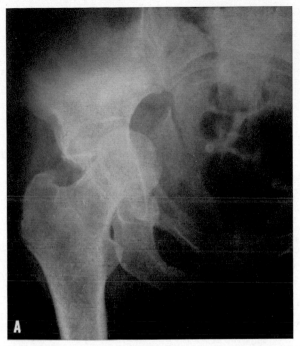

Fig. 15—(A) Intrapelvic dislocation of hip in female of 34.

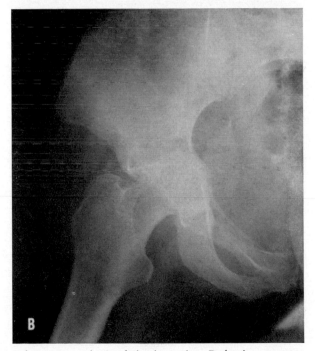

Fig. 15—(B) After two weeks in skeletal traction. Reduction was not maintained.

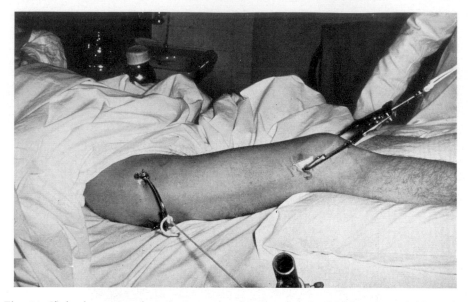

Fig. 16—Skeletal traction for attempts at reduction of central dislocation of hip. Wire through lower end of femur and a second wire through greater trochanter applying traction laterally.

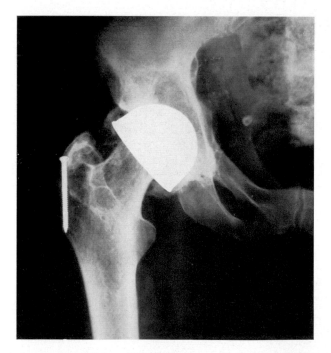

Fig. 17—Case shown in figures 15 and 16. Primary vitallium cup arthroplasty. Over-sized cup prevented intrapelvic displacement. Follow up six years showed almost complete return of normal function.

shaft of the femur should immediately make the observer suspect a co-existing dislocation of the hip (fig. 18 B). In any case, a severe fracture of the shaft of the femur should be suspected as having an associated dislocation of the hip.

In the treatment of this combination of injuries, it is essential that the dislocation of the hip be reduced first, since the insertion of an intramedullary

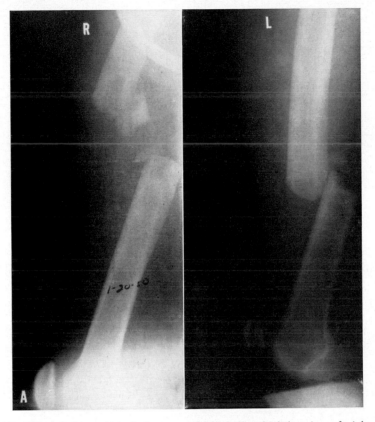

Fig. 18—(A) Bilateral femoral shaft fractures associated with dislocation of right hip. The marked distraction of fragments of shaft of right femur suggests ipsolateral dislocation of hip.

rod in the femur or other means of treatment is difficult to achieve until the dislocation is reduced. If there is a fracture of the acetabulum with or without sciatic nerve involvement, the dislocation of the hip is reduced by open operation through the posterior approach. If there is no fracture of the acetabulum, the hip joint may be reduced as follows:

The patient is placed on the sound side, and the fracture of the shaft of the femur is exposed as is usually done for the insertion of the Küntscher nail. A Kirschner wire is then inserted through the distal end of the proximal

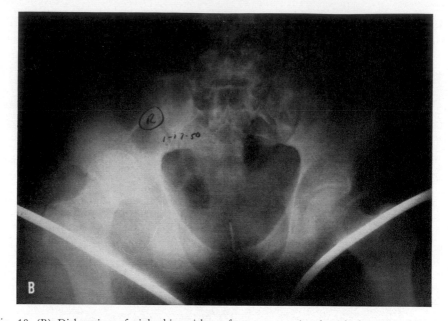

Fig. 18—(B) Dislocation of right hip without fracture, associated with fracture of femoral shaft. This is the same case as fig. 18 A.

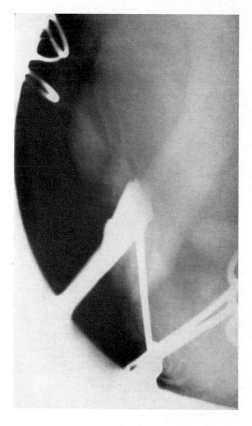

fragment, and a traction bow applied. By this means, firm control of the proximal fragment is then achieved, and the reduction may be accomplished by flexion of the hip and traction in the line of the long axis of the shaft (fig. 19). With the hip reduced, the Küntscher nail is then inserted as usual. The guide wire comes out through the buttock on the affected side. The Küntscher nail is then driven down through the proximal fragment until it appears at the fracture site. The guide wire is then removed and inserted through the Küntscher nail from above downward until it, too, appears at the fracture site. The fracture is then reduced, and the guide wire driven into the distal fragment down to the

Fig. 19—Kirschner wire through distal end of proximal fragment with spreader for traction to reduce dislocation.

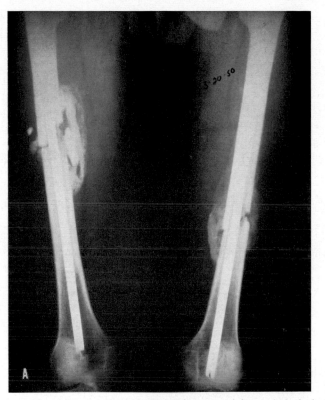

Fig. 20–(A) After bilateral Küntscher nail fixation of femoral shaft fractures.

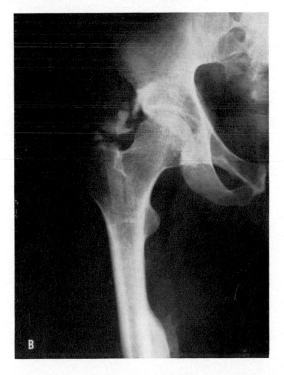

Fig. 20–(B) One year follow up
of dislocated hip. Note calcific
deposit above trochanter. Little
limitation of motion.

femoral condyles, and the Küntscher nail is then driven home into its position in the femoral condyle. The guide wire is then removed, and the wound is closed. If there are no other concomitant injuries, the patient is allowed to be ambulatory early, just as in the case of a pure dislocation of the hip or a fracture of the shaft of the femur treated by the Küntscher nail as has been described in previous chapters. In the case illustrated, a myositis ossificans occurred (fig. 20 B) and may be seen in the x-ray superior to the greater trochanter. In this case the result achieved was almost perfect, as the patient had a very slight limitation of motion. It is now six years since the accident occurred, and there has been no evidence of aseptic necrosis of the head, nor traumatic osteoarthritis of the hip joint.

References

[1] Böhler, L.: Treatment of Fractures. New York, Grune & Stratton, 1956, vol. I.

[2] Campbell, W. C.: Posterior dislocation of the hip joint with fracture of the acetabulum. J. Bone & Joint Surg. *18*: 842, 1936.

[3] Judet, J., and Judet, R.: Technique and results with an acrylic head prosthesis. J. Bone & Joint Surg. *34 B*: 173, 1952.

[4] Key, J. A., and Conwell, H. E.: Fractures, Dislocation and Sprains, St. Louis, C. V. Mosby Co., 1956.

[5] Moore, A. T.: The self-locking metal hip prosthesis. J. Bone & Joint Surg. *39 A*: 811, 1957.

[6] Smith Petersen, M. N.: Evolution of mould arthoplasty of the hip joint. J. Bone & Joint Surg. *30 B*: 59–83, 1948.

[7] Watson-Jones, R.: Fractures and Joint Injuries. Edinburgh, E. & S. Livingstone, Ltd., 1955.

CHAPTER 41

INTRACAPSULAR FRACTURES OF THE NECK OF THE FEMUR

Preston A. Wade, M.D.

Intracapsular fractures of the neck of the femur usually occur in elderly people, especially women, who fall in a trivial accident such as a slip on a rug or a misstep off a curb. Since there are usually no concomitant injuries and very little trauma to soft parts, accompanying shock is rare. The patient lies on the ground and is unable to arise, assuming the typical position of external rotation of the foot and shortening of the limb. She is usually unable to rotate the foot internally or to raise the limb from the ground.

Classification

The most important classification of intracapsular fractures has to do with the site of the fracture and the impaction of the fragments. The type of treatment and the results are entirely different in each instance. Differentiation is made primarily by x-ray, but can also be made by clinical examination.

Impacted Valgus Fracture (Abduction Type)

In this fracture (fig. 1 A and B) the displacement of the distal fragment is in abduction and the traumatizing force firmly impacts the two fragments so that the head is in the valgus position. In many instances it is difficult to see the fracture line, and the valgus deformity of the head may be the most important primary diagnostic sign in the x-ray. These patients may have considerable pain in the hip and may be unable to walk, but in many instances the pain is not severe enough to prevent them from weight-bearing, and often the fracture is not recognized. If the patient is allowed to continue walking with this type of fracture, within the period of three weeks absorption at the fracture line takes place, he may suddenly fall to the ground with pain in the hip, and examination will show a displaced fracture, with the fragments in a varus position. It is therefore very important that these cases be diagnosed early and treated properly.

Any elderly patient who has had a fall and complains of pain in the knee or hip may be suspected of having a fractured hip and deserves an x-ray examination.

It is not necessary to apply traction or splinting to the impacted type of fracture for transportation.

559

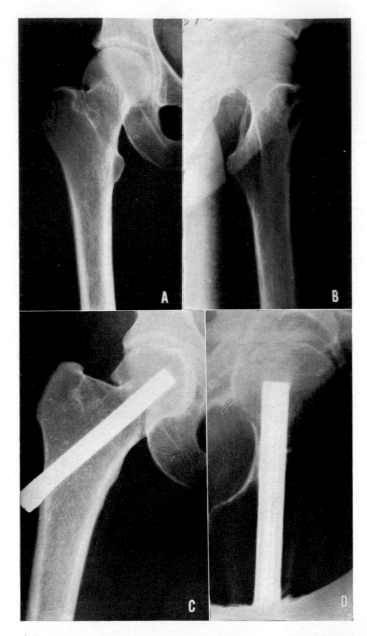

Fig. 1—(A and B) Intracapsular fracture of neck of femur — impacted in valgus position (abduction type). (C and D) Internal fixation by Smith-Petersen nail. Nail should be inserted near the calcar and either in center of neck in lateral view or just posterior to center.

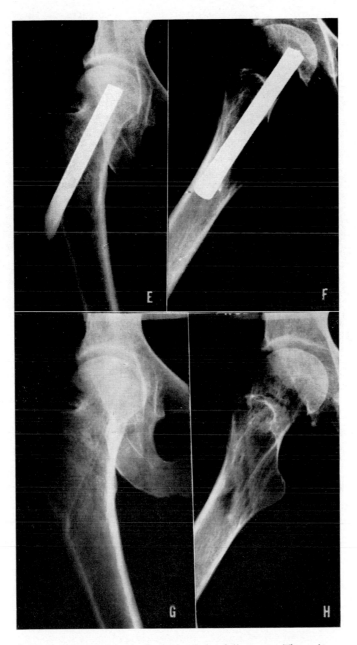

Fig. 1–(E and F) Fracture has united. Six months follow up. There is some increased density of femoral head which suggests avasular necrois. (G and H) One year follow up. Nail has been removed. Density of femoral head is more apparent and avascular necrosisis present. No symptom at this time.

Displaced Varus Fracture (Adduction Type)

More than 90 per cent of the intracapsular fractures of the neck of the femur are of this type (fig. 2 A), and the typical displacement of shortening and external rotation of the leg usually make the diagnosis easy. X-ray examination is necessary to confirm the diagnosis. The patient with a displaced fracture of the femoral neck should be transported in a Thomas splint with moderate traction. If this is not available, the two limbs should be bound together.

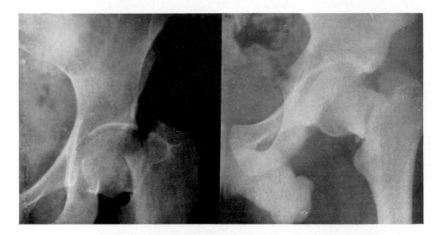

Fig. 2–(A) Displaced varus type of intracapsular failure of femoral neck (adduction type). Note upward displacement, varus deformity and rotation of head. (B) Base of neck fracture of femoral neck in child of 15. Not a common fracture and rate of nonunion is high.

Treatment

Impacted Valgus Fracture

It is well known that this type of fracture heals readily and bony union may be expected in almost every case. However, there is considerable disagreement as to the proper treatment.

The patient may be treated by bedrest for three or four weeks and be allowed ambulation with crutches for four months until the fracture is healed.

The author agrees with many other surgeons in advocating that these cases should be immediately subjected to nailing so that the fragments cannot be disimpacted, and the patient may then be allowed to walk within a period of a few weeks before the fracture has been healed. In any case, the most important consideration is the recognition of the fracture so that either one of the two forms of treatment may be instituted. If the fracture is not recognized, the results may very well be serious and disability may result. If the fracture is treated either by bedrest and protected weight-bearing or by nailing, the result should be excellent.

In our clinic we use either the Smith-Petersen nail (fig. 1) or the multiple nails of Austin-Moore (fig. 3). The advantage of the latter is that one is less likely to disimpact the fragments while inserting the nail.

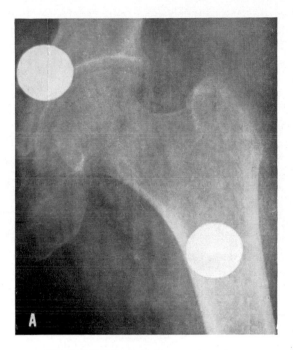

Fig. 3—(A) Impacted fracture in valgus.

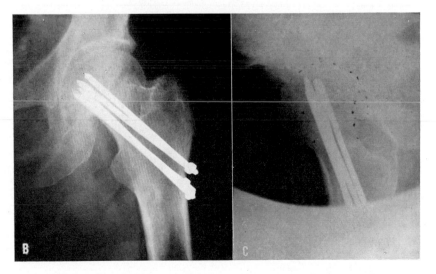

Fig. 3—(B and C) Internal fixation by means of 4 Moore nails.

Avascular necrosis: In spite of the fact that the impacted fracture heals readily in almost every instance, there still remains the complication of avascular necrosis which occurs in about 20 per cent of the cases (fig. 1 F and G). The necrosis may occur in a period of six months to a year or may be slow in appearing and cause no symptoms for two or three years. Despite the presence of this condition, many elderly patients are able to ambulate well with little pain for many years after x-ray evidence of necrosis is apparent. In others, the disintegration of the head is rapid, the disability of the hip severe, and some form of operative reconstruction or femoral head replacement is necessary.

Displaced Varus Type of Fracture

Results of the treatment of this type of fracture have been so poor that many methods have been tried with various claims as to results.

The Whitman abduction method, in which an attempt is made to reduce the fracture by means of traction, abduction, internal rotation and immobilization in a plaster spica, was popular for over half a century, and the reported success varied from 100 to 10 per cent bony union. It is now recognized that the treatment was not only difficult, uncomfortable and undesirable, but gave almost as high a rate of nonunion as if no treatment were given.

With the advent of the Smith-Petersen nail described by Smith-Petersen and Cave in 1925, the surgeon has been given an opportunity to reduce and fix the fracture by mechanical means. We now consider this to be the best method of treatment. We believe that every intracapsular fracture of the neck of the femur should be operated on, and the fracture reduced and the nail inserted, and that no other treatment is indicated except in a few instances. If the patient is *in extremis* or has a severe complication such as marked cardiac decompensation, it may then be advisable to make no attempt to fix the fracture. On the other hand, the fact that the patient has other pathologic lesions as a result of his senility or debility, or that he is 80 or 90 years old, does not in any way contraindicate the operation.

There is considerable difference of opinion concerning the wisdom of using primary femoral head replacement in this type of fracture. We believe that we are able to obtain primary bony union in about 50 per cent of cases of the intracapsular fracture of the neck of the femur. We therefore feel that except in unusual circumstance, such as Parkinson's disease, an attempt should be made to nail the fracture. In the 50 per cent failures, the secondary operation may be done when nonunion is inevitable.

Avascular necrosis occurs in about 25 per cent of these cases, and at present there is no means of predicting which patients will develop avascular necrosis and which will not. It seems obvious that the fate of the femoral head is decided at the time of the trauma, and it may be only after a period of a year or two that one is able to make the diagnosis.

The Pauwell's classification of the hip fractures is considered by many to be important in prognosticating the possibility of union or nonunion. This classification is based on the measurement of the angle in the anterior-posterior x-ray between the line of fracture and the horizontal. An angle of 30 degrees or less (Classification 1) is considered to indicate a good prognosis; from 30 to 70 degrees (Classification 2) a fair prognosis; 70 to 90 degrees (Classification 3) a very poor prognosis because of the fact that there is a shearing force at the fracture line which prevents impaction of the fragment. Lately there has been evidence to indicate that this classification is not necessarily a good aid to prognosis, and in our clinic we are much more concerned with accurate reduction and proper fixation by the nail than we are with the obliquity of the fracture line.

Time of Operation

An elderly patient who has sustained an intracapsular fracture of the neck of the femur should immediately be transported to the hospital in a Thomas splint, and x-rays should be taken on arrival. After diagnosis is made by x-ray, the patient may be taken to his bed and temporarily placed in Russell's traction (fig. 4). This type of traction is most comfortable for the patient and

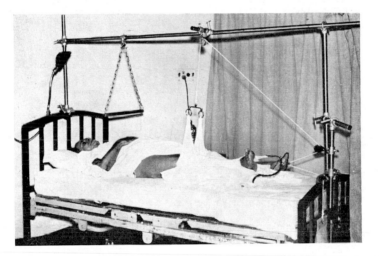

Fig. 4—Russell traction for patient during preoperative period.

tends to reduce a displaced fracture during the waiting period before operation. Russell's traction is not without its dangers, the most important being peroneal nerve palsy and resulting foot drop due to external rotation of the limb against the sling. If the patient is put in Russell's traction with at least 45 degrees flexion of hip and knee, external rotation will be more easily overcome than if the knee and hip are more extended. After application of the traction if there is a tendency for the limb to rotate externally, this may be corrected by means of a roll of ace bandage wrapped about the lower limb and extended over the overhead traction with a weight of 1 or 2 pounds (fig. 5).

The patient is properly examined and evaluated and the necessary treatment instituted to prepare her for operation. She is hydrated and if there is cardiac decompensation, it is treated. If she has diabetes, it is brought under control. The examination and preliminary preoperative treatment may take two or three days. In any case, the patient should be operated on as soon as

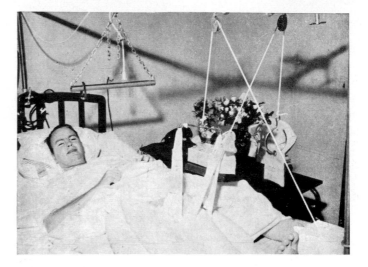

Fig. 5—External rotation of leg in Russell traction may be prevented by Ace bandage about lower leg extended over pulley on overhead traction frame.

possible after admission, but not before proper evaluation. We ordinarily operate on our patients within 12 hours after admission to the hospital, but we do not hesitate to delay the operation 12 or 24 hours if it is necessary. However, unnecessary delay will invariably cause complications and add to the mortality and morbidity. We do not believe that the patient should be operated on immediately after arrival at the hospital and taken directly from the admitting room to the operating room.

Anesthesia

We prefer general anesthesia for our patients, particularly if there is marked displacement of the fracture fragments and reduction is necessary. However, if indicated we will use local anesthesia. In some instances spinal anesthesia in elderly patients may be indicated, but we prefer not to use it.

Technic of Operation

The patient is placed on the fracture table (we prefer the Bell type table, fig. 6) and great care is taken to pad the sacral region so that the prolonged supine position does not cause pressure area on the sacrum. After the patient

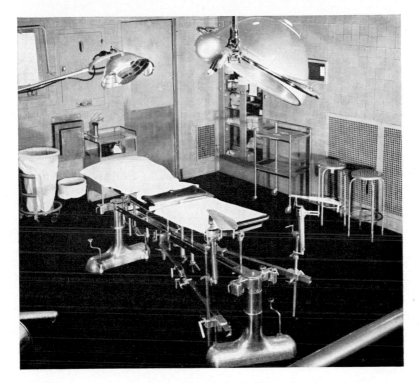

Fig. 6—(A) Bell traction table. Flat sole plates facilitate fixation of foot to traction apparatus.

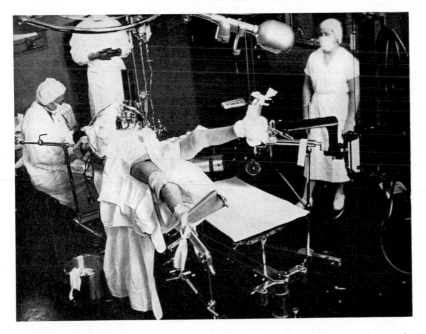

Fig. 6—(B) Patient on Bell table with feet attached to traction plates. Note cone of portable x-ray in place for lateral x-ray. Right leg is in internal rotation and abduction after reduction.

is anesthesized, the perineum is brought snugly against the perineal post and the sound limb fixed to the foot piece on the traction bar with very little traction. The leg is elevated with enough flexion of the hip so as to accomodate the cone of the portable machine which is put in place at this time for the taking of the lateral x-ray. The injured limb is then immediately fitted to the foot piece of the traction bar if there is no displacement of the fracture

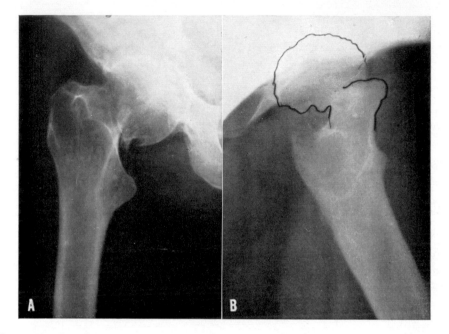

Fig. 7–(A) Anterior-posterior view of displaced intracapsular fracture of femoral neck.
(B) Lateral view shows angulation and displacement of femoral head.

fragments. However, if there is the usual upward displacement of the shaft (fig. 7) and external rotation, the operator reduces the fracture by means of gentle, continuous steady traction directed in the long axis of the limb. As the upward displacement is felt to be reduced, the limb is gradually abducted about 20 degrees and internally rotated fully. The foot is then fixed to the foot plate on the traction bar and anteroposterior and lateral x-rays are taken. Reduction should easily be accomplished with little force.

At this point a metal object such as a penny is placed over the middle of Pouparts ligament and a second penny over the anterior surface of the thigh about 2 inches below the upper end of the greater trochanter so that these points may serve as land marks in inserting the guide wires (fig. 8). The skin is marked with Gentian Violet at the site of the placement of the pennies.

The AP and lateral x-rays are taken, and if the reduction is not satisfactory, the limb is removed from the traction and manual reduction is again attempted by means of traction with the hip in extension or by means of the

Leadbetter maneuver [9] in which the hip and knee are flexed and traction is exerted upward.

A second x-ray is taken, and if the reduction is satisfactory the limb is placed on the foot piece of the traction bar with only enough traction to immobilize it.

If reduction cannot be accomplished by closed means, the operator then proceeds to open the hip joint and reduce the fracture and insert the nail, while visualizing the fracture site.

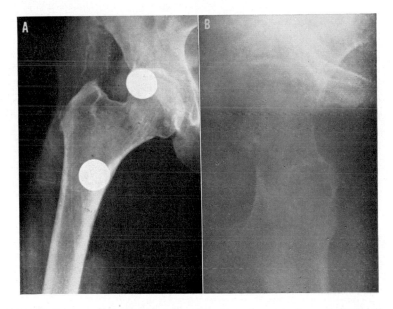

Fig. 8—(A) Anterior-posterior view of reduced fracture shown in figure 7. Reduction accomplished by gentle traction, internal rotation and slight abduction. Pennies placed over middle of Pouparts ligament and over anterior thigh 2 inches below greater trochanter serve as landmarks for insertion of guide wire. (B) Lateral view after reduction.

If the fracture is properly reduced, the area of the hip, upper thigh and abdomen is suitably cleansed, properly prepared with zephrin and drapes are applied.

We use silk to suture the drapes to the skin so that the x-rays are not cluttered with silhouettes of clamps and towel clips. The area is draped so that the portable x-ray machine for the lateral x-ray can be placed permanently under the drapes and does not have to be replaced after each exposure.

An incision of at least 6 inches in length is made from a point just below the tip of the greater trochanter down the lateral surface of the thigh. It is not necessary to insist on a very small incision, since it often interferes with the proper placement of the nail. The incision is deepened to the tensor fascia lata, and towels are draped about and sutured to the edges of the wound. The tensor fascia is incised, and the vastus lateralis muscle is either reflected anteriorly or split at its middle. By means of insertion of Bennett tibial retractors, tension may be placed on the muscle as it is split so that the two or three groups of lateral circumflex femoral vessels may be visualized, clamped and divided between clamps.

The shaft of the bone is exposed below the greater trochanter, and after the operator refers to the guide x-ray a point is chosen on the lateral cortex of the femur which seems a proper site for the insertion of the guide wire.

A hole in the cortex is started with a very sharp Steinmann pin. A large-sized drill is then used to drill a hole through the cortex in the direction the guide wire is expected to take. The hole is larger than the guide wire so that the position of the wire may be changed as it is inserted.

The guide wire is then inserted through the hole in the cortex into the neck and head of the femur. It is not drilled into the neck but is pushed manually and guided by "feel" into the neck. This allows the operator to feel the course of the nail as it enters the neck and head, and if it strikes the hard cortex of the bone, it may then be shifted to find the intramedullary canal.

Since we insert the Smith-Petersen nail over the guide wire, we feel that it is essential that the latter be made of good stainless steel and should never be notched, since the entering nail may bend the wire at a notch and snap it off, leaving the distal end within the bone. The ideal placement of the guide wire should be along the calcar and into the head at its middle or just inferior to the middle of the neck in the AP view (fig. 9 A). In the lateral view the

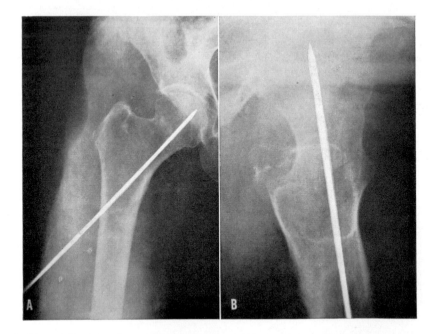

Fig. 9—(A and B) After insertion of guide wire. Note wire is inserted along the calcar in anterior-posterior view. The end of the nail is near the center of the head. In the lateral view the wire is just posterior to center of head.

guide wire should be either exactly in the middle of the neck or just posterior to the middle of the neck (fig. 9 B). It should never be placed anterior to the middle of the neck, since this may allow the nail to extrude as the leg externally rotates.

If the guide wire is not in perfect position, it is left *in situ* and a second drill hole made. Using the first wire as a guide, a second wire is then inserted into its proper position in the head. We believe it is unwise to remove the

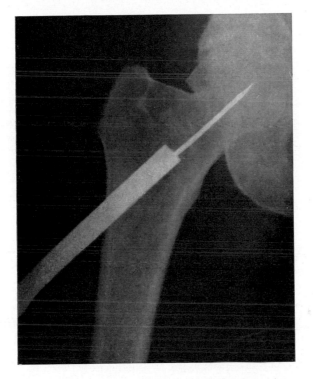

Fig. 10—X-ray check as nail is being driven over the guide wire. This x-ray is necessary to prevent bending or breaking of wire if nail does not follow the wire accurately.

original guide wire and try to replace it by memory. If it is left in place and a new hole made for the second wire, there is less danger of error.

When the guide wire is properly in place, the cortex is prepared by a bore and a small osteotome is used to fashion slots into which the flanges of the Smith-Petersen nail insert.

The length of the nail is then determined by measurement of the guide wire. One should be careful to allow for the head of the nail to extrude slightly from the bone. It is acceptable to have the nail ¼ inch too long, but it cannot be ¼ inch too short.

The nail is then inserted over the guide wire (fig. 10), care being taken to prevent sciving or splitting of the cortex as the nail is driven through it.

It is helpful to have an assistant push against the Smith-Petersen nail from above downward on the cortex as it is being driven in, so as to prevent sliding upward along the bone. It is most essential that the nail be properly measured before insertion. If it is of improper length and is pulled out and a second nail inserted, the hole in the cortex of the shaft of the femur is enlarged so it does not secure the nail well, and it is very apt to extrude later. The nail should be driven well within the head of the bone and up to within $1/8$ inch of the cartilage (fig. 11). If the fracture disimpacts slightly

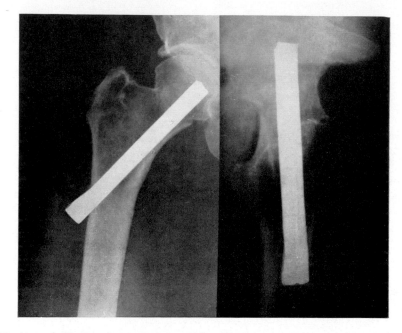

Fig. 11–(A and B) Anterior-posterior and lateral views of nail after insertion into the head. Note slight disimpaction of head fragment.

at the time of the insertion of the nail, it is unwise to attempt to impact it by means of the impactor at the fracture table. It is much better to allow the patient to stand on the limb a day or so after the operation, thus impacting the fragments more satisfactorily than one can do by driving an impactor against the shaft of the bone.

After the nail has been properly inserted, and x-ray check shows it in proper position, the guide wire is removed and the wound is closed in layers.

Postoperative Care

The patient is returned to his bed, and as soon as he awakens is moved about and is sat up in bed immediately. He is allowed out of bed within the first 24 hours and is asked to stand, if possible, in a walker or with crutches and is encouraged to ambulate.

Many elderly patients are unable to stand and use crutches or the walker, and in many cases partial weight-bearing is allowed in order to encourage ambulation.

The patient is kept in the hospital only as long as is necessary for his general care. If the fracture is impacted in valgus position, we allow some weight-bearing within two weeks and full weight-bearing within three or four weeks if the patient is able to do so without pain.

If the fracture is the displaced varus type, we do not allow full weight-bearing for four months, as the fracture is not expected to heal before this period. If x-ray examination shows the fracture line to be filled in with the lines of bony trabeculi crossing the fracture line, it may then be considered healed, and the patient is allowed full weight-bearing. If, on the other hand, the fracture line is distinct or widened, the patient is continued on crutches until healing is evident. This period may be anywhere from four to twelve months. If during this period it is quite obvious that nonunion is inevitable, as evidenced by marked widening of the fracture line or displacement or extrusion of the nail, then no time should be lost in embarking on an operative procedure to correct the disability.

The technic just described is insertion of the conventional Smith-Petersen nail and has been the practice in our clinic for many years. There are other types of fixation for this fracture, and one that we have used with great success is the multiple Moore nail fixation [2] in which four Moore nails are inserted across the fracture line in such a way as to prevent rotation of the fragment (fig. 2). The insertion of these nails is not difficult and has an advantage in that the bulk of the nail is small and does not tend to rotate

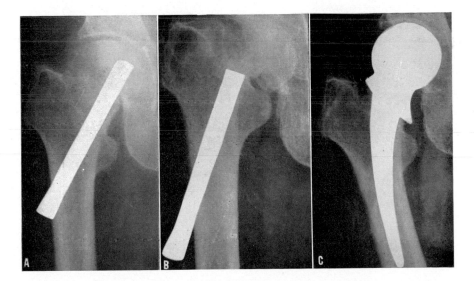

Fig. 12—(A) After nailing of intracapsular fracture by Smith-Petersen nail. (B) Extrusion of nail eight weeks after operation. Note marked absorption of femoral neck. (C) After femoral head replacement by Frederick Thompson prosthesis.

the head of the bone on insertion. These nails are also useful in treating fractures in children.

The Smith-Petersen nail often extrudes due to avascular necrosis of the head or obvious nonunion at the fracture site (fig. 12). If when the nail is inserted, the hole in the cortex is enlarged by splitting or because the nail is removed and replaced, the nail is more apt to extrude because the fixation in the head is not enough to prevent slipping. Since this has occurred in some of

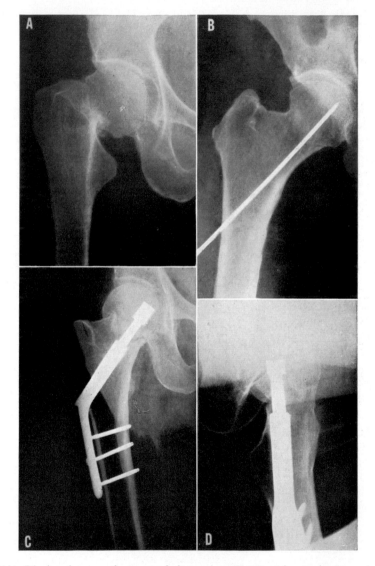

Fig. 13—(A) Displaced varus fracture of femoral neck. (B) After reduction of fracture and placement of guide wire. (C and D) After insertion of Ken-Pugh nail. The nail is fixed at 135 degree angle. Note size of tri-phalanged end of nail.

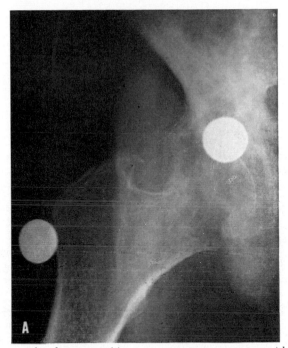

Fig. 14—(A) Intracapsular fracture (adduction type) after reduction with metal landmarks in place.

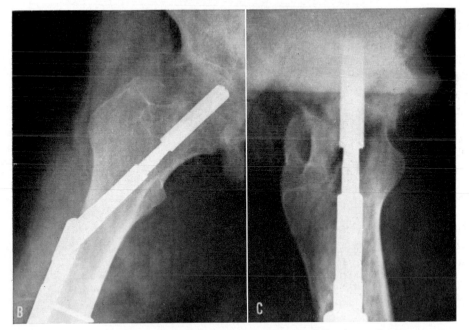

Fig. 14—(B and C) After insertion of Massie nail. Angle of nail fixed at 150⁰. This necessitates low entrance of nail in femoral cortex. Note longer segment of triphalanged nail end.

our cases, we have recently used a means to prevent extrusion either by means of the Jewett nail or one of its modifications. When the Jewett nail is used, and there is the usual shortening of the neck, the nail is apt to extrude through the head into the acetabulum. Because of this, collapsible nails have been devised. The Ken-Pugh (fig. 13) and the Massie nail (fig. 14) are both satisfactory. The Massie nail being manufactured only with a 150 degree angle is more difficult to insert than the Pugh, which is manufactured in 135 as well as 150 degree angles.

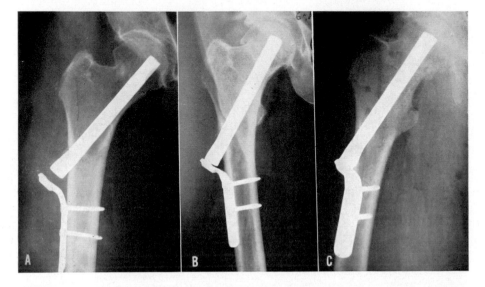

Fig. 15—(A) "Back-out" plate. After conventional Smith-Petersen nailing, a short plate is applied to femoral shaft, bent to allow a fourth of an inch space between nail and end of plate. (B) After 1 month neck absorbs and nail extrudes toward plate. (C) After 8 weeks neck absorbs further and nail impinges against plate, preventing further extrusion.

We have used a more simple method which serves the same purpose. After insertion of the Smith-Petersen nail, an ordinary 3-hole Thornton plate is applied to the shaft of the bone with the upper end bent away from the end of the Smith-Petersen nail so that it is separated from the nail by a space of ¼ inch (fig. 15). The plate is fixed to the shaft, and in the convalescent period when the neck shortens and the nail extrudes, it is allowed to extrude for ¼ inch and is then held firmly against the "Back-out" plate. The fact that the plate is easily applied and serves the same purpose as the collapsible nails has made it useful in our clinic.

Nonunion

As soon as nonunion is found to be inevitable as evidenced by aseptic necrosis of the head or widening of the fracture line or extrusion of the nail, an operative procedure should immediately be performed before there is shortening and upward displacement of the shaft and contraction of the muscles about the hip.

MacMurray Operation

The MacMurray operation (fig. 16) is a most satisfactory one for nonunion. However, it presupposes the viability of the femoral head and necessitates at least eight weeks of immobilization in plaster. It does, however, give very

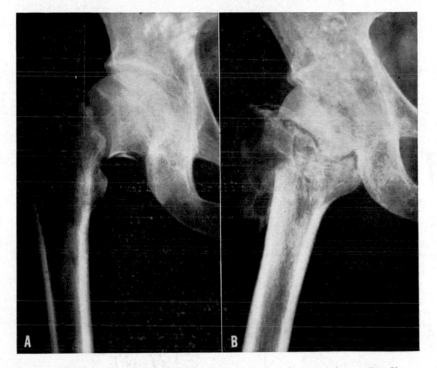

Fig. 16—(A) Nonunion of femoral neck fracture 3 months postinjury. (B) Six months after MacMurray osteotomy. Fracture line still visible.

satisfactory results, but cannot be used in older patients who cannot stand immobilization in plaster.

In order to obviate the necessity for postoperative immobilization in plaster, one may use internal fixation to hold the fragments in position after a MacMurray operation. Such a case is illustrated in figures 17 A—E. In this patient, a 25 year old nurse, the MacMurray operation was performed and the fragment fixed by means of the Lorenzo screw and plate (fig. 17 B). The osteotomy site healed rapidly as did the intracapsular fracture site, and the patient did well although evidence of aseptic necrosis of the head developed after several years (Fig. 17 D). The nail was removed, and seven years later the patient was without symptoms, but x-rays showed evidence of aseptic necrosis of the head (fig. 17 E).

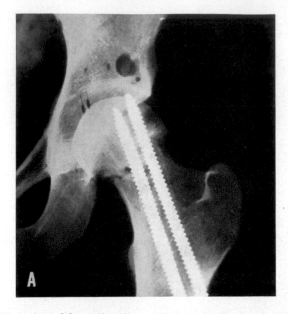

Fig. 17–(A) Nonunion of femoral neck in a 25 year old female after screw fixation.

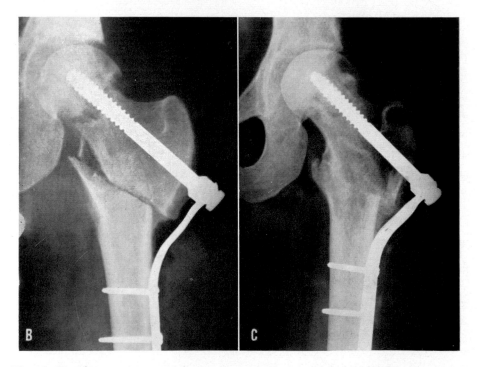

Fig. 17–(B) After osteotomy and fixation by Lorenzo screw and plate. (C) Six months post-operation. Osteotomy site and fracture healed. Evidence of relative increased density of head suggesting avascular necrosis.

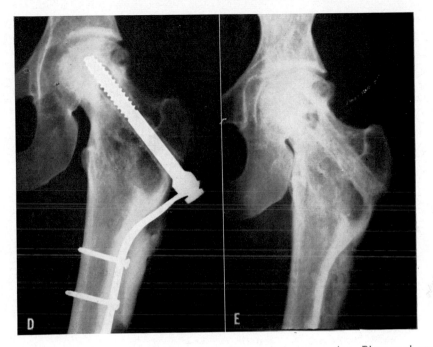

Fig. 17–(D) Two years postoperative. Avascular necrosis progressing. Plate and screw removed. (E) Five years postoperative. Narrowing of joint space, increased density of head with lytic areas in head. Patient has excellent function and no pain as yet.

Replacement Prostheses

The most popular and probably the most suitable reconstructive operation for nonunion of the neck of the femur is the femoral head replacement by means of a metal prosthesis. The two most popular prostheses are the Frederick Thompson (fig. 12) and the Austin-Moore (fig. 18). We prefer the Austin-Moore prosthesis in this clinic because the intramedullary stem is somewhat broader than the Thompson and thus prevents rotation in the shaft, and the holes in the stem tend to be filled in by bone after some time and thus fix the prosthesis more firmly in place. The small hook on the upper end of the prosthesis also facilitates its removal when one is testing the size of the intramedullary canal.

Both the anterior and the posterior approach (southern exposure of Austin-Moore) have been used in our clinic with considerable success. We now prefer the posterior approach because it provides easier exposure of the capsule and the joint and because of the fact that as the patient lies in bed in the postoperative period, the leg naturally falls in external rotation and there is less chance of dislocation. After insertion of the prosthesis and relocation of the head within the acetabulum, if the reduction seems secure, no external immobilizing apparatus is applied, and the patient is allowed up within a week or ten days. Weight-bearing is permitted as soon as the patient is able to do so without pain.

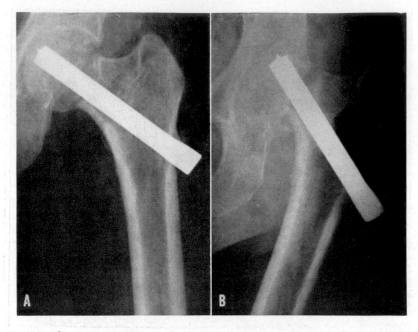

Fig. 18–(A) After conventional Smith-Petersen nailing of femoral neck fracture. (B) Six months postoperative. Head and neck absorbing, nonunion is obvious.

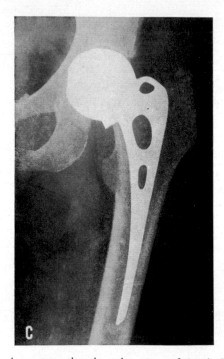

Fig. 18–(C) Replacement arthroplasty by means of Austin-Moore prosthesis.

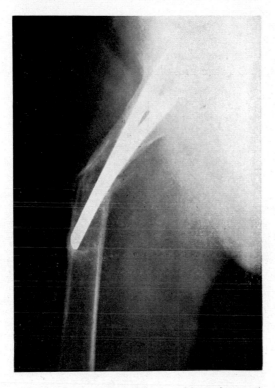

Fig. 19—(A) During reduction of Austin-Moore prosthesis after replacement, the femoral shaft was fractured. Nonunion resulted. Note marked decalcification of femur.

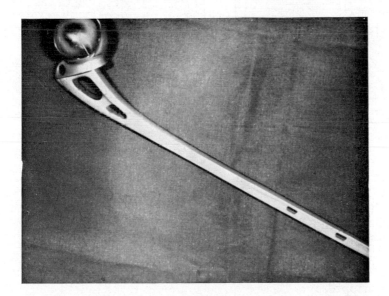

Fig. 19—(B) Long stem intramedullary vitallium prosthesis.

Complications

During the insertion of the prosthesis, there are several complications to be avoided. While the medulla of the femur is being prepared for the stem of the prosthesis, great care must be taken that the gouge does not traverse

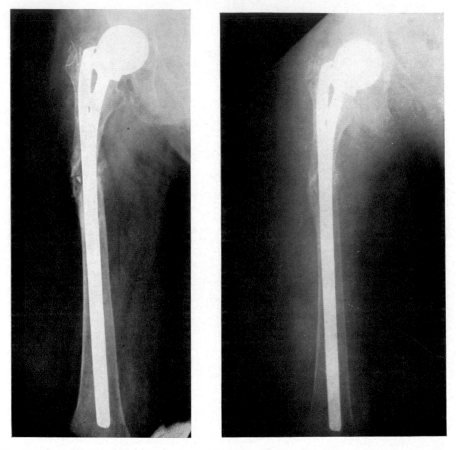

Fig. 19–(C) Two months after insertion of long stem prosthesis, replacing conventional type. (D) One year postoperative. Fracture united. Patient 85 years old, is now walking well with return of function.

the tract of the Smith-Petersen nail which has been removed. If this does occur, the prosthesis will be improperly placed across the shaft of the bone rather than into the intramedullary canal, and the greater trochanter can easily be snapped off during the procedure.

After the prosthesis has been inserted into the shaft, it must be reduced into the acetabulum with great care to avoid undue leverage on the brittle cortex of the shaft of the femur. If leverage is applied to the shaft, the cortex may be snapped, thus causing a fracture and necessitating a long period of immobilization. If such an accident does occur, a long-stem prosthesis may be made to extend past the fracture site into the shaft of the femur, thus combining the usefulness of the prosthesis with the immobilization afforded by a Küntscher nail (fig. 19).

References

[1] AUSTIN-MOORE, A. T.: Fracture of the hip joint — a new method of treatment. Internat. S. Digest 19: 323, 1935.

[2] —: The self-locking metal hip prosthesis. J. Bone & Joint Surg. 39 A: 811, 1957.

[3] BÖHLER, L.: The Treatment of Fractures. New York, Grune & Stratton, Inc., 1958.

[4] BOYD, H. B., and GEORGE, I. L.: Complications of fractures of the neck of the femur. J. Bone & Joint Surg. 29: 13, 1947.

[5] CAMPBELL, W. C., ORR, H. W., and OSGOOD, R. B.: Report of a commission appointed by the Am. Orth. Assoc. to study end results of intracapsular fractures of neck of femur. J. Bone & Joint Surg. 12: 966, 1930.

[6] HAMPTON, O. P.: Wounds of Extremities in Military Surgery. St. Louis, C. V. Mosby Co., 1951.

[7] HERMANN, O. J.: The MacMurray osteotomy for non-united hip fractures. New England J. Med. 232: 186, 1945.

[8] JEWETT, E. L.: Rigid internal fixation of intracapsular femoral neck fractures. Am. J. Surg. 91: 621 (April) 1956.

[9] KEY, J. A., and CONWELL, H. E.: The Management of Fractures, Dislocations and Sprains. St. Louis, C. V. Mosby Co., 1951.

[10] LEADBETTER, G. W.: A treatment for fracture of the neck of the femur. J. Bone & Joint Surg. 15: 931, 1933.

[11] MAHONEY, J. W., MULHOLLAND, J. H., JOHR, J. and DOOLING, J. A.: Immediate Moore prosthetic replacement in acute intracapsular fractures. Am. J. Surg. 95: 577 (April) 1957.

[12] MITCHELL, J. I.: Fracture of the neck of the femur in children. J. A. M. C. 107: 1603, 1936.

[13] PAUWELS, F.: "Der Schenkelhalsbruch, ein mechanisches Problem." Stuttgart, Enke, 1935.

[14] PUGH, W. L.: A self-adjusting nail-plate for fractures about the hip joint. J. Bone & Joint Surg. 37 A: 1085, 1955.

[15] SMITH-PETERSEN, M. H., CAVE, E. F., and VAN GORDER, G. W.: Intracapsular fractures of the neck of the femur. Arch. Surg. 23: 715, 1931.

[16] THOMPSON, F. R.: Two and a half years experience with a vitallium intramedullary hip prosthesis. J. Bone & Joint Surg. 36 A: 489, 1954.

[17] WATSON-JONES, R.: Fractures and Joint Injuries. Baltimore, Williams and Wilkins Co., 1955.

[18] WILSON, J. C.: Fractures of neck of femur in childhood. J. Bone & Joint Surg. 22: 531, 1940.

CHAPTER 42

INTERTROCHANTERIC FRACTURES
OF THE FEMUR

CARLETON M. CORNELL, M.D. and RENDEL LEVONIAN, M.D.

When intertrochanteric fractures occur in old age, they are a major disaster. These fractures are most common in the 70 to 90 year age group, in contrast to intracapsular fractures which predominate in the age group 15 years younger. The frequency in women is as high as nine times greater than in men. Old age is a period of serious degenerative change. To quote Cleveland, "These patients are a veritable museum of pathologic changes, antedating their trauma."

With increased life expectancy, the growing number of people living beyond 65 is creating formidable problems in geriatrics, one of them, a continuing rise in the number of intertrochanteric fractures. With the osteoporotic changes of old age, the femoral cortex thins and the cancellous bone becomes rarefied and brittle. The trochanteric region, which is subjected to severe stress of body weight and divergent muscle forces, is most vulnerable to fracture. These fractures usually result from indirect trauma such as is caused by misstepping, forceful twisting or tripping. Open fixation of these fractures has replaced conservative treatment and has reduced the mortality from about 30 per cent to 12 or 15 per cent (table 1).

TABLE 1–*Intertrochanteric Fractures*
(Second Surgical Division [Cornell] Bellevue Hospital)
Period from 1940—1955

NONOPERATIVE

	CASES	DEATHS	MORTALITY PERCENTAGE
1940—1945	62	19	30.6
1945—1950	39	8	20.5
1951—1955	40	15	37.5
Totals	141	42	29.8

OPERATIVE

1940—1945	8	0	0
1945—1950	43	6	14.00
1951—1955	100	14	14.00
Totals	151	20	13.2

Anatomy

Intertrochanteric or trochanteric fractures involve the extracapsular portions of the proximal femur from the base of the neck to the upper femoral shaft through the lesser trochanter. Figure 1 shows the head, neck and trochanteric region in half-section. The body weight is transmitted from the superior roof of the acetabulum through the femoral head, to the inferior portion of the cervical neck, to the shaft of the femur. The cortex along this stress line is thickened and dense, and is called the *calcar femorale*. From this cortex inward, there is a unique architectural arrangement of cancellous bone (lamellae) for the greatest strength. The capsule encloses the head and most of the neck. The ligaments of the hip joint are attached to the rim of the acetabulum and insert in a broad area about the distal femoral neck proximal

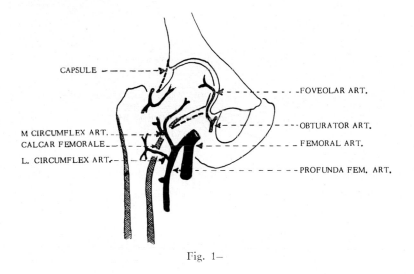

Fig. 1–

to the trochanters. The blood supply to this region is illustrated. The head receives a scant supply by the nutrient artery, a branch of the obturator artery, and from the capsule. The intracapsular portion of the neck and the trochanteric region receive intraosseous and ligamentous branches of the medial and lateral circumflex vessels of the deep femoral artery. There is collateral circulation with the superior and inferior gluteal vessels.

Figure 2 A shows the shaft neck angle of the femur. This varies from 110—140 degrees. Figure 2 B is a view of this region from above, showing that the anterior inclined angle of the neck axis is about 12 degrees when the femoral condyles are horizontal. With the leg in external rotation, this angle is close to 30 degrees. These angles are all important in understanding the technique of the open fixation of both intracapsular and extracapsular fractures. By eliminating the anteriorly inclined angle through internal rotation of the leg, the axis of the neck is horizontal, the floor is now in a common plane with this axis. The neck shaft angle thus becomes the only adjustable factor necessary when inserting the guide wires and pin. The crescentic greater trochanter serves for attachment of the gluteus media and gluteus minimus muscles. Their action is abduction and to some extent external rotation. The short, heavy quadratus femoris, the obturator internus abdominis, and the gemelli are the powerful external rotators and adductors

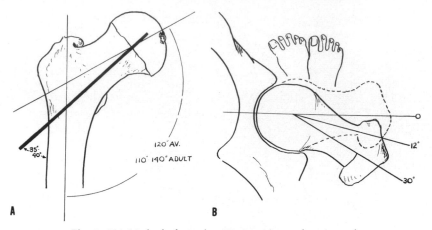

Fig. 2—(A) Neck shaft angle. (B) Anterior neck axis angle.

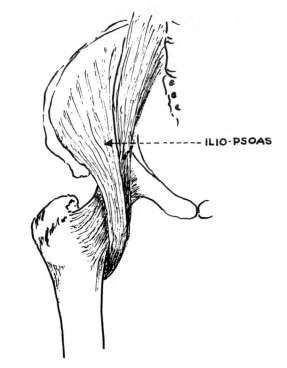

Fig. 3—To show iliopsoas insertion into lesser trochanter.

attached to the posterior intertrochanteric ridge. These muscles cause the characteristic displacements of the trochanteric fractures.

Figure 3 shows the iliacus and psoas muscles emerging from the pelvis passing over the head and neck to insert in the lesser trochanter. Their action is a powerful medial and upward pull and accounts for typical deflection of an avulsed lesser trochanter.

Classification of Trochanteric Fractures

Anatomically it seems logical to classify fractures of the hip as *intra-capsular* and *extracapsular* fractures. The extracapsular are true trochanteric fractures and in turn are classified by *stability* and *region*. Stability depends on the integrity of the *calcar femorale*. Overlapping or comminution of this cortex causes instability and leads to typical coxa vara deformity. About 21 per cent of extracapsular fractures are unstable.

Pertrochanteric fractures (fig. 4 A and B) are those which involve the base of the femoral neck, site of the ligamentous attachment of the hip joint and may or may not involve the lesser trochanter. They are extracapsular and not to be confused with neck or intracapsular fractures (Böhler). The leg is externally rotated and the lesser trochanter radiographically prominent. The neck is displaced anteriorly. There is shortening and coxa vara.

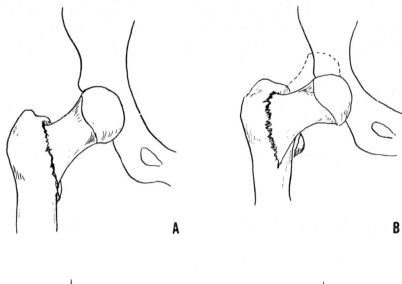

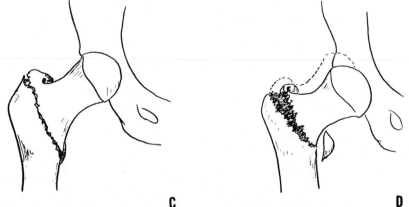

Fig. 4—(A) Stable pertrochanteric. (B) Stable intertrochanteric. (C) Unstable pertrochanteric. (D) Unstable intertrochanteric.

The intertrochanteric type (fig. 4 C and D), involves both the greater and the lesser trochanters. They may be extensively comminuted and unstable or they may be simple, impacted fractures making clinical and x-ray recognition difficult. Usually the leg is externally rotated, the fracture line is open superiorly, and the neck is in a mild coxa vara.

In the subtrochanteric fracture (fig. 5 A), the line of fracture traverses the intertrochanteric region and involves the upper shaft and the lesser trochanter. The lesser trochanter may remain with the distal fragment. When the obliquity of the fracture line is reversed to run upward and medially, the

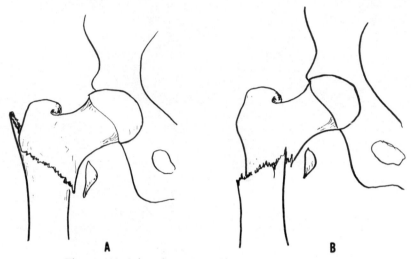

Fig. 5—(A) Subtrochanteric. (B) Reverse subtrochanteric.

fracture is a reverse intertrochanteric fracture (fig. 5 B). These are apt to be severely comminuted and unstable, and are likely to result in a final coxa vara deformity.

Clinical Aspects

Extracapsular as well as intracapsular fractures usually cause complete disability, with pain in the hip. Deformity occurs with the leg adducted, externally rotated and shortened. Prominence and local tenderness of the hip are more marked in extracapsular fractures. Diagnosis of the type of hip fracture will seldom be made except by x-ray.

Reaction of the patient varies. Shock, although not usual, may follow. Because of systemic senile conditions associated with this age group, cardiac decompensation, urinary retention or bronchopneumonia may supervene with the early development of electrolyte imbalance, acidosis and azotemia.

Treatment

Prompt and aggressive emergency treatment is necessary to forestall these complications. Demoral is given for analgesia in anticipation of shock. A

Thomas splint is properly applied prior to moving the patient. Care in padding the ankle and application of traction is essential.

On admission to the emergency room, fluid replacement therapy is started and the extremity is re-examined for circulatory embarrassment due to traction. Before the patient is transferred to his bed, diagnostic x-rays are taken. Anteroposterior views are the only necessary ones, and will not require removal or loosening of the splint. Lateral views of the hip will be taken in the operating room, with the patient under anesthesia. Both pre- and postreduction films are taken at that time.

The patient is then placed in Russell's or Buck's traction and immediately evaluated. A thorough physical examination should always take into account the possibility of pathologic fracture. Studies of cardiorespiratory and renal systems are made with chest x-rays, electrocardiographs and blood and urine analyses. If there are abnormal findings of any magnitude, it is wise to enlist the help of an internist.

Most trauma surgeons are agreed that early open fixation of both intra-capsular and extracapsular fractures results in the lowest mortality. The 24 to 48 hour period is ideal, though hasty emergency surgery does not allow sufficient time to evaluate the patient. Survival is not quite the problem with intracapsular fractures as it is with the extracapsular types.

Early operation reduces mortality and postoperative morbidity. Most patients tolerate carefully planned surgery. Many patients on whom open fixations have been performed have previously sustained cerebral accidents or have had coronary artery disease with occlusion. Many have diabetes mellitus.

Operation

Internal fixation of these fractures, particularly the unstable types, is often a challenge to the operator's ingenuity. The object of surgical fixation is to obtain accurate reduction with restoration of the extremity length, correction of varus deformity and the maintenance of reduction by an adequate appliance. It has been our experience that a Smith-Petersen nail or a Lorenzo screw with femoral bar is suitable for most of these fractures. However, appliance failures are of the greatest significance in causing coxa vara in the unstable types. The major shearing force is located at the junction of the nail and bar. It is at this point that bending or breakage occurs. Even the screw may loosen and give way. Of the available appliances, the Jewett nail, a one-piece nail and bar, though more difficult to handle, will provide the greatest strength for severely comminuted types.

Anesthesia

Since most patients are in the geriatric group and these people tolerate little anesthetic agent, the anesthesiologist should be consulted. Sodium pentothal hypnosis together with a curare-like drug provides sufficient relaxation to apply traction and to obtain proper positioning of the patient on the orthopedic table. The patient is maintained on nitrous oxide and oxygen supplemented by procaine infiltration of the operative area. With such a regimen, the patient can be held in a light plane of anesthesia, circulatory depression can be avoided and early reaction made possible.

Procedure

Following induction, the patient is placed on an orthopedic table equipped with AP and lateral radiographic cassette holders. No manipulation or strenuous maneuver is necessary or desirable. Gentle traction with slight abduction and external rotation is applied, and the leg is then brought into neutral position and internally rotated. The extremities are maintained in the leg extension pieces. If reduction has not been accomplished by this, it can be accomplished under direct vision. This is particularly true in the unstable types of fractures. After preparing and draping the patient, a Michel clip or a penny is placed midway between the antero-superior spine of the ilium and the pubic tubercle. This represents the midpoint of the head of the femur. Some surgeons employ another Michel clip in the subtrochanteric region as an additional guide. At this time, scout AP and lateral x-ray films are taken.

Incision

A horizontal incision from the greater trochanter down over the femoral shaft is made and carried through the tensor fascia and the vastus lateralis muscle. The subtrochanteric region and the upper shaft of the femur are exposed subperiosteally. Direct manipulation of the fracture may now be necessary to effect a reduction by exposing the fracture site. There are those in which the proximal fragment will remain in a posterior or externally rotated position despite a reduced distal fragment. The proximal fragment is rotated into position by inserting the wires into the fragment and manually rotating it anteriorly into proper position with the distal fragment. The nail or screw may then be inserted and the bar properly applied.

Trochanteric fractures are particularly suited to fixation because the neck provides excellent purchase for the nail or screw.

Using the Michel clips as guides, an 8 inch wire is inserted from a point about 1½ to 2 inches below the trochanter and driven inward to a point just above the middle of the femoral head. The exposed pin will form an angle of from 35 to 40 degrees (fig. 2 A) with the femoral shaft. Four inches of the pin are driven in. AP and lateral x-rays are then taken. The optimum position of the nail is in the lower or inferior half of the neck, with the end just above the midpoint of the femoral head and in the posterior half of the neck. The appropriate length of screw or nail is determined and, after removing the cortical bone about the wire with osteotome and burr, the nail or screw is placed over or alongside the wire and inserted. A plate of suitable length is attached to the end of the screw or nail and then fixed to the upper femoral shaft with Collison screws. Great care must be taken to set the screw attaching the nail and bar. The length of the femoral bar or plate will depend on the type of fracture. Unstable fractures require longer plates.

During the procedure, blood and water replacement are carefully adjusted to balance estimated losses. Overhydration will upset a precarious fluid equilibrium and may precipitate water intoxication with pulmonary edema and cardiac decompensation. It is, therefore, far safer to underhydrate the patient.

Postoperative Care

The reaction of these patients may vary from a very benign to a stormy postoperative course. Analgesics and sedation are given in minimal doses. These elderly patients develop senile psychoses rapidly as well as the systemic decompensations and must, therefore, be mobilized within the first 48 hours. A great deal is achieved toward this end by getting the patient up in a chair and commencing rehabilitation exercises. Ambulation on crutches is begun after two weeks, although this is frequently impossible for these people without some weight-bearing. Weight-bearing will depend on the stability of the fracture, the success of accurate fixation in good valgus position, and x-ray evidence of callus. In the stable types this is usually possible in 8 to 10 weeks; in the unstable types 10 to 12 weeks with the appearance of good healing by x-ray.

Complications

Factors most frequently complicating extracapsular fractures of the femur on the Second Surgical Division (Cornell) of Bellevue Hospital from 1940 to 1950 are shown in table 2.

TABLE 2—*Most Common Factors Complicating 144 cases of Extracapsular Fractures 1940 to 1950*

1. Decubitus Ulcers	54
2. Hypertensive cardio-vascular disease with decompensation	37
3. Bronchopneumonia	32
4. Arteriosclerotic heart disease with coronary insufficiency	30
5. Other fractures	21
6. Psychoses	21
7. Diabetes mellitus	11
8. Generalized arteriosclerosis	10

Operative Mortality

The postoperative causes of death in these fractures on the Cornell Division of Bellevue Hospital from 1950 through 1955 are indicated in table 3.

TABLE 3—*Postoperative Causes of Death in Intertrochanteric (Extracapsular) Fractures, Second Surgical Division (Cornell) Bellevue Hospital 1940–1955*

1. Arteriosclerotic heart disease with failure	5
2. Pulmonary embolism	3
3. Pneumonia	3
4. Generalized arteriosclerosis with cerebral vascular accident	3
5. Coronary occlusion	2
6. Uremia	2
7. Pyelonephritis	1
8. Carcinoma of the stomach	1
Total	20

All cases were complicated by other disease processes which contributed to death. A higher mortality occurred when operation was delayed beyond the first 48 hours of admission.

There were 20 deaths of a total of 151 open fixation procedures. The outstanding cause of death was arteriosclerotic heart disease with failure. Most deaths occurred within the first postoperative week; others died after a protracted decline. It is significant that a majority of deaths were in that group of patients in whom surgery was delayed beyond 48 hours after admission. This is the experience of most clinics and indicates the necessity for early open fixation.

Complications of Treatment

Most fractures will go on to firm union if the patient survives. By far the greatest problem is the development of *coxa vara* deformity, principally in the unstable types. This deformity occurs in about 20 per cent of the healed fractures. Bending, loosening of the screw or breakage of the pin shaft junction allows this deformity to develop. Premature weight-bearing will bend or break any appliance now in use.

Case 1: An 85 year old white woman having acquired hemolytic anemia controlled by cortisone therapy for two years, sustained a subtrochanteric fracture of the left femur. Open fixation was done with a Lorenzo screw and McLaughlin bar. Despite "no" active weight-bearing, coxa vara developed within one month as shown in figure 6.

Hematoma of the wound is certainly common and emphasizes the necessity for careful hemostasis. Bleeding must be recognized early and the clot evacuated. The rare complication of *nonunion* occurs in the comminuted unstable types of pertrochanteric and subtrochanteric fractures. *Infection* most certainly is a predisposing factor. The following case illustrates this.

Case 2: A 38 year old white man sustained serious injuries consisting of fractures of the skull, ribs and comminuted unstable subtrochanteric fracture of the right femur. Admitted to another hospital, he was of necessity treated by Russel traction. When no callus developed in three months, internal fixation with nail and plate was performed. The operative wound became infected and osteomyelitis developed. The hardware was removed. The patient was admitted to Bellevue Hospital nearly two years later with obvious nonunion and a draining wound. The infection was controlled and the wound healed. At this time there was marked deformity and four inches shortening. Osteotomy and Smith-Petersen nail and bar was performed. Infection recurred and again the hardware was removed (one year later) in a Veterans Administration Hospital. Three years later, fully six years after the initial injury, he was readmitted to Bellevue Hospital with nonunion and marked shortening due to coxa vara and bone loss (fig. 7 A and B). The wound was now well healed. Again, open operation was done. The bone ends were freshened, a Küntscher nail employed as internal splint, and bone chips packed about the fracture site (fig. 7 C). Within five months, there was firm bony union and the patient was ambulant without the aid of crutch or cane. The patient had some restriction of motion at the hip joint and some shortening of the leg.

Another interesting case of nonunion is shown in figure 8. This 60 year old white man was admitted to Bellevue Hospital with an unstable severely comminuted extracapsular fracture involving the intertrochanteric and pertrochanteric region of the right femur. He was treated for 12 weeks in Russell's traction. Abundant callus was apparent by x-ray, and weight-bearing with a cane was allowed. An excellent range of motion of the hip was present. Eight months later when the patient complained of severe pain and disability, it

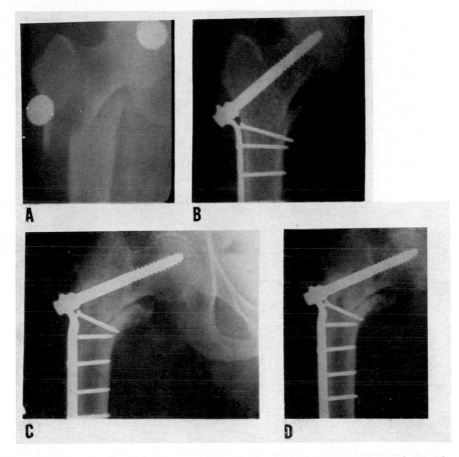

Fig. 6—(A) Prereduction. (B) Postoperative. (C) One month postoperative and (D) Three months postoperative x-rays showing development of coxa vara deformity.

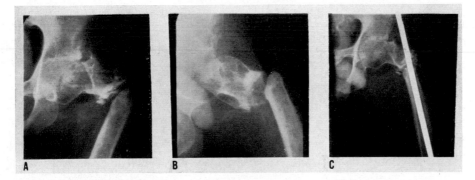

Fig. 7—Final preoperative and postoperative x-rays. (A and B) Preoperative. (C) Final postoperative.

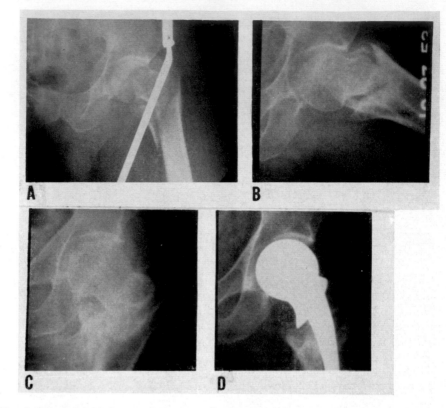

Fig. 8—(A) Original fracture. (B) Lateral view 13 months. (C) A–P view 13 months. (D) Thompson prosthesis inserted.

was recognized that he had nonunion with coxa vara deformity. The patient was operated on and the head and neck of the femur removed and a Thompson prosthesis inserted. The patient did extremely well for five months, walking unaided and having a full range of motion in the hip. However, by 14 months he complained of pain in the hip though x-rays remained essentially unchanged. Obturator neurectomy has afforded some relief from pain.

Although the following case is not a complication of treatment, it is interesting as a problem of treatment. This patient had widespread metastatic lesions from a clear cell carcinoma of the kidney. She had undergone nephrectomy and bilateral adrenalectomy. X-rays revealed a metastatic focus in the subtrochanteric region of the left femur. Despite irradiation over a four month period, the lesion remained unchanged and one day she felt sudden pain on moving in bed. X-rays disclosed a fracture at the site of the lesion. This was treated by internal fixation by means of a Küntscher nail, although a nail and bar might also have been used. The patient was afforded pain-free movement of the extremity. Anticipation of pathologic fracture and early fixation is a sound principle in the treatment of fractures.

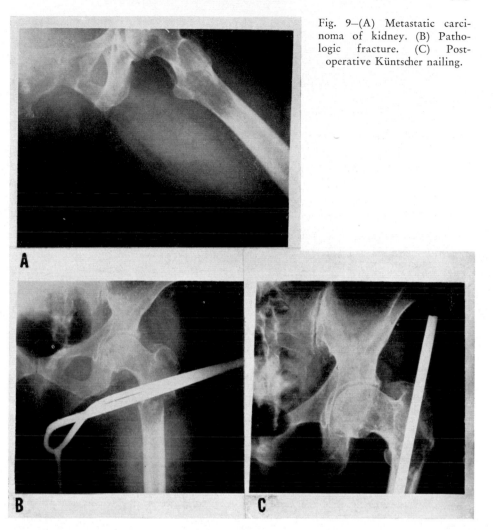

Fig. 9–(A) Metastatic carcinoma of kidney. (B) Pathologic fracture. (C) Postoperative Küntscher nailing.

References

[1] BICKEL, W. A., and JACKSON, A. E.: Intertrochanteric fractures of the femur. Surg. Gynec. & Obst. *91*: 14, 1950.

[2] BÖHLER, L.: The Treatment of Fractures. ed. 4 (English). From Ernest W. Hey Groves: ed. 4 (Rev. German). Baltimore, Wood, 1936.

[3] CLEVELAND, M., BOSWORTH, D. M., and THOMPSON, F. R.: Intertrochanteric fractures of the femur. J. Bone & Joint Surg. *29*: 1049, 1947.

[4] EVANS, E. M.: The treatment of trochanteric fractures of the femur. J. Bone & Joint Surg. *31 B*: 190–203, 1949.

[5] HAMMOND, G., and LADY, J. B.: Medical risks in intertrochanteric fractures. Surg. Clin. N.A. 1371, (Oct.) 1948.

[6] LEVENTHAL, G. S.: Intertrochanteric fractures. Surg. Clin. N.A. 1559, (Dec.) 1953.

[7] NEER, C. S.: The surgical treatment of the fractured hip. Surg. Clin. N.A. 499–512, (April) 1951.

[8] Practitioner's conference: Fractures of the hip. *XII*: Feb. 20, 1956.

[9] WATSON-JONES, R.: Fractures and Joint Injuries. *II*: 4th edition 685. Williams & Wilkins, Baltimore 1955.

CHAPTER 43

FRACTURES OF THE FEMUR

Preston A. Wade, M.D.

The femur is the largest, thickest, longest and strongest bone in the body, and the violence involved in its fracture often causes multiple injuries to the other parts of the body, and usually considerable injury to the soft parts of the thigh involved. A patient with a fracture of the femur must therefore be examined very carefully for concomitant injuries. There is no other fracture in which the emphasis on the patient as a whole is more necessary.

A study of multiple injuries involving the shaft of the femur shows a certain pattern of occurrence which is quite consistent. The most common coincident injuries associated with the fracture of the femur are those involving the knee, hip and spine. Because the pain and obvious deformity and disability of the fractured femur are so predominant, the injuries to the other areas may often be overlooked. The most commonly overlooked coincident injury is that sustained to the hip, in which the hip joint is dislocated or in which there is an intrapelvic dislocation or a subluxation with a fracture of the posterior lip of the acetabulum. If these injuries are not recognized at the time of the accident, their discovery may be delayed for weeks or months, thus preventing the reasonably good return to function which one may expect from prompt treatment. Fractures of the patella and other injuries to the knee involving the ligaments may also be overlooked. It is wise, also, to instruct the young surgeon that not only must the knee, hip and spine be carefully examined at the time of the accident, but that some time during a reasonable period in the first few days after the accident, all of these areas must be x-rayed.

A patient with a fracture of the femur should be considered a good candidate for shock if he is not already in shock at the time of the accident. Several pints of blood may be lost within the confines of the muscles of the thigh, and this may occur hours after the original accident. Preparation for the treatment of shock must be made when the patient is admitted to the hospital, before any effort is made to carry out x-ray examination.

First Aid

The first dictum of the Trauma Committee of the American College of Surgeons has always been, "splint 'em where they lie." In no fracture is this more important than in that of the femur. All of these should be splinted at the site of the injury before the patient is transported. The most efficient and best method of splinting is the traction splint. The Thomas splint (fig. 1), if available, is the most efficient, but care should be taken to see that the binding of the ankle does not interfere with circulation of the foot. If a

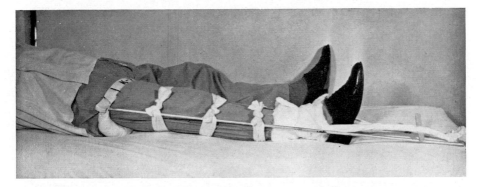

Fig. 1—Conventional Thomas splint for transportation of fracture of femur.

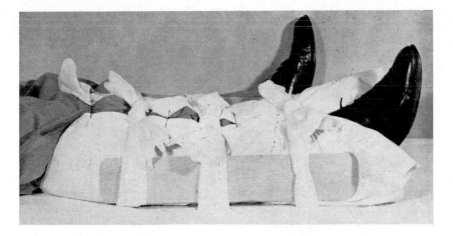

Fig. 2—Pillow board splint for immobilization of fractures about the knee as well as those of lower leg.

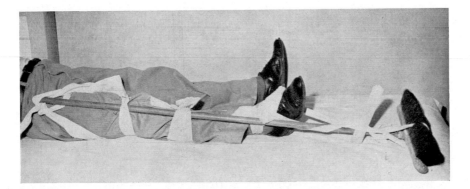

Fig. 3—Makeshift traction splint. Note sling in groin into which broom stick is inserted. Sling tied to ankle and over end of broom can be twisted to exert traction.

Thomas splint is not available (and one must realize that in times of mass casualties they will not be available in sufficient numbers), it is necessary to use a substitute. The simplest method is to use the sound limb as a splint, strapping and binding the affected limb to it. A lateral board splint is a satisfactory means of splinting, and lower third fractures may be well supported by means of a pillow board splint, as is recommended for fractures of the lower leg (fig. 2).

A simple method of using a board one or two feet longer than the injured extremity as a traction splint should be taught to all first aid groups. This makes a most efficient type of splint and is easily applied even by the amateur (fig. 3). This principle involves only a sling in the groin into which the upper end of the board or stick is inserted, and a rope or cloth sling applied to the ankle. This latter sling is attached to the opposite end of the board and traction may be applied by means of a Spanish windlass maneuver, using a stick to twist the rope or sling attached to the foot. The board may then be quickly and easily bound to the injured limb by wrappings of cloth, clothing or other bandaging material.

Open Fractures

As in open fractures in any part of the body, those of the femur are surgical emergencies, but because of the serious injuries that may be associated with the latter, a delay in débridement may be justified. A patient with a brain injury, crush injury to the chest or a severe injury to the abdomen may need treatment of these lesions before the open fracture is treated. Treatment of within-out puncture wounds of the thigh may well be delayed for days if the conditions so demand. There is no other open fracture in the body in which operative procedure in treatment is more difficult. The area must be exposed by means of a proper vertical incision, and the devitalized and obviously dead tissue must be excised and removed along with the foreign material and obvious contamination. However, one must not attempt to excise such wounds *en bloc,* as the integrity of the circulation may be jeopardized. One must use judgment in cleansing all dead and dying tissue and foreign material from the wound, protecting all vital structures. It is essential to be exceedingly conservative in excising skin. Maintenance of skin coverage and preservation of bone are most important in treating open fracture of the femur.

Fractures in Children

Fractures of children have recently assumed much greater importance than in the past, when most fractures were treated by closed methods. The reason for this change in attitude is that nowadays most doctors and even lay people have knowledge of the improved technics in the operative treatment in fractures in adults and expect to apply these principles to fractures in children. Children's fractures, particularly those of the femur, have been overtreated in many instances, and operative procedures which are unnecessary and indeed harmful are sometimes performed. A fracture of the shaft of the femur with the usual 2 or 3 cm. overriding may be expected to result in perfect restoration of function by simple closed reduction and immobilization in plaster, even though perfect reduction of the fractures is not achieved (fig. 4). The simple skin traction methods, such as Bryant's traction for younger children (fig. 5)

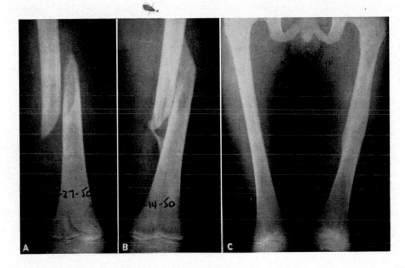

Fig. 4—(A) Oblique fracture of femur in child of 6. Typical "bayonet" displacement. Treated by traction for 6 weeks. (B) Eight weeks postinjury. Note displacement unreduced by traction. Fracture solidly united by abundant callus. (C) Two and one half years postinjury. Legs are equal in length. Growth rate of epiphyses stimulated by fracture and displacement.

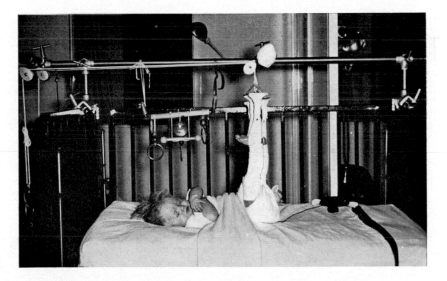

Fig. 5—Bryant's traction for fracture of shaft of femur in infant. Note both lower extremities are suspended in traction. Plaster traction strips extend as high as possible on thigh. Weight sufficient to just lift buttock from bed.

or Russell's traction (fig. 6) for children over 5 may be expected to result in rapid and sound healing with complete return to normal. These methods do not immediately and completely correct the shortening, but they achieve proper alignment and correction of rotation. The temporary shortening

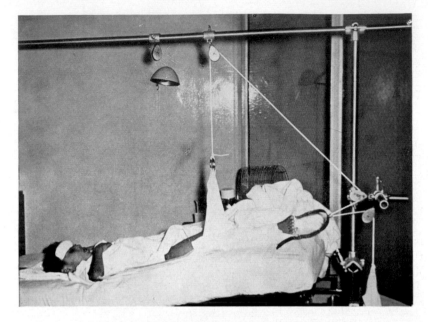

Fig. 6—Russell's traction for older children.

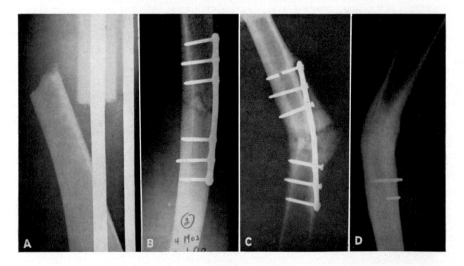

Fig. 7—(A) Fracture of shaft of femur in child of 13. (B) Four months after plate and screws applied. Note fracture line is still apparent. (C) Sixteen months later. Nonunion with breaking of screws and loosening of plates. (D) Prompt union in 3 months after removal of metal.

stimulates epiphyseal growth so that the shortened bone very soon reaches the exact length of the sound limb. On the other hand, if one corrects the overriding by surgical means, nature stimulates an overgrowth of the injured limb to correct the orginal shortening, so that with the added stimulation of

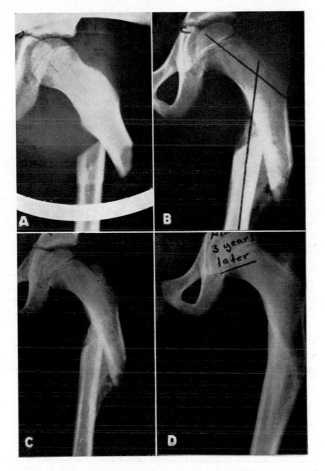

Fig. 8—(A) Fracture of upper third of shaft of femur in child of 6. (B) After seven weeks in traction. No improvement in position of fragments. Solid union with abundant callus. (C) After 12 weeks. (D) After three years. No shortening. Angulation and deformity almost entirely disappeared.

the operative intervention, a further lengthing results in a longer limb on the injured side. It is therefore incorrect to assume that one may safely operate on a fractured femur in a child in order to achieve immediate perfect reduction. It does not follow, however, that if there is no displacement of the fracture, a displacement should be encouraged. Nature is wise in that there is no increase in the rate of growth in the undisplaced fracture, but there is a very definite increase in one which is displaced. It is also a fact that children's fractures do not accept metal well, and nonunion and delayed union may result from the application of plates and screws. The single case of delayed union of a fracture of the shaft of the femur in a child in our records at The New York Hospital is one in which a plate was applied at another hospital (fig. 7). The case came to us 16 months later, ununited, and a union was promptly obtained when the plate was removed.

An example of healing of a fracture of the shaft of the upper third of the femur in a child is shown in figure 8.

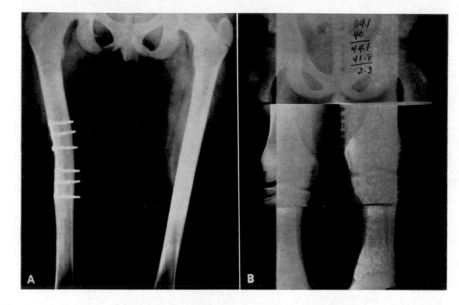

Fig. 9—(A) Fracture of femoral shaft in boy of 7 fixed by plate and screws. (B) Five years later. 2.3 inches lengthening on affected side.

A fracture of the shaft of the femur in a child of seven was operated upon and a plate applied, resulting in lengthening of two and one-half inches on the affected side five years later. The result of an operative procedure is shown in figure 9.

Fractures in Adults
Treatment by Means of Russell Traction and Skeletal Traction

We emphasize the fact that traction is still a very simple, safe, and good method for the treatment of a fracture of the shaft of the femur. Particularly in the young person or in the patient with the shattered femur, it is much wiser to use the well tried and satisfactory treatment of Russell's traction (figs. 10 and 11) or skeletal traction through the tibial tubercle (figs. 12–14). We prefer the threaded Kirschner wire or Steinmann pin inserted through the tibial tubercle rather than through the lower portion of the femur because the nail or wire tracts are more distant from the fracture site and joint

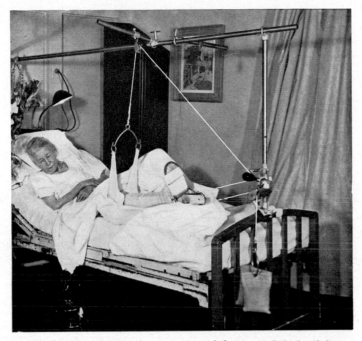

Fig. 10—Russell's traction for comminuted fracture of shaft of femur.

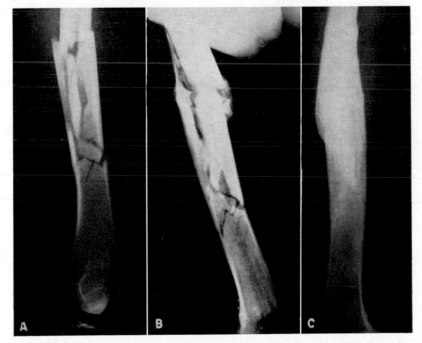

Fig. 11—(A) Comminuted fracture of femoral shaft in male of 28 treated by Russell traction.
(B) After 8 weeks in traction. (C) Follow up one year later.

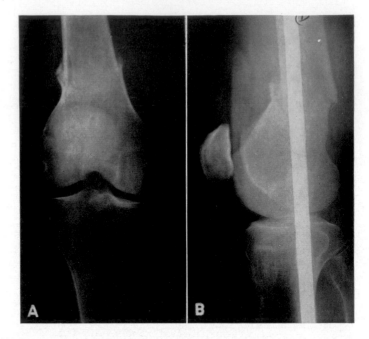

Fig. 12–(A) Fracture of femoral shaft, lower third, treated by skeletal traction with wire through tibial tubercle. (B) Lateral view showing posterior angulation at fracture site.

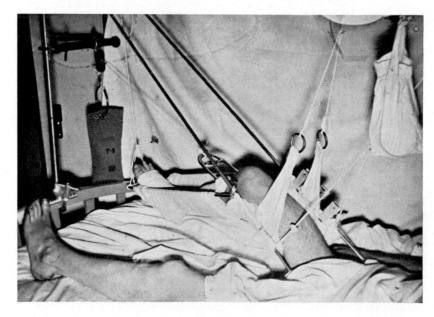

Fig. 13–Photograph of case show in figure 12. Note sling under fracture site to correct posterior angulation.

capsule and do not transfix the muscles on the lateral and medial surfaces of the femur. We do not believe that traction on the tibial tubercle for a period of several weeks causes traction injury to the knee joint because all of the thigh muscles are attached to the tibia. The pull on the tibia causes a traction on the muscles of the thigh not on the knee joint structure. By means of traction, a perfect result should be achieved in almost every young patient. Therefore, no chance should be taken with any operative procedure which might result in a complication.

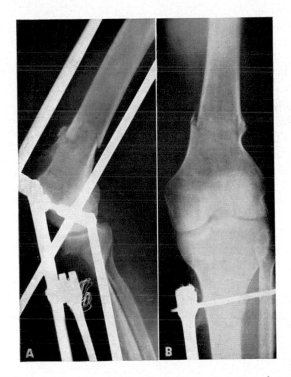

Fig. 14—(A and B) Same case as figures 12 and 13. Note correction of posterior angulation.

In the older patient, however, the long immobilization and confinement to bed may cause complications which we believe are more dangerous than those which might be expected to result from treatment by the means of intramedullary rod.

The duration of the traction will depend on the type of fracture, age of patient and evidence of healing as shown by x-ray. In children, five or six weeks immobilization is all that is necessary and after removal from traction, plaster is necessary for only two or three weeks. The longer immobilization in children's fractures is unnecessary.

In the adult, traction must usually be maintained for twelve weeks. Occasionally, if the x-ray shows rapid healing and clinically the fracture is solid, the immobilization may be removed in eight or ten weeks.

After removal from traction the patient is allowed to move about in bed and within a week or ten days he may be ambulated with crutches. The use of an ischial weight-bearing brace as a routine means of treatment of femoral shaft fractures is to be deplored. The brace is not effective in preventing angulation or refracture, and it is uncomfortable and expensive and delays the progress of muscular rehabilitation in the affected limb.

Intramedullary rods

The treatment of fractures of the shaft of the femur in adults has been revolutionized in the past few years through the use of the intramedullary nail. The older methods of traction or operative procedures, utilizing plates and screws and necessitiating long periods of hospitalization and immobilization in plaster, often resulted in permanent stiffening of knee and ankle, particularly in older patients. Some of the most serious disabilities resulting from a fracture of the shaft of the femur were these resulting joint disabilities. With the intramedullary rod, the patient's stay in the hospital is shortened, there is no immobilization of knee and ankle, rehabilitation is greatly hastened, and the end result is much better than that achieved by the older methods. The most important advantage is in the comfort to the patient of being ambulated early (within a week or two) and of having no immobilization of his joints. The shorter period of hospitalization is also of great importance, particularly in the older patient. The decrease in the cost to the hospital, the patient and the insurance companies may be a secondary advantage, but it is still very important. There are, of course, complications which may result from the use of intramedullary rods, but if the operation is properly done, the incidence of infection and technical complications, as well as fat emboli and pulmonary emboli, is little greater than that which may be associated with other means of treatment.

Fractures of Middle of Shaft

The middle two quarters of the shaft of the femur is that area in which a fracture is best treated by the intramedullary rods (fig. 15). In these cases, fixation is sure, firm and permanent, and the patient may be expected to be ambulated early, and to be allowed early weight-bearing. The insertion of the nail seems to produce an earlier and more abundant production of external callus then other means of treatment (fig. 15 E). Union is quicker and much surer and obvious in the x-ray.

We use the open method of insertion of the nail and believe that it is a much more sensible and realistic approach to the problem than the closed method advocated by Böhler and Küntscher. This latter method is much more difficult technically and involves the use of the fluoroscope, which we believe is exceedingly dangerous to patient and operating staff. We open the fracture site and insert the guide wire into the proximal fragment until it extrudes at the buttock. A cloverleaf nail is then inserted over the guide wire until it appears at the fracture site. The guide wire is then removed, replaced into

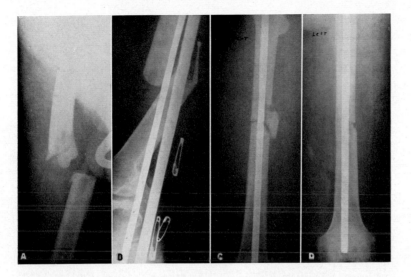

Fig. 15–(A and B) Bilateral femoral shaft fracture in male of 24. (C and D) After internal fixation of both femurs. Right femur (A) operated upon 8 days postinjury. Left femur (B) operated upon 15 days postinjury.

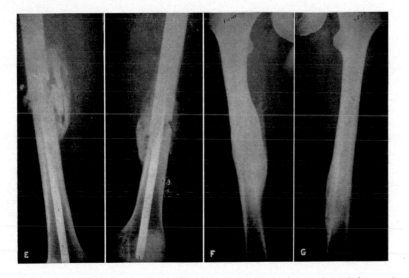

Fig. 15–(E) X-ray showing excessive callus formation 8 (right) and 7 (left) weeks post-operative. (F and G) After removal of nails. Two year follow up.

the nail, then into the distal fragment after reduction of the fracture. The nail is then driven over it until it is seated properly into the intercondylar region of the femur. The guide wire is removed, and the wound is closed. Careful estimate of the length of the nail and the width of the intramedullary canal will usually provide for perfect placement of the nail. The nail should be inserted with the apex of the cloverleaf anterior so that the anterior cortex of the femur is not perforated by sharp edges, a result which might ensue if the nail were placed in the reverse position. We use a 9, 10 or 11 mm. reamer to make sure that the intramedullary canal is prepared for the proper size for the chosen nail. In the older patient, in whom the intramedullary canal is very wide, it may be necessary to use two nested nails to fill the canal with the rods (fig. 16). On occasion in the elderly patient, we have

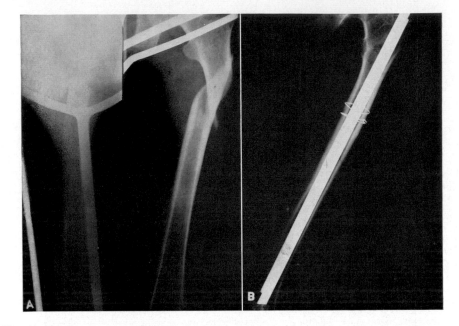

Fig. 16—(A) Fracture of upper third of femoral shaft in patient of 80. Note wide intra-medullary canal. (B) After operative reduction and internal fixation. Two nested Küntscher nails of 12 mm. diameter filled the 16 mm. canal so as to fit snugly.

found it necessary to use some means to prevent rotation of the lower fragment when the fit of the nail was not accurate owing to a very large intramedullarly canal. We find that within two weeks the fragments become set, and rotation thereafter does not occur.

Upper Third Fractures

Fractures of the upper third of the femur are difficult to treat by means of traction because of the displacement of the upper fragment which flexes, abducts and externally rotates. We have used the usual intertrochanteric nail and plate with considerable success in these upper third fractures. There are certain transverse fractures of the upper third which are slow to heal and which may be treated by the intramedullary rod, utilizing the principle of compression. Illustrated in figure 17 is a fracture of the upper third treated by means of Jewett nail. Figure 18 illustrates the use of a long slotted plate only. Figure 16 shows a case in which the intramedullary rod is used. We have been able to use the intramedullary rod within 3 inches of the greater trochanter in spite of the fact that the intramedullary canal expands at its upper end because the nail is firmly fixed in the greater trochanter as it enters the bone. This fixes the upper fragment quite firmly.

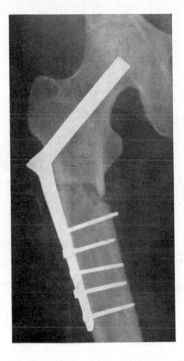

Fig. 17—Fracture of upper third of femoral shaft treated by Jewett nail. This site heals slowly and distraction at fracture site is unfavorable for healing. This case went on to nonunion.

Fractures of the Lower Third of the Femur

Fractures of the lower third of the femur cannot be as easily or as efficiently immobilized by means of intramedullary rods as those above, because the expanding intramedullary canal does not allow for proper fixation of the distal fragment. We have used the method of fixation by the use of the Rush pins on a few occasions in the supracondylar type of fracture, but we have not found it to be as successful as the blade plate or angle plate (fig 19). In the older patient, in whom this fracture most commonly occurs, great care must be taken that the cortex is not damaged by internal fixation. The internal fixation may not be effective because of the relatively thin cortex in these elderly patients. However, if operative intervention of lower third fractures is possible, it is preferable to long immobilization in plaster or traction.

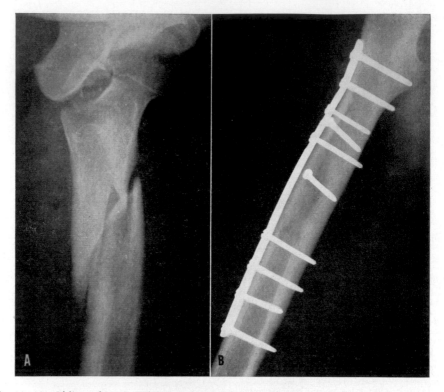

Fig. 18—(A) Oblique fracture of upper third of femoral shaft in female of 24. (B) Operative reduction and immobilization by means of 8 hole vitallium plate and 2 cross fixation screws.

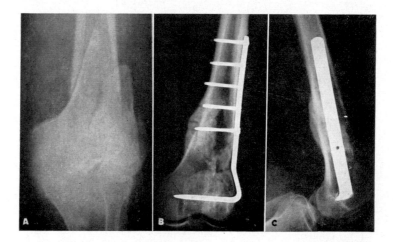

Fig. 19—(A) Supracondylar T-fracture of femur. (B and C) After operative reduction and immobilization by means of Austin Moore plate and screws. One year follow up. Excellent function.

Segmental Fractures

Segmental fractures are much more easily reduced and more firmly fixed by intramedullary fixation than by other means of treatment (fig. 20). Comminuted fractures may also be best handled by rods with the addition of bands or wires.

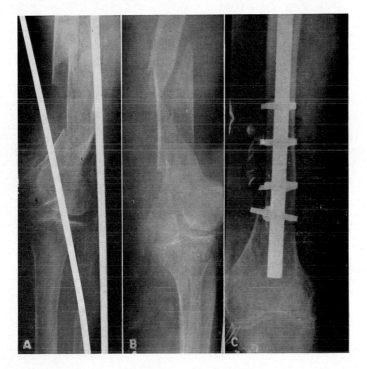

Fig. 20—(A) Segmental fracture in elderly patient. (B and C) Fixation by Küntscher nail and Parham bands.

Pathologic Fractures

A pathologic fracture of the shaft of the femur is an indication for intramedullary fixation. Even though the patient has an incurable disease as the result of carcinoma of the breast, hypernephroma or other malignancy, the intramedullary rod may be expected to give striking relief from pain. The patient may usually be ambulated, whereas otherwise he might be confined to bed for the rest of his life. We do not hesitate to use intramedullary rods in the fixation of pathologic fractures of the femur in almost every case. We have come to the point where we use prophylactic intramedullary nailing in those cases in which a fracture is inevitable. It is most amazing that in some of these cases, the area involved becomes solidified by bone consolidation after intramedullary nailing (fig. 21).

Fear that the tumor may be spread down the intramedullary canal by means of the nail being driven through the involved area has not been

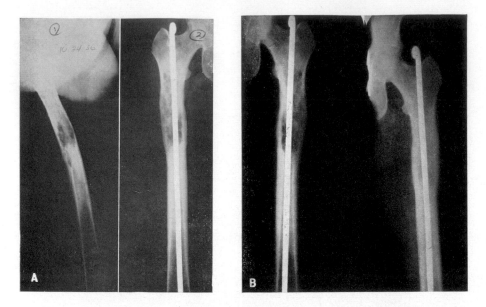

Fig. 21–(A) *Left*. Metastatic lesion in femoral shaft. Carcinoma of breast. Fracture is inevitable. *Right*. After prophylactic nailing by means of Rush nail. (B) *Left*. One month postoperation. *Right*. One year postoperation. Note that lytic lesion has been filled in by new bone. No other treatment.

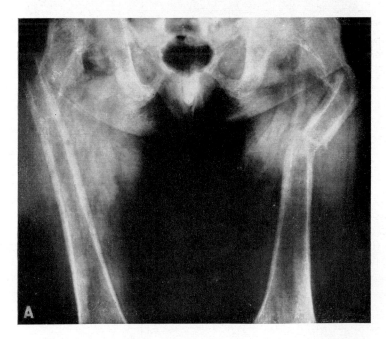

Fig. 22–(A) Multiple fractures of femoral shafts in advanced hyperparathyroidism. Treated in bilateral Russell's traction.

justified in our experience. If it is at all possible, closed nailings should be done in pathologic fractures since opening into the involved area may cause spread of the tumor in the wound, and in some cases, particularly hypernephromata, hemorrhage may be a serious complication.

Pathologic fractures occuring in advanced hyperparathyroidism are difficult to treat because of the marked fragility of the bones. It is necessary to treat these fractures by simple traction (fig. 22), until the parathyroid tumor is removed. Thereafter rapid and sound healing may be expected as the calcium is redeposited in the bone.

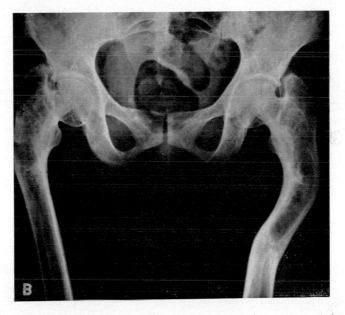

Fig. 22—(B) After removal of parathyroid tumor healing was prompt and femurs became solid one year after operation.

Fractures in the Aged

Fractures in the shaft of the femur in the aged are often seen as the result of a minor trauma, particularly in those individuals with a pre-existing knee or hip disability. The limitation of motion in the knee or ankle causes an unnatural leverage at the supracondylar region and a fracture through the weakened cortex results. These patients are often very difficult to handle because of their complicating pathologic conditions and because of the thin, brittle cortex of their bones. Intramedullary rods may be used with great success in the elderly (fig. 23), but great care must be taken because the nail may be easily driven through the thin cortex of the shaft (fig. 24). Fixation material, such as plates with bolt, and angle plates used for supracondylar fractures, may easily break through the cortex of the femur when applied (fig. 25). The results of the early ambulation and early joint motion in the elderly quite justify the use of early operative procedures.

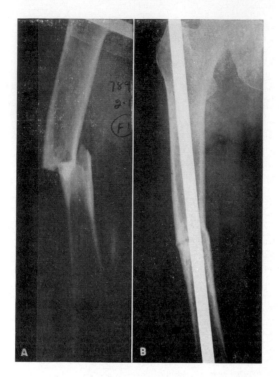

Fig. 23.—(A) Fracture of femoral shaft in male of 85. Note wide intramedullary canal. (B) One month postoperative. Two nested Küntscher nails. Patient was ambulated in four days and weight-bearing in three weeks.

Fig. 24.—(A) During insertion of Küntscher nail into distal fragment of femoral shaft fracture, the nail penetrated the thin anterior cortex of shaft. (B) Nail was withdrawn to fracture site and guide wire inserted distally into lower fragment and x-ray shows position satisfactory. (C) First nail driven over guide wire into position in lower fragment. Guide wire withdrawn and second nested nail driven into lower fragments. Two nails necessary to fill canal and stabilize fracture.

↓

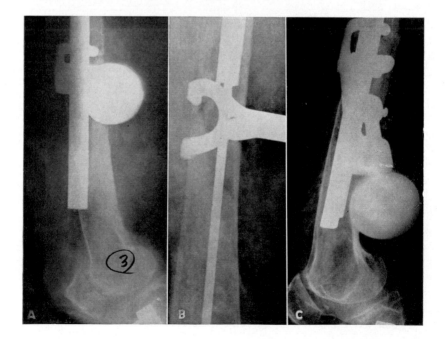

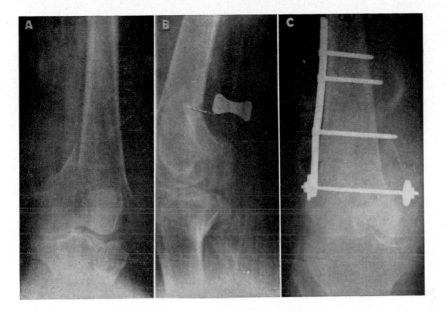

Fig. 25–(A and B) Supracondylar T-fracture in female of 88. Note decalcified bone and very thin cortex. (C) After attempt at internal fixation. Note that bolt and washer have been drawn through the cortex of the condyle.

Summary

1. Fractures of the shaft of the femur are often associated with multiple injuries and with severe soft part injuries of the involved limb.

2. Patients sustaining fractures of the shaft of the femur are often subject to shock, either at the time of the original trauma or in the hours afterwards while being transported or after being admitted to the hospital.

3. Accompanying injuries most likely to be overlooked are those involving dislocation or subluxations of the hip with or without fractures of the posterior lip of the acetabulum and injuries to the knee and to the spine.

4. Fractures in the femur in children should rarely be operated upon and should never be immobilized by means of internal fixation. Shortening up to 2 cm. due to the fracture of the shaft of the femur is usually corrected by increased rate of growth of the injured limb. Operation and internal fixation are apt to result in delayed union or lengthening of the affected leg.

5. Fractures of the shaft of the femur in adults in most instances are best treated by intramedullary rod. Transverse fractures of the middle two quarters of the femur and in many instances comminuted and oblique fractures may well be treated by this method. Fractures of the upper third of the femur within three or four inches of the greater trochanter may best be treated by the intramedullary rod.

6. The rod is indicated in pathologic fractures and may be used as a prophylactic measure to prevent inevitable fractures.

7. Fractures of the lower third of the femur are best treated by internal fixation by means of angle plate or bolt and plate.

8. Fractures of the shafts of femurs in the elderly involve, for the most part, the supracondylar region and are usually associated with limitation of motion due to pre-existing knee or hip disability. Internal fixation in the elderly is a great advantage because of the early ambulation and the freedom of motion of knee and ankle joint.

References

[1] BLOUNT, W. P.: Fractures in Children. Baltimore, Williams and Wilkins Co., 1955.

[2] BÖHLER, L.: The Treatment of Fractures. New York, Grune & Stratton, Inc., 1958.

[3] CHARNLEY, J.: The Closed Treatment of Common Fractures. Baltimore, Williams and Wilkins Co., 1950.

[4] HENRY, A. K.: Extensile Exposure, ed. 2. Baltimore, Williams and Wilkins Co., 1957.

[5] KEY, J. A., and CONWELL, H. E.: The Management of Fractures, Dislocations and Sprains, ed. 6. St. Louis, C. V. Mosby Co., 1956.

[6] KÜNTSCHER, G.: Die Marknagelung von Knochenbrüchen. Arch. klin. Chir. 200: 443, 1940.

[7] McKEEVER, F. M.: Fracture of the shaft of the femur in adults: Evaluation of methods of treatment. J.A.M.A. 128: 1006, 1945.

[8] RUSSELL, R. H.: Fracture of the femur. A clinical study. Brit. J. Surg. 11: 491, 1942.

[9] WATSON-JONES, R.: Fractures and Joint Injuries. Baltimore, Williams and Wilkins Co., 1955.

CHAPTER 44

INJURIES TO THE MENISCI AND THE LIGAMENTS OF THE KNEE JOINT

FREDERICK LEE LIEBOLT, M.D.

Rupture of the medial meniscus is the most common of the serious injuries to the knee joint. The medial meniscus is injured more frequently than the lateral meniscus because, being attached to the tibial collateral ligament, it cannot rotate with the tibia as freely as the lateral meniscus which is unattached to the fibular collateral ligament. The author's statistics reveal tears of the medial meniscus to be six times more common than tears of the lateral meniscus. Other reports vary between 1.7–1 (Smillie [13]), 2.6–1 (Dunn [6]), 3.7–1 (Dickson [5]), 5.1–1 (Bristow [3, 4]) and 37–1 (McMurray [12]).

Tears of the meniscus may be of many types, and not necessarily longitudinal, as is commonly thought. Although longitudinal ruptures are the most common, there may be tears which are transverse, oblique, horizontal, incomplete, tabs, fringes, stretching or tearing of the attachments and combinations of the above. In the author's first 111 consecutive cases, the above types of tears were present in 18 different positions, with longitudinal tears taking precedence over the next most common transverse tears in the ratio of 8.7 to 1.

Injuries to the medial meniscus occur in various ways and many explanations are given to account for them. All agree that the most common cause is the force that is applied when the foot temporarly is fixed at the time the knee is driven inward. Most reports, however, state that the meniscus is trapped and crushed between the condyles. Nevertheless, the author believes that as the femur rotates internally, the femoral attachment of the tibial collateral ligament also is rotated internally and posteriorly, and this fixes and immobilizes the meniscus because the latter is attached to the ligament. Then if the tibia is in external rotation, undue stress in placed on the anterior attachment of the meniscus; if in internal rotation, undue stress is placed on the posterior attachment, and if in neutral position, undue stress is placed on the peripheral attachment. Such forces initiate the injury, but the degree of violence determines the type; a lesser force loosens, stretches or tears the attachments, while a greater force splits the meniscus longitudinally or jerks it in two transversely.

The sensations of weakness, slipping, instability or the actual giving way of the joint, are the most common symptoms of a torn meniscus and are much more usual than locking. These sensations are due to the torn portion of the cartilage moving under the pressure of the femoral condyle on the tibial condyle. Such knees are prone to injury, and each time the knee gives way or locks, pain, swelling and temporary disability occur. Each additional injury produces minimal trauma which is accumulative and which, over a period of years, produces osteoarthritic changes in the joint. Persons with torn menisci do not like to walk over rough terrain or down steps, and are fearful of any motion which produces internal rotation of the knee joint. Finally the patient develops great fear of instability and seeks aid in the form of elastic bandages, braces or surgery.

Thus the history obtained from the patient is of great importance, and from it the proper diagnosis can be made. No other feature of the work-up is as important. Without a proper and detailed record of all past events, an accurate diagnosis is impossible. Frequently, patients are seen during an interval period when there are no positive physical findings and yet, from the history alone, the diagnosis can be established.

In acute injuries of the menisci, the synovial fluid often is mixed with fresh unclotted blood; in chronic recurrent injuries, the fluid is clear yellow and contains no blood. In either case, the joint is swollen. With experience the examiner can differentiate by palpation between bloody effusion and synovial effusion, and confirmatory evidence can be gained through aspiration of the joint. The degree of effusion is determined by using the ballottement sign, which is performed by placing the leg in extension and using one hand to press downward on the suprapatellar pouch to force the fluid into the joint while using the fingers of the other hand to tap the patella to cause it to strike against the femoral condyles. The presence of swelling will not interfere with making the diagnosis of an injured cartilage and will not prevent a thorough examination of the joint for other conditions, such as injury to the condyles, strain of the collateral ligaments, rupture of the cruciate ligaments and x-ray determination of loose bodies and fractures.

The principal positive physical finding is tenderness localized to the joint line. Such tenderness must be differentiated from tenderness of the collateral ligaments, and careful palpation is necessary to determine this; in fact, the areas of tenderness involving the ligament or the meniscus may approximate each other so closely that surgery may depend on the width of one finger; that is, tenderness of the ligament indicates conservative treatment while tenderness of the meniscus one finger's width away indicates operation. The frequency of negative findings in exploratory arthrotomies is due to this point, i.e., the failure to determine accurately before operation the principal and maximal site of tenderness.

Additional information is gained through six signs. Of the five by the author, the first three are for the menisci directly and are based on the fact that the menisci are pressed between the femoral and tibial condyles only upon hyperextension and upon hyperflexion. The last two are to differentiate between injuries of the menisci and the collateral ligaments. The signs are (1) the passive snapping of the knee into hyperextension by the examiner, which produces pain localized to the medial meniscus, or to the lateral joint line for injuries to the lateral meniscus; (2) the passive forcing of the knee into hyperflexion, which produces pain localized to the affected meniscus; (3) the active snapping of the knee into hyperextension by the patient, which produces protective limitation of motion of the affected knee; (4) the forceful abduction and forceful adduction of the knee, which produce pain referred to the opposite collateral ligament and indicates a ligamentous rather than a cartilaginous injury; (5) the sharp internal rotation of the tibia by a quick twist of the ankle, which produces sudden pain localized to the medial joint line as the tibial collateral ligament tugs on the injured meniscus. If the latter sign produces pain at the tibial collateral ligament instead of the medial joint line, a ligamentous injury must be considered. It can be used also in a reversed manner for injuries to the lateral aspect of the knee, but is less specific because the fibular collateral ligament is not attached and does not tug on the lateral meniscus. The examiner should be ready to interpret this sign at the time it is performed because it produces exquisite pain and the patient will not allow it to be repeated; (6) the McMurray [12] sign consists of an auditory or palpable click in the knee joint when the leg is rotated back and forth, with the knee in maximum flexion (heel to thigh) and again in 90 degrees flexion (right angle). According to McMurray, this sign is useful only for injuries from the middle to the posterior attachment of either cartilage, and "is of little value when the lesion is anterior to the midline of the joint."

The above signs are helpful but all are rarely present in one patient, and in many cases of proved torn menisci, none of the signs is positive. They are useful, however, but not to be depended upon entirely for diagnosis.

The term "locking" needs to be defined, since some reports state that locking occurs in practically every case of injury to the meniscus while others state with equal emphasis that locking is rare. The difference rests on the definition of the term. It is true that a 25 degree flexion deformity, with inability to reach complete extension, does exist in all acute injuries of the menisci, but such failure of extension is functional rather than mechanical and is due to pain, spasm and effusion. True locking is a mechanical defect caused by one of the following: the inner portion of a longitudinally torn cartilage shifts to the midline of the condyles or beyond to the intercondyloid fossa; a transversely torn cartilage is caught between the condyles anteriorly; or a loose body is trapped between the condyles. In such instances, as the joint is closed in extension, the offending structure mechanically prevents the rolling together of the condyles, much the same as a stick prevents the rolling together of the hinges of a closing door.

Locking of the joint does not always occur. In fact, there are more torn cartilages which do not lock the knee joint than there are those that do. Although locking may occur at the time of the original injury, generally it becomes much more frequent long afterwards, when the inner fragment becomes more hypermobile and slips back and forth with ease across the tibial condyle. Over a period of time, patients learn to unlock their knee but in a first injury and in displacement of a longitudinal fragment beyond the midline of the joint, it becomes necessary for the physician to employ reduction measures. The methods used vary with different surgeons and

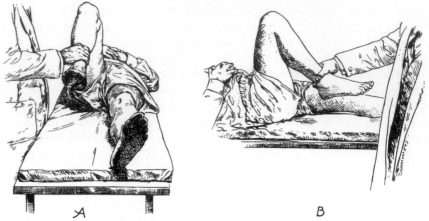

Fig. 1—First maneuver of author's technique for unlocking the knee joint. Note in front view (A) and side view (B) that calf of leg is forced firmly against the thigh.

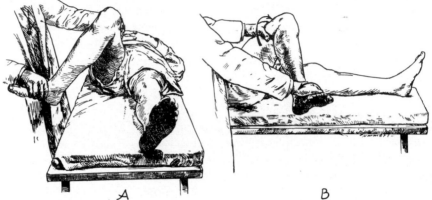

Fig. 2—Second maneuver of author's technique for unlocking the knee joint. Note in front view (A) and side view (B) that the femur is firmly rotated internally and the tibia is firmly rotated externally.

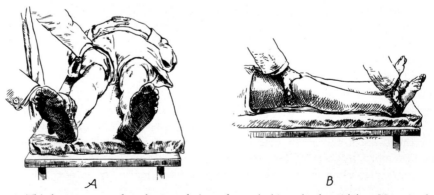

Fig. 3—Third maneuver of author's technique for unlocking the knee joint. Note in front view (A) and side view (B) that the knee slowly is extended while the femur is held in internal rotation and the tibia in external rotation.

consist of manipulation under anesthesia, traction to the leg, shaking and rocking of the joint, abduction and adduction of the tibia and open operation.

The following method devised by the author for unlocking a knee joint has been used sucessfully to date. It is performed without anesthesia. The patient is placed in a supine position and the calf of the leg is forced up against the thigh (fig. 1). Then with the femur held internally rotated and the tibia markedly rotated externally (fig. 2), the knee slowly is extended (fig. 3). Such a manipulation generally causes the inner fragment of the meniscus to slip back into its normal position along the periphery of the joint. Should the manipulation be unsuccessful after two or three attempts, as demonstrated by the Jones[7] sign in which the leg fails to extend 180 degrees, surgery by open operation is indicated, rather than further manipulation under anesthesia.

In 1909 Sir Robert Jones[7] established the current conservative surgical viewpoint when he stated, "I refuse to operate in any case I see early, the subject of a first derangement." In order to follow the previous advice and to give the patient the benefit of the doubt in the hope that the first injury may not be a tear of the meniscus, or if it is that it may heal, as some believe, the patient is treated by aspiration, a roller elastic bandage, ice packs and rest, followed after 48 hours by heat, massage and ambulation. The author does not subscribe to the use of plaster casts because they are cumbersome, incapacitating, produce limitation of motion and have no bearing on the healing of a torn cartilage in that to date no satisfactory evidence has been offered that torn cartilages heal even peripherally at the site of blood supply.

All patients will recover from the first injury whether or not the meniscus is torn. However, when instability, slipping, giving way, locking and recurrent injuries occur, arthrotomy for removal of the medial meniscus is indicated. The procedure should be performed under tourniquet control for visibility and for the prevention of added trauma by constant sponging.

For acute injuries, there is no need at any time to make long incisions or widely to expose the knee joint. Normal anatomic conditions preclude the use of long incisions because the tibial condyles, and medially the infrapatellar branch of the saphenous nerve, prevent the use of an incision below the joint line; the bellies of the vastus medialis and lateralis muscles limit the proximal extent of the incision. McMurray has reported two cases in which long incisions produced dislocations of the patella. Only in other conditions such as knee fusion or synovectomy are large incisions necessary or indicated.

Adequate exposure of the medial meniscus is gained by a well placed, longitudinal, anteromedial incision extending proximally from the joint line for not more than 6–8 cm. Through such an incision the entire joint can be visualized except for the suprapatellar pouch which is best investigated by the palpating finger. This is the only time, however, when it is necessary or proper to place a finger in the joint. Should physical findings or exploration reveal the necessity of approaching the opposite aspect of the joint, a similar incision is made.

It must be remembered that one of the greatest factors in successful knee joint surgery is to prevent surgical trauma or to keep it to a minimum. Bruising of the articular cartilages by knife cuts, instruments, excessive sponging and retractors is unforgivable. The incision, of course, should be adequate, but such additional trauma as incising normal muscle tissue, cutting sensory nerves, dissecting the capsule from its normal attachments, incision into the suprapatellar pouch, sectioning ligaments and displacing the patella for exposure, are all unnecessary and are to be emphatically condemned.

After detailed exploration of the joint the medial meniscus should be detached anteriorly, excised both from the coronary and medially from the tibial collateral ligaments, and removed as far posteriorly as possible through one incision. Forty years ago Sir Robert Jones[7] advocated the removal only of the torn portion of the cartilage, but today this is considered to be an unsound surgical procedure. In three patients operated upon recently by the author, complete relief of symptoms was obtained by removing peripheral portions of normal, unregenerated, menisci left behind by other surgeons. However, this statement should not be interpreted to mean that it is necessary to remove the posterior portion of the meniscus, as advocated by Bosworth[1] and others, because there is adequate evidence that the proper removal of a cartilage anteriorly does not produce additional symptoms. Furthermore, the author is aquainted with one case operated on by another surgeon in which the popliteal artery was injured, requiring amputation of the leg.

Passive motion is started the day after operation and active motion the third day. On the sixth or seventh day after operation, the patient is allowed up wearing a 4 inch roller all-cotton elastic bandage, and is discharged from the hospital without crutches or cane. The sutures are removed the tenth day after operation. The author's postoperative regimen for meniscectomy of the knee joint has been given in detail in another publication.[9] A plaster cast after operation is not necessary and definitely is contraindicated because of the stiffness of the knee which follows. Casts and unnecessary trauma at operation have been the cause of the firm feeling and well taken stand of laymen and many physicians, that operation on the knee joint should not be performed because of the great danger of stiffness and immobility.

Much confusion exists as to the prognosis following removal of the menisci. Physicians, laymen, athletes, compensation courts, athletic directors and army officers frown on the procedure. Almost every person knows of a case that has not turned out well. The general feeling is that once the knee is operated upon, the joint never again will be the same. There is adequate reason for this belief. Improper diagnosis, inadequate surgery, poor operative technic, infection and immobilization, are the causes of poor results.

With the above factors eliminated, however, there still remains the fact that many patients cannot return to full activity. On this question hinges the great difference of opinion. The error is made in grouping together all cases of meniscus injury without separating the pure meniscus injuries from those complicated by other injuries to the knee joint. For example, if a torn anterior cruciate ligament exists in conjunction with a torn meniscus, obviously the removal of the meniscus will not return the joint to normal. It is patently unfair to blame the disability from a torn ligament on the fact that the meniscus is removed or that the knee is operated on. Without any of the above complications, the removal of a torn cartilage results in a normal patient who can return to full activity.

In regard to the ligamentous injuries of the knee joint, the structure most frequently involved is the tibial collateral ligament. Forces applied to the lateral aspect of the knee joint or the abduction of the leg on the thigh produce stretching of the tibial collateral ligament on the medial side.

Contrary to general opinion, rarely is the ligament actually ruptured. In the author's experience, the ligament has been found to be interrupted only in violent injuries and in surgical accidents incurred at the time the medial meniscus is being excised. The frequent reports of rupture are believed to be based on the degree of lateral relaxation, rather than on the actual interruption of the ligament. Such a viewpoint is possible, because there is a wide range of normal lateral relaxation of the knee joint, plus a wide range in the degree of traumatic stretching of the ligament.

The author's sign to determine integrity of the tibial collateral ligament is to flex the knee, place the heel of the same leg on the table on which the patient is sitting and then internally rotate the thigh until the knee reaches the table. In this position the ligament is made taut, and adequate palpation can be performed.

In injuries to the tibial collateral ligament, tenderness and swelling are found to be localized to the ligament. This is the only differential point between injury of the ligament and injury of the medial meniscus. Strain of the ligament most often is interpreted as a tear of the medial meniscus, and is responsible, more than any other reason, for the numerous operations performed for a torn meniscus which reveal that the meniscus is normal. Rupture of the ligament is present when the medial femoral and tibial condyles separate, and only when the joint space definitely separates, should surgical repair be undertaken.

Tear of the fibular collateral ligament is nearly as frequent as tear of the tibial collateral ligament. The injury follows a direct blow or force applied to the medial aspect of the knee joint which, in turn, separates the lateral condyles and stretches the adjacent ligament.

The author's sign for injury to this ligament is to place the heel of the affected leg on the opposite knee in the sitting position and to palpate the matchlike round ligament on the lateral aspect of the joint. The maneuver places the ligament under tension and, if injured, specific tenderness with or without swelling will be localized to the structure. When rupture is present, medial relaxation is increased.

Many methods have been devised for the surgical repair of the collateral ligaments. The surgeon should be familiar with the various technics and apply the method most suitable to the condition encountered. Following surgery a long-leg plaster cast with the knee flexed 10 degrees is applied and worn for eight weeks.

Rupture of the patellar ligament is rare but does occur. It is produced when direct violence, such as a gunshot wound or a blow of the patellar ligament against a relatively sharp surface, interrupts the ligament with or without lacerating the skin. In complete tears the quadriceps muscle contracts and separates the interrupted ends, making surgical repair imperative. Interruptions which are fresh may be repaired by regular sutures or by living sutures made from strips of fascia lata; interruptions which are old may be repaired by a segment of calcaneal tendon placed through the patella and tibia, in an effort to establish a new tendon of sufficient strength to resist the powerful contraction of the quadriceps muscle. A long-leg plaster cast with the knee at 180 degrees extension is used for eight weeks.

In avulsion of the tibial tubercle the patellar ligament holds and the tibial tubercle is jerked away from the bone. The condition results from the stumbling of older persons in whom the tibia is soft and decalcified, and often weakened by Paget's disease. Surgical repair is indicated by screwing or suturing the tibial tubercle into place. A long-leg plaster cast with the knee at 180 degrees is applied for eight weeks.

Tear of the posterior cruciate ligament is extremely rare and occurs only with extreme violence, as when the knee is dislocated. Surgical procedures for replacement of the torn ligament are on record, but the occurrence of the lesion is so rare that the author never has found it necessary to employ them.

The anterior cruciate ligament frequently is stretched or torn by one of the following: a force producing internal rotation of the knee joint, a force producing hyperextension of the knee, a force applied anteriorly to the femur at the same moment a force is applied posteriorly to the tibia, or by dislocation of the knee. The diagnosis is established by the gliding forward of the tibia on the femur.

In some instances the ligament may hold under injury and tear off the area of the tibial spine at the site to which it is attached. In such cases the fragment of bone containing the ligament should be brought down to its bed in the intercondylar fossa of the tibia and should be reattached by a wire suture which is placed about the fragment of bone and then drawn distally through two oblique drill holes in the tibia, at which point the two ends of the wire are tied.

Inasmuch as medial meniscus tears almost always are associated with injuries of the anterior cruciate ligament the torn medial meniscus should be excised, at which time an attempt may be made to suture the interrupted ligament. However, suturing of the ligament is very difficult if not impossible, because it is inaccessible in its deep position in the intercondylar fossa; because rarely can the ends be approximated even in the fresh state; because such tears are not clean cut, frequently being ragged and irregular; because the sutures will pull through the strands of ligament; and because if operation is performed late the interrupted ends will be found to be absorbed, degenerated or absent.

It is not recommended that all absent cruciate ligaments be replaced surgically, or that they be replaced in those with little disability or in those who perform strenuous activity, such as playing football. However, when severe instability is present, a new ligament may be inserted by one of several methods.

References

[1] BOSWORTH, D. M.: Operation for meniscectomy of knee. J. Bone & Joint Surg. *19*: 1113–1116, 1937.

[2] BRANTIGAN, O. C., and VOSHELL, A. F.: The mechanics of the ligaments and menisci of the knee joint. J. Bone & Joint Surg. *23*: 44–66, 1941.

[3] BRISTOW, W. R.: Internal derangement of the knee joint. J. Bone & Joint Surg. *17*: 605–626, 1935.

[4] —: Internal derangement of the knee joint. Am. J. Surg. *43*: 458–465, 1939.

[5] DICKSON, F. D.: Injuries of the knee joint. J.A.M.A. *110*: 122—127, 1938.

[6] DUNN, N.: Observations of some injuries of the knee joint. Lancet *1*: 1267–1274, 1934.

[7] JONES, R.: Notes on derangement of the knee. Ann. Surg. *50*: 969–1001, 1909.

[8] KING, D.: The healing of semilunar cartilages. J. Bone & Joint Surg. *18*: 333–342, 1936.

[9] LIEBOLT, F. L., and STEIN, J. J.: Physical reconditioning of the knee following removal of menisci. Arch. Phys. Med. *27*: 413–416, 1946.

[10] LIEBOLT, F. L.: Tears of the medial meniscus. Surg. Clin. N. A. *30*: 555—562, 1950.

[11] —: Injuries of the medial meniscus. Clin. Orthopedics *3:* 48—55 (May) 1954.

[12] McMURRAY, T. P.: The semilunar cartilages. Brit. J. Surg. *29*: 407—414, 1942.

[13] SMILLIE, I. S.: Injuries of the knee joint. Edinburgh, E. & S. Livingstone, Ltd., 1946.

CHAPTER 45

FRACTURES OF THE KNEE

FREDERICK LEE LIEBOLT, M.D.

Supracondylar and Intercondylar Fractures

Supracondylar and intercondylar fractures of the lower end of the femur (the most common fractures of this bone) are produced by indirect forces such as occasioned by falls from a height when the victim lands on either the foot or the knee joint as well as by torsion injuries and by direct forces such as in automobile and industrial accidents.

In supracondylar fractures the line of interruption may be transverse, oblique or comminuted. The proximal end of the distal fragment is displaced posteriorly by the pull of both heads of the gastrocnemius muscle. The distal fragment is also displaced slightly upward, causing shortening of the extremity. Also, the proximal fragment may be displaced slightly medially due to the pull of the adductor magnus muscle. In intercondylar fractures the line of interruption may be vertical or T-shaped separating the medial and lateral condyles, or either condyle may be fractured. The vertical fracture line commonly extends through the intercondylar fossa but rarely through the articular surfaces. In some cases the distal end of the proximal fragment may be wedged between the condyles.

The clinical findings at the fracture site include swelling, pain and point tenderness localized to the femoral condyles, marked limitation of motion of the knee joint, irregular contour of the thigh due to displacement, shortening of the limb, and extensive and exquisitely tender swelling of the knee joint due to intra-articular hemorrhage. In the more severe injuries, sensation of the leg may be diminished or absent owing to pressure, stretching or tearing of the popliteal and tibial nerves. Also, the leg may be cold and the dorsalis pedis and posterior tibial pulsations may be absent because of impairment of the popliteal artery by pressure from the distal bone fragment, pressure from extensive swelling of the knee joint or rupture of the vessel. Lesser complications may include injury to the cruciate ligaments, the collateral ligaments or the menisci.

The objectives of the treatment are to prevent possible gangrene by immediate aspiration of the swollen knee joint to relieve pressure on the popliteal artery, and by immediate traction to reduce the fragments sufficiently to preserve arterial function; to align and reduce the fragments so as to avoid shortening and to preserve the articular surfaces in order to obtain a stable, movable, painless, weight-bearing joint.

First aid consists of immobilization either with two splints, one extending from the groin to the foot and the other extending from the axilla to the

626

foot or by placing a rolled blanket between the legs from the groin to the feet and strapping both extremities together with cloth strips.

Conservative treatment consists of immobilizing the extremity in a long-leg plaster cast with the knee flexed slightly. With displacement in supra-condylar fractures, reduction may be obtained by manipulation or by traction. Reduction by manipulation is performed under local, general or spinal anesthesia. Traction is applied to the leg as in fractures of the shaft of the femur, and the fragments are molded together by pressure posteroanteriorly beneath the distal fragment, and pressure laterally over the proximal fragment, following which the leg is immobilized in a single plaster spica with the knee flexed. Reduction by traction is accomplished by placing a Kirschner wire through the upper end of the tibia and applying a Thomas splint with a Pearson attachment to flex the knee. Motion should not be instituted until bony union has taken place.

For displaced intercondylar fractures, open reduction is advised. To reduce the separated condyles a fixation bolt is placed transversely through the fragments. A plaster cast is unnecessary, and early motion should be instituted.

The time of immobilization should be eight to twelve weeks except when a fixation bolt is used in intercondylar fractures. In this last instance, crutches may be used but weight-bearing should not be allowed for 8 weeks.

For supracondylar fractures the prognosis is good, provided there is accurate reduction and proper immobilization, but for intercondylar fractures the prognosis is only fair because the fracture enters the joint.

Medial and Lateral Condyle Fractures

Fractures of the medial and lateral condyles of the femur are fairly common. They are caused by indirect forces such as those exerted when the patient falls from a height and lands on the feet, when torsion is applied to the leg by direct forces such as a blow either to the lateral or medial aspect of the distal end of the femur, or by a crushing injury in which the knee is caught between two objects.

The fracture line may be vertical or oblique and comminution may occur. Displacement is not common because of the ligamentous attachments about the condyles of the femur. When present, however, the displacement is downward in fractures of the lateral portion, forward into the knee joint in fractures of the posterior portion, and downward when either the medial or the lateral ligament has avulsed the bone. Joint hemorrhage occurs but varies in degree.

Clinical findings include the distention of the knee joint with fluid and blood, false motion, tenderness localized to the fracture and limited motion of the knee with or without locking of the joint.

In treatment, the objective is to obtain accurate anatomic replacement of the fragment in an attempt to prevent limitation of motion, pain, instability and arthritis. For first aid the thigh and leg are immobilized with two splints extending from the hip to the foot and held together with cloth strips. Under conservative treatment the knee should be aspirated for the removal of fresh blood. When displacement is not present, the knee joint is immobilized for eight weeks in a plaster cast extending from the groin to the toes. In cases of minimal displacement the fragment can be manipulated into good position by digital pressure, by a carpenter's clamp or by abduction or adduction of the knee, following which a long-leg plaster cast is applied for eight weeks. With greater displacement, open reduction is performed by the use of screws through the fragment, or by a bolt through the femoral condyles. A plaster cast is not necessary when a bolt is used and may not be necessary when screws are used.

The complications of such fractures are limitation of motion of the knee joint from improper reduction, stiffening of the knee joint following plaster immobilization, infection of the knee joint after internal fixation and lateral relaxation of the knee joint.

The time of immobilization should be eight weeks. When only crutches are used, weight-bearing should be avoided for eight weeks, but complete healing does not occur for twelve weeks. The prognosis is good except when the fracture line extends across the articular surface.

Epiphyseal Separation

Epiphyseal separation of the lower end of the femur results indirectly from extreme hyperextension or torsion applied to the knee joint, and directly from a blow to the distal one-third of the femur while the foot is fixed. The injury is rare except in children whose knee joints are fused. It occurs mostly among boys, especially between the ages of 8 to 14 years.

Pathologically, the separation may be either incomplete or complete, depending on the traumatic force applied to the area. The displacement usually is forward and upward, although in some cases of direct violence the epiphysis may be displaced laterally or posteriorly. In the latter instance, the popliteal vessels may be compressed, stretched, or torn.

Clinical signs include marked swelling above the knee joint, obvious deformity of the leg and shortening of the affected leg. Palpation may reveal the diaphysis to be in the popliteal space.

The objective of treatment is to obtain accurate reduction to prevent growth disturbance. In first aid, the leg should be immobilized as indicated in the first aid treatment for supracondylar fractures of the femur. Without displacement, conservative treatment consists of immobilizing the extremity for six weeks by a long-leg plaster of Paris walking cast. With displacement, the incomplete anterior dislocations may be reduced by gentle traction, with the knee flexed 45 degrees, followed by slight anteroposterior pressure applied to the epiphysis. The leg is immobilized as mentioned above. The complete anterior dislocations are reduced by strong traction with the knee flexed 45 degrees and by firm anteroposterior pressure to the epiphysis, following which the leg is flexed to 90 degrees to gain anatomic position. A long-leg cast is applied as above. The complete posterior dislocations are reduced by strong traction with the knee flexed 45 degrees, while at the same time the epiphysis is pulled forward and the knee extended. The leg is immobilized as stated above. Surgical treatment rarely is necessary.

The time of immobilization is six weeks and healing requires eight weeks. The only complication is that occasionally there may be a slight deformity of the knee joint due to an irregularity in growth at the epiphyseal line. With anatomic reduction the prognosis is excellent.

Patella Fractures

Fractures of the patella occur through the indirect forces caused by a sudden strain from jumping or falling from a height or from lifting with the knee semiflexed; and through a direct force, such as that which occurs in an auto accident in which the knee of the occupant is brought violently against the instrument panel — the so-called "dash-board" fracture. The injury is rather frequent in adults, but rare in children and adolescents.

In cases due to indirect violence, the patella is usually fractured transversely in the lower one-half, with or without a small amount of comminution. There may be no separation of the fragments and only slight tearing of the quadriceps expansion; usually, however, the bone fragments are pulled apart, with tearing of the anterior capsule and lateral expansion of the quadriceps tendon. The upper fragment tends to be drawn proximally by the quadriceps muscle and the lower fragment remains *in situ* due to its close anchorage to the tibia by the patellar ligament, although occasionally it may be found to be tilted forward. When the fragments are widely separated, the tear of the capsule may extend to the region of the collateral ligaments.

When the injury is the result of direct violence, there is relatively little separation of the fragments and no tearing of the capsule unless force has been applied to the leg after the patella has been fractured. The lines of the fracture may run in any direction, but are rarely longitudinal. Fractures by direct violence are apt to be compound.

The clinical findings reveal the knee to be markedly swollen and the joint to be distended with fluid, usually blood. False motion of the patella can be demonstrated by moving the fragments independently. If the fracture is incomplete, active extension of the leg will produce great pain and if the fracture is complete, active extension of the leg is lost.

The x-ray examination should include anteroposterior, lateral and supero-inferior views of the patella.

The objective of treatment is to obtain perfect anatomic alignment and union of the fragments in order to regain full function of the quadriceps muscle and full motion of the knee joint and to re-establish the smooth gliding articular surface of the patella. First aid immobilization is by a posterior splint extending from the midthigh to the heel. Conservative treatment involves aspiration, when necessary, to relieve extreme distention and pain. When there is no displacement of the fragments, the extremity is immobilized by a long-leg plaster cast, extending from the groin to the toes, with the knee in complete extension. Surgical treatment should be open reduction when there is a definite separation of the fragments. The methods of operative treatment are four: Kirschner wires drilled percutaneously through the fragments in crucial fashion, suturing of the fragments and the quadriceps expansion, with the admonition that firm suturing of the quadriceps expansion is a more important than suturing of the fragments; partial excision of the patella with suturing of the quadriceps tendon to the remaining fragment and complete excision of the patella in severely comminuted fractures. The disadvantages of patellectomy are the removal of the normal protection of the femoral condyles, the elimination of the normal pulley action of the patella during active extension of the knee, and the loss of the last 10 degrees active extension of the knee joint.

When the fracture is open, infection of the knee joint may occur. Late complications of patellar fractures include nonunion due to incomplete approximation of the fragments or to active motion too early, refracture a few months after the original fracture, especially when flexion has remained limited and malunion producing an irregular articular surface, resulting later in osteoarthritic changes.

With conservative and open reduction methods, immobilization should be for eight to ten weeks, with complete healing requiring twelve weeks. With removal of either the fragments or the entire patella, immobilization and healing require only six weeks. The prognosis in most cases is excellent, but there may be slight limitation of motion at extreme flexion of the knee joint.

Tibial Condyle Fractures

Fractures of the tibial condyles result indirectly from falls from heights and from twisting injuries, and directly from a violent blow above or below the knee joint, or from the front or from the side with the leg extended. Inasmuch as most blows are received from the lateral side of the knee, the lateral tibial condyle is injured more frequently than the medial condyle. The injury is fairly frequent in adults but quite rare in children.

There are five types of fractures of either condyle (The head of the fibula may also be fractured with the lateral condyle except in type 5.):

Type 1. — Fragment displaced outward.
Type 2. — Depression of the condyle.
Type 3. — Oblique fracture and depression of the weight-bearing surface with only a
    small portion of the condyle retaining a normal level.
Type 4. — Fracture and depression of the posterior portion of the condyle.
Type 5. — Fracture and depression of the anterior portion of the condyle.

There are three variations in fractures of the head of the tibia: the inverted T-shaped fractures, the inverted V-shaped fractures and the inverted Y-shaped fractures. The fragments usually are displaced distally and either laterally or medially, depending on which condyle is injured. It must be remembered that the menisci may be torn or detached, and that the fractures produce marked hemarthrosis.

The clinical findings are marked distention of the knee joint due to hemorrhage, painful passive lateral motion, limited extension and flexion of the knee joint, tenderness at the site of the injury, and sensitivity of the entire anterior portion of the condyle to pressure and palpation.

The x-ray examination requires anteroposterior, lateral and oblique views to establish the diagnosis. Often the comminution is much more extensive than the films indicate.

Complications to be considered are hemorrhage sufficiently severe to obliterate the popliteal artery and embarrass or occlude the circulation to the leg. Fractured fragments also may be displaced sufficiently to obliterate the popliteal artery. In addition examination should be made for involvement of the peroneal and tibial nerves, but generally these latter are not involved.

The immediate objective of treatment is to preserve the circulation of the lower extremity and, later, to obtain a stable and functioning knee joint. For first aid the leg should be immobilized by applying boards from above the knee to beyond the ankle joint, or by tying the two extremities together.

The earliest treatment should be aspiration. This is essential in all condyle fractures because bloody effusion is marked and is a constant finding. When minimal or no displacement is present, immobilization is accomplished with a plaster cast extending from the upper thigh to the toes, with the knee in slight flexion. When there is distinct displacement of the lateral condyle, the leg is adducted on the femur under general anesthesia, and with the use of a carpenter's clamp or Bochler's vise, the condyles of the tibia are compressed strongly and the clamp is removed. A plaster cast is applied carefully from the upper thigh to the toes with the knee in slight flexion. Should the x-ray show good reduction, the cast is left on for eight weeks. After the cast is removed, the patient should not bear weight on the leg for at least one month. When the medial condyle is displaced, the leg is abducted on the femur and the same treatment is rendered as for fracture of the lateral condyle. Surgical treatment varies. The removal of the meniscus is indicated when it is torn, loose or detached. A bone bolt may also be placed transversely after the fragments are elevated into anatomic position. No cast is applied, and early motion is instituted. When a fragment is large enough, it may be elevated into anatomic position and fixed by a pin, placed transversely, which is incorporated into the plaster cast for rigid fixation. Lastly, a Kirschner wire may be placed to lever the fragments into anatomic position.

With or without a plaster cast, weight-bearing on the injured leg should be prohibited for eight weeks. Healing requires twelve weeks. As a rule the prognosis is poor. The collateral ligaments are stretched, and this, plus fragment inability to realign and to elevate completely the depressed condyle, produce permanent instability of the knee. With time, traumatic arthritis develops. Motion invariably is limited regardless of the form of treatment. In compound fractures, infection may add to the destruction of the knee.

Tibial Spine Fractures

Fractures of the spines of the tibia result from an indirect force through simultaneous blows to the anterior aspect of the lower thigh and to the posterior aspect of the upper tibia with forcible rotation. Fractures of the tibial spines due to direct force do not occur.

Pathologically, the anterior tibial spine is displaced posteriorly due to the pull of the anterior cruciate ligament. However, in cases where the anterior cruciate ligament itself is torn, the spine then may be displaced in any direction depending on the force causing the fracture. The posterior tibial spine rarely is fractured, and the posterior cruciate ligament rarely is torn.

The clinical findings include swelling of the knee as a result of bloody effusion, marked limitation of motion; and abnormal anteroposterior mobility.

The objective of treatment is to obtain an accurate reduction of the tibial spine in order to gain a stable knee joint. For first aid the knee is immobilized by use of wooden splints applied to both sides of the leg. The conservative treatment for incomplete and undisplaced fractures is to immobilize the knee in extension by a long-leg plaster cast for six weeks. When displacement is present, open reduction is performed through a longitudinal incision on the medial aspect of the knee, which is extended downward and curved outward to the crest of the tibia. Two holes are drilled obliquely upward through the tibia to the base of the tibial spine. A thin, stainless steel wire is inserted into one hole, identified within the knee joint through the medial incision, passed through the cruciate ligament above the fractured fragment and directed back down the outer hole in the tibia; the two ends are then twisted together, thus pulling the fragment into place. The leg is immobilized by a plaster cast extending from the groin to the toes. When union is complete, within six to eight weeks, the wire may be removed through a small incision under local anesthesia by cutting one end and pulling on the other. When satisfactory reduction is not accomplished and motion is blocked at the anterior portion of the knee joint, the fragment should be removed and the cruciate ligament reattached; the latter, however, is difficult and rarely successful.

Immobilization should be for six to eight weeks. Healing requires eight weeks. When properly reduced the tibial spine heals with a good result. Should union fail to occur, anterior relaxation of the knee joint and permanent deformity of a moderate degree follow. Oftentimes there is added damage to the articular cartilage which may leave a degree of residual disability.

Tibial Tuberosity Fractures

Fracture of the tibial tuberosity may be caused indirectly by a violent contraction of the quadriceps extensor muscle, such as seen in jumping from a height and landing on the ground with the knees slightly flexed. These fractures may also be caused directly by a blow to the region of the tuberosity of the tibia. The injury is rare.

The signs, symptoms and disability are the same as those of a ruptured patellar ligament: acute pain, localized swelling and inability to extend the knee. The avulsion occurs often in association with Paget's disease.

The condition must be differentiated from Osgood-Schlatter's disease, an osteochrondritis of childhood which is thought to be due to avulsion of the tibial tuberosity but which actually is due to growth factors affecting the tibial tuberosity. In this condition, there is a limp but no actual inability to extend the leg; the tuberosity is intact and not torn away from the tibia; calcifications and ossifications are present both posterior to and within the patellar ligament. These factors serve to differentiate an osteochondritis of the tibial tuberosity from an acute, avulsed fracture of the tuberosity.

The clinical findings are swelling and tenderness localized to the tibial tuberosity. In complete avulsions the patella is found more proximal than normally and the extension of the knee is lost, while in incomplete avulsions there is pain on extension and flexion of the knee joint. The objective of treatment is to gain good apposition and union in order to restore the function of the quadriceps muscle. For first aid, the leg is immobilized by two splints (one on either side) extending from the upper thigh to the ankle. An additional method is to strap the two extremities together. In incomplete fractures without displacement, immobilization of the knee joint by a long-leg plaster cast is sufficient to effect a cure. In incomplete fractures with displacement, surgery is necessary either to pull down the fragment in conjunction with the patellar ligament and to anchor it to the original site by a metal screw, or to remove the bone fragment and reattach the patellar ligament to the tibia by chromic catgut sutures. Plaster cast immobilization should be used for six weeks. There are no complications. Healing requires eight weeks. The prognosis is excellent.

Fibula Fractures

Fractures of the upper end of the fibula occur indirectly as a result of torsion, often in association with fractures of the tibial condyles and the lower tibia, and rarely alone. Seldom is direct violence the cause. The fracture line may be either oblique or transverse, with minimal displacement.

The symptoms and signs of a fibular fracture are: swelling and tenderness over the affected area, pain produced by rotation of the foot with the knee fixed in flexion and by flexion of the knee against resistance. Anteroposterior and lateral x-ray views are sufficient for diagnosis but because such fractures frequently are associated with fractures of the lower tibia, full-length views of the leg should be obtained.

With or without displacement, conservative treatment is to immobilize the leg in a walking plaster cast extending from the midthigh to the base of the toes. The cast should fit snugly around the knee joint and be worn for four weeks, after which time the patient may walk on the leg. In the rare instances in which the proximal fragment is displaced upward and backward due to the contraction of the biceps femoris muscle, the fragment is reduced by direct digital pressure and the leg is immobilized in flexion to maintain the loose fragment in good position. Walking, except with crutches, is not permissible for six weeks. Open reduction is necessary only when the displacement is great or is producing peroneal nerve symptoms.

The complications of the fracture may be an injury to the peroneal nerve in the portion that curves around the neck of the fibula. Treatment depends on the condition of the nerve. When the nerve is contused or crushed, the foot should be supported in a position of dorsiflexion to place at rest the peroneal, anterior tibial and long toe extensor muscles. Should the nerve be interrupted, neurorrhaphy is necessary. Later the nerve may become involved by scar tissue or callus formation, producing a gradual onset of paralysis some weeks after the accident. Treatment for this is neurolysis.

Immobilization is for four weeks in nondisplaced and for six weeks in displaced fractures. Healing requires eight weeks in both types. The prognosis is excellent if there is no injury to the peroneal nerve.

Reference

[1] LIEBOLT, F. L.: Illustrated Review of Fracture Treatment. Los Altos, California, Lange Medical Publications, 1954.

CHAPTER 46

TREATMENT OF TIBIAL SHAFT FRACTURES

Rolla D. Campbell, Jr., M.D.

Introduction

Fractures of the tibial shaft, with or without fractures of the fibula, are common injuries sustained at all ages and seem particularly frequent in the young adult, who is apt to suffer leg trauma in athletics or heavy work as well as from the fast-moving automobile. Because the tibia is a subcutaneous bone, its fracture is often complicated by an open wound, which adds to the difficulties of treatment. Furthermore, the tibia is one of the few bones in the human skeleton in which delayed or nonunion frequently may occur, particularly at the junction of the lower and middle thirds, where its blood supply is often less than adequate for bone healing even without loss of soft tissue covering.

Because of the frequency with which fractures of the tibia are seen by trauma surgeons, and because of the relatively high potential for complications peculiar to this bone when injured, specific considerations must be outlined and discussed in this section.

Organization of Immediate Care for the Patient

The patient's general condition determines the immediate treatment of fractures of the leg, which would receive attention secondarily to acute emergencies involving the central nervous and cardiorespiratory systems.

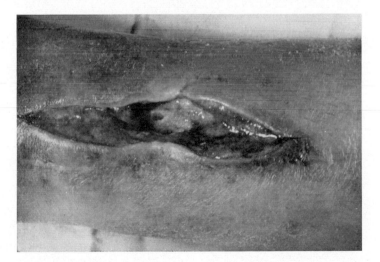

Fig. 1—Late results to tight wound closure.

As soon as permissible, however, the tibia should be splinted by Thomas splint-sling traction, or by long leg posterior plaster or lateral plaster with the knee in flexion of at least 30 degrees. An exception is a fracture of the junction of the upper and middle thirds or of the upper third of the shaft, in which the architecture of the obliquity presents the proximal fragment anteriorly. Too much flexion of the knee in these cases would cause anterior displacement of the proximal fragment due to pull of the patellar tendon.

Immediate arterial repair is mandatory; nerve repair can be postponed. Wound débridement should be carried out on an emergency basis with major emphasis on obtaining relaxed primary closure by relaxing incisions and sliding flaps as needed (fig. 1). If bone coverage cannot be gained primarily without tension, split thickness skin grafting is usually well received in the fourth to seventh day after injury. Soft tissue coverage of bone is of prime

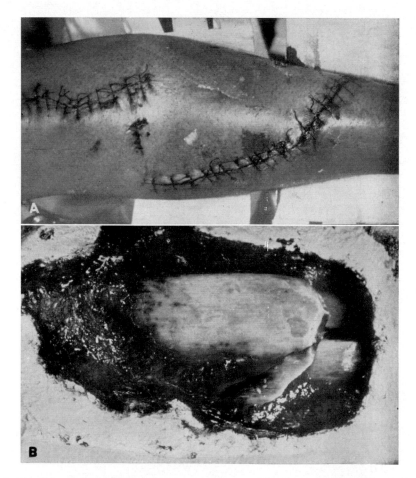

Fig. 2–(A) After initial closure of an open fracture. This leg is in os calcis traction on a Böhler frame. (B) Three weeks later; wound breakdown occurred from motion of unstable fragments. Note the exposed bone.

importance, and all attention must be directed to this initially; leaving bone exposed invites infection and seriously curtails bone repair.

Traction

If the fracture is unstable and exposure of the badly traumatized soft tissue is necessary, os calcis traction with the patient on a Boehler frame or in a flexed Thomas splint suspension will not delay union, according to Boehler, [2] if the traction does not exceed 6 or 7 pounds. Plaster splints may be applied to aid in immobilization. If the knee is flexed, the plaster splints should not go above the knee for the traction to be effective. There should be frequent x-ray examination, and wedging may be needed to improve the position of the fragments even if the patient is in traction. Usually traction may be discontinued at three or four weeks, but sometimes it takes longer for the fracture site to become "sticky" so that casting may be done without loss of reduction. It is very important that distraction be avoided.

All too often, however, unstable open fractures, even in traction in a plaster shell on a Boehler frame, will not be sufficiently immobilized to permit wound healing, and even closed unstable fractures may cause skin necrosis from within outward (fig. 2 A and B). This problem may be especially noted if the fracture consists of long, sharp fragments in the middle

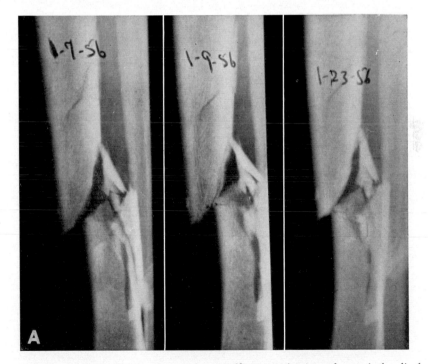

Fig. 3–(A) Views of leg in traction without sufficient reduction of anteriorly displaced upper fragment until after it had eroded through the skin from within outward. (Courtesy Am. J. Surg. April 1958, Wade and Campbell.)

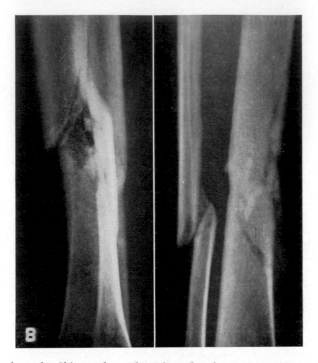

Fig. 3—(B) Final result. Skin grafts and prolonged soft tissue care eventually made up initial losses due to inadequate early control of fragments. (Courtesy Am. J. Surg., April 1958, Wade and Campbell.)

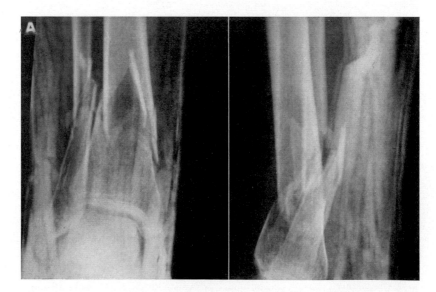

Fig. 4—(A) Inadequate reduction by cast methods alone of comminuted fractures of the lower third of the tibia and fibula. (Courtesy Am. J. Surg., April 1958, Wade and Campbell.)

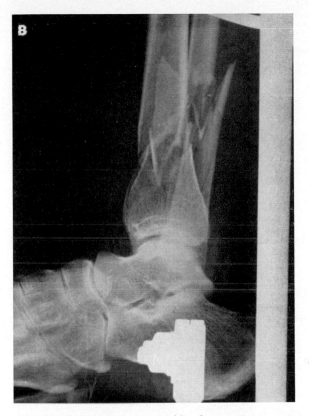

Fig. 4–(B) Good alignment by traction on a Boehler frame. (Courtesy Am. J. Surg., April 1958, Wade and Campbell.)

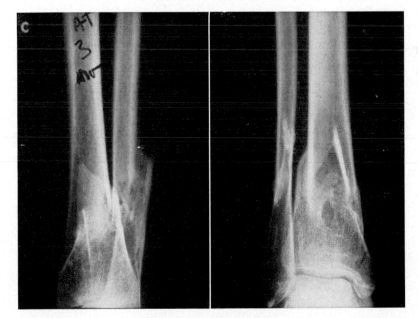

Fig. 4–(C) Result at three months, when leg was clinically solid. (Courtesy Am. J. Surg., April 1958, Wade and Campbell.)

third of the tibia (fig. 3 A and B). Much can be said, therefore, in defense of primary internal fixation or transfixation of such fractures. However, the more comminuted fractures and those lower in the tibia are more easily controlled by os calcis traction (fig. 4 A–C).

Principles of the Long Leg Cast

Cast treatment for the fractured tibial shaft should extend from the toes to a point just below the groin. A short leg cast is never indicated except when the patient is in traction on a Boehler frame. If the cast does not cause the patient to complain that it is too high, it is usually too short. If the cast does not extend almost to the groin, the soft tissues of the thigh allow the femur to move the knee too easily and so disturb the upper fragment of the tibia.

The knee should be flexed at least to 30 degrees to relax the cruciates and medial and lateral ligaments and thus to minimize rotary motion of the proximal tibia by the femur. Later when weight-bearing is permitted in the cast on a fracture already secured by early callus, the knee may be straightened.

Because of the shape of the upper articular surface of the talus, which is broader in front than behind, the ankle should be dorsiflexed to 95 degrees, if possible, both to prevent equinus stiffness later and to give firmer lateral stability to the lower tibia. However, recurvatum of a low shaft fracture may result from this maneuver, so that temporary relative equinus at the ankle may be necessary for fractures in the lower third of the shaft.

The cast should be snug, preferably skin tight over stockinette, with thin felt padding over the malleoli and dorsal foot prominence. When a walking heel is applied, it should be in the anterior line of the tibia and built up behind to be parallel with the floor rather than with the bottom of the cast, and sharp edges of the heel should be trimmed off to prevent tripping. Putting the heel on with its backside forward helps in this regard. The opposite shoe may be built up proportionately to help the patient clear the casted foot in walking.

Windowing a snug cast often results in soft tissue ballooning into edema at the opening unless the extremity is kept elevated, and this may occur even with elevation. If skin exposure is necessary, bivalving and the use of very guarded half-shell or three-quarter posterior shell splinting is preferable.

Open VS. Closed Methods of Treatment

Open VS. Closed Fractures

Since reports of large series of closed and open fractures uniformly show that regardless of the method of treatment employed, closed fractures heal faster than open fractures treated similarly, [15, 19] one can argue that to open the fracture risks some prolongation of bone-healing time. Seldom does one find a problem of nonunion of the normal tibial shaft in a closed fracture which has received careful conservative (closed) treatment. An exception to this occurs in the problem of very unstable fractures which might cause skin breakdown if not fixed internally or transfixed.

Internal Fixation in Open Fractures

Certainly, a minimum of contamination, soft tissue damage and time after injury may combine occasionally to permit primary internal fixation of open fractures of the tibia if the fracture is so unstable that soft tissue damage without internal fixation cannot be prevented (fig. 5 A–C). With antibiotics

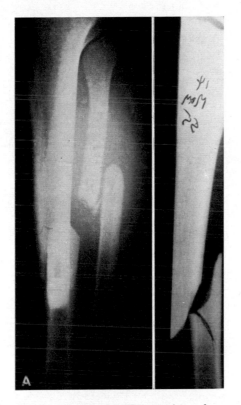

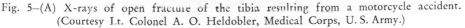

Fig. 5–(A) X-rays of open fracture of the tibia resulting from a motorcycle accident. (Courtesy Lt. Colonel A. O. Heldobler, Medical Corps, U. S. Army.)

and thorough surgical cleansing, the "golden period" of primary internal fixation may only rarely extend to eight or ten hours. In unstable fractures which have not responded satisfactorily to traction and/or cast methods of treatment, the alternative is delayed primary internal fixation after the wounds of compounding have healed.

Benefits of Internal Fixation

What are the arguments for open reduction and internal fixation for the tibia? Of course, the reasons vary somewhat with the architectural type of fracture, but in general they include the purported gains of (1) better reduction of the fragments, (2) more secure fixation (both factors supposedly en-

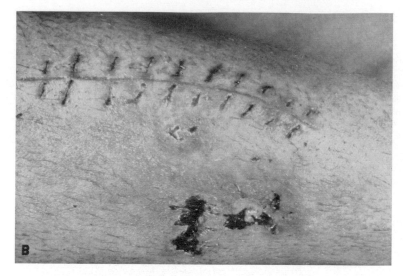

Fig. 5—(B) Incision for internal fixation was based laterally in healthy tissue; a minimum of surgical trauma was added to the wounds of compounding, which were débrided and loosely closed. (Courtesy Lt. A. O. Heldobler, Medical Corps, U. S. Army.)

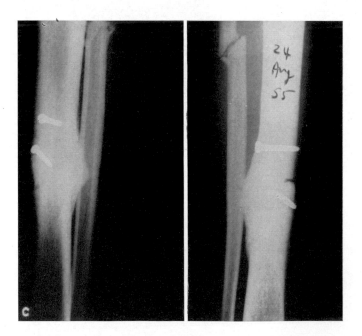

Fig. 5—(C) Bone healing at three months after internal fixation by two screws. (Courtesy Lt. Colonel A. O. Heldobler, Medical Corps, U. S. Army.)

couraging faster bone union) and (3) less need for lengthy cast immobilization which might cause joint stiffness and osteoporosis.

Segmental and Large Butterfly Fragments

If these fractures are unstable or displaced, and cannot be reduced and held securely by closed methods with or without the use of traction, open

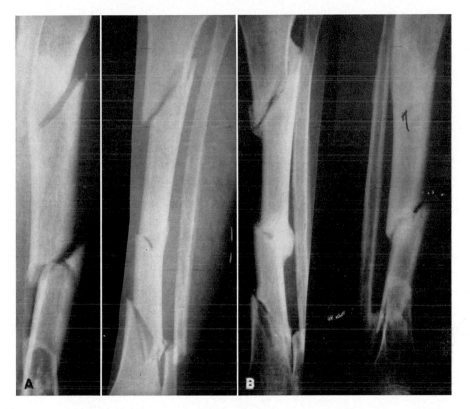

Fig. 6—(A) Closed segmental fractures in an elderly man. Any method of internal fixation of these fractures would have presented disadvantages mechanically and physiologically. (B) Fortunately, cast methods alone sufficed, and the leg was not opened. The patient walked without support at seven months. (Courtesy Am. J. Surg., April 1958, Wade and Campbell.)

reduction and fixation by intramedullary nail with or without Parham bands or screws is indicated if the soft tissues are in good health. Early use of such internal fixation may help protect the soft tissues from further injury by unstable bone fragments. Occasionally, however, a segmented fracture will respond well to closed methods of treatment, which would then be the method of choice (fig. 6 A and B).

Oblique-Spiral Fractures

One occasionally may need to use internal fixation at the fracture site in oblique spiral fractures of the tibia. Shortening can often be prevented, however, simply by applying the cast with the knee flexed, and molding it snugly with slight traction at the ankle by the sling method of Wilson [22, 23] and Carpenter [3] (fig. 7 A–C) or with the use of temporary transfixion

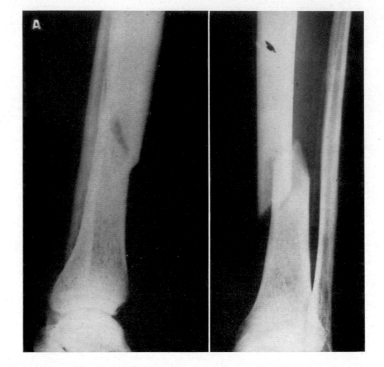

Fig. 7–(A) Closed fracture of the tibia alone.

wires through the os calcis and proximal tibia (fig. 8 A–J). A most convenient apparatus is that of Watson-Jones [20] which provides a saddle for the thigh at the flexed knee while the lower (leg) part of the cast is applied. Too much effort should not be expended in lining up the fracture *by x-ray* in regard to rotation. Attention should rather be paid to the general attitude of the leg, ankle-to-knee-to-pelvis, with the other leg usually displaying the amount of tibial torsion that is normal for the individual. Angulation can be easily corrected by wedging if care is taken to leave lateral struts, and if one does not try to wedge in more than one direction at a time (fig. 9 A and B). However, in contradiction to the conservative policy just outlined in regard to oblique spiral fractures, is the fact that these unstable fractures are usually more easily handled if fixed primarily by screws (fig. 10 A–C).

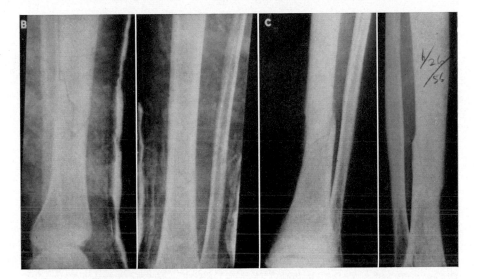

Fig. 7—(B) Well reduced by closed methods. (C) Healed at four months. The intact fibula undoubtedly contributed to the stability of this fracture.

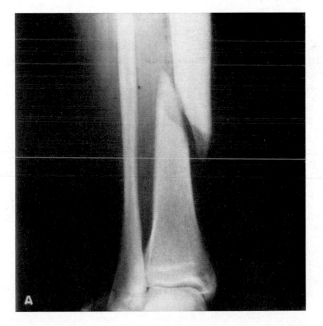

Fig. 8—(A) Open unstable tibial fracture which patient incurred while ice skating.

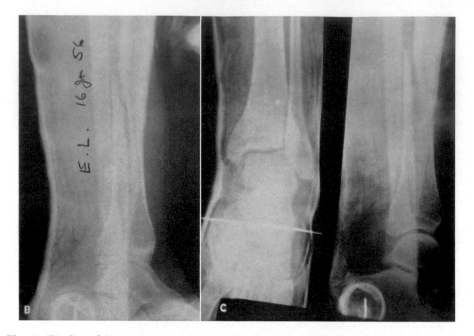

Fig. 8—(B) Os calcis traction on Watson-Jones apparatus, plus direct pressure over the proximal fragment, gained reduction after débridement and wound closure. (C) Initial good reduction.

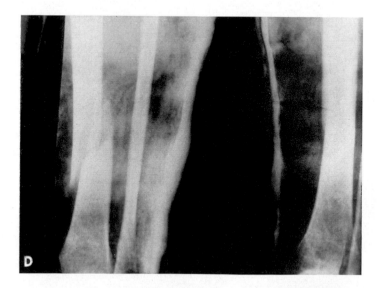

Fig. 8—(D) Slipping out of reduction occurred even with the wire above, transfixing the tibia as well as os calcis transfixion, both incorporated in the long leg cast.

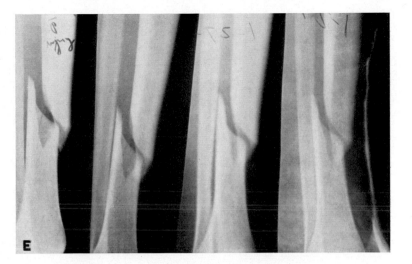

Fig. 8—(E) Better reduction attempted by controlled rotation of the lower fragment.

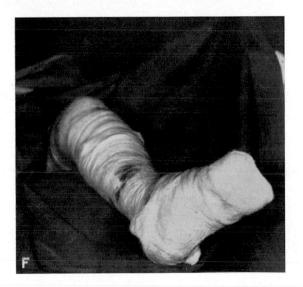

Fig. 8—(F) The cast after manipulation seen in Figure 8 E.

Transverse Fractures

Conservative principles apply all the more to transverse fractures where reduction usually is easy to obtain and to maintain. Operation is seldom necessary. Earlier weight-bearing is permissible in these stable fractures. In a small series at Valley Forge the use of the Lottes nail seemed to give faster healing of transverse fractures. Plates are contraindicated in principle for transverse fractures because of their action of holding the bone ends apart after initial absorption of the fracture site (fig. 11 A—C).

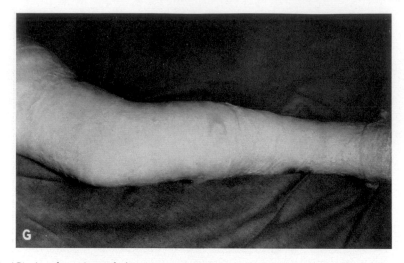

Fig. 8—(G) Another view of the same cast. Note where the transfixion wires are wrapped into the plaster.

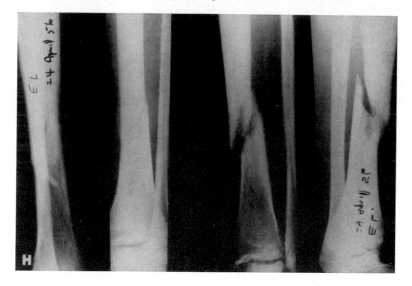

Fig. 8—(H) Deceptive appearance of solid healing suggested by anteroposterior and lateral views at four months (on left). Oblique views showed true status of delayed union (on right).

Comminuted Fractures

According to Urist's review [16, 17] of nonunions of the tibia, the more extensive the comminution, the more contraindication there is to opening the fracture site or attempting internal fixation (fig. 12). Even Vom Saal,[18] an advocate of intramedullary nailing, agrees with this principle because of the disastrous effect of adding to the problem of avascular necrosis of fragments

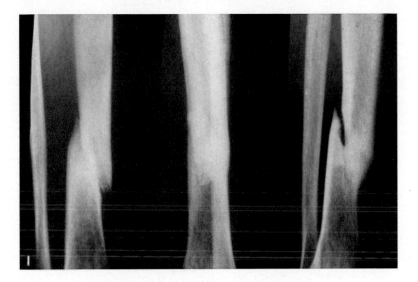

Fig. 8—(I) X-rays at ten months after injury.

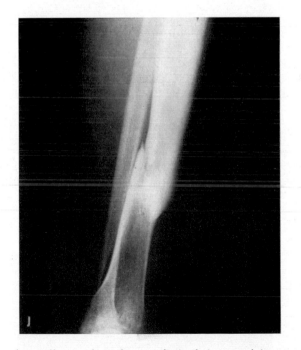

Fig. 8—(J) Although excellent end result was obtained, it seemed in retrospect that much time would have been saved by primary screw fixation.

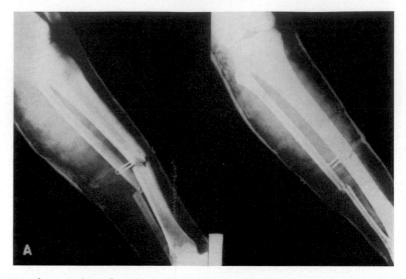

Fig. 9–(A) If a metal marker is taped on the cast before x-rays are taken and this spot is identified by a pencil line, the exact level of the fracture can be ascertained for wedging.

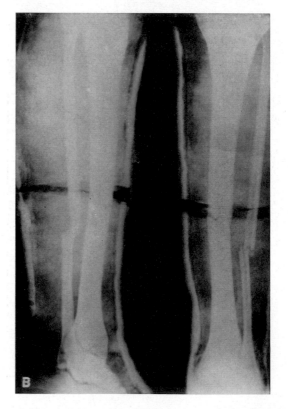

Fig. 9–(B) After wedging. Another adjustment of alignment by wedging was needed a few days later. The fracture site was maintained thereafter in good position.

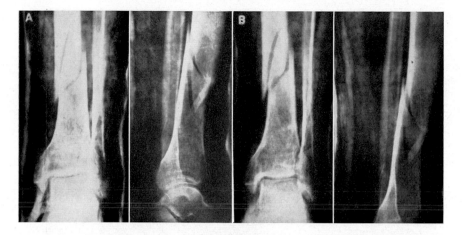

Fig. 10–(A) A well reduced fracture; leg was held in a snug cast from the toes to the groin. (B) Slight slipping at three days.

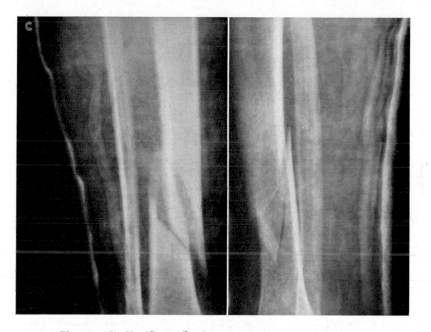

Fig. 10–(C) Significant further position loss at seven days.

by the exposure and fixation manipulations of surgery. However, blind Lottes nailings without opening the fracture site can help a great deal in very unstable comminuted fractures in the middle one-third of the shaft of the tibia.

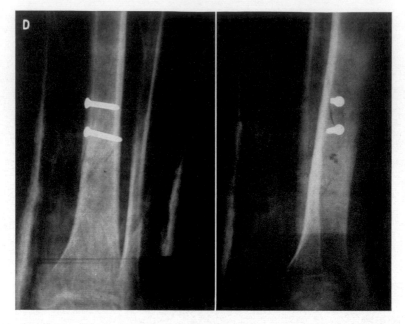

Fig. 10—(D) Screw fixation could not be avoided. This method was elected instead of the use of os calcis traction.

Indications and Limitations of the Several Types of Internal Fixation Materials

Using the Minimum of Internal Fixation

Urist has shown microscopically that the zone of bone necrosis around metal internal fixation device is 2 mm. around each screw. The same reaction also occurs adjacent to plates and nails. Healing time can only be delayed by manipulation of loosened fragments, which may further separate them from soft tissue attachment, and by the extensive periosteal stripping needed in applying plates (fig. 13).

Limitations of Various Devices of Internal Fixation

Screws should be limited to use in obliquities which are long enough to take two screws placed at least 2 cm. apart. They should be inserted *transversely to the long axis of the shaft* so that stress will achieve compression rather than separation of the fracture site, as shown by the work of Arzimanoglou and Skiadaressis.[1] However, if a very guarded postoperative course is followed and the patient is not allowed up until a tight, light long leg cast has been applied with proper flexion of the knee, a single screw as internal suture in a shorter obliquity may serve useful purpose (fig. 14 A–C). Occasionally, one must place the screw at right angles to the *obliquity of the fracture* to gain adequate purchase. Rarely, screws may suffice to hold

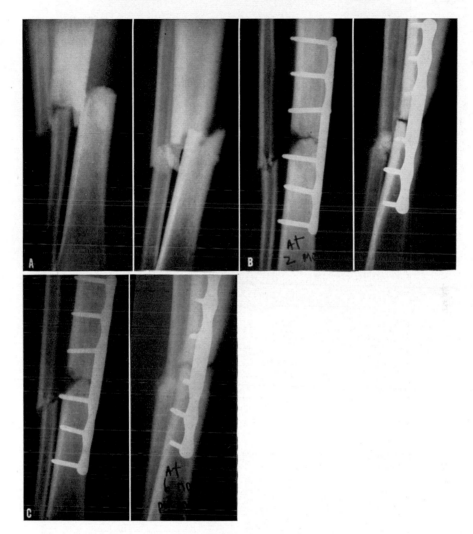

Fig. 11–(A) Original fractures. (B) Two months postoperatively. Note the gap at the fracture site. There was no infection to blame for this defect. (C) Four months later. This tibia did not heal until after removal of plate and screws, and grafting. Perhaps this problem could have been avoided if a sliding plate technique had been used. (Courtesy Am. J. Surg., April 1958, Wade and Campbell.)

both ends of a segmental fracture (fig. 15 A and B). Frequently, they may be ideal for converting a large, loose, displaced butterfly fragment to an onlay graft, and even sometimes used at angles around an intramedullary nail (fig. 16 A–D). For the best tightening effect, a drill of larger bore than the screw should be used for the cortex adjacent to the screw's head and a drill of smaller bore than the screw tip for the cortex in which the tip

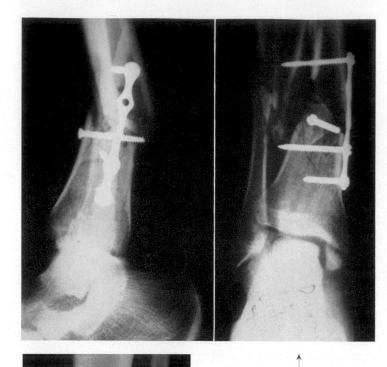

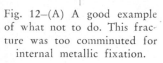

Fig. 12–(A) A good example of what not to do. This fracture was too comminuted for internal metallic fixation.

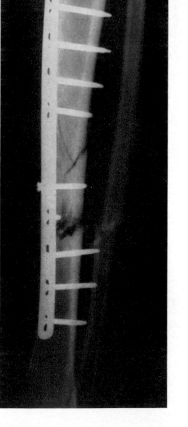

Fig. 13–Another metallic insult to the vascularity of the tibia. This massive application of hardware was associated with wound breakdown and followed by nonunion. A Lottes nail would have served the purpose of internal fixation much better and could have been applied with a small incision and much less periosteal stripping.

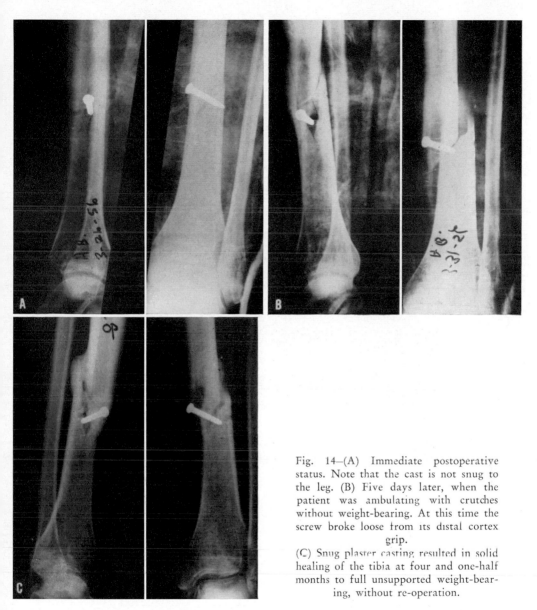

Fig. 14–(A) Immediate postoperative status. Note that the cast is not snug to the leg. (B) Five days later, when the patient was ambulating with crutches without weight-bearing. At this time the screw broke loose from its distal cortex grip.

(C) Snug plaster casting resulted in solid healing of the tibia at four and one-half months to full unsupported weight-bearing, without re-operation.

gains securement. Screws placed from the medial side rather than from the lateral aspect of the shaft are easier to locate and remove later through stab wounds, and require less periosteal stripping for exposure. Even when placed medially, screws seldom cause irritation to the skin before their purpose has been served, and countersinking of the heads is not only unnecessary but is dangerous because it weakens the subadjacent bone cortex.

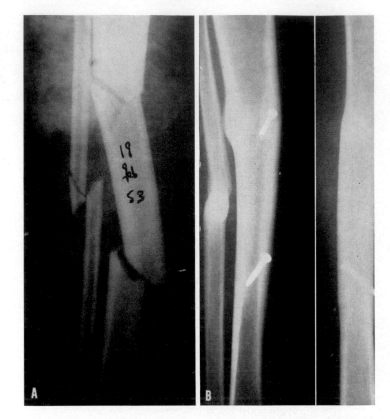

Fig. 15—(A) Segmental fracture of the tibia which required open reduction and internal fixation. (B) Two small incisions and a minimum of periostal stripping were required for fixation by single screws. Careful postoperative cast splitting resulted in prompt healing in good position at four months.

Parham Bands: These circumferential bands are enjoying a new popularity, especially in ski country. They can be used almost with the same indications as for screws and are useful when fragmentation is greater than anticipated and screws do not suffice. If needed to hold long oblique fragments around an intramedullary nail, the bands should be applied first so that a tighter nailing can be obtained (fig. 17 A–C). Special apparatus for tightening is necessary for good application of the bands, but care should be taken not to tighten the bands too tightly and thus cause bone necrosis. Most surgeons who employ the bands plan to remove them at six to eight weeks to prevent ring sequestri, although there is no assurance that this criterion is clearly defined by well substantiated studies (fig. 18).

Transfixion Wires: Kirschner wires crisscrossed through an obliquity may be useful in the absence of better equipment to hold the fragments while a long leg cast is applied (fig. 19 A and B). In such circumstances they could

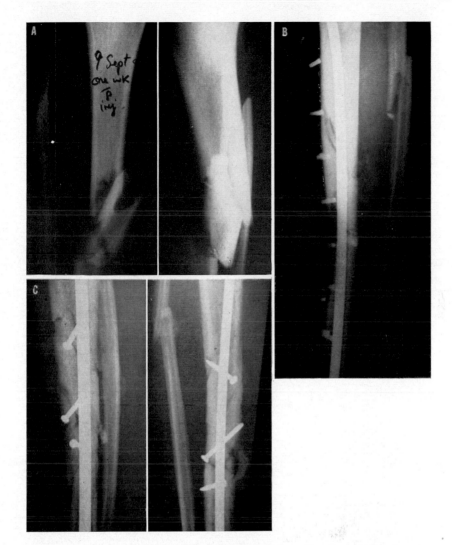

Fig. 16—(A) Segmental fracture not responding satisfactorily to os calcis traction and closed reduction. (B) During operation: A large anterior butterfly fragment became completely detached. Note where it is missing from the anterior cortex. (C) This loose butterfly fragment was screwed back into place.

be cut off beneath the skin. However, such wires may easily migrate out of the bone before healing is sufficient to prevent displacement of the fracture. Two Kirschner transfixion wires used proximally and two distally through the tibia incorporated in the cast are adequate to hold a very unstable fracture from shortening, angulation or rotation in instances where there has been too much contamination or comminution at the fracture site to permit the

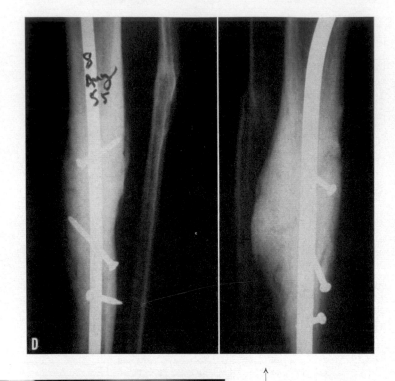

Fig. 16–(D) Solid healing resulted with patient taking full weight-bearing at four months. (Courtesy Lt. Colonel A. O. Heldobler, Medical Corps, U.S. Army.)

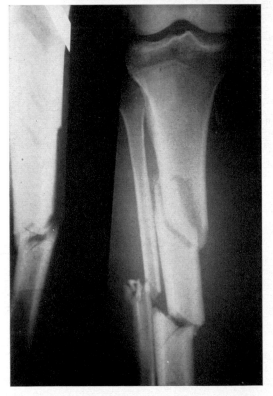

Fig. 17—(A) Original views of segmental fracture problem. (Courtesy Am. J. of Surg., April 1958, Wade and Campbell.)

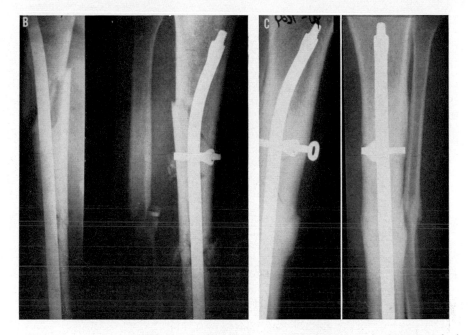

Fig. 17–(B) Lottes' nail was not sufficient because of the type of obliquity of the fracture at the junction of the upper and middle thirds, allowing anterior displacement of the proximal fragment. A Parham band held this reduction. (C) Appearance at two years. The patient had refused to have the band removed. (Courtesy Am. J. of Surg., April 1958, Wade and Campbell.)

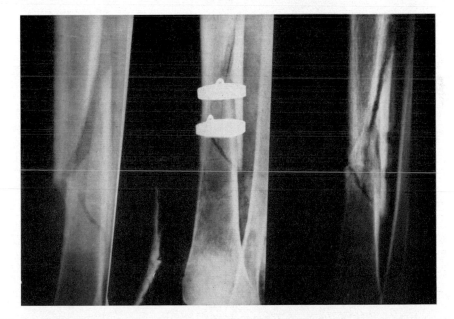

Fig. 18–(A) This group shows the appearance of the original fracture problem, the use of Parham bands at open reduction, and the status of healing at two and one-half months after removal of the bands. Note the deep groove cut by the bands into the butterfly fragment. Unfortunately, this patient developed nonunion. (Courtesy Am. J. of Surg., April 1958, Wade and Campbell.)

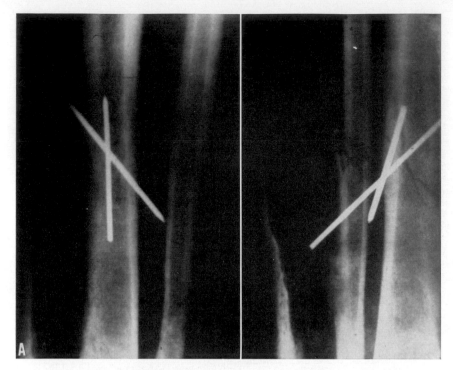

Fig. 19–(A) Kirschner wires holding an unstable fracture.

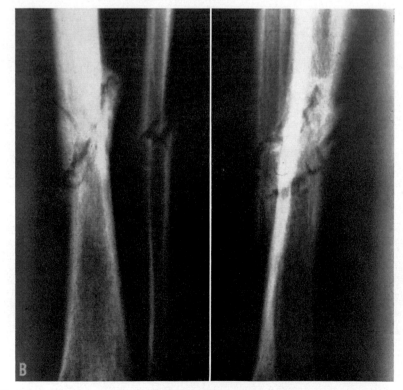

Fig. 19–(B) Appearance after removal of wires at eight weeks. The patient was healed to full weight-bearing at four months.

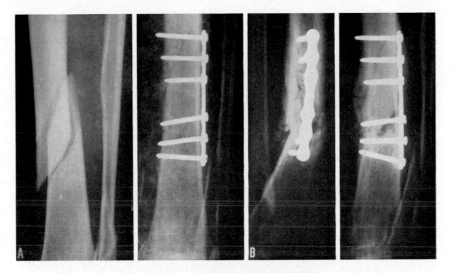

Fig. 20—(A) Plate well applied from the lateral cortex. Postoperative view and original fracture are shown. (Courtesy Am. J. of Surg., April 1958, Wade and Campbell.) (B) Non union at ten months. Screw fixation alone would not have involved as much periosteal stripping or foreign body opposition necrosis as resulted from plating. (Courtesy Am. J. of Surg., April 1958, Wade and Campbell.)

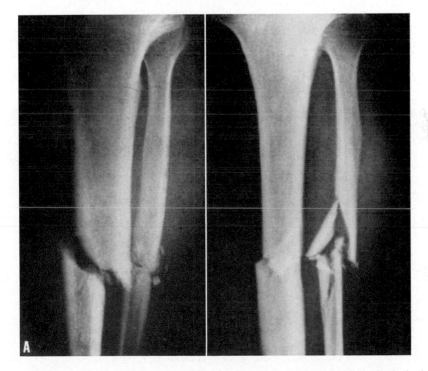

Fig. 21—(A) Unstable fracture not suitable for screw fixation. Closed methods had not been successful in holding a satisfactory reduction.

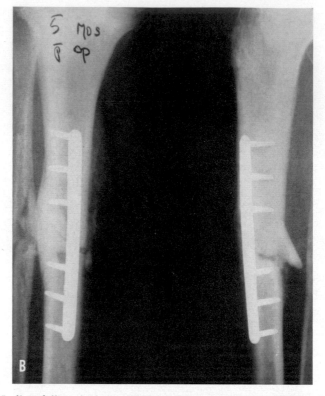

Fig. 21–(B) Healing followed plating. However, this fracture would have been ideal for internal fixation by Lottes' nail, which probably could have been inserted without the necessity of opening the fracture site.

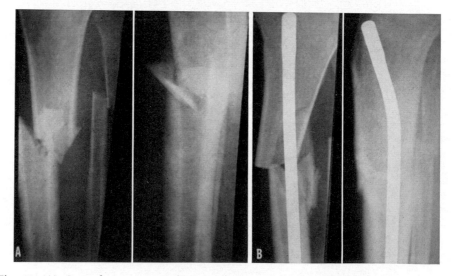

Fig. 22–(A) Open fracture responding poorly to os calcis traction. (B) Angulation after delayed primary nailing. The nail failed to hold the proximal fragment. (Courtesy Am. J. of Surg., April 1958, Wade and Campbell.)

presence of metal there. Transfixion of the os calcis with another transfixion strong single wire above the fracture in the tibia will usually prevent shortening and rotation but not always angulation, even in a snug plaster.

Plates

Plates are occasionally indicated for internal fixation of fractures with short obliquities or for small butterfly fragments; not elsewhere! Even in

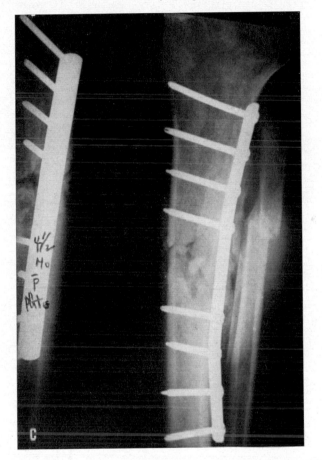

Fig. 22–(C) Final good result after plating (Courtesy Am. J. of Surg., April 1958, Wade and Campbell.)

these fractures other methods are preferable (fig. 20 A and B). Even slotted plates do not permit enough consistent impaction of the fracture to make them applicable for transverse fractures, because the plate holds the fragments apart after initial absorption at the fracture site. If possible, plates are better applied on the lateral aspect of the tibia where they will not complicate soft tissue healing over the fracture (fig. 21 A and B). Screws used with plates should not approach nearer than 0.5 cm. to the fracture site because of the problem of pressure necrosis of bone around screws as well as under the plate. Double plates are never indicated.

Nails

Intramedullary nails, when diamond shaped, fit the interior of the tibia tightly in the middle third, but a single round nail provides no stability against rotation. This problem also exists for the diamond shaped Lottes nail when attempts are made to use it for fractures in the proximal or lower third of the tibial shaft where the medullary canal is much larger than the nail (fig. 22 A–C). Likewise, the Lottes nail, with its posterior convexity,

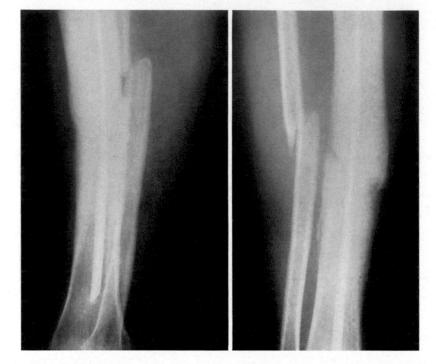

Fig. 23—Ten months after application of single Rush nail; nonunion has resulted. This poor selection of internal fixation was complicated by inadequate postoperative splinting, which permitted short leg cast beginning at two months.

invites some recurvatum of the fracture, which is worse for the lower fractures, and this problem has not been as easy to correct by delayed manipulations of the fragments as Lottes has indicated.[10, 11] Single Rush nails in the tibia are not adequate to prevent angulation, displacement, and rotation (fig. 23). Nonunions may occur from dependence on such inadequate internal support, and, therefore, the Rush nails should be used in pairs, so that three-point pressure of the curved nail is applied from both sides. The nested U-nails of Vom Saal are driven down through the proximal fragment, spread and retracted into the proximal fragment, before being driven distally, to prevent motion. In the application of any of these nails, the knee should be flexed to thin out soft tissues over the proximal knee joint. Distal insertion of the nails proximally is not practicable because of the dorsiflexed position of the ankle and thinness of the subcutaneous tissues over the malleoli, as well as the disengagement effect of gravity on the nails in ambulation. In pounding the nails down the operator should beware of the hazard of going

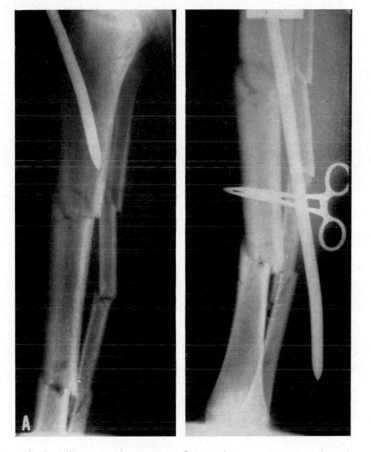

Fig. 24—(A) Blind nailing seen in process of posterior cortex penetration due to wrong direction of initial insertion, which was not flat enough to the long axis of the tibia. Also, the middle third fragment is not displaced somewhat posteriorly to receive the nail.

through the opposite (posterolateral) cortex of the proximal fragment as well as that of knocking off a large butterfly fragment, usually there or at the anterior cortex of the lower fragment. Blind nailing, which is desirable in obviating the need for opening the fracture site, presents these problems, although experienced nailers have great confidence. In attempting a blind nailing of a fracture of the junction of the upper and middle thirds of the tibial shaft, the lower fragment is best displaced slightly posteriorly on the proximal fragment to avoid posterior disengagement of the nail (fig. 24 A).

However, if the fracture is at the junction of the lower and middle thirds, to engage the nail most easily, the lower fragment should be displaced slightly anteriorly to the upper fragment and in some recurvatum (fig. 24 B and C). These principles apply to the Lottes nail only (fig. 25).

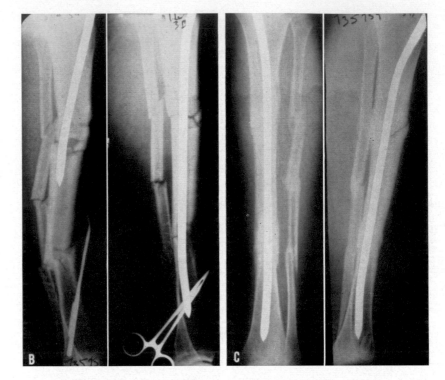

Fig. 24–(B) Proper alignment of the nail at its insertion and slight posterior displacement of the middle third fragment resulted in successful blind nailing. Note that the lower third fragment was easily engaged by the nail, because of this fragment's position of slight anterior displacement and some recurvatum. (C) Successful healing in good alignment.

Comparison of Healing Times

Internal Fixation Alone

Using internal fixation, McLaughlin in 1949 [15], found healing time for closed fractures to be 4.6 months for 63 patients, with no nonunions, and 7.7 months for 74 patients with open fractures, with 6 nonunions. Failures were blamed on defective technic and on postponement of operation until after other methods had failed.

Closed Methods Alone

Depending on temporary sling traction for immediate closed reduction and casting, Carpenter in 1952 [3] had just as fast healing (3.0 months for 19 closed noncomminuted fractures and 5.2 months for 32 closed comminuted fractures, averaging 4.3 months) and faster healing (5.5 months) for 41 open

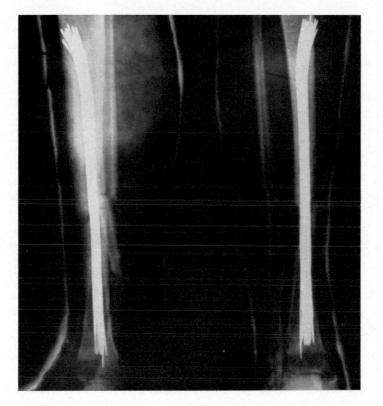

Fig. 25—This collector's item shows a determined intramedullary fixation by eighteen Kirschner wires. Final result is not known, but one hopes that the wires did not migrate.

comminuted cases than McLaughlin. In the open cases, Carpenter had three nonunions, or 7 per cent, which is also about what McLaughlin reported (8 per cent). Carpenter's work brought serious question to the need for internal fixation at the fracture site in tibias. Lottes' paper in the same year [10] reporting conservative treatment in a control group (casts, or K-wires and casts if unstable) of 65 patients, found that healing in the closed fractures was 7.2 months, and in open fractures 10 months, with 6 nonunions for the entire group (11 per cent). Although Boehler's group insists that nonunions do not occur in their patients who receive three weeks of light traction on a frame for unstable fractures and then begin immediate weight-bearing in a skin tight long leg cast for a total of ten weeks or three months, all types of fractures included, they did admit to 3½ per cent incidence of union delayed beyond six months. [2]

Different Types of Internal Fixation

Plates and Screws: Lottes reported the use of plates in a control group of 49 cases, with 10 months average healing time in the closed fracture and 11.8 months in the open fractures, with an incredible incidence of nonunion of 45 per cent (11 cases) in the whole group.[12] This report of Lottes on the results of use of plates is about twice as bad as McLaughlin's cases in respect to healing time for both open and closed fractures, and at least five times as bad in regard to nonunions.

Screws Alone: White et al.,[21] using primary screw fixation when indicated, reported in 1953 on 51 patients who had healing in 5.2 months and on 11 others with some delay beyond this time, including 4 nonunions (6.5 per cent), 3 due to osteomyelitis. This was about the same incidence as McLaughlin and Carpenter experienced with open fractures only.

Intramedullary Nails: In 1952 Vom Saal [18] reported that 34 patients, in whom nested U-nails had been used predominantly, had a very fast average healing time of 3 months, comparable to the closed methods of Boehler. Lottes' much larger series of 102 nailings took a little longer than Vom Saal's, with average healing in five months for the closed fractures and six months for the open cases, but like his, contained no instances of nonunion.

Appreciation of the Presence of an Intact Fibula

In fresh fractures of the tibia, an intact fibula is of great help in holding reduction of the tibia. Review of the Valley Forge cases showed overall reduction in healing time when the fibula was intact.[19] Of course, in nonunion of the tibia, osteotomy of the fibula may be needed for impaction of the tibial fracture or for insertion-synostosing to the tibia. Intramedullary nailing of the fibula, which is usually easy to do from the lateral malleolus with a Rush pin if there is an adequate fibular intramedullary canal, is often of value in helping to stabilize extensively comminuted and contaminated fractures of the lower one half of the tibia.

Definition of Delayed and Nonunion

Although solid bone union by x-ray of amount sufficient to fill a gap of cortex of 5 mm. may take a year, and remodeling the intramedullary canal even longer, the patient can conservatively be said to have delayed clinical union if motion can be demonstrated at the fracture site at ten weeks, and grafting should be considered if this condition persists beyond four months. Nonunion has occurred in the presence of sclerotic bone ends which seal off the intramedullary canal at the fracture site and where motion is demonstrable clinically. Usually, ten months to a year are necessary for such bone changes at the fracture site to be well defined.

Evaluation of Methods of Treating Nonunion

Urist in 1954 [17] summed up this problem by stating that healing time in the tibia is proportional to the length of the shaft damage and to the separation of the fragments. Other factors adding to the incidence of nonunion were surgical dissection of the fracture site, exposed bone, sepsis and the implantation of metallic appliances for internal fixation. In transverse and oblique spiral fragments, if at least 50 per cent contact exists, healing will average from 6 to 9 months for disappearance of the fracture line and restoration of the intramedullary canal by x-ray. The use of internal fixation did not change this time requirement for the better but caused further delay if done poorly. Comminuted fractures were only made worse by open reduction. Usually, 9 to 18 months were found to be required to remodel the shaft after a simple wedge fracture, and from 12 to 24 months if 1 cm. of the shaft in width and length has been comminuted.

The big difference in Urist's healing times and those reported by the many other authors above is that he insists on absolute bone remodeling union by x-ray instead of what is felt clinically to be solid and considered sufficiently safe by x-ray for unsupported weight-bearing. Undoubtedly, differences of opinion on the latter will always exist.

Healing Times from the Combined Fracture Service of The New York Hospital—Hospital for Special Surgery

Table 1 is a summary of the healing times for recently reviewed cases of fractures of the tibia shaft from the New York Hospital—Hospital for Special Surgery combined Fracture Service.[19] It was established on the basis of the time when the patient was successfully permitted unsupported weight-bearing. If x-ray criteria for union had been severe enough to require remodeling of the tibia shaft or very dense callus, each category quoted above would have been anywhere from one to four months longer. In deciding when the patient could safely be allowed unsupported weight-bearing, it was necessary that the fracture site be painless to reasonable manual stress and longitudinal contusion as well as to progressive weight-bearing. A certain amount of evidence of bone union as seen by x-ray was required but this varied greatly with the individual cases.

TABLE 1—*Healing Times of The New York Hospital Cases*

Method of Treatment	Total	Closed	Healed	Open	Healed	Overall Healing
Screws	32	25	4.0 mo.	7	4.3 mo.	4.2 mo.
Plates	21	11	4.6 mo.	10	4.6 mo.	4.6 mo.
Nails	19	15	5.3 mo.	4	4.1 mo.	4.8 mo.
Bands	4	4	3.7 mo.			
Traction	17	8	5.5 mo.	9	6.5 mo.	6.0 mo.
Casts	34	21	3.6 mo.	13	6.0 mo.	5.1 mo.

Table 2[19] summarizes complications according to the method of treatment. The large incidence of complication with plates helps to explain the present tendency to resort to the use of plates in fractures of the tibia only when no other method will possibly suffice, which is rare indeed.

In an effort to gain more numerical significance, the complications from

TABLE 2.—Summary of Complications According to Method of Treatment (New York Hospital)

Method of Treatment	No.	Closed	Complications	Non-Unions	%	Open	Complications	Non-Unions	%	Total Non-Un.	%
Screws	32	25	2, 1 delayed union by poor mechanics; 1 nonunion with infection	1	4	7	1 infection healed in 6 months	0	0	1	3
Plates	21	11	2, 1 delayed union in trans. fracture; 1 nonunion with infection	1	9	10	7 all nonunions including 3 infections (with 1 amputation)	7	70	8	38
Plates *	18	11	2, 1 delayed union in trans. fx.; 1 nonunion with infection	1	9	7	4 all nonunions without infection	4	57	5	27
Nails	19	15	2, 1 death, embolism; 1 angulation failure	0	0	4	None	0	0	0	0
Bands	4	4	1 nonunion without infection	1	25	0		0	0	1	25
Traction	17	8	1 nonunion without infection	1	12.5	9	1 infection healed in 6 months	0	0	1	5.9
Casts	34	21	None	0	0	13	1 nonunion with infection; severe soft tissue injury	1	7.6	1	2.9

* Excluding 3 cases of open fractures plated elsewhere and admitted to The New York Hospital with infection which eventually were classified as nonunion.

TABLE 3—Complications from the Combined Fractures Service of New York Hospital— and the Valley Forge Army Hospital.

Method of Rx.	Total	Closed	Complications	Non-Union %	Open	Complications	Non-Union %	Total Nonunion %
Screws	58	44	4 1 Delayed union (poor mechanics) 1 Nonunion without infection (too early wt. bearing) 2 Nonunion with infection	3—6.8%	14	1 Infection; healed at 6 months	0—0	3—5%
Plates	44	25	3 1 Delayed union (transv. fx.) 1 Nonunion without infection (oblique fx.) 1 Nonunion with infection	2—8%	19	9 4 Nonunions without infection: 2x transv. fx. 1x comminuted fx. 1x obliq. spir. fx. 5 Nonunions with infection	9—47%	11—25%
Nails	30	19	2 1 Death (thromboembolic) 1 Angulation failure	0—0	11	1 Nonunion with single Rush nail	1—9%	1—3.3% all nails 0% Lottes nails
Traction Transfixion	20	8	1 Non-union (over-pull)	1—12%	12	1 Infection; Healed at 9 months	0—0	1—5%
Bands	4	4	1 Nonunion without infection	1—25%	0	0	0—0	1—25%
Casts	82	38	0	0—0	44	7 2 Delayed unions 5 Nonunions with infections after extensive soft tissue loss & contamination	5—11%	5—6.5%

the above hospitals were combined in table 3.[19] The misfortunes resulting from the use of plates remained significantly frequent. The experience with traction is misleading in regard to closed cases because of the limited experience. In other categories, as noted in the review of literature mentioned previously, the instance of complications is not extraordinary.

References

[1] ARZIMANOGLOU, A., and SKIADARESSIS, G.: Study of internal fixation by screws of oblique fractures in long bones. J. Bone & Joint Surg., *34 A*: 219–223 (Jan.) 1952.

[2] BÖHLER, L., and BÖHLER, J.: Fracture Course. Phila. Committee on Trauma. Philadelphia Am. Coll. Surg. (April) 1955.

[3] CARPENTER, E. B., DOBBIE, J. J., and SIEWERS, C. F.: Fractures of shaft of tibia and fibula; comparative end results from various types of treatment in teaching hospital. Arch. Surg. *64*: 443 (April) 1952.

[4] ELLIS, H.: Speed of healing after fracture of the tibia. J. Bone & Joint Surg. *40 B*: 42 (Feb.) 1958.

[5] FREEMAN, W. A., and GARNES, A. L.: Open tibial shaft fractures — Immediate soft tissue cure. Am. J. Surg. *95*: 415 (March) 1958.

[6] GRUNDMAN, G., and LINKE, V.: Therapy of fractures of the shaft of the tibia. Arch. Orthop. u. Unfall-Chir. *47*: 489, 1955.

[7] HAMILTON, R. L., and JAHNA, H.: Simple proven method for treatment of shaft with or without fracture of fibula. Am. J. Surg. *88*: 218, 1954.

[8] KING, T.: Compression of the bone ends as an aid to union in fractures. A report of 49 ununited and 4 recent fractures. J. Bone & Joint Surg. *39 A*: 1238 (Dec.) 1957.

[9] KÜNTSCHER, G.: Medullary nailing of shaft fractures. Arch. klin. Chir. *276*: 217, 1953.

[10] LOTTES, J. O.: Intramedullary fixation for fracture of shaft of tibia. South. M. J. *45*: 407, 1952.

[11] —: Report of 300 nailings for fractures of shaft of tibia. J.A.M.A. *155*: 1039, 1954.

[12] —, HILL, E J., and KEY, J. A.: Closed reduction, plate fixation and medullary nailing of fractures of both bones of leg; comparative end result study. J. Bone & Joint Surg. *34 A*: 86, 1952.

[13] MAKOWSKY, L.: Nailing of complicated fractures of shaft of tibia with rigid Küntscher nail; experience and problems. Monatsschr. Unfallh. *48*: 267–270, 1955.

[14] MARSHALL, D. V.: Three-side plate fixation for fractures of the femoral and tibial shafts. J. Bone & Joint Surg. *40 A*: 323 (April) 1958.

[15] McLAUGHLIN, H. L., GASTON, S. R., NEER, C. S., and CRAIG, F. S.: Open reduction and internal fixation of fractures of the long bones. J. Bone & Joint Surg. *31 A*: 94–101 (Jan.) 1949.

[16] URIST, M. R., MAZET, R., and McLEAN, F. C.: The pathogenesis and treatment of delayed union and non-union. J. Bone & Joint Surg. *36 A*: 931–968 (Oct.) 1954.

[17] URIST, U. H.: End result observations influencing treatment of fractures of shaft. J.A.M.A. *159*: 1088, 1955.

[18] VOM SAAL, F.: Intramedullary fixation of the tibia. Bone & Joint Surg. *34 A*: 86–95 (Jan.) 1952.

[19] WADE, P. A., and CAMPBELL, R. D., Jr.: Open versus closed method in treating fractures of the leg. Am. J. Surg. *95*: 599–616 (April) 1958.

[20] WATSON-JONES, R.: Fractures and Joint Injuries. Baltimore, William & Wilkins, 1955, pp. 802–803.

[21] WHITE, E. H., RADLEY, T. J., and EARLEY, N. N.: Screw stabilization in fixation of the tibial shaft. J. Bone & Joint Surg. *35 A*: 749–755 (July) 1953.

[22] WILSON, P. D., and COCHRANE, W. A.: Fractures and Dislocations. Philadelphia, J. B. Lippincott Co., 1928, pp. 656–657.

[23] —: Management of Fractures and Dislocations. Philadelphia, J. B. Lippincott Co., 1938, pp. 628–630.

CHAPTER 47

WOUNDS OF EXTREMITIES, CROSS-LEG FLAPS OTHER RECONSTRUCTIVE PROCEDURES ON THE SOFT TISSUES

HERBERT CONWAY, M.D.

The surgeon responsible for treating the effects of trauma is particularly interested in the management of wounds of the extremities. Their successful handling demands the ultimate in knowledge of the principles of cleansing, débridement, wound healing, combating infection and the covering of open defects. Effective employment of such knowledge is rewarded by diminished period of morbidity, prevention of deformity and, in many cases, avoidance of amputation of the damaged extremity. Statistics gleaned from both World Wars show that wounds of the extremities make up the largest single anatomic group (45 per cent) of all war wounds. Inaccurate management—often resulting from evacuation problems rather than from surgical failure—accounts for the popular image of the wounded soldier: lameness, casts, crutches. In civilian life, the injured are rapidly taken to a hospital in which completely adequate facilities and equipment are available, and it remains only for the surgeon to employ them effectively.

Perhaps in no group of selected traumatic cases is the exercise of sound principles of surgery so richly rewarded as in wounds of soft tissue of the extremities whether they be limited to those structures, or associated with fractures of the underlying bones (open fractures). Though no statistics are available to me, it is my feeling that nonunion of open fractures of the lower tibia and fibula is more frequently the result of failure to effect primary healing of the wound (or wounds) of soft tissue than of failure to reduce the fractures effectively. Primary wound healing can be attained only if dirty, devitalized and contaminated soft and bony tissues are removed in the technic of operative débridement. This procedure commonly results in a defect of soft tissue the margins of which cannot be approximated by suture lest undue tension result in gangrene and infection of the closed wound. If the surgeon errs in judgment and closes under tension, he may create circumstances provocative of suppuration with attendant "osteomyelitis from without in," (in contrast to the classic type of nontraumatic hematogenous osteomyelitis). Moreover, anaerobic infection (tetanus, clostridial myositis or gas gangrene) may be precipitated by undue tension as well as by failure to excise necrotic tissue during débridement.

Given before the Annual Fracture Trauma Course of the American College of Surgeons held at The New York Hospital, Hospital For Special Surgery and Cornell University Medical College.

673

Toward the objective of primary healing of wounds of soft tissue of the extremities, the details of management now will be elucidated. Again, it is emphasized that wounds of soft tissue *alone* may be sufficient to cause serious complication or crippling deformity.

Principles of Soft-Tissue Wound Healing

Controlling influence should be exercised in the management of fresh wounds of the extremities by (1) débridement of the wound, (2) rest of the affected extremity, (3) careful consideration of blood supply and tissue tension, (4) attainment of complete hemostasis and (5) prevention of infection. The principles of surgery remain constant; only the technic whereby they are put into effect is altered or improved from time to time.

Débridement

Careful débridement is basic to the care of fresh traumatic wounds. The late Mont Reid,[36] my mentor, who wrote a classic monograph on this subject 20 years ago, stated that it is doubtful whether the presence or absence of bacteria is of greater importance in wound healing than the persistence of debris and devitalized tissue, or attention to other aspects of the healing process. The dictum of Pare,[33] over 400 years ago, that the gentlest cleansing of wounds with ordinary soap and water gives the best wound healing has been reaffirmed only this year by an exhaustive study which was presented by Blocker, Lewis, Pomerat and their co-workers.[4]

Dirt, grease and foreign bodies should be removed from the depths of the wound and from the neighboring skin by gentle cleansing, using a detergent if necessary. Dead tissue, or tissue into which foreign material has been imbedded should be excised by scalpel. Often this means the excision of a margin (one-quarter inch or so) of the skin edges. Viable muscle can be distinguished from nonviable by the fact that the former contracts when cut or pinched, whereas the latter does not. Necrotic muscle, fascia or tendon should be excised.

The objectives, then, at the time of emergency surgery, are to rid the wound of foreign material, to remove devitalized tissues (avascular segments of muscle—significantly cyanotic or ischemic flaps of soft tissue), to excise contaminated or completely loosened bony fragments (provided their removal does not result in loss of continuity of the involved long bone) and to effect closure of the surface defect. This last recalls the Trueta [41] treatment, advanced during the 1930's by that famous surgeon of the Spanish Civil War. The unusually difficult evacuation problems during that conflict bar all criticism of the Trueta regimen, but its use dooms the extremity to osteomyelitis of bony fragments (even though this may not be extensive) and condemns the subject to prolonged convalescence. Moreover, there is increased probability of all of the undesired sequellae: nonunion of the fragments, osteoporosis of structures distal to the fractures and even proximal to them, atrophy of soft tissues, causalgia and ankylosis. Certainly preferable is the ready closure of the wound by one of two technics: either advancement of a regional flap of soft tissue to cover the bony fragments—and closure of the defect from which the flap was created (over muscle bellies or other soft tissues) by free graft of skin or, in difficult local presentations, the use of a free skin graft directly over the exposed bones.

Rest of the Affected Extremity

Billroth [2] emphasized that rest of the injured part is of the greatest importance in wound healing. Reid [36] stated, "Injurious substances are taken from the wound into the blood; hence every muscular movement and every consequent congestion of the wound, may eventually prove injurious." Reid and Carter [37] state that there is not yet a complete recognition of the fact that rest, insured by complete immobilization, is just as valuable in the treatment of wounds of soft tissue as in dealing with injuries involving bony structures. This principle is too often ignored. Its application will be rewarded by kind healing of extensive wounds of soft tissue.

Blood Supply and Tissue Tension

The location of the wound, the age of the patient, his general health, the presence and degree of sclerosis of the arteries and arterioles, the presence of old scars such as those following varicose ulcers and finally, the degree of tension on the sutures, all have significant effects on the blood supply of a wound. The circulation of the lower leg is jeopardized easily because it is terminal circulation at the greatest distance from the cardiac pump. This is magnified in those instances in which the injury has caused mass destruction of a significant percentage of the combined calibers of the blood vessels of the involved extremity, and in people of the older age groups whose collateral circulatory reserve is diminished by regional arteriosclerosis.

The problem of tension in a healing wound is directly related to its blood supply. The thoughtful surgeon may anticipate passive congestion, edema or ischemia so that one wound might be positioned in elevation (in relation to the level of the heart) while another might be put in the horizontal position or even in slight dependency. The oscillating bed helps to provide *passive* aid to the filling and emptying of the capillary bed of an extremity under the duress of difficult healing. Whenever primary suture cannot be accomplished without undue tension on the margins of the wound, the surgeon must use a flap of tissue or a free graft of skin. These technics will be discussed later. There is no question that the accuracy with which a surgeon judges the efficiency of circulation in the repair of a given wound is a direct gauge of his skill. With good débridement and closure without tension, ideal healing may be anticipated; with incomplete débridement and/or suture under questionable tension, the surgeon must anticipate regrettable complications. Serious sequellae are preventable if the surgeon will combat tension by the use of flaps and/or grafts of skin at the time of the emergency surgery.

Hemostasis

Hematoma produces inordinate tension and thus interferes with blood supply of flaps and even may obstruct the circulation of the extremity by annular compression of a dangerous degree. Thus, the attainment of a dry wound through accurate clamping and ligature is of the utmost importance in the achievement of primary healing of the traumatic wound. Bleeding points should be clamped accurately, the hemostat compressing a minimum of tissue. Ligatures should be of the finest plain catgut which is practicable. Hemostasis should be followed by flooding the wound with warm, physiologic saline solution, to rid it of invisible bacteria.

Prevention of Infection

Reid and Carter [37] have pointed out that fresh wounds, either superficial or traumatic, are seldom, if ever, absolutely free of bacteria; their sterilization is relative. However, healthy living cells have a remarkable power of combating bacteria, whereas dead or devitalized tissues are powerless against them. The prevention of infection thus depends on accuracy of débridement, avoidance of hematoma and suture of the wound without tension. After thorough cleansing of the wound and its adjacent skin as outlined above, the skin should be sterilized by painting it with a solution which is bactericidal but not injurious to living cells. At The New York Hospital a colorless, stainless, aqueous solution of benzalkonium chloride (1: 1000) is used. There is no need either to suffuse the open wound with this solution or to use antibiotics locally. Alcoholic solutions such as tincture of iodine are contra-indicated because the alcoholic base acts exactly like a fixative to living tissue.

Types of Wounds

Subcutaneous Lacerations

Relatively small lacerations of the skin may be surface manifestations of much more extensive subcutaneous lacerations in which hematoma of the areolar tissue overlying the fascia of the muscles is quite extensive. Subcutaneous laceration and hematoma result from shearing injuries of the extremity. In this situation the visible laceration of the skin must be elongated by incision, often in more than one direction, to permit excision of hematomatous areolar tissue and ligation of distant bleeding points.

Avulsion Flaps of Soft Tissue

This is a common injury, usually caused by a shearing tear. Because the blood supply of skin and soft tissues of the extremities is delivered by perforating endarterial tufts of vessels to blocked areas about 3 inches square, the avulsion of a flap larger than this will be followed by slough of the soft tissues incorporated in the flap. Manchot [24] demonstrated the anatomy of this complication in 1889, and today his diagrams stand as a classic contribution (fig. 1). A traumatic avulsion flap usually is cyanotic, and its cutaneous

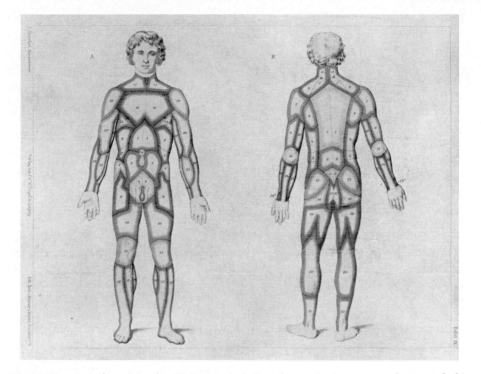

Fig. 1—Drawings from Manchot [24] (1889) depicting that author's concept of areas of skin which are supplied with an endarterial circulation. To form pedicles of large dimension several of these areas must be brought into circulatory balance by collateral circulation. Thus, larger flaps require development by successive surgical incisions (delay procedures).

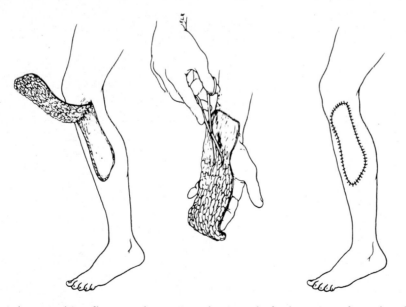

Fig. 2—A large avulsion flap must be amputated, trimmed of subcutaneous fat and replaced as a free skin graft. This will more certainly insure primary wound healing with a minimum of complications.

surface commonly is the site of severe abrasion with indriven dirt or grease. As the surgeon cleanses such a flap, he is sorely tempted to replace it by gentle suture at its margin. This procedure is a mistake if the flap is larger than 3 inches in its long dimension—gangrenous slough with needless subsequent infection, delay in rate of recovery, and mandatory grafting of skin are the inevitable sequellae. The proper procedure is to amputate such a large avulsion flap, trim the specimen of subcutaneous fat and replace the skin as a free graft. Marginal sutures of silk are required. To provide postoperative pressure the tails of these are left long, to be tied firmly over a generous bolus of cotton waste (mechanic's waste). The necessary postoperative immobilization is achieved by the application of a padded plaster cast.

Open Fracture of Tibia and Fibula with Loss of Overlying Skin and Subcutaneous Fat

Reduction of Fracture: Once débridement and closure are accomplished, the reduction of the fracture is the chief problem. Often this may be accomplished by operative manipulation of the fragments at the time of débridement. If fragments can be engaged effectively, casting is the procedure of choice for immobilization, care being taken to mark out or to cut a generous window so that the wound can be inspected regularly and diligently. If fragments cannot be held in apposition satisfactorily, traction must be employed. Just

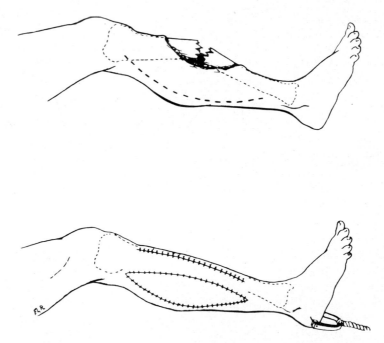

Fig. 3—The bipedicled flap provides a satisfactory means by which proper surface coverage and primary wound healing can be obtained following compound fracture associated with soft tissue loss.

as the failure to attain primary healing of the wound has an unfavorable effect on the healing of the fracture, so the failure to reduce the fracture results in passive congestion, excessive ecchymosis and obstructing edema.

The Bipedicled Flap: In this circumstance the surgeon must be familiar with the technic of the double-pedicled flap of skin and fat (fig. 3). Loss of

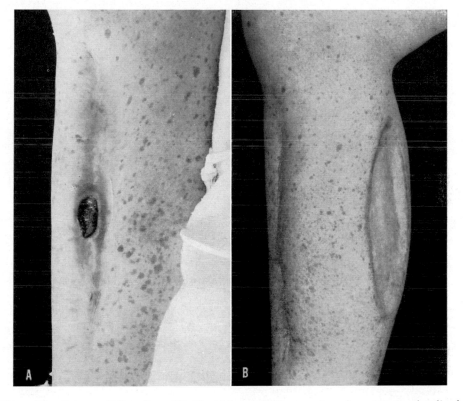

Fig. 4—Bipedicle or sliding flap. (A) Unstable pretibial scar, site of an inactive localized osteomyelitis. (B) Following excision of unstabled scar a bipedicled flap was utilized for surfacing of the defect. A skin graft was placed posteriorly.

soft tissue is commonly anterior, *i.e.*, over the crest of the tibia. Vertical incision is made over the dorsal aspect of the leg, at least 2½ inches and preferably 3 inches away from the margin of the wound. In the average extremity this means that the incision is at or near the Achilles tendon. The skin and fat between this incision and the wound are dissected carefully from the fascia of the musculature, thus creating a flap which is left contiguous with adjacent soft tissue superiorly and inferiorly. Because such a flap has two attachments, it is classified as *bipedicled.* It is a simple maneuver to slide this flap anteriorly to permit good soft tissue coverage of the bony structures as the margins of the wound are approximated by interrupted silk sutures *without tension*. The defect over the posterior calf, elliptical in contour, is then surfaced by a thick-split graft of skin, readily obtained from the lower abdomen. This donor site is preferred, for with one extremity already damaged, it is unwise to apply surgery to the other. The simple cutting of a split graft of skin has caused the reawakening of an old thrombophlebitis. If, for any reason, it is necessary to use the thigh as a donor site, the dressing over this area should not be annular in type. It is desirable to cover the donor site with gauze impregnated with xeroform ointment (bismuth tribromphenate). This agent is bacteriostatic and mildly astringent. Pressure may be obtained by the use of elastic adhesive (elasto-plast). The dressing over the donor site should not be disturbed for 14 days, at which time epithelization should be complete. The skin graft should be secured with interrupted marginal sutures of silk, the tails of which are not cut off. Xeroform gauze is placed over the graft, and on top of that, a thick bolus of cotton waste. Suitable pressure is applied to the graft by crisscrossing the long tails of the sutures as they are tied over the bolus of cotton waste. The entire extremity may then be encased in a padded plaster cast, a window being cut for observation of the healing of the wound.

Reconstructive Surgery of the Soft Tissues of the Extremity

Too frequently, the plastic and reconstructive surgeon sees those cases in which failure to execute the above principles has resulted in a crippled extremity which exhibits extensive superficial and deep scar, nonunion of the fractured tibia, osteoporosis, atrophy of the soft tissues and often, partial or complete ankylosis of the joints. There may be surface osteomyelitis with draining sinuses, and the roentgenogram may show sequestration in addition to the nonunion and decalcification. The plastic surgeon must replace the scarred area with healthy skin and subcutaneous fat, since it is not possible to execute a bone graft — in repair of the nonunion fracture — through tissues which are anything other than healthy, with good circulation. In such a reconstructive problem, free grafts of skin are not adequate for replacement of scar tissue, for the surgeon cannot successfully place a bone graft through an area of thick-split skin overlying nonunion of bones. Because two tissues are needed, skin and fat, the graft is a compound graft and a nutrient pedicle is required for its survival as it develops its new circulation.

The Tubed Pedicle

Reconstructive surgery of soft tissues was dominated in the 23 year interval between the two world wars by the use of the tubed pedicle. The popularity of the tubed pedicle was due to the fact that the development of this type of transplantation mechanism during World War I (Gillies [16] and Filatoff [14]) represented a distinct advance in technique of soft-tissue transfer. The tubed pedicle provided a cleanly healed, sausage-like mass of tissue. This was an advance over the open pedicles previously used, where under surfaces suppurated frankly. This degree of infection occasionally militated against the success of the migration of tissue. During World War II, as the burden of myriad cases with massive defects descended on military surgeons, it became apparent that the tubed pedicle actually was a limiting mechanism which provided only a meagre amount of soft tissue for ultimate transfer.

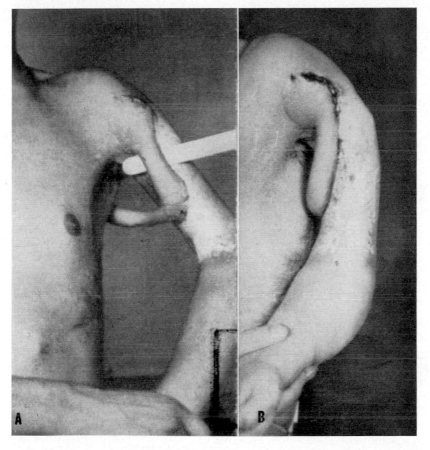

Fig. 5—Extensive scar of the arm with nonunion of the humerus following gas gangrene and treatment by tubed pedicle in preparation for bone graft. (U.S. Army Lovell General Hospital case, 1942.) (A) The mid-portion of the pedicle has been set into the mid-arm as a bridge to insure adequate circulation for the final division of the pedicle. (B) A thoracic tubed pedicle has been prepared and migrated to the upper arm.

Moreover, such pedicles, if constructed on the thigh, required multiple transfers with successively lower implantations on the extremity until the required soft tissue finally could be inset as replacement for the scarred area over the tibia. Thus, the period of convalescence, in a patient already chronically ill and crippled, was prolonged inordinately.

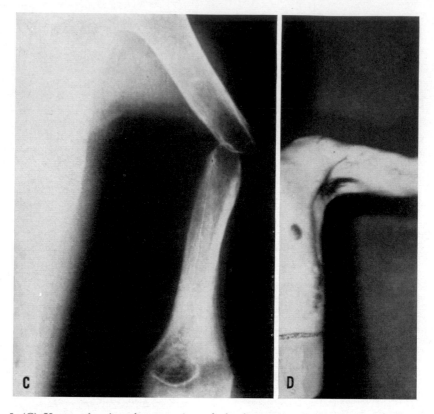

Fig. 5–(C) X-ray showing the nonunion of the humerus. (D) At the fourth operation the pedicle was divided from the thorax, scar excised from the arm, and the pedicle inset.

The Broad-based Flap

The ready procurement of free-skin grafts through the development of new instruments for the cutting of grafts (Padgett dermatome,[30] Reese dermatome,[35] Barker vacutome,[1] electrodermatome,[26] to name a few) made it practicable to construct large, broad-based flaps and to transfer them without the old problem of infection of their undersides. The raw areas were "closed" by free grafts of skin.[23] This development revolutionized the reconstructive surgery of soft tissues. Its superiority to the tubed pedicle lay in the facts that more generous amounts of tissue could be migrated, fewer operative stages were required, and the period of convalescence was shortened significantly. Figures 5 and 6 demonstrate comparable case problems handled by the tubed pedicle and by the "closed" flap technics. The saving of time and numbers of operative procedures is impressive.

The Cross-Leg Flap

History: Celsus[8] was the first surgeon to employ the bipedicled, sliding flap in covering an adjacent defect. This technic became known as the

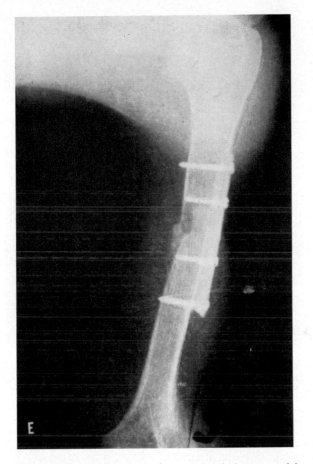

Fig. 5—(E) x-ray showing the onlay type of bone graft which was used by the orthopedic service of the Lovell General Hospital to effect union of the ununited fracture. Six operations were required over a period of eight months. The procedures were successful but the number of operations and the period of morbidity is to be compared with the management of the case reported in figure 6.

"French method" of soft tissue transplantation because it was so frequently used by the French surgeons, Nelaton and Ombredanne. [28] It was used widely during the first World War. Imre, [18] an ophthalmologist, first advocated the rotation flap for the correction of soft tissue defects of the eyelids. The first cross-leg flap procedure was performed in 1854 by Frank H. Hamilton, [17] of Buffalo, New York, for the treatment of a chronic ulcer of the leg. Hamilton realized the adjunctive value of the nourishing pedicle of soft tissue in the healing of nonunion fracture of the tibia. In 1885 Maas [22] published the report of a cross-leg flap executed successfully by Billroth in 1874. In that early period the pedicle had been left attached for only 17 days, and the report stated that the flap was secure one year later. He reported a similar case by Czerny, and three cases of his own.

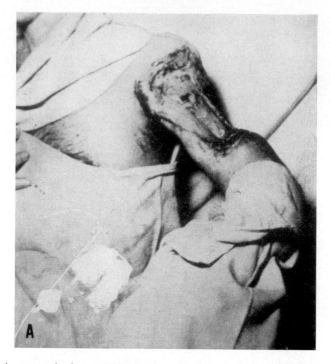

Fig. 6—Extensive wound of arm with loss of continuity of humerus treated by preliminary split skin graft followed by broad based pedicle from thorax in preparation for bone graft. (A) Appearance of the arm six days after grafting at which time this wounded soldier was transported to the United States by air. (B and C) Appearance of the arm after reconstruction by broad based thoracic pedicle and subsequent bone graft. Photographs C and D were supplied by Dr. T. G. Blocker, Jr., of Galveston, Texas, on whose service at Wakeman General Hospital of the U.S. Army this phase of the surgery was carried out. Three operations completed this reconstruction in a period of 11 weeks. This case record is to be compared with that presented in figure 5. The two case reports demonstrate the advances in reconstructive surgery brought out by the burden of great numbers of cases and the magnitude of the wound problems during World War II.

In 1919, Davis [13] stated, "pedunculated flaps . . . give the best results . . . in exposed positions . . . In using a flap from a distant part every effort should be made to place the patient in a comfortable position." He suggested that the leg casts be made before operation, removed for the execution of the procedure, and reapplied after operation. He concluded, however, that the success of such casts was a questionable matter. In 1942, Padgett [29] stated, "For . . . direct coverage of bone, as following a radical operation for osteomyelitis of the tibia, a skin flap is preferable to a skin graft." He advocated the use of a pedicled flap for wounds of the sole of the foot, in areas where deep tendons were exposed, where bone was denuded and if a joint had been opened. He further advocated such a pedicled flap for areas of deficient blood supply or for areas which must withstand considerable trauma. Morley,[27] in 1942, felt that pedicled flaps were preferable over amputation stumps and

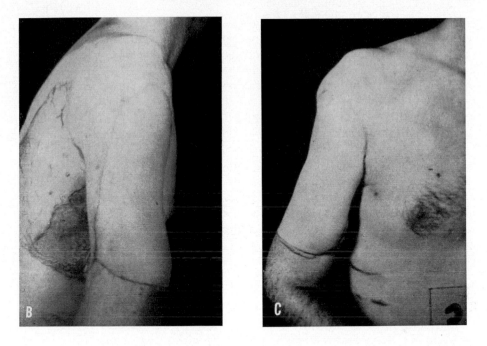

for coverage of areas to be submitted to future operation. D. O. Brown,[6] writing in 1943, stated that he preferred cross-leg flaps to partial-thickness grafts of skin because the latter had a poor chance of success over areas of fibrosis; they were not durable over bone, cartilage and tendons; their contraction militated against the motion of joints; they did not serve as a good operative field for subsequent nerve, tendon and bone operations, and their appearance was "indifferent."

Ghormley and Lipscomb[15] published a report on a series of 33 cross-leg flaps and 15 cross-thigh flaps in 1944. Padgett and Gaskins[31] reported a series of 58 cases of cross-leg flaps in 1945. In 1948, Lewin[20] reported on 33 cross-leg flaps. White[42] transplanted a series of 70 cross-leg flaps directly without preparing the pedicle in stages with a solitary failure. In 1950 Jayes[19] reviewed his series of 60 cross-leg flaps. In 1952 Stark[40] reported upon a series of 43 cross-leg and cross-thigh flaps without a failure. In 1955 Cuthbert[12] reported 9 consecutive cases in which he performed a bone graft in conjunction with the transplantation of a cross-leg flap. The cross-leg and cross-thigh flaps have undergone gradual technical evolution which has led to increased safety in their transplantation. This evolution is evidenced by improvements in the technic of preparation of the pedicle, in choice of the donor site, in design of the pedicle and in the device for postoperative immobilization.

Necrosis following the immediate transplantation of a cross-leg or cross-thigh flap has led to the more cautious plan of preparing the pedicle in two or more preliminary operative stages. This plan allows for augmentation of collateral circulation. Hamilton (1854) [17] according to his historic account, outlined his pedicle in a preparatory operation prior to transplantation. Reich (1917) as quoted by Perthes, [34] advocated outlining the pedicle surgically prior to its transplantation. Perthes (1917) compressed the perimeter of his pedicles between two long darning needles so that collateral circulation was encouraged to flow through the base of the pedicle. The fact that slough of the pedicle (if it were to develop) would be quantitatively less and also more superficial if the flap were outlined in stages, was recognized by Blair [3] in 1921. To this Lexer [21] agreed in 1929. Brown and Cannon, [7] in 1944, suggested that the first outlining of the pedicle should be along two sides with undermining through-and-through, and that the ends should be incised at a second operation. They stated that to outline and undermine a pedicle completely in one procedure was not to delay the flap but to delay the *use* of the flap. Mathews [25] stated in 1943 that he always prepared his pedicle in stages on the lower extremity if the length-to-width ratio was greater than one-to-one. From vascular injection studies on cadavers Stark (1948) [38] concluded that pedicles based on the medial calf, the anterior or medial thigh, possessed the best arteriolar blood supply, and hence had the best chance of success. Technical refinements include those of Macomber and Rubin (1947) [23] who pointed out that the under surface of the base of the pedicle could be converted into a closed wound by surfacing it with a thick-split graft of skin. This represented a significant forward step, since the broad-based flap, which makes it possible to transplant more generous amounts of tissue than the tubed pedicle, now could be executed without the disadvantages of open wounds which required frequent dressing care, and sometimes went on to develop infection. Braithwaite and Moore (1949) [5] covered this exposed under surface of the pedicle by turning back an adjacent flap of normal tissue and suturing it to the raw under surface of the flap. Others have turned back the scar for this purpose.

Technic

Preparation of the Pedicle: The cross-leg flap procedure is one in which every stage is planned in advance. The medial calf and the anteromedial thigh have been shown to be the richest in vascularity. On the medial calf the posterior tibial, the saphenous and the medial inferior geniculate arteries are contributory arteries; the third perforating branch of the deep femoral artery, and the highest geniculate supply the medial and anterior thigh. Also, these areas are the most accessible as donor sites which can afford comfortable cross-leg positions. Without manipulating the extremities into positions of torture, it is possible to transplant a pedicle from the medial calf, or from the anterior and medial thigh to any area of the foot and leg. For cosmetic reasons one is loath to use the calf as a donor site in a female patient. The donor site, which is surfaced with a thick-split skin graft, results in moderate deformity of contour and appearance.

To plan this type of transplantation with precision, one outlines the perimeter of the wound with dye or ink, allowing an ample margin. Then one works backward through the various stages of the transplantation of the pedicle. A pattern of the area to be covered by the distal tip of the pedicle is cut from a transparent material such as vinylite. The greatest vertical measurement of the defect becomes the smallest horizontal dimension of the proposed flap. The edge of the pattern nearest the opposite extremity is extended with gradually increasing width until it reaches the donor leg, when

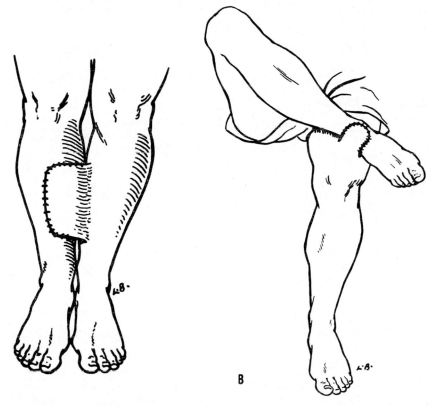

Fig. 7—Illustrations of typical cross-leg flaps. (A) "Book flap" modification of cross-leg procedure where a short, broad pedicle is required. (B) Distally based anterior thigh flap.

the two legs are held in the contemplated juxtaposition. By this technic, one can tell whether or not the defect can be approximated closely enough to the donor calf or thigh to permit the suture of the planned flap to the recipient defect without tension or torsion. The most comfortable position of the patient must be achieved. When one of these areas appears as a likely and comfortable donor site, the proximal half of the pattern is held on the donor area. The recipient limb is abducted and the distal end of the pattern is allowed to fall into position around the partial circumference of the donor leg and is outlined where it comes to rest. The recipient extremity is then put into the proposed cross-leg position, and it can be seen whether or not the distal tip of the pattern of the proposed pedicle will lie on the recipient area without tension. Thus, the shape and size of the defect and the pedicle, as well as the post-operative position of the extremities, are planned prior to the first operative step.

A pedicle from the medial calf will supply comfortably almost any area on the leg or foot, with the possible exception of the posterior leg. This can

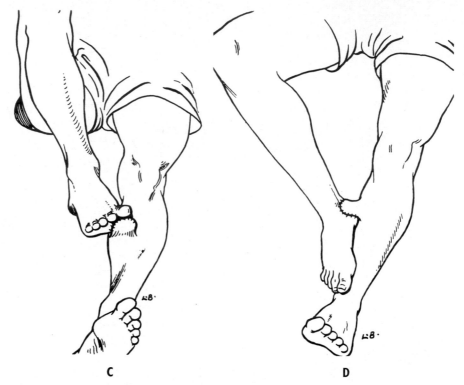

| C | D |

Fig. 7–(C) Distally based medial calf flap. (D) Proximally based pedicle from the medial calf. (Reproduced with permission of R. B. Stark and journal from Plast. and Reconstruct. Surg. 9: 73, 1952.)

be most effectively surfaced with a flap from the anterior thigh. All pedicles from the medial calf can be planned so that their bases are proximal, with the exception of those to the plantar aspect of the foot and to the lateral aspect of the leg. Pedicles from the anterior thigh will comfortably surface the ankle and leg as well as some areas of the foot. Areas to be covered on the posterior leg can be surfaced with proximally based flaps from the thigh, whereas areas to be covered on the anterior leg must be covered with flaps based distally.

Immediate pedicled flaps of limited size can be applied to the foot and leg, but the more conservative procedure is that of delayed transplantation. If the pedicle to be transplanted is as broad as it is long and if it is based proximally, it may be transplanted without preliminary operative preparation. However, if these ideal measurements do not prevail or if the pedicle must be based distally, preparation of the pedicle should be carried out in stages. If it is decided that delayed transfer is to be effected, it is best to outline the pedicle first by two parallel incisions at the sides of the proposed flap, undermining between them. The distal end of the pedicle should not be incised until the second operation. Approximately 10 to 14 days should be allowed between stages.

Migration of the Cross-Leg Flap: At the time of transplantation of the cross-leg flap the defect to be surfaced is the fixed objective, the pedicle has

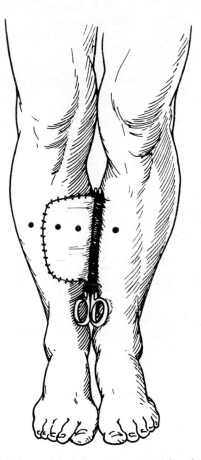

Fig. 8—The blood supply of the pedicled flap is measured by the histamine wheal test. A rubber-shod clamp is applied to the base of the pedicle, and histamine is applied to the scarified areas marked in the drawing. The relative vascularity of the normal leg and that of the pedicle are compared. If a wheal forms as rapidly upon the pedicle tissue as upon the control area, the base of the pedicle may be transected with safety. By the use of this test the period of hospitalization is minimized and the pedicle may be divided at the earliest safe date. (Reproduced with permission of journal from Ann. Surg. 1956, January *143:* 37. Conway and Stark [10].)

been prepared previously by operative incision and suture, and the post-operative position has been determined at the time of selection of the donor site. The flap must be finally migrated from its planned donor site in pre-ordained position to the fixed objective on the opposite extremity. Therefore, with the pattern of movement rigidly determined, the pedicle can be migrated

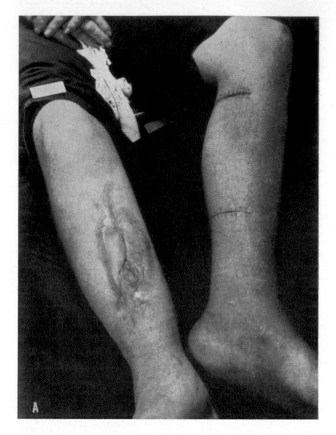

Fig. 9—(A, B and C) Long defect requiring a short, broad pedicle. The "book flap" modification of the cross-leg procedure provides satisfactory cover of this type of defect. (Reproduced with permission of author and journal from Plast. and Reconstruct. Surg. 9: 173, 1952.)

to the opposite extremity. Plaster of Paris is the material of choice with which to immobilize the heavy extremities. The technic for applying this type of immobilization has been described in detail.[39] The author agrees with Padgett and Stephenson [32] who state, "When transferring a flap from one leg to the other the proper application of the cast is really the *sine qua non* of the procedure."

Other technical details pertinent to the transfer of the pedicle should be mentioned. The secondary defect which results from elevation of the pedicle should be surfaced with a free thick-split graft of skin taken preferably from the abdomen rather than from the thigh, so that the dressing to the donor site may not cause embarrassment of the circulation to an extremity. The graft should be secured with a tied-on bolus-type dressing. Sufficient free graft should be taken to close the under surface of the pedicle, so that a completely closed wound is effected. In the transfer, the pedicle should be

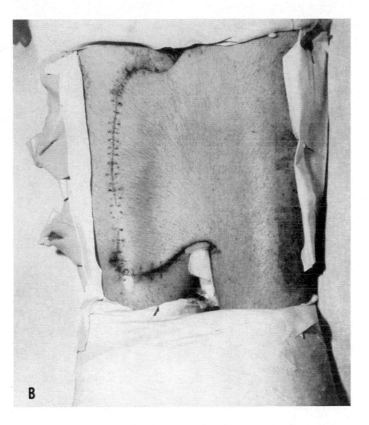

elevated first at its distal end. The color of the pedicle and of the bleeding from the marginal vessels must be observed carefully. Persistent venous bleeding, cyanosis or blanching of the pedicle, ivory-mottled or blue-mottled coloration are indications for the postponement of the transfer (Climo [9]). Usually the patient is uncomfortable for three to five days after operation. The severity of discomfort is directly proportional to the degree of flexion of the knees. Dry heat and massage to the area of the hips may allay local pain and promote the patient's comfort. An ounce of whiskey every four hours will reduce discomfort in older patients. Vasodilators such as Priscoline or papaverine may be of aid. If the immobilization device is suspended from a Balkan frame with counterweights, the patient can move about in the bed with relative ease. After a week's time, the patient may be allowed in a wheelchair for short periods, care being taken that the legs are horizontal rather than dependent. He may use the toilet with the casts extended horizontally onto the seat of his wheel chair. Chemotherapy is maintained throughout the period of transfer. Cross-leg flaps which exhibit any of the signs of circulatory embarrassment may be aided by the passive vascular exercise afforded by the use of the oscillating bed.

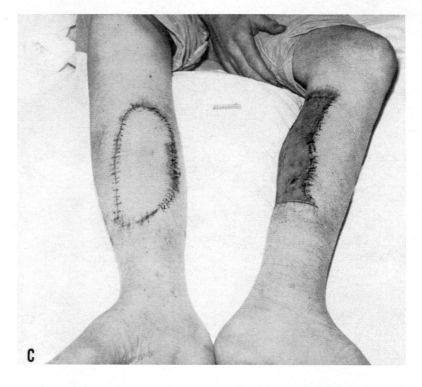

Severance of the Cross-leg Flap: Plastic surgeons wait for varying periods of time between transfer and severance of the pedicle. By experience, it is known that three weeks is sufficient time for establishment of adequate circulation between the recipient area and tip of the pedicle. Usually, the base of the pedicle can be severed safely at that time, but this is not always true. In many instances, the pedicle can be severed sooner. To reduce the number of hospital days and to preclude the danger of detaching a pedicle before it is capable of survival in its new location, a number of tests have been described to evaluate the efficiency of the circulation. Of all of these, I find the histamine wheal test [11] which R. B. Stark, D. Joslin and I originated the most practical. A rubber-shod clamp is used to tourniquet the pedicle at its base. The test consists of applying histamine to scarified areas on the pedicled tissue and on the legs adjacent. Appearance of a wheal in eight minutes indicates vascular sufficiency. This test helps the surgeon choose the earliest time which is safe for detachment of the pedicle. Partial severance of the pedicle at successive intervals is a conservative method of handling the problem, but has the disadvantage of loss of time and additional

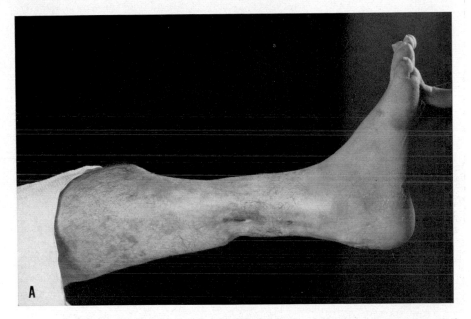

Fig. 10—Atrophic conditions of lower leg with annular scar following débridement and the inadvertent removal of the middle third of the tibia. (A and B) Patient was casualty in the Korean Conflict.

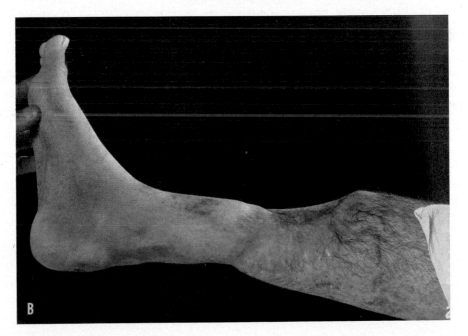

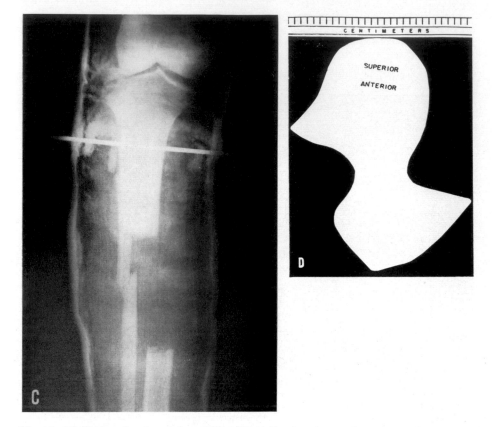

Fig. 10–(C) X-Ray showing defect to the tibia following the overly-zealous débridement of bone. (D) Pattern of the extent of the scar tissue which indicated that it was necessary to transplant a section of tissue measuring 20 cm. in one direction and 34 cm. in the other.

trips to the operating room. Once the base has been severed, the flap must be set into the damaged extremity. If more than minimal trimming of the pedicle is necessary, it is safer to do this several days after severance.

Massage and dry heat applied to the joints which have been immobilized will minimize disability. Ambulation should be started progressively, but only after application to both extremities of tailored elastic stockings. The patient should wear this external support for one year following surgery. Until full sensation returns to the pedicle and to the free graft on the donor site, these transplants should be protected from extremes of heat and cold.

Mustarde Flap

In the management of defects of extremities of the leg, the ingenious flap developed by Mustarde has been found to be very useful. By this technic a broad-based flap is attached to the forearm and, by the use of free grafts, a pocket-like cavity is developed underneath the large block of tissue to be

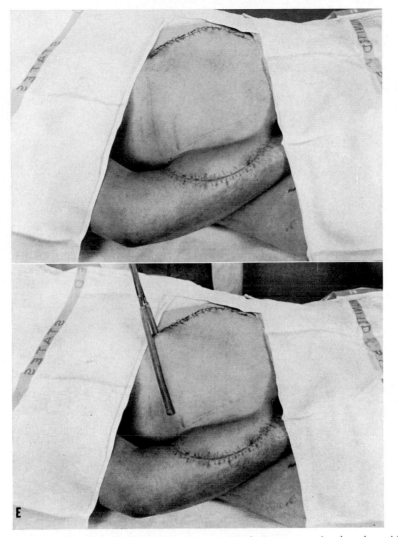

Fig. 10 (E) *Top.* The necessarily generous amount of tissue was developed rapidly by the technique of the Mustardé flap. This first-stage operation shows the outlined tissue attached by wicket-shaped flap to the forearm. The planned transplant has been isolated by dissection of the skin and subcutaneous fat from the abdominal fascia. At this first operation, skin grafts were applied to the fascia and also to the fat on the underside of the flap so that the sutured incision buries a broad cutaneous pocket. Bottom. As an adjunct to the rapid development of collateral circulation from the arm, rubber-shod clamps are inserted for thirty minutes three or four times a day.

migrated. The details of the flap—which represents the height of achievement as far as rapidity of transfer and surface area of pedicled tissue are concerned—are brought out in the case which is illustrated in figure 10.

Results: In a previous report, R. B. Stark and I[10] recorded 78 cases in which cross-leg flaps had been employed to provide adequate soft-tissue

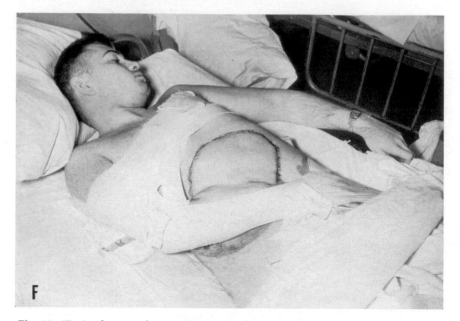

Fig. 10—(F) At the second operation, incisions were made to further outline the flap.

coverage for the lower leg and foot. Seventy-six of these flaps were successful. The two failures were due to improper inset of the flap and to infection, respectively. Forty-three of these cases were the original cases of Stark.[40] I now report that reconstructions of the lower leg have been carried out in a total of 92 cases. Success was achieved in 90 of these, the failures being the two reported previously and referred to above. This is the method of choice for the correction of the usual post-traumatic scarred defects of the lower leg in preparation for definitive surgery on the bones. More extensive procedures such as the Mustarde flap are required for problems involving larger areas.

Summary

The principles of the management of wounds of soft tissue of the extremities have been set down. The importance of the management of the wounds of soft tissue in cases with associated fractures (open fractures) is emphasized. In complicated cases of nonunion with infection or scarring, adequate coverage with skin and subcutaneous tissue is necessary before bone grafting or other reconstructive surgery can be undertaken. In order to transplant such tissue, a pedicled flap is necessary. Details of the technic of transplantation of tissue to a lower extremity by the cross-leg flap technic as well as by other transplantation procedures are described.

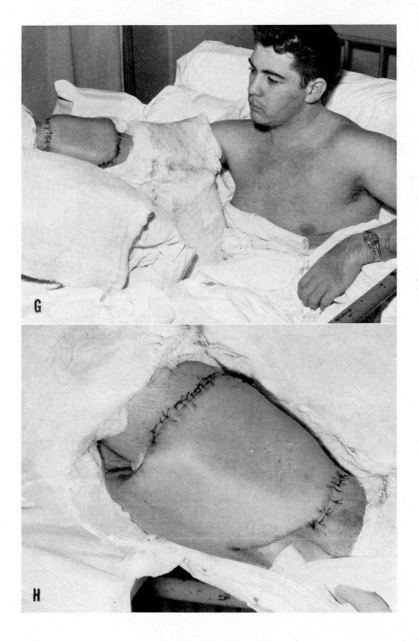

Fig. 10—(G) At the third operation the flap is elevated from the abdomen, migrated to the lower leg and sutured into the leg following excision of the scar. (H) Close-up view of the flap showing its inset into the leg.

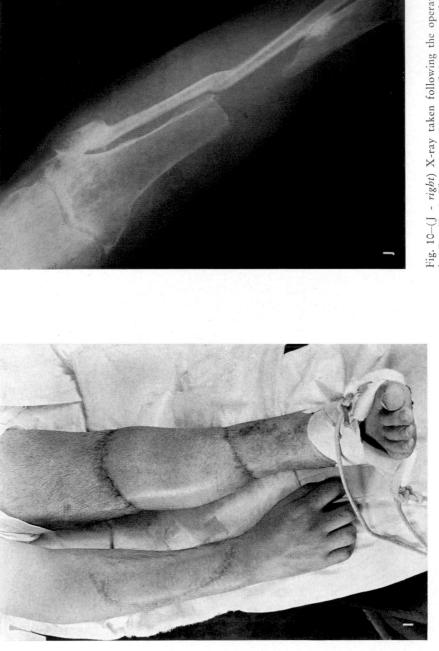

Fig. 10—(J - *right*) X-ray taken following the operation performed by Dr. T. C. Thompson, Director of Surgery at the Hospital For Special Surgery. Synostoses of the upper and lower fragments of the tibia to the fibula were carried out. This orthopedic procedure was successful and the patient has been walking on the leg for the past three years. The Mustarde flap made it possible to reconstruct this leg by reason of the fact that it allowed for the transfer of a very generous amount of tissue in a limited period of time and with a limited number of operative procedures (five in all).

Fig. 10—(I - *left*) Appearance of the transplanted tissue following its inset over the lower extremity. Note that the forearm which served as a carrier shows only a curved scar as a result of this technic.

References

1 BARKER, D. E.: Vacutome-a new machine for obtaining split thickness skin grafts. Plast. & Reconstruct. Surg. *3*: 492—501, 1948.

2 BILLROTH, R.: Die allgemeine chirurgische Pathologie und Therapie. Berlin, 1863.

8 CELSUS, A. C.: The delayed transfer of long pedicle flaps in plastic surgery. Surg. Gynec. & Obst. *33*: 261—272, 1921.

4 BLOCKER, T. G., Jr. et al.: Microbiological and histological studies in wound healing. Presentation before American Association of Plastic Surgeons Meeting, Dallas, Texas, May 23, 1958.

5 BRAITHWAITE, F., and MOORE, F. T.: Skin grafting by cross-leg flaps. J. Bone & Joint Surg. *31 B*: 228—235, 1949.

6 BROWN, D. O.: Repair of limb wounds by the use of direct skin flaps. Brit. J. Surg. *30*: 307—314, 1943.

7 BROWN, J. B., and CANNON, B.: The repair of surface defects of the foot. Ann. Surg. *120*: 417—430, 1944.

3 CELSUS, A. C.: De Medicina, etc., 1750. (Found in Davis — Plastic Surgery — p. 10.)

9 CLIMO, S.: Dermal bleeding and delay operation. Plast. & Reconstruct. Surg. *8*: 59—63, 1951.

10 CONWAY, H., and STARK, R. B.: Soft tissue coverage for injuries to the foot and leg. Ann. Surg. *143*: 37—48, 1956.

11 —, and JOSLIN, D.: Cutaneous histamine reaction as a test of circulatory efficiency of tubed pedicles and flaps. Surg. Gynec. & Obst. *93*: 185—189, 1951.

12 CUTHBERT, J. B.: The "marsupial" skin flap. Brit. J. Plast. Surg. *2*: 125—131, 1949.

13 DAVIS, J. S.: Plastic Surgery. Philadelphia, Blakiston Co., 1919, p. 693.

14 FILATOV, W. P.: Plastike na Kruglem Ctebe. Vestnik oftalmologii, Nos. 4—5, 1917.

15 GHORMLEY, R. K., and LIPSCOMB, P. R.: The use of untubed pedicle grafts in the repair of deep defects of the foot and ankle. J. Bone & Joint Surg. *26*: 483—488, 1944.

16 GILLIES, H. D.: The tubed pedicle in plastic surgery. New York J. Med. *III*: 1—4, 1920.

17 HAMILTON, F. H.: Elkoplasty or Anaplasty Applied to the Treatment of Old Ulcers. New York, Holman, Gray and Co., 1854.

18 IMRE, J., Jr.: New principles in plastic operations of the eyelids and face. J.A.M.A. *76*: 1293—1297, 1921.

19 JAYES, P. H.: Cross-leg flaps: A review of sixty cases. Brit. J. Plast. Surg. *3*: 1—5, 1950.

20 LEWIN, M. L.: Resurfacing procedures in compound injuries of lower extremities. Ann. Surg. *128*: 66—79, 1948.

21 LEXER, E.: Lehrbuch der Allgemeinen Chirurgie, Verlag von Ferdinand Erika in, Stuttgart, *I*: 123, 1929.

22 MAAS, H.: Über Plastik mit frischen gestielten Lappen aus entfernteren Koerpertheilen, Arch. klin. Chir. *31*: 559—589, 1885.

23 MACOMBER, W. B., and RUBIN, L. R.: Late repair of massive tissue defects by split skin-lined flap grafts. Am. J. Surg. *73*: 564—567, 1947.

24 MANCHOT, D.: Die Hautarterien des menschlichen Körpers. Leipzig, F. C. W. Bogel, 1889.

25 MATHEWS, D. N.: The Surgery of Repair. Springfield, Ill. Charles C Thomas, 1943, p. 143.

26 MELOY, W. C., and LETTERMAN, G. S.: The Electro-Dermatome. Plast. & Reconstruct. Surg. *6*: 84—87, 1950.

27 MORLEY, G. H.: Cooperation with orthopedic surgery. Proc. Roy. Soc. Med. *35*: 762—763, 1942.

28 NELATON, C., and L. OMBREDANNE: Les Autoplasties. Paris, G. Steinheil, 1907.

29 PADGETT, E. C.: Skin Grafting. Springfield, Ill., Charles C Thomas, 1942.

30 —: The calibrated skin graft — a new principle and a new type of graft. Surg. Gynec. & Obst. *69*: 779—793, 1939.

[31] —, and GASKINS, J. H.: The use of skin flaps in the repair of scarred or ulcerative defects over bone and tendons. Surgery *18*: 287—289, 1945.

[32] —, and STEPHENSON, K. L.: Plastic and Reconstructive Surgery. Springfield, Ill., Charles C Thomas, 1948, p. 777.

[33] PARE, A.: Oeuvres Completes d'Ambroise Pare. Paris, J. B. Bailliere, 1840.

[34] PERTHES, G.: Lappenvorbereitung in situ. Ein neuer Weg zur Bildung langer plastischer Lappen ohne Gefahr der Nekrose. Zentralbl. Chir. *44*: 641—644, 1917.

[35] REESE, J. D.: Dermatape: a new method for management of split-skin grafts. Plast. & Reconstruct. Surg. *1*: 98—105, 1946.

[36] REID, M. R.: Some considerations of the problems of wound healing. New England J. Med. *215*: 753—766, 1936.

[37] —, and CARTER, B. N.: The treatment of fresh traumatic wounds. Ann. Surg. *114*: 4—18, 1941.

[38] STARK, R. B.: Blood supply of cross-leg pedicle flaps. Plast. & Reconstruct. Surg. *3*: 694—699, 1948.

[39] —: Pre-operatively applied, mated, plaster of Paris casts as an aid in the migration of open-pedicle cross-leg flaps. Plast. & Reconstruct. Surg. *2*: 433—438, 1947.

[40] —: The cross-leg flap procedure. Plast. & Reconstruct. Surg. *9*: 173—204, 1952.

[41] Rueta, J.: Principles and Practice of War Surgery. St. Louis, C. V. Mosby Co., 1943.

[42] WHITE, M. F.: Personal communication.

CHAPTER 48

INJURIES OF THE ANKLE

Robert L. Patterson, Jr., M.D. and Paul W. Braunstein, M.D.

The ankle plays a most important role in weight-bearing and walking. In the spectrum of injury patterns the joint is subjected to many variations of stress which lead to many different types of fractures. Injuries to the ankle may vary from very minor ones, such as sprains, to more serious types, such as comminuted, displaced fractures. There are, however, several types of injuries which are most commonly encountered, and the diagnosis and treatment of these will be emphasized in this chapter.

Ankle Fractures in Children

True displaced ankle fractures are extremely rare. Much more commonly one encounters separation of the distal tibial epiphysis caused by acute trauma.

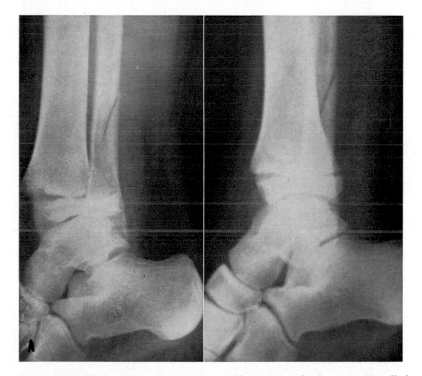

Fig. 1—(A) A distal tibial epiphyseal separation with posterior displacement is well demonstrated (*left*). On the right, postreduction films reveal adequate restoration of anatomical continuity. The oblique fracture of the fibula remains undisplaced both before and after reduction.

Figure 1 A (lt.) illustrates such an injury with posterior displacement of the distal tibial epiphysis at the epiphyseal line. There is also a longitudinal oblique fracture of the fibula. Figure 1 A (rt.) reveals perfect anatomic reposition, the reduction having been obtained by closed means with traction

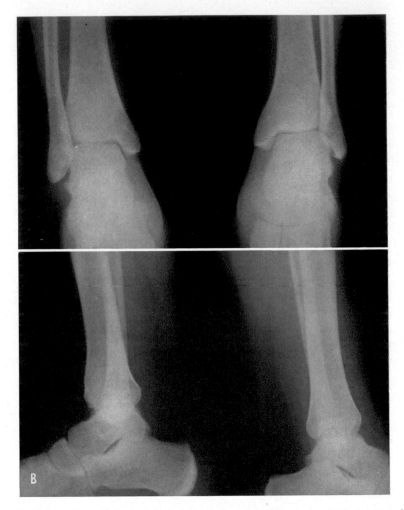

Fig. 1—(B) Restoration of the epiphyseal separation has been accomplished. Growth lines are normal and no disturbed anatomy has resulted.

and dorsiflexion. Figure 1 B, taken several years later, demonstrates that there is no gross anatomic change in the ankle joint. Aitken has demonstrated that the classical horizontal epiphyseal injury seldom leads to any serious gross disturbance. It is rather the vertical or perpendicular epiphyseal injury that traverses the epiphyseal line which can lead to gross disturbances at a later date, with changes in the normal weight-bearing or carrying angle of the extremity. Malleolar fractures in children are rare. When these injuries are sustained, the child is normally considered a young adult and is treated accordingly.

Ankle Injuries in the Adult

Sprain

The usual sprain is incurred by an inversion type of injury with tearing of the fibulocalcaneal ligaments. The severity of this injury can vary from the very minor sprain in which there is simply pain and slight swelling, to one which completely disables the patient. Treatment consists of immobilization according to the degree of injury suffered. A very minor sprain is amply immobilized by simple Ace bandaging or by strapping. More serious injuries without bony damage or loss in integrity of the ankle mortise should be immobilized for a period of four to six weeks either by posterior splinting or by a walking cast. Immobilization should be continued until pain, swelling and disability have subsided. It has not been our practice to inject procaine into sprained ankles and to permit the patient to return to normal activity. We feel, rather, that the sprain will heal more firmly and more satisfactorily if the injured part is rested until the ligaments have repaired by fibrous

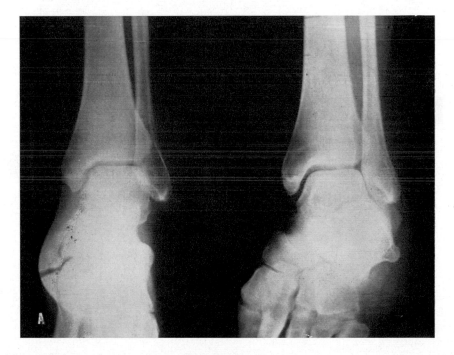

Fig. 2—(A) Here normal AP films and internal rotation films fail to reveal any soft tissue or bony abnormality.

union. Figure 2 A exhibits AP and slight internal rotation views of the ankle with a perfectly normal appearing mortise. There is some slight increase in the soft tissue shadow over the lateral malleolus. However, inversion stress films (fig. 2 B) reveal definite tilt of the talus which must be due to fairly severe and complete injury of the fibulocalcaneal ligaments traversing the lateral aspect of the ankle. The usual treatment of this injury is immobilization without operative intervention. Immobilization must be complete and must

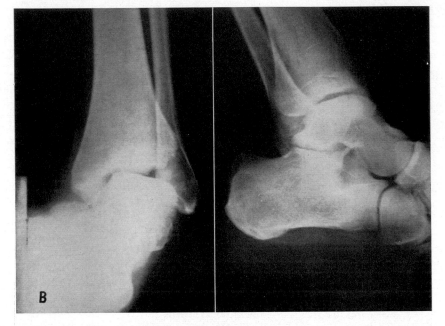

Fig. 2—(B) An inversion stress film of the ankle demonstrated in figure 2 A reveals weakness of the fibulotalar ligaments with inward rocking of the talus and therefore instability of the ankle joint.

be maintained for a period of 12 weeks. If the injury is diagnosed immediately, operative repair of the torn lateral collateral ligaments can be performed.

Fractures of the Ankle in Adults

A first degree fracture of the ankle is usually characterized by a break of one of the component bones of the joint without displacement or tear of associated ligaments. In the most common injury, fracture of the lateral malleolus, an eversion or external rotation type of injury usually causes an oblique rotation fracture of the fibula. There may be slight backward displacement of the distal fragment with the minimal angulation at this site. There is no widening of the ankle mortise, nor is there any tenderness, swelling or deformity of the uninjured medial malleolus. The medial malleolus can occasionally be fractured by direct trauma without displacement of this bone fragment. However, lateral malleolar injuries usually involve minimal talar displacement and resulting impairment of the normal ankle mortise. The usual treatment for undisplaced ankle fractures is first to ascertain by x-ray and physical examination whether there is no more serious injury with loss of the mortise and tenon relationship of the ankle. Should the injury prove to be a severe single malleolar fracture, a short leg cast and immobilization for a period of seven to ten days without weight-bearing is perfectly satisfactory. If the injury is of a lesser degree of severity, immediate weight-bearing in a walking plaster may be permitted. In the severe case, after the period of immobilization without weight-bearing there is a six week period of immobilization in a walking plaster and finally removal of the plaster and immediate unprotected weight-bearing. Almost all types of these injuries are amenable to this therapy and almost all will heal with excellent results. No operative intervention is indicated in such injuries.

Second Degree Injuries

Second degree injuries of the ankle include such fractures as bimalleolar fractures, fractures of the lateral malleolus with associated deltoid ligament tears, and trimalleolar fractures. All these injuries are characterized by involvement of the normal tibiotalar relationships with consequent disruption of the mortise and tenon joint of the ankle and widening of joint space. Severe consequences may result from lack of correction of this abnormality of the ankle joint and are of utmost importance in the final recovery of the patient. A joint which heals with a widened mortise will certainly lead to an unstable ankle and will go on to a classical traumatic arthritis of the ankle joint. Figure 3 A reveals a bimalleolar fracture with loss of the normal tibiotalar relationships. The medial malleolus has been displaced laterally, the tibial plafond is no longer resting on the gently curved articular surface of the talus. Note, as well, that the lateral malleolar fragment is displaced laterally. Such classic malleolar fractures are seldom associated with severe muscle or nerve injuries, but the amount of hemorrhage accompanying them can present a problem. Therefore, it is most important to care for the soft tissue by wrapping them adequately with pressure bandages as soon as the patient has been examined and x-rayed. Application of ice packs and elevation of the extremity until definite therapy can be carried out are rules. Should bleb formation take place, there is always a serious possibility that a closed fracture may be converted to an open one owing to skin necrosis. Bimalleolar fractures are frequently amenable to closed reduction. The reduction must be carried out under general anesthesia with the patient completely relaxed so that muscular spasm does not interfere with the achievement of adequate reduction. Whether closed or open, reduction must be perfect. Complete restoration of the normal ankle anatomy is essential and any procedure must be directed towards this end. In figure 3 A, the previously described bimalleolar fracture is shown following primary closed reduction. There has

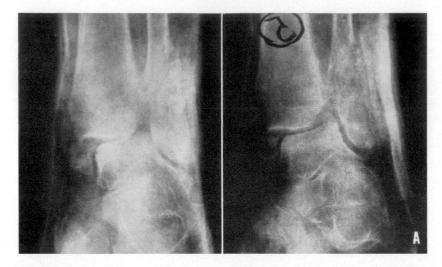

Fig. 3–(A) Following an attempt at reduction, there is complete loss of the normal mortise and tendon relationship in this ankle joint. Such a result, if left uncorrected, will be disastrous to future function in the ankle joint.

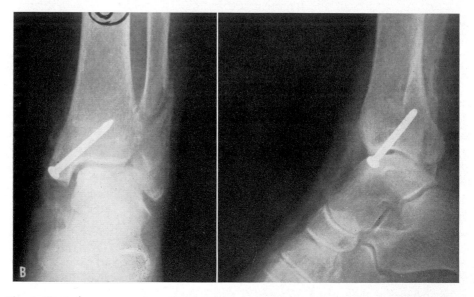

Fig. 3–(B) A fracture poorly reduced such as in figure 3 A has been adequately reduced by open reduction and internal fixation. One medial malleolar screw has restored the normal ankle anatomy and has led to an adequate anatomic and functional result.

been loss of the adequate reduction with lateral displacement of the talus, a situation which would certainly lead to serious dysfunction at a later date. Figure 3 B shows that this displacement has been corrected by the use of a medial malleolar screw. Note that the normal relationship of the tibia with the talus has been corrected, though there is slight loss of normal anatomical continuity of the fibula. A Collison screw placed through the medial malleolus via a very small curvilinear medial incision has adequately reduced the ankle and will hold it until healing can occur. Figure 4 A illustrates a rotation type of injury of the ankle with a bimalleolar fracture. There is lateral displacement of the medial malleolus and lateral and posterior displacement of the lateral malleolus. Closed reduction of this fracture led to adequate realignment of the fracture fragments, as can be seen in figure 4 B. However, figure 4 C, taken seven days later, shows that there is again inferior displacement of the medial malleolus, slight lateral displacement of

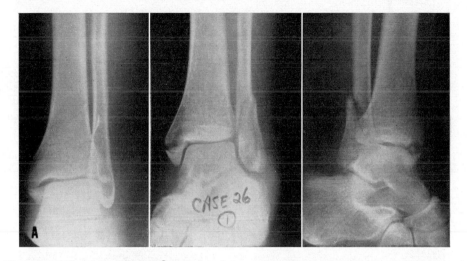

Fig. 4—(A) Here a rotational bimalleolar fracture has led to distraction and slight lateral displacement of the talus and attached malleolar fragments.

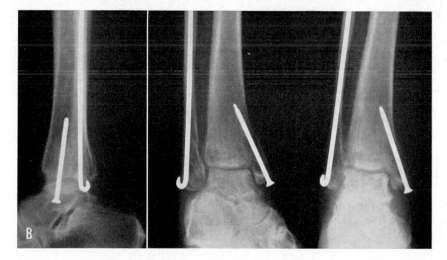

Fig. 4—(B) Closed reduction has returned the ankle to normal anatomic alignment.

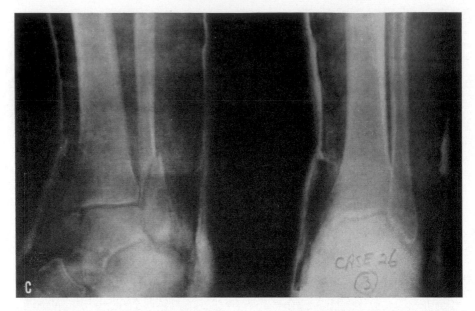

Fig. 4–(C) Seven days later, despite external plaster immobilization, displacement of the medial malleolus distally and displacement of the lateral malleolus laterally has occurred.

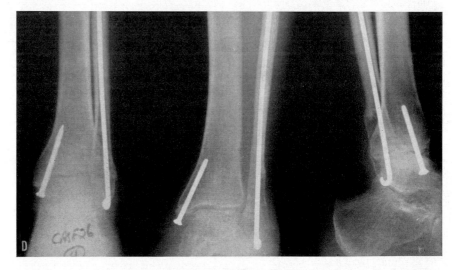

Fig. 4–(D) Operative reduction has restored the medial and lateral malleolus fragments to their normal position.

the lateral malleolus and slight shift of the talus laterally. This was considered completely unacceptable and operative reduction was carried out, placing a Collison screw through the medial malleolus and a Rush pin up the fibula to insure fixation of this rather unstable fracture, as shown in figure 4 D. It has been our policy to attempt closed reduction. If the closed reduction has been carefully observed to assure that no shift has occurred from the fifth to the twenty-first day, when the plaster may loosen because of the loss of edema or of excessive movement of the leg and ankle, then fibrous and bony union may occur without complication. Should closed reduction prove unsatisfactory, open reduction is immediately undertaken, with internal fixation, usually by Collison screw fixation of the malleolus with or without accompanying Rush pin fixation of the lateral malleolus. This rather recent innovation has led to marked stabilization of the fracture site so that actually the period of external plaster immobilization has been markedly shortened. While, in the past, external immobilization associated with Collison screw fixation or closed reduction was maintained as long as twelve weeks, the addition of Rush pin fixation has decreased the period of immobilization

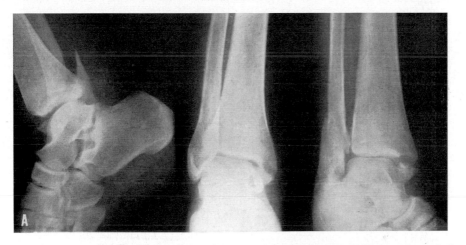

Fig. 5—(A) Here a bimalleolar fracture has occurred with moderate displacement of the medial malleolus but marked displacement of the lateral malleolar.

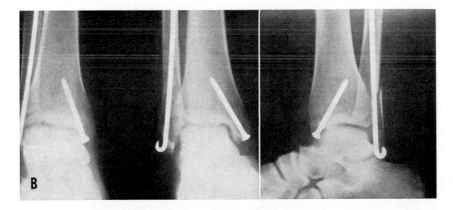

Fig. 5—(B) More adequate and stable reduction in this fracture was obtained by both medial malleolar Collison screw fixation and lateral malleolar Rush pin fixation. Note the return of normal lateral malleolar anatomy by Rush pin fixation.

to a point where six or eight weeks, or even four weeks, have proven satisfactory for complete stabilization of this injury. Figure 5 A demonstrates a
case of rather marked displacement of the lateral malleolus which was not
completely corrected by simple medial malleolar screw fixation. Accordingly,
Rush pin fixation was performed, placing the lateral malleolus in a much
more favorable anatomic position and leading to a more rapid recovery of
the patient to complete weight-bearing and full function (fig. 5 B). It should
be stressed that whether closed or open reduction is utilized, the patient must
be observed frequently and carefully for signs of "slipping" of the fracture

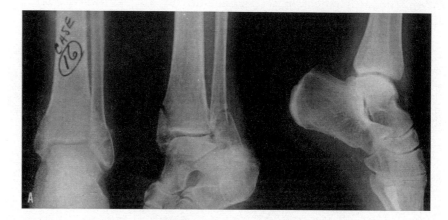

Fig. 6–(A) This bimalleolar fracture is minimally displaced laterally; hence closed reduction
seemed feasible.

fragments to their original position of displacement. Should "slipping" of
a fracture go unnoticed until healing has occurred, it may be necessary to
resort to osteotomy to correct this malunion, or the patient may go on to
eventual traumatic arthritis and a useless, painful ankle. Figure 6 A demonstrates a laterally displaced talus in a bimalleolar fracture. Closed
reduction of this fracture was considered adequate, as noted in figure 6 B
which shows good alignment of the tibial plafond and the talus. The external
malleolus also appears well aligned. Figure 6 C shows that two months later,
however, because the patient had received infrequent roentgenographic examinations, the talus had shifted laterally, had become tilted and was no
longer in alignment with the tibia. It was necessary to correct this malalignment operatively by using screw and plate fixation of the fibula to
the tibia following mobilization of the medial malleolus by means of medial
incision. The final result reveals a four-hole plate holding the fibula in
place with return of normal tibiotalar relationships (fig. 6 D). This extensive
surgery could have been avoided had the patient been adequately observed
and open reduction carried out as soon as "slipping" had occurred.

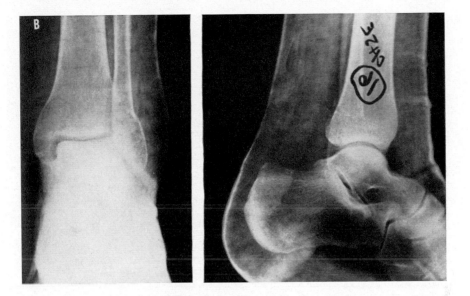

Fig. 6—(B) Closed reduction and external plaster fixation has produced a very adequate realignment of the tibial plafond and talus.

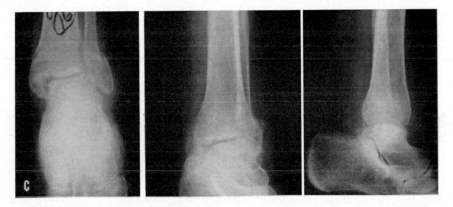

Fig. 6—(C) Two months later, after a period of relatively infrequent observation, the talar tilt and lateral displacement has recurred.

Another second degree injury of note is rupture of the deltoid ligament occurring with a lateral malleolar fracture. The most important point to be stressed in the diagnosis and care of this injury is that these injuries can be missed in routine examination if stress films are not procured. If the patient exhibits medial malleolar tenderness or swelling, if there is any deformity of the ankle or if there is suspicious widening of the joint space between the medial malleolus and the talus, one should always take stress films, with eversion and lateral stress being placed on the foot and ankle while the leg

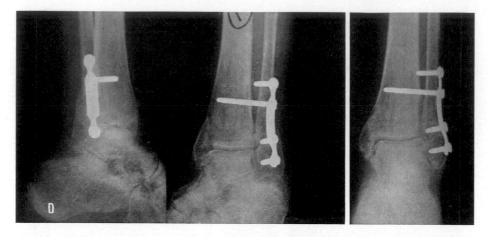

Fig. 6–(D) Plate and screw fixation have realigned this relatively neglected fracture. More careful observation by x-ray may have prevented this large amount of surgery.

has stress placed on it medially. Figure 7 A demonstrates a deltoid ligament tear with marked displacement of the talus laterally. Figure 7 B shows that following operative reduction and plaster of Paris immobilization, the talus has returned to the normal tibiotalar relationship, and that there is no widening of the joint space. We have resorted to operative reduction of these injuries because with closed reduction we can seldom be clinically certain that there is not some incarceration of fragments of the deeper portions of the deltoid ligament into the tibiotalar portion of the ankle joint. Accordingly, we have resorted to primary open reduction in many instances of complete

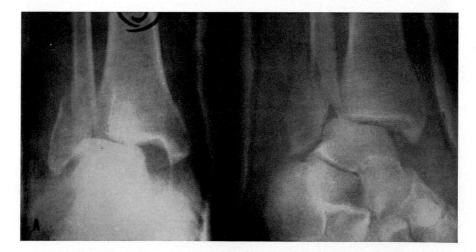

Fig. 7–(A) Despite an attempt at reduction, the laterally displaced talus has remained because the tear of the deltoid ligament has led to instability and this has not been corrected prior to immobilization.

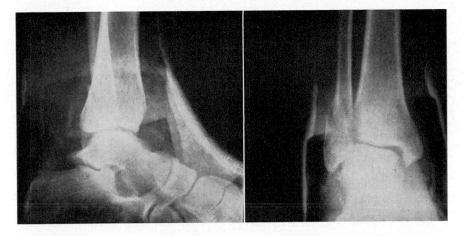

Fig. 7—(B) Operative reduction with suture of the deltoid ligament and external plaster immobilization has led to return of normal ankle anatomy.

tear of the deltoid ligament. It should be stressed that it is extremely easy to overlook deltoid ligament tears, as demonstrated in figure 8 A. The usual ankle views taken at the time of injury reveal a low lateral malleolar fracture with a suggestion of lateral displacement of the talus but no obvious loss of the anatomic relationships of the ankle. However, stress films (fig. 8 B) reveal a rather marked tilt of the talus as well as complete loss of the integrity of the deltoid ligament with widening of the joint space between the medial malleolus and the talus. The stress film establishes the diagnosis and gives adequate indications for necessary therapy.

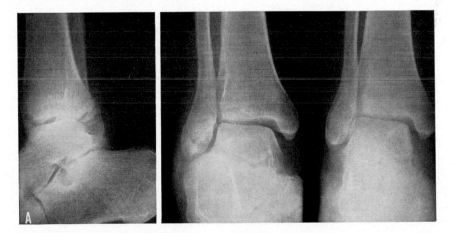

Fig. 8—(A) Normal ankle roentgenograms taken on a patient following injury reveal a lateral malleolar fracture but no grossly displaced medial malleolar fracture or loss of normal tibiotalar relationship.

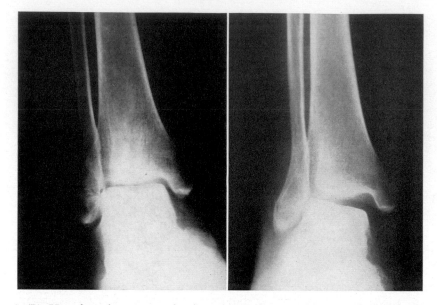

Fig. 8–(B) Here lateral stress on the foot and medial stress upon the fibula reveals a talar tilt and widening of the tibiotalar interval, diagnostic of deltoid ligament rupture.

Trimalleolar fractures are defined as those fractures of the ankle in which the medial malleolus and lateral malleolus are fractured; in addition, the posterior lip of the tibia is fractured and displaced upward and posteriorly. These fractures are more serious than others because the posterior dislocation of the talus is extremely difficult to handle without adequate replacement of the posterior lip of the tibia. In a recent series of 57 trimalleolar fractures studied by us, only 11 required posterior lip fixation because of the majority of the posterior lip fragments comprised less than one-third of the tibial articular surface. If the posterior lip fragment was more than one-third of the articular plate, it was frequently adequately reduced either by closed reduction, or by open reduction when fixation of the medial malleolus and lateral malleolus was carried out. With trimalleolar fractures, displacement can be of extreme degree. Figure 9 A reveals complete posterior dislocation of the talus on the tibia with a relatively small posterior lip fragment. Figure 9 B shows that though operative reduction was carried out, the posterior lip of the tibia was not fixed, simple medial malleolar and lateral fixation proving adequate to return the talus to its normal anatomic position. Even though closed reduction is attempted in a great many trimalleolar fractures with marked displacement, we frequently resort to open reduction to assure anatomic restoration of the joint. Figure 10 A demonstrates a tri-malleolar fracture with a larger posterior lip fragment. Again there is posterior displacement of the talus on the tibia, and in this case the surgeon carried out reduction by internally fixing the posterior lip fragment of the tibia, as shown in figure 10 B. There was complete restoration of the normal

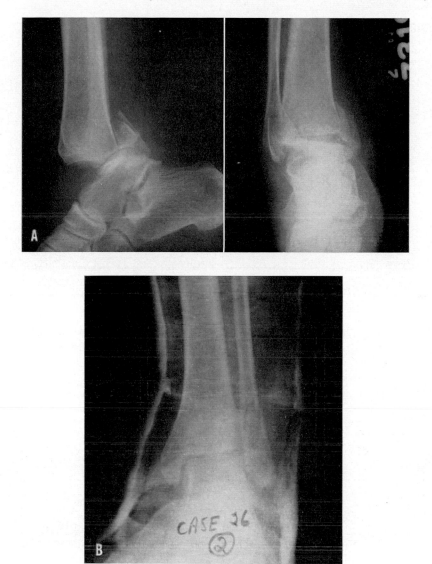

Fig. 9—(A) Trimalleolar fractures, even with small posterior lip fragments, may exhibit posterior dislocation of the talus because lateral and posterior displacement may occur permitting the talus to dislocate without actual large loss of posterior tibial articular surface.
Fig. 9—(B) Though posterior dislocation of the talus has occurred, the posterior lip fragment is small. Therefore, adequate reduction of the medial and lateral malleoli has led to normal tibiotalar relationships. The small posterior lip fragment is inconsequential in determining the final result.

anatomy of the ankle joint, and though osteoporosis of disuse is evident in the postreduction film, the normal anatomy has been restored.

Our approach to trimalleolar fractures is first to attempt closed reduction. Should perfect reduction not be obtained, we resort very early to open

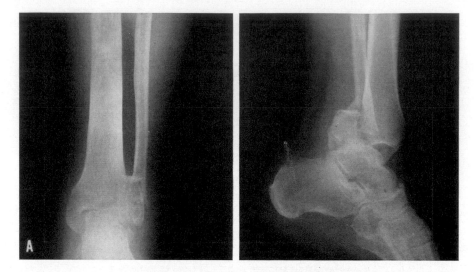

Fig. 10—(A) A large posterior lip fragment is demonstrated associated with posterior talar dislocation.

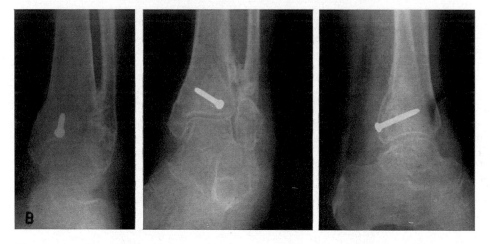

Fig. 10—(B) Here perfect anatomy has been restored by simple posterior lip fixation. Should one-third or more of the posterior tibial articulation be fractured and displaced, adequate reduction by closed or open methods is mandatory.

reduction with internal fixation. The usual type of reduction employed in treatment of the fracture is demonstrated by figure 11 A and B. Figure 11 A shows a trimalleolar fracture with a large posterior lip fragment which has been displaced upwards. There is mild, slight, posterior dislocation of the talus on the tibia. This amount of dislocation, while not strikingly evident, is completely unacceptable. The talus must be placed into its normal anatomic position to prevent very serious consequences in the near or distant future. In this case classical reduction has been carried out with internal fixation of the posterior lip and the medial malleolus by Collison screw fixation, as demonstrated in figure 11 B.

Though it is seldom employed, another method is used in those injuries where either a closed or an open procedure is incapable of producing normal reduction of the ankle. Figure 12 A reveals a markedly comminuted, displaced

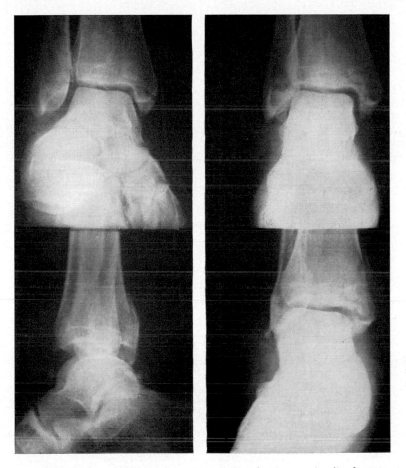

Fig. 11—(A) The lateral view in this fracture reveals a large posterior lip fracture (approximately one-third of the tibial articular surface). Note there is minimal but very definite posterior talar subluxation.

trimalleolar fracture of the ankle. It was impossible to reduce this fracture by closed reduction, and because of poor skin condition, open reduction could not be attempted. Accordingly, os calcis traction by the use of a Kirschner wire was carried out with very satisfactory reduction of the fragments, as shown in figure 12 B. Though some posterior displacement of the distal portion of the lateral malleolus remains, a perfectly satisfactory tibiotalar relationship has been maintained by the use of traction; figure 12 C reveals

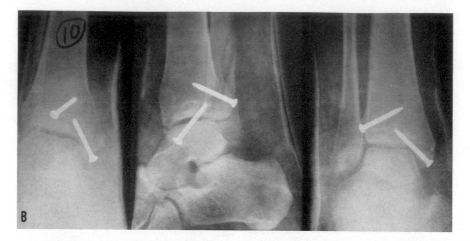

Fig. 11—(B) Perfect anatomical continuity has been restored by medial malleolar and posterior malleolar screw fixation. While displacement in this case was minimal, perfect replacement of the posterior lip was again essential.

normal restoration of the ankle joint following removal of the os calcis traction six weeks later. We have seldom resorted to this procedure in treating ankle fractures, but it is one which can frequently be of great use should more conservative methods fail to achieve adequate reduction, or should the general condition of the patient prevent any operative intervention. Tibiofibular diastasis, that is, fractures or injuries of the ankle which involve tear of the tibiofibular ligaments with extreme widening of the tibiofibular interval, have been encountered only occasionally in our series of cases treated in The New York Hospital. The usual reduction in a closed fracture

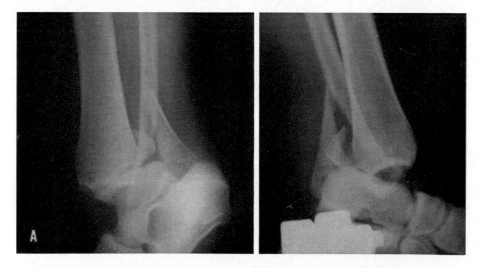

Fig. 12—(A) Here is demonstrated a severely displaced trimalleolar fracture with a small posterior lip.

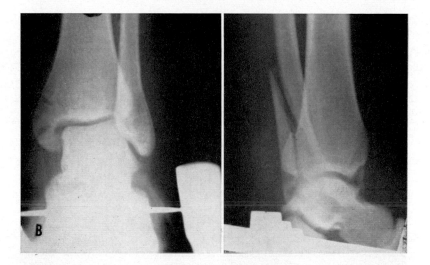

Fig. 12–(B) Os calcis traction by the use of Kirschner wire has restored relatively normal tibiotalar continuity.

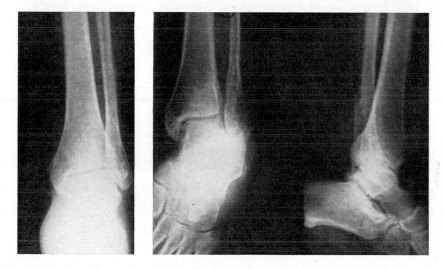

Fig. 12–(C) Several months later, following removal of all traction devices, a normal ankle has been obtained with a very satisfactory result.

of this type, using external plaster mobilization, has been satisfactory to reduce the spread of the tibia and fibula caused by loss of the tibiofibular ligament distally. Occasionally, screw or bolt fixation of the tibia to the fibula is necessary. Because the talus is wide anteriorly and narrow posteriorly, it is imperative that during tightening of the tibiofibular bolt, the foot be held at 90 degrees of dorsiflexion so that the widest portion of the talus is presented. If this is not done, dorsiflexion postoperatively will be difficult or impossible. Such tibiofibular diastasis is demonstrated in figure 13 A where an open fracture of the medial malleolus of the ankle is associated with the tibiofibular diastasis. Here débridement and simple medial malleolar screw fixation gave adequate reduction, and fixation of the medial malleolus prevented spread of the ankle mortise, as figure 13 B demonstrates. A bolt fixation of the tibia and fibula has led to satisfactory results, but it should be remembered that the tibiofibular joint is a movable joint and that permanent solid fixation of the tibia and fibula will lead to eventual breaking

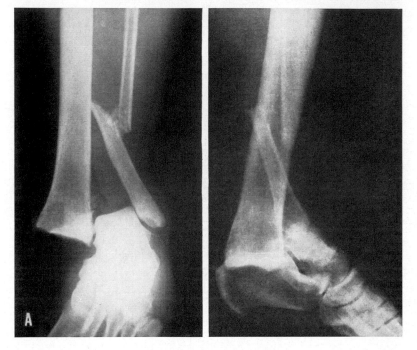

Fig. 13—(A) This markedly displaced open fracture exhibits medial malleolar fracture and lateral malleolar fracture associated with complete tibiofibular diastasis.

of the internal fixation apparatus. We have seen occasional cases of fractures through Collison screws or tibial bolts which have been placed through a tibiofibular joint for a protracted period of time.

There have been only rare examples of serious, severe comminuted fracture of the ankle on the Fracture Service. These have usually responded to closed reductions or preferably to open reduction with screw fixation. A study at The New York Hospital of unstable bimalleolar and trimalleolar fractures, and deltoid ligament tears showed that while a great number of closed reductions were adequate, open reductions were far more satisfactory. It is well to realize that this study was performed in a hospital which has adequate facilities and that the criteria used for the diagnosis of "slipping" were extremely rigid. The same study revealed that in all those fractures which required further therapy following a reduction, the majority redisplaced significantly before the eleventh day, and only five slipped after the twelfth day. Therefore extreme vigilance is employed during the first two weeks following reduction. It is questionable whether "slipping" will occur after that time if external or internal mobilization is carried out satisfactorily.

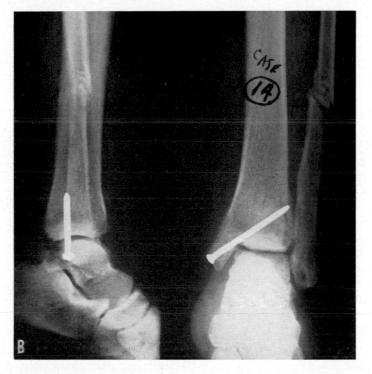

Fig. 13–(B) Simple medial malleolar screw fixation without internal or external repair of the tibiofibular ligament has led to adequate realignment of the ankle joint. In those cases with tibiofibular diastasis not amenable to this type of treatment, either external plaster immobilization or tibiofibular "bolting" is sufficient to overcome the tibiofibular diastasis.

Summary

The greatest number of ankle fractures can be adequately treated by careful diagnostic measures and external plaster immobilization following reduction. Occasional unstable fractures of the ankle will require open reduction, and occasional closed reductions which fail to maintain alignment will require open reduction for adequate alignment. It is extremely important to adequately replace the normal ankle relationships. A widened tibiofibular mortise, a displaced malleolus, an unreduced deltoid ligament, can lead to disastrous short or long term results. With these criteria in mind, the ankle can be approached with good hopes for satisfactory therapeutic results in a relatively short time.

CHAPTER 49

FRACTURES AND DISLOCATIONS OF FOOT AND TARSUS

Howard Balensweig, M.D.

Bonnin [1] has carefully catalogued and classified all types of injuries which are possible in this area and the various mechanisms involved in them. The most common injury of the foot is a fracture of one of the toes. The most important industrially is fracture of the os calcis. The average percentage disability resulting from a fracture of the os calcis is one-third of the foot; this not infrequently means that the patient can no longer return to his former occupation. This fracture has caused an incalculable loss of man hours and the problem of its treatment has not yet been solved. Injuries to other bones of the foot and tarsus are relatively rare or produce minor disability.

The Os Calcis

Following fracture of the os calcis it is difficult to correlate the x-ray and clinical appearance of the foot with the percentage disability. Apparently trivial fractures may result in a large percentage disability, while a completely crushed, widened and misshapen os calcis may give no symptoms and an excellent end result.

Objectively, there are certain results of injury which can logically be blamed for disability. Distortion of the subtalar joint with resultant arthritic changes does produce marked restriction or elimination of subtalar joint motion with altered mechanics of foot motion. The arthritic changes can be productive of constant pain and peroneal spasm. Loss of the Böhler angle with resultant shortening of the Achilles tendon weakens the latter and reduces or eliminates the ability of the patient to push-off. The injury to the soft tissues following a compression injury from below up to the specialized septate pad of the heel produces fibrosis and presumably can be a cause of pain. The fracture may result in an alteration or even subluxation of the calcaneocuboid joint which may be productive of pain.

Triple arthrodesis or subtalar fusion is a common orthopedic procedure for various foot deformities and muscle weaknesses. When these procedures are performed correctly, there almost never is pain as a result of loss of subtalar motion. There may be some loss of push-off, but this rarely interferes with gait to any significant extent. Though subtalar fusion or triple arthrodesis performed as a late procedure following fracture of the os calcis successfully eliminates subtalar motion, it is not outstandingly successful in eliminating complaints of pain.

The author has had the opportunity to evaluate the late results among workers as compensation cases and among seamen. My clinical impression is that there is a better correlation between the percentage loss of use of the foot and the patient's personality and racial background along with incentive for monetary gain than there is between the pencentage loss of use and the x-ray appearance of the foot. One occasionally sees a patient with a healed fracture of the os calcis who was never treated because the fracture was not recognized. In general, this group has shown the best clinical results.

Warrick and Bremner [2] reviewed 300 cases of fracture of the os calcis and classified them into types. In their article one will see a demonstration of all the major types of fracture in atlas form.

Type of Fracture

Isolated fracture anterior end, otherwise called fracture of the anterior process of the calcaneus: 40

Isolated fracture sustentacelum tali: 1

Fracture of tuberosity 4 beak type and 31 vertical type: 35

Compression Shearing Fractures: 172. In general the fracture line runs from the medial posterior to lateral anterior. Two main fragments only in 86. Diminution of the tuber angle with fracture line not running through an articular surface in 49. Fracture line involving posterior facet without displacement in 28. Fracture line involving posterior facet with lateral displacement of lateral portion in 9.

Two Main Fragments with Comminution of the Lateral Fragment: 128.

Essex-Lopresti [3] concerned himself with the shearing compression type with comminution and classified it into two main types; one the joint depression type, referring to the posterior subtalar joint and two, the tongue-type. He visualizes the mechanism after landing on the foot as follows: the os calcis everts and the sharp downward angled taloid spur strikes the lateral buttress of the os calcis or thickened area along the lateral superior portion of the body. This causes a vertical fracture line through the body at this point. With this area giving way, the force then shifts medially, shearing off the medial joint of the os calcis including the sustentaclum tali. The fracture line runs medial posterior and lateral anterior, either entering the posterior subtalar joint or running alongside it, but most often running through its midportion. With further compression, there is a third horizontal line of cleavage which may extend all the way back to the tuberosity or may extend only behind the posterior subtalar joint. With this horizontal line running back to the tuberosity, the tongue type develops with a seesaw action, the posterior subtalar joint being depressed and the superior half of the posterior portion of the body and tuberosity elevating. In the joint depression type, which is the more common, the posterior subtalar joint along with a variable portion of the superior portion of the body depresses between the medial and lateral walls of the body of the os calcis (fig. 1).

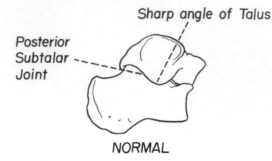

Sharp angle of Talus

Posterior
Subtalar
Joint

NORMAL

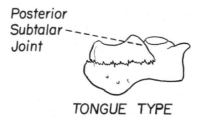

Posterior
Subtalar
Joint

TONGUE TYPE

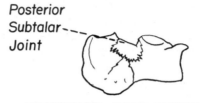

Posterior
Subtalar
Joint

POSTERIOR JOINT DEPRESSION

Fig. 1.

Treatments of Fractures of the Os Calcis

Treatment of fractures of the os calcis has varied from ambulation as tolerated with a compression bandage up to fusion and even excision of the os calcis. The standard treatment for many years followed the precepts of Boehler, who recommended reduction by compression of the sides of the os calcis, then immobilization for 8 to 12 weeks, sometimes preceded by a period of traction. Because of dissatisfaction in this country and in England with the indifferent results from this procedure many other methods have been tried.

Essex-Lopresti[3] surveyed a series of patients and tried to evaluate the relationship of the type of fracture to the end result and also the age to the end result. He concluded that fractures not involving the subtalar joint occurred in 25 per cent of fractures of the os calcis, and 93 per cent of these had no symptoms or trivial symptoms subsequent to the injury. Ninety-three per cent returned to work within six months when treated by exercise therapy alone and 92 per cent returned to work when immobilized and then allowed to gradually exercise.

When he concentrated on the fractures involving the subtalar joint the figures were much less favorable. In patients over 50, exercise therapy without attempts at reduction gave better results than attempts at reduction whether successful or unsuccessful. In patients under 50 years old, successful reduction gave better results than exercise therapy. In his hands, in a small series, successful reduction in people under 50 resulted in 80 per cent returning to work in under 6 months and having few to trivial symptoms. When reduction was unsuccessful, 70 per cent were disabled for work or play. His recommended method of treatment for patients under 50 years old with fractures involving the subtalar joints, was reduction using a Steinmann pin to impale the tongue-type fracture fragment, and then manipulatively reducing the fracture and applying a plaster shoe incorporating the pin. Subsequent to this he prescribed exercises of the ankle and toes. In cases with a depressed fracture of the posterior subtalar joint, he recommended open reduction, then maintaining the bone in reduced position with the Steinmann pin and a plaster shoe.

Ivar Palmer [4] reported 23 cases on whom he performed an open reduction for fractures involving the subtalar joint with displacement, elevating the depressed joint surface and placing a piece of bone beneath it. All of these patients returned to work within four to eight months. He stated that they had some limitation of motion of the joint and he felt that he had had remarkably favorable results. There was no statement in the article about the percentage of patients having pain.

A few authors have recommended immediate or very slightly delayed subtalar fusion or triple arthrodesis, but these series have not been sufficiently large to provide statistics.

In the recent literature there is a tendency to recommend some form of early mobilization, with or without plaster without attempts at operative reduction. L. Barnard and J. Odegard [5] recommend treating a patient in a walking plaster with the foot held in equinus and a foam rubber pad under the heel which allows them to wear the plaster for six weeks before discarding it. Other proponents of the early mobilization school recommend application of compression dressings, elevation and ice bags for three to four weeks in bed with exercises of foot and ankle, and then mobilization as tolerated by the patient.

On review of cases treated by many methods we find that the worst results have been in cases immobilized in plaster without weight-bearing or with very limited weight-bearing for three months without any real attempt at reduction. Those patients whose fractures have been essentially ignored because of other associated injuries have had favorable end results. Occasional selected cases that have had open reduction have had good results. In those cases where attempts at open reduction were not successful, the results have been extremely poor. Late subtalar fusion or triple arthrodesis has seemed to benefit the patient very little. We therefore feel that unless one finds from careful review of the x-rays that an open reduction has a fair chance of success, we would recommend early mobilization with or without plaster preceded by bed rest and exercises with application of compression dressings until the swelling has reduced sufficiently to allow mobilization. Palmer's technique of open reduction can produce excellent results in selected cases in young adults. The after-care is more important than the initial care. The patient should be provided with a high laced shoe with elevated heel and some form of soft mold for the foot, and compression dressings of one form or another to discourage edema. Occasionally, injection of Hydrocortone into the subtalar joint will relieve peroneal spasm and allow the patient more activity and therefore promote subsidence of edema. Once chronic edema of the foot is permitted with resultant fibrosis of the various joints of the tarsus, the results are either prolonged or permanent disability. The operation of excision of the os calcis is an admission of failure and should only be considered for those cases which are otherwise totally disabled. If fusion is the operation of choice in the opinion of the surgeon, it should be performed early. If performed initially, it should be undertaken before the foot has become tense with blood. At the time when the foot is very tense and misshapen, we recommend molding the os calcis as well as possible with the use of hands alone, immobilization in a light padded plaster, and then fusion after edema has subsided. This usually takes place three weeks later, by which time the fragments have molded together somewhat and the anatomy can be more easily determined. A precaution which should always be observed is in some way to push in or replace the lateral wall of the body of the os calcis in order to maintain the normal free space between the lateral border of the os calcis and the tip of the fibula through which the peroneal tendons run. A common cause for prolonged disability is peroneal spasm, often due to narrowing of this space or even irregularity of the floor of the peroneal sheath. One almost unnecessary bit of advice is always to x-ray the opposite foot. It is fruitless to attempt to restore a normal Böhler angle in a person who is congenitally flatfooted.

Fractures of the Forefoot and Toes

The most common fractures of the foot involve the toes. These also are the most commonly maltreated. The oblique fracture through the proximal phalanx of the fifth toe, occurring when walking barefoot and striking a piece of furniture with the foot, is by far the commonest fracture of the toes seen in private practice. Treatment of this fracture is best performed by placing a small piece of gauze between the fourth and fifth toes and then taping them together. The patient should then walk in a shoe which is cut out around the fifth toe or loose enough to prevent pressure over it. The sole should be rigid or made rigid by the application of an extra sole or by placement of a metatarsal bar. The ideal shoe for women is a platform sole shoe of the wedge type. The ideal treatment for men is to add an extra sole to the shoe along with a metatarsal bar and to release the leather along the fifth toe. These patients can then return to their former occupation within a day or two and provide themselves with excellent physiotherapy by walking.

The same type of treatment as outlined above can be applied to fractures of the outer four toes. Tape the affected toe either to the nearby one or the two nearby ones and then stiffen the sole of the shoe. If the injury was of a crushing type and there is blood under the nail, always release the blood. Injuries to the big toe cause more difficulty in walking and at times it is advisable to apply a cast with a walking heel for this type of injury.

Undisplaced fractures of the metatarsals can be treated simply by application of a metatarsal bar to a firm shoe. It is sometimes advisable to strap the foot in addition and to place a small metatarsal pad against the foot with the strapping. A displaced fracture of one metatarsal can be treated with a walking plaster. Walking will tend to mold the fracture back into place and it will heal without event. Occasionally, displaced fractures of the first metatarsal, especially if accompanied by a great amount of swelling and soft tissue injury, may need a period of hospitalization for elevation of the foot before starting weight-bearing. Attempts at manipulative reduction are successful in some, but many cannot be so reduced. When this is so, satisfactory results are often obtained by accepting the position and allowing early ambulation in plaster. If there is dorsal displacement of the first metatarsal, this can and should be reduced. There are occasional indications for open operation.

Fracture dislocations involving the bases of the metatarsals, usually the five or the outer four, often require open reduction. Not infrequently, the dorsalis pedis vessel is the main vessel supplying the forefoot and this can become compressed by hematoma or even cut. It is far better to openly reduce this sort of fracture and at the same time release the hematoma and prevent prolonged disability from the hematoma and even breakdown of the skin. At times, one will be surprised to find a tendon interposed between the fracture fragments. We have seen these fracture dislocations treated by early ambulation with surprisingly excellent results, but if one elects this sort of treatment, one should first make sure that the circulation is adequate.

Fractures of the Midtarsal Bones

Fractures of the scaphoid, cuboid and cuneiforms are rare when seen alone. In most instances, treatment by immobilization until the patient is comfortable and then commencing mobilization out of plaster will suffice. Occasionally, fractures of the scaphoid will be comminuted and flattened so that there is an ugly dorsal prominence. This type of injury should be treated by open reduction with the main object of removing the bony prominence. This bony prominence will produce a long term disability because of rubbing on the shoe. It is also cosmetically unsightly. At the time of open operation, one may elect to fuse the taloscaphoid joint if this is grossly involved. Fractures of the other bones mentioned above require only symptomatic care and as rapid mobilization as allowed by the patient.

Fractures of the Talus and Subtalar Dislocations

The last World War provided an unsolicited fund of talus fractures, primarily from airplane accidents. Mr. Coltart [6] collected 228 injuries to the talus occurring in the Royal Air Force between 1940 and 1945. Seventy per cent of these occurred from serious plane accidents while the rest occurred from ground accidents.

Classification of Type

1. Chip and avulsion type, 56 cases. Most of these were minor and a few required removal of a large chip which interfered with motion of the ankle.
2. Compression of head of the talus, 6 cases, occurring when the foot was plantar flexed and the force was directed along the neck of the talus.
3. Fractures of the body, 15 cases.
4. Fractures of the neck, 37 cases.
5. Fractures of the body associated with subtalar dislocation, 7 cases.
6. Fractures of the neck associated with subtalar dislocation, 38 cases.
7. Fractures of the neck associated with posterior dislocation of the body of the talus, 31 cases.
8. Subtalar dislocations, 18 cases.
9. Complete talar dislocation, 9 cases. All of these went anterolaterally and apparently occurred when the foot was forcibly plantar flexed and inverted with force continuing.
10. Unclassified, 11 cases.

In his late follow-up of a large series of cases, he noted that fractures of the neck of the talus heal in about eight weeks.

Aseptic necrosis of the body of the talus did not occur when there was fracture of the neck or the body of the talus alone. It occured in cases of fracture of the body of the talus with subtalar dislocation in 5 out of 7 cases. It occured in fracture of the neck of the talus with subtalar dislocation in 12 out of 38 cases. It occurred in fracture of the neck of the talus with dislocation, posteriorly, of the body of the talus in 14 out of 31 cases. It occurred in one case of total dislocation of the talus, while 7 totally dislocated tali were removed and one was replaced and did not have vascular necrosis.

His recommendations for treatment were: For chip fractures, little to no immobilization unless the fragment was large and then remove the fragment. For undisplaced neck fractures, immobilization in a plaster boot for 8 weeks. In those cases with displacement, reduce by placing the foot in equinus for 4 weeks and then place the foot in neutral position for a further 4 weeks. In cases with fractures of the neck or body and subtalar dislocation, there were 45 cases and 9 good results. The rest required eventual subtalar fusion.

Illustrative Cases

Case 1: E. P., a 65 year old female, who was involved in an accident when an automobile ran into an embankment. The driver was killed. This patient and her husband both sustained injuries to the feet. She sustained an anterior and lateral dislocation of the talus from the ankle joint along with a fracture of the os calcis and reversal of the Boehler ankle. There was loss of skin over the anterior portion of the talus presenting in the lateral border of the foot. The patient developed an osteomyelitis with, in addition, aseptic necrosis of the body of the talus (figs. 2 and 3). Patient was seen by the author

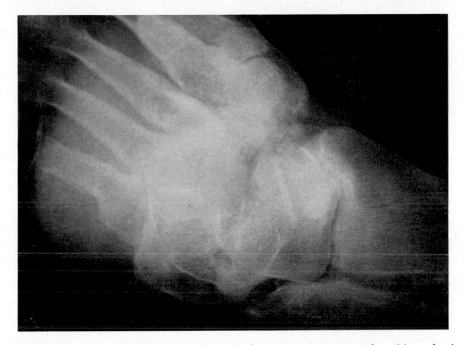

Fig. 2–Case 1. Anteroposterior view of ankle showing apparent normal position of talus in the mortise with rotation of the os calcis laterally.

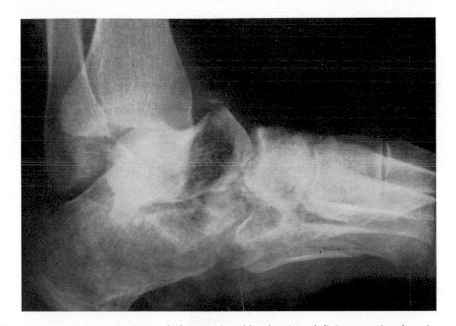

Fig. 3–Case 1. Lateral view of foot and ankle showing definite anterior luxation of talus with the anterior portion of the talus projecting superiorly and marked disturbance of the talo-navicular joint.

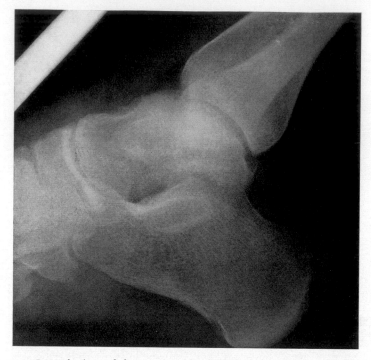

Fig. 4—Case 2. Lateral view of foot and ankle showing apparent normal position of the talus. On close inspection a fracture through the neck of the talus could be seen and there is a disturbance of the subtalar joint relationship only seen by blurring of the subtalar joint in this view.

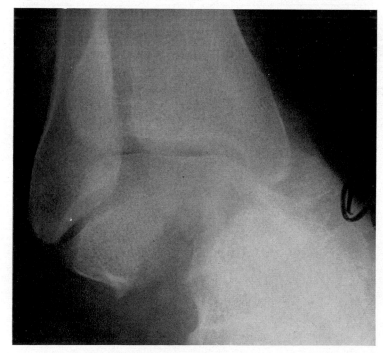

Fig. 5—Case 2. Anteroposterior view of ankle showing the medial subtalar dislocation taking with it the distal half of the talus.

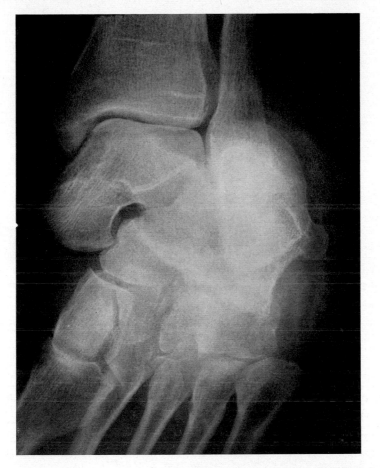

Fig. 6–Case 3. Anteroposterior view of right ankle demonstrating complete lateral subtalar dislocation of the foot beneath the talus with medial rotation of the talus.

three weeks postinjury, at which time osteomyelitis had already become established, and treatment consisted of conservative débridement and plaster immobilization for four and one-half months. Follow-up examination, 9 months postinjury, revealed few complaints, namely 10 degrees of ankle motion, patient bearing full weight on foot with a small residual sinus.

Case 2: A. M., age 27, sustained injury to the right ankle in an automobile accident. Diagnosis was fracture-dislocation of the talus with medial subtalar dislocation. She fortunately was seen the same day and a closed reduction was performed. The foot was placed in equinus and inversion. The cast was removed two months after reduction, and the patient allowed gradual weight-bearing. Follow-up examination one year postinjury, revealed some sclerosis of the talus, indicating early traumatic arthritic changes and limitation of dorsiflexion of ankle. The only complaint was slight pain on prolonged weight-bearing (figs. 4 and 5).

Case 3: E. H., age 63, sustained injury to the right ankle, stepping out of her car backwards and twisting her right ankle when she stepped on a stone. She sustained a lateral subtalar dislocation with simple fracture of cuboid. An attempt was made to do an

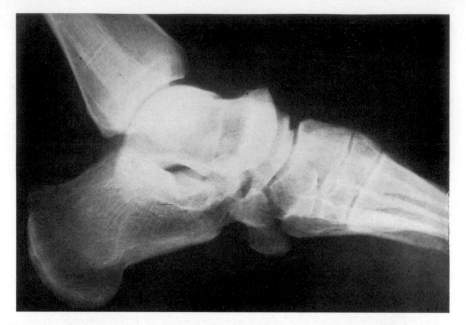

Fig. 7–Case 3. Lateral view of foot and ankle demonstrating overlapping of shadows of the head of the talus and the scaphoid, alteration in subtalar joint alignment and the fracture through the mid-portion of the cuboid bone.

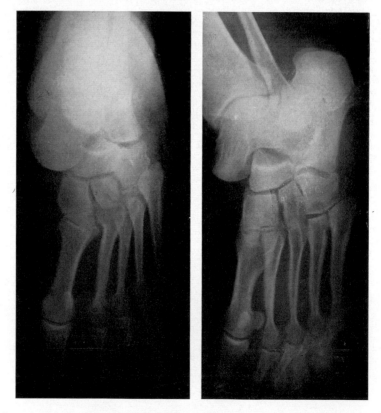

Fig. 8–Case 3. Anteroposterior and oblique views of right foot demonstrating how the foot along with the navicular cuboid and os calcis shift laterally underneath the talus.

emergency closed reduction without anesthesia. Twenty-four hours after injury, a closed reduction under general anesthesia was successfully performed. The patient was maintained in plaster for two and one-half months. Follow-up examination one year later revealed some complaints of pain in foot, particularly on prolonged standing, and about 50 per cent defect of inversion and eversion. The foot was normally outlined (figs. 6–8).

References

¹ BONNIN, J. G.: Injuries to the Ankle. London, Wm. Heinemann, Ltd., 1950.

² WARRICK, C. K., and BREMNER, A. E.: Fractures of the calcaneum. J. Bone and Joint Surg. B 35: pp. 33—45 (Feb.) 1953.

³ ESSEX-LOPRESTI, P.: The mechanism, reduction, technique and results in a fracture of the os calcis Brit. J. Surg. 39: 395—419, 1952.

⁴ PALMER, I.: Mechanism and treatment of fractures of the calcaneus. J. Bone & Joint Surg. 30 A: No. 1, January 1948. Pages 2–8.

⁵ BARNARD, L., and ODERGAARD, J.: Conservatice approach in the treatment of fractures of the calcaneus. J. Bone & Joint Surg. 37 A: 1231—1236 (Dec.) 1955.

⁶ COLTRART: "Aviators Astragalus", J. Bone and Joint Surg. B 34: pp. 545—566 (Nov.) 1952.

CHAPTER 50

AMPUTATIONS

T. Campbell Thompson, M.D.

Amputation is the ultimate (and sometimes the best) result that can be obtained in the treatment of fractures and trauma. Certainly amputation is not recommended as the primary treatment of any extremity that has been the subject of severe trauma, but in many instances it is inevitable. If it is, the sooner it is done the better. Every part of the human body has a definite function, and if an extremity or part of an extremity cannot carry out this function, it is useless and is often better amputated. This is especially true when retention of the part interferes with the function of the other parts of the body. This applies particularly to a badly injured finger. If the blood supply has been completely cut off, the digit will become gangrenous and will have to be amputated or will slough off spontaneously. If the blood supply is intact, the finger should be saved only if it can serve a useful function. To do this, it must have (1) motion in the joints, (2) muscle power through the tendons and (3) sensation through the nerves. One of these three functions can be restored by a bony operation on a joint, or a tendon repair or graft or a nerve suture. If two of these three functions have been lost, the patient is much better off without the finger so that the remaining fingers can function normally. One stiff, painful finger can cripple a hand completely, while an actively functioning hand missing one finger is no real hardship.

In the upper extremity the usual rule is to save as much length as possible. In the hand this is especially true of the thumb. In the lower extremity, the decision to amputate or not to amputate should depend on whether or not the patient will ever be able to walk on the extremity. The purpose of the lower extremity is to bear weight. If it cannot do this, the patient is better off without it. If the foot has good circulation, normal sensation and no deformity, amputation should not be considered. The patient can be fitted with a weight-bearing brace even though there may be nonunion of the tibia or femur or gross knee instability. If the tough skin on the sole of the foot has been lost, or if the foot is deformed, painful or completely anesthetic, the patient is usually better off with an amputation below the knee.

After a severe injury to the foot or ankle, a Syme's amputation should be performed if there is enough plantar skin on the foot to cover the ends of the tibia or fibula. If the foot or skin of the sole of the foot has been hopelessly damaged, amputation below the knee at the "site of election" should be done. This site of election is based on the fact that the best below-knee stump is about 4 or 5 inches below the knee joint. At this site healing should be by first intention. Longer below-knee stumps are subject to circulatory trouble and ulceration and are rarely satisfactory. An amputation immediately following trauma is usually merely a débridement of an extremity that has already been amputated by the original injury. The wound is usually contaminated, so débridement and application of skin traction is the best treatment.

If a clean amputation can be performed well above the injury at the site of election, it is sometimes indicated as a primary procedure. Following trauma a simple débridement is usually the treatment of choice.

Secondary closure of an open amputation is rarely indicated. Although this is an excellent method of obtaining early healing in an open wound, the resulting scar is usually rough and irregular and cannot stand the pressure of a prosthesis. Almost all open amputations require revision, and this is best done many weeks after the original amputation, when healing is complete, where there is no edema or infection, and where a complete excision of scar tissue is possible. Then after careful plastic closure has been done, a well-formed stump with nonadherent skin over it will result if primary healing occurs. This is the only type of stump that can be depended upon not to give trouble when fitted with a prosthesis.

Summary

1. In any severe extremity injury, complete examination to test the function of the vessels, nerves, tendons and bones should decide the necessity for, the possibility of and the desirability of amputation.

2. If amputation is inevitable or advisable to eliminate a part that will be useless, the sooner it is done the better. X-rays should be taken, but the decision as to treatment should be based on the condition of the circulation, the soft part injury, the sensation and muscle power.

3. In cases of doubt, careful and thorough débridement is the best primary treatment.

4. In open amputations, skin traction is vital and should be instituted at once and continued as long as necessary.

5. Late revision of open amputations is far superior to early secondary closure which rarely produces a satisfactory stump.

6. The stump should be covered with good, normal skin (rather than a skin graft) and the scar should not be adherent to the bone.

7. Fitting of the patient with a satisfactory prosthesis and instruction in its use is the responsibility of the surgeon who amputates.

8. Rehabilitation of an amputee is easier than that of a patient with a deformed, painful or paralyzed extremity.

CHAPTER 51

PERIPHERAL NERVE INJURIES

Howard S. Dunbar, M.D.

Injuries to peripheral nerves are common in civilian accidents. Because these accidents frequently involve bones, major blood vessels and viscera, the injury to a peripheral nerve may be overlooked while all attention is focused on treatment of the part of the injury which is an immediate threat to life. In addition, emergency bandages and splints often cover the injured extremity so that only a hand or a foot is available for examination. It is especially important to recognize an associated nerve injury before attempting reductions or manipulations of fractures. Approximately 20 per cent of fractures of long bones have a concomitant nerve injury, so that this is a matter of some importance.

The diagnosis of nerve injury is actually a simple affair requiring little time and no special equipment. The great majority of nerve injuries can be diagnosed by a few simple tests of the hands and feet.

Radial Nerve

This nerve is the most frequently injured of all peripheral nerves. Its intimate relationship to the middle and lower portion of the humerus makes it particularly liable to injury in fractures in this area. If the lesion is at midhumerus, there is loss of dorsiflexion at the wrist and metacarpophalangeal joints. In addition, there is failure of the brachioradialis to contract with forceful flexion at the elbow, and the thumb cannot be extended and abducted in the plane of the palm (fig. 1). If the site of injury is higher still, the triceps will also be paralyzed.

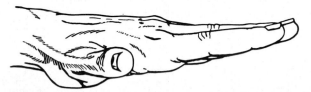

Fig. 1—Full abduction of the thumb in the plane of the palm depends on the abductor pollicis longus and the extensor pollicis brevis supplied by the radial nerve.

The area of sensory loss after radial nerve injury is unreliable but may be a variable field over the dorsum of the webbing between the thumb and index finger.

736

Ulnar Nerve

The ulnar is injured frequently in fractures and dislocations at the elbow and by penetrating wounds at the wrist. Its important supply is to the small muscles of the hand, including all the interossei, the third and fourth lumbricales, and the adductor pollicis. It also supplies the medial half of the flexor digitorum profundus and the flexor carpi ulnaris. The area of total sensory supply is to the tip of the fifth finger, and this area will be totally

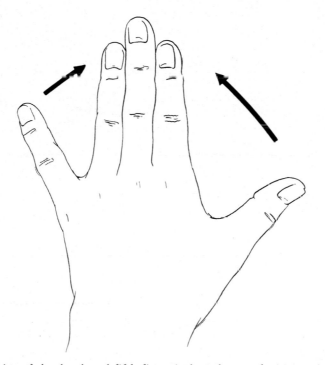

Fig. 2—Adduction of the thumb and fifth finger is dependent on the interossei and adductor pollicis supplied by the ulnar nerve.

anesthetic in interruption of the ulnar. Motor function can be simply tested by having the patient attempt to spread the fingers and then bring them together. This motion depends entirely on the ulnar nerve (fig. 2).

Median Nerve

The median nerve is injured rather infrequently. The usual site of injury is at the wrist or in the forearm. It supplies the flexors of the fingers, primarily the first three. It is concerned also in the important function of apposition of the thumb. Its absolute sensory area is the tip of the index finger, which is totally anesthetic in median nerve interruption. Motor function may be easily ascertained by testing flexion of the distal phalanx of the index finger (figs. 3 and 4).

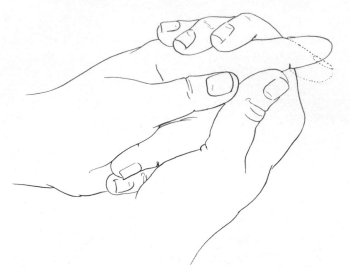

Fig. 3—Flexion of the distal phalanx of the index finger is a function of the flexor digitorum profundus supplied by the median nerve.

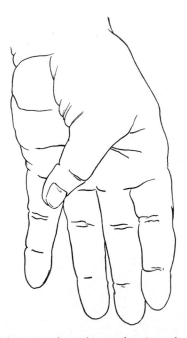

Fig. 4—Rotation of the thumb across the palm so that its volar surface contacts the base of the fifth finger. Produced by the opponens pollicis, flexor pollicis brevis (superficial head) and the abductor pollicis brevis, all supplied by the median nerve.

Tibial Nerve

This nerve supplies flexors of the toes and foot and its loss makes any plantar motion of the toes impossible (fig. 5). In addition, there is a wide absolute sensory supply to the plantar surface of the foot and plantar surface of the toes.

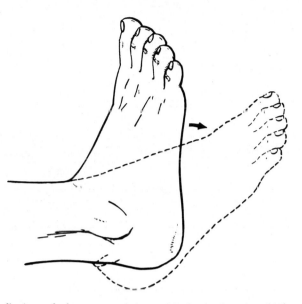

Fig. 5—Plantar flexion of the toes and foot completely lost in tibial nerve injury. The gastrocnemius tibialis posterior and flexors of the toes are paralysed.

Common Peroneal Nerve

This is the most frequently injured nerve in the lower extremities, both from fractures of the upper portion of the fibula and from pressure against the bone by casts, splints, traction devices and under knee rolls. It supplies the extensors of the foot and toes and injury produces the familiar "drop foot" (fig. 6). Injury to this nerve is very frequently overlooked.

Injuries to other peripheral nerves are relatively infrequent in civilian practice. For those particularly interested in a full description of all nerve injuries, the text of Haymaker and Woodhall [1] is recommended.

Treatment

Closed Injuries: This refers primarily to nerves injured in association with fractures or dislocations. It is impossible to determine at the time of injury if a nerve is physically divided or is anatomically intact but not functioning. There is seldom justification for immediate surgery. Many of these nerve injuries will recover spontaneously. One should follow recovery of function very carefully. If recovery is not proceeding satisfactorily, one should not hesitate to explore. It is seldom justified to wait more than six to eight

47*

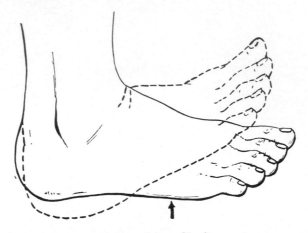

Fig. 6—Foot drop in common peroneal nerve injury. The foot and toes cannot be dorsiflexed because of paralysis of the tibialis anticus and the extensors of the toes.

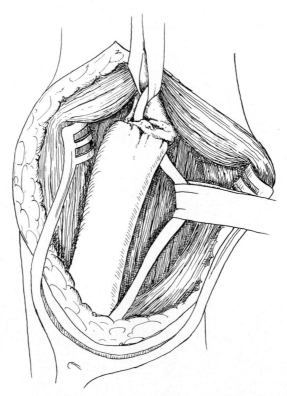

Fig. 7—Radial nerve caught in fracture site. No return of function twelve weeks.

weeks if the nerve shows no signs of recovery. With present surgical technic, the operative risk is small. If the nerve is found intact, no great harm has been done. If the nerve has been caught between bone fragments, or compressed by displaced fragments, or caught in callus, it can be freed or transplanted as necessary. If the nerve has been divided or crushed beyond recall, it can be repaired and a good deal of time saved that might have been spent debating over electric tests for regeneration and their interpretation.

Open Injuries: Some of these injuries occur with compound fractures or penetrating missiles, and are associated with extensive damage to soft parts including major blood vessels. Under such conditions a proper primary suture of a divided nerve is rarely possible.

Occasionally, a stab wound may involve a nerve with little damage to other structures. In such special situations emergency nerve repair is indicated.

Admittedly, there are many times when it is difficult to make a decision. For the most part, when in doubt delay and repair the nerve later under ideal conditions. On the other hand, long delays of months are not justified. Excluding emergency suture, all evidence indicates that the earlier the nerve repair, the better the final result.[4] Therefore, as a general rule, all nerves should be repaired as soon as local and general conditions permit.

Compression Injuries: Most of these injuries occur while the patient is under anesthesia and are all too well known. The brachial plexus is often injured by shoulder braces used in deep Trendelenburg position for operations in the pelvis. The radial, peroneal and ulnar nerves are also frequently injured by pressure from stirrups, tourniquets and arm board during anesthesia. Fortunately, most of these recover spontaneously. Such injuries can be avoided or at least minimized by proper padding. In addition, the peroneal and ulnar nerves are often injured by repeated trauma from leaning on the elbows or crossing the legs. The median nerve is occasionally compressed at the wrist by the transverse carpal ligament.

Technic of Nerve Repair

The skin of the extremity should be in good condition and entirely free of blisters and superficial infection. To operate through a poor field hoping that antibiotics and chemotherapy will prevent infection is inviting disaster. Actually, antimicrobials are seldom necessary in peripheral nerve work unless one is attempting primary suture.

The extremity should be draped so that the nerve in question may be exposed for as far as might be necessary. The initial incision should provide adequate exposure. If possible, the operation should begin with local anesthesia. When the nerve is exposed, it can be tested by pinching it below the neuroma. If the patient feels pain, some sensory fibers are functioning. The nerve may be stimulated electrically with any kind of current. One may determine the current strength by first getting a response from muscle and then raising the strength three or four times. This should give an immediate response in the muscles supplied when applied to the nerve above the point of injury if the fibers are intact. In actual practice, it is usually no problem to determine visually whether a nerve has been divided or is intact.

Once a decision has been made to resect the nerve, general anesthesia may be used for the rest of the procedure, especially if a wide dissection is necessary. In extending incisions, do not cross flexion creases. Orientation sutures are placed so that the nerve is not twisted during suture. The neuroma is then divided and, if possible, one can estimate about how much slack will be needed to allow suture without tension. The neuroma is then trimmed off with a razor blade until healthy nerve bundles are seen at both ends of the nerve. There should be absolute hemostasis. Usually, a little light pressure will stop any oozing from the cut ends. The nerve should be freed up as far as necessary in both directions so that there will be no tension on the suture line. Branches may be stripped with the back of a scalpel to provide more length. In some areas, it is possible to transplant the main nerve trunk. Finally, the adjacent joints can be flexed. By these means, three inch gaps may be overcome in most major nerve trunks.

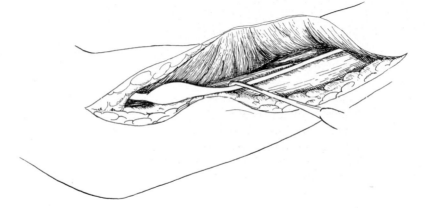

Fig. 8–(A) Neuroma ulnar nerve ten weeks after injury.

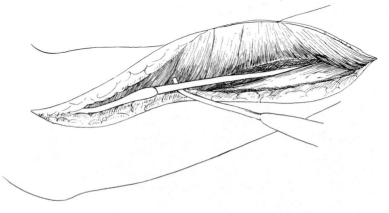

Fig. 8–(B) Neuroma resected and nerve sutured.

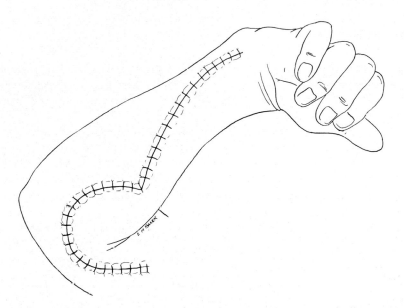

Fig. 8–(C) Final result showing extent of skin incision and position of elbow and wrist to be held in plaster.

The epineurium should be approximated with fine suture material—00000 silk or fine tantalum wire is satisfactory. The extremity should be restrained in proper position by a plaster cast properly padded. One should expect and allow for some postoperative swelling. For a detailed description of incisions and the operative approach to peripheral nerves, the text of Seletz [2] is recommended.

Postoperative Care

The cast should be removed in three to four weeks and the extremity slowly brought to full motion in another three to four weeks. Proper splints should be used as necessary to prevent deformities. Physiotherapy should begin as soon as possible. This should include daily electric muscle stimulation as well as the usual measures to prevent contractions and deformities. A variety of tests have been devised to determine return of function and prognosis of nerve injuries.

Tinel's sign is perhaps the oldest and most widely employed. It consists of the production of tingling in the distribution of nerve when a part of the nerve distal to the site of injury is tapped gently. It supposedly is produced by stimulation of regenerating unmyelinated sensory axons. In practice, it is a reliable sign if the tapping of the nerve is done carefully with a small blunt object such as the end of a pencil. Of course, one should begin distally and work back toward the suture site.

Another test is direct intraneural stimulation using fine needles introduced directly into nerve trunks. This is particularly valuable in following regeneration in predominantly motor nerves.

Electromyography and chronaxia are also employed in the study of peripheral nerve injuries and may provide valuable information. These procedures should be done and interpreted only by one skilled in their use and especially familiar with the equipment necessary.

In spite of all these tests, it is sometimes impossible to be certain of the exact status of the nerve. If there is any question of the integrity of the suture line, one should not hesitate to re-explore the nerve. Regeneration occurs at about 1 mm. per day with a good deal of individual variation. If at any time, regeneration has stopped short of an acceptable result, the nerve should also be explored.

Results

All peripheral nerves can be repaired and will regenerate. This includes the digital nerves as far distal as the first interphalangeal joint. A 75 per cent return of function is about the best we can anticipate. In general, the results are good with primarily motor or sensory nerves. For example, suture of the radial nerve in the arm is rewarded with a very high percentage of acceptable results. On the other hand, results of ulnar or sciatic nerve suture high in the extremity commonly leave a good deal to be desired. In addition, the distance regenerating axons must travel has a direct bearing on the outcome. The greater the distance from injury site to end organ the poorer the final result.

The results of procedures such as freeing an intact nerve from scar and callus or releasing the nerve from compressing ligaments or bone fragments are infinitely better than nerve suture. Therefore, one must be very conservative regarding resection and suture if there is a chance that the nerve is intact.

Finally, if the result of nerve surgery is unsatisfactory, tendon transplants, proper fusion of joints and fitting of permanent prostheses are helpful ancillary procedures and should not be neglected.

Causalgia

This poorly understood syndrome occurs following penetrating injuries of mixed peripheral nerves. It consists primarily of burning pain over the distribution of the involved nerve. As time goes on, the pain spreads to involve the entire extremity. The extremity is usually warm at first but later becomes cold, often with increased sweating. The extremity is held absolutely still. Touching the skin or air moving over the skin causes excruciating pain. There is marked atrophy of the skin, nails and muscles.

Often, the actual nerve injury is trivial although causalgia may occur after complete nerve section. The pathogenesis of this peculiar syndrome is not clear; various theories have been proposed, none of which is satisfactory. The median and tibial nerves are most frequently involved. Rarely the syndrome disappears with repair or neurolysis of the involved nerve. It may be mild and regress spontaneously. Occasionally, repeated sympathetic blocks are helpful. Sympathectomy is successful in about 80 per cent of cases.

References

[1] HAYMAKER, W., and WOODHALL, B.: Peripheral Nerve Injuries. Philadelphia, W. B. Saunders Co., 1953.

[2] SELETZ, EMIL: Surgery of Peripheral Nerves. Springfield, Ill., Charles C Thomas, 1951.

[3] Peripheral Nerve Injuries; Med. Research Spec. Report Series 282, H. J. Seddon, Ed. London, Her Majesty Stat. Office, 1954.

[4] WOODHALL, B. B., and BEEBE, G.: Peripheral Nerve Regeneration: A follow-up study of 3,656 World War II injuries. V. A. Medical Monograph. Supt. of Documents, U. S. Gov't. Printing Office, Washington, D. C.

CHAPTER 52

ACUTE ARTERIAL INJURIES

Jere W. Lord, Jr., M.D.

An acute arterial injury may be inflicted with a small, penetrating object such as a bullet, ice pick or knife, in which case there is little associated injury to the adjacent soft parts, and the point of entrance (and occasionally exit) is small. On the other hand, the injury may be caused by a piece of shrapnel or an automobile accident and may result in badly displaced fragments of fractured bone or dislocation of a knee, elbow or shoulder joint, all associated with damage to the soft parts. The status of the collateral circulation will depend to a great extent on the type of trauma sustained.

A second consideration is the manner in which the artery may be injured. A partial tangential laceration of an artery may produce a gaping hole which cannot close spontaneously and from which bleeding will cease only if the pressure of the blood in the surrounding tissues equals that within the artery, an unlikely condition if the soft part wound has a large opening to the outside. However, if the artery has been completely severed, the ends can retract and the adventitial coat of loose fibrous filaments will close over the open end which is narrowed as vasoconstriction takes place. Thrombosis usually ensues and hemorrhage ceases.

An artery may be traumatized directly by a blunt force or indirectly from violence in a neighboring area. In the latter there may be merely spasm with temporary (or occasionally permanent) cessation of blood flow through the involved segment. If contusion of the wall has occurred, the damage may involve all coats of the artery including the endothelial lining, and this may lead to occlusion by thrombus.

The effects of disruption in the flow of blood through a major artery to an extremity depend on the extent and integrity of the collateral circulation. For example, there is a poor collateral circulation at the level of the external iliac artery, whereas the collateral circulation is excellent in the region of the superficial femoral artery in the midthigh. However, a large cavitational wound involving marked loss of the soft parts in the midthigh region plus severance of the superficial femoral artery could so damage the collateral circulation that ligation of the femoral artery would be followed by gangrene of the extremity. The writer treated one patient who sustained a small penetrating injury which resulted in contusion with thrombosis of the superficial and profunda femoral arteries. The associated soft part injury was not great, but gangrene of the leg would have followed if restoration of blood flow had not been effected through a vein graft sutured to the healthy ends of the superficial femoral artery.

Not always does loss of tissue follow the interruption of a major artery. Usually, however, there is some functional impairment when exercise demands a rapid inflow of oxygenated arterial blood. Occasionally conservative therapeutic measures will lead in time to the development of a rich arterial collateral circulation which is adequate for all functional needs.

Trauma to an artery may also occur in the operating room, either accidentally during an operative procedure having nothing to do per se with the arterial tree, e.g. hernioplasty, bowel resection, radical lymph node removal in the cervical, axillary and inguinal regions. Further, with the recent trend towards radicalism in the surgical approach to the eradication of cancer, neoplasms formerly deemed inoperable because of encroachment on or encirclement of an artery, more recently have been handled by resection of the artery in continuity and restoration of blood flow by venous or arterial grafts.

Diagnosis

The diagnosis of an acute arterial injury is readily made if shock is not profound. In the absence of shock, pulsations should be present in the extremity beyond the point of injury. If they are absent and the distal part of the extremity is cold and anesthetic, then major arterial occlusion has occurred. Locally marked hemorrhage usually follows a major arterial injury unless the skin wound is small, whereupon examination might reveal a pulsating hematoma. If contusion with thrombosis has occurred, then hemorrhage would be of smaller moment unless a large vein had been severed. Marked spasm alone without serious bleeding is sometimes responsible for the local changes observed in the distal part of the extremity.

Treatment

In most injuries to a major artery, hemorrhage is marked and if it is not controlled, death may rapidly occur. The best method for the control of hemorrhage from either a small or a large wound of the soft parts associated with the arterial injury is by a pressure dressing. It should be firmly applied and when traction of the extremity is possible (Thomas splint), the combination will control hemorrhage in the vast majority of patients. A tourniquet should never be applied unless the extremity is so badly mutilated as to eliminate all consideration of arterial repair and the need for immediate amputation is clear. The only exception to the above principle is the inability to apply an effective pressure dressing. Control of hemorrhage should be paralleled by immediate restoration of the circulating blood volume by whole blood. Only when blood is not available should plasma and plasma substitutes be used. Finally, as a poor but temporary stopgap until blood has been made available, one may use physiologic saline. Although shock may not be evident, whole blood should be available and administered if it is thought that blood loss has been significant. The patient in shock should have the head placed lower than the rest of the body in the absence of severe

Vein grafts are suitable, however, only in arteries of the extremities when the surrounding tissue can be used for support. Within the thorax and abdomen, arterial defects should be bridged either by arterial grafts or by prosthetic devices. Homologous arterial grafts preserved by any one of a variety of methods will be useful. These grafts serve simply as struts or conduits which are gradually covered by the host's endothelium and invested with the host's fibrous tissue. A viable graft which will live permanently in its new environment would be a highly desirable thing but at present has not been developed.

Recent studies by Voorhees, Jaretski and Blakemore, and Hufnagel suggest that plastic materials such as Vinyon "N" cloth and Orlon fashioned into tubes function beautifully as permanent conduits of arterial blood and hence may ultimately become the ideal "graft" to bridge gaps in the aorta and other large arteries within the thoracic and abdominal cavities. Studies in our laboratory suggest that Dacron may be the most suitable plastic. The Edwards woven Texon tube has been reported upon favorably and is commercially available. Knitted crimped Dacron prostheses are satisfactory and available. *

The technics of suturing grafts are identical to those of suturing arterial anastomoses. The grafts should be under "physiologic" tension and not permitted to angulate or buckle. Excessive longitudinal tension must be avoided. All writers agree that the grafts should be carefully covered by pleura or peritoneum.

Conservative Measures

In the occasional case of arterial injury wherein restoration of continuity is not possible for one of several reasons, then so-called conservative or medical measures may be of considerable value in developing an adequate collateral circulation to save the extremity. The proper use of gravity is of extreme importance in the management of the limb which must survive on its collateral arterial circulation. The blood pressure is usually low in these small vessels and elevation of the foot or hand 12 inches above heart level may render it ischemic. On the other hand, by placing the foot or hand 6 inches *below* heart level, the collateral flow readily fills the capillaries and veins. The most satisfactory way to elevate the bed is to place 6 inch blocks under the posts at the head and to allow the patient one pillow. A position such as "high Fowler's" is deleterious since the venous pressure is elevated to such an extent that the poor arterial flow will be further hampered. "Gatching" the bed by bending the hips and knees interferes with arterial and venous flow.

Abolition of vasomotor tone is most helpful in improving the collateral arterial blood flow. Tobacco is completely eliminated from the patient's routine because of its constricting effect on the small blood vessels. Reflex vasodilatation is valuable and encouraged by placing an electric pad or warm

---

* Pilling Co., Philadelphia, Pa.

water bottle on the abdomen either continously or for one hour four times a day. No heat in any form is applied to the extremity, a cradle is used to prevent trauma from the bed clothes and the foot or hand is wrapped in cotton for protection, for the containment of whatever warmth the part may have and finally, to avoid the vasoconstricting effect of chilling drafts.

Anticoagulant therapy may be of genuine value in the conservative management of an arterial injury. There is a threefold purpose in lessening the tendency of the blood to clot, namely the avoidance of thrombosis in the small arterial collateral vessels, in the main artery proximal and distal to the site of occlusion, and finally, to avoid the devastating effect of a deep venous thrombosis which is prone to occur when the arterial flow is sluggish. Heparin and/or Tromexan or Dicumarol may be employed depending on the facilities available for their careful control.

Vasodilating drugs such as Priscoline, Papavarine, Etamon, alcohol, and a host of other agents are worth very little. Our experience with the intra-arterial use of histamine and Priscoline has been disappointing for the most part.

In summary, the important factors in the conservative management of arterial injuries are (1) the proper use of gravity, (2) the elimination of vasomotor tone and (3) the judicious use of anticoagulant therapy.

CHAPTER 53

RUPTURES OF TENDONS AND MUSCLES

J. Paul Harvey, Jr., M.D.

Trauma usually causes fractures or contusions. Severe muscular activity itself can fracture bones. Occasionally, trauma in the form of a sharp blow can rupture a muscle or tendon, and acute muscular contraction or a force applied counter to an acute muscular contraction will cause a separation of the musculotendinous junction, the origin, or the insertion of a muscle. Though this muscular injury is seen infrequently compared to the large numbers of fractures commonly treated, it must always be kept in mind by the examining physician.

Rupture of some portion of the muscle is rare and it is thought to be usually attributable to some predisposing weakness. It has been a clinical impression that rupture of contractile muscular substance is more likely to occur in young people while tendinous rupture is more common among the elderly. The aging process in areas of scant blood supply causes loss of resiliency and consequent loss of strength. Also, those tendons which slide through bony channels (the long head of the biceps in particular) are subjected to fraying action and irritation with resultant rupture. Elsewhere, as a result of fractures and mal-position, bony prominences are projected against tendons and rupture may occur. This is particularly true in the wrist, where after mal-union of the Colles' fracture, the extensor pollicis longus or rarely other tendons may rupture.

Data on the comparative frequency of rupture of various tendons and muscles depends on the author quoted. The following lists are arranged in order of most frequent to least frequent.

Table 1.—*Comparative Frequency of Rupture of Tendons and Muscles*

Conwell and Aldredge	Waugh's Review of Literature	Waugh's Series	Boyd in Campbell's Operative Orthopedics
muscles of calf	calf muscles	biceps brachii	supraspinatus tendon
extensors of leg	extensors of leg	muscles of calf	extensor of knee
biceps brachii	biceps brachii	Achilles tendon	biceps brachii
Achilles tendon	Achilles tendon	supraspinatus tendon	Achilles tendon
extensor of thumb	extensor of thumb and fingers	extensors of leg	extensor pollicis longus
abductors of thigh	supraspinatus tendon	extensors of thumb and fingers	extensor digitorum communis
triceps brachii	rectus abdomini	triceps brachii	
	abductors of thigh		
	triceps brachii		
	pectoral muscles		

It is evident that, in general, extensors of leg — both quadriceps mechanism or patellar tendon, and calf muscles including Achilles tendon, are most frequently affected, along with biceps brachii, supraspinatus and extensor digitorum communis. Ruptures of the remaining muscles and tendons occur rarely. The rectus abdominis has been reported as rupturing in pregnancy, and thigh abductors have been reported ruptured among equestrians.

The principles of treatment of these injuries are (1) to approximate the separated tissue, (2) to hold this approximation without tension until healing has taken place, (3) to prevent scar formation between injury site and surrounding tissues and (4) to reactivate the muscle and mobilize the joint to preinjury status.

In fresh injuries the approximation can be done after freshening the edge of rupture and removing tags of tissue and the rough edge. Interrupted silk sutures (mattress type) can be used to obtain anatomic apposition. In instances where the defect has existed for a period of time, contracture of the muscle causes formation of a gap which must be bridged by some fascial material such as free graft of fascia lata, portion of the tendon itself as in Achilles tendon, free graft such as palmaris longus for extensor pollicis longus, or muscle transplant such as extensor indicis proprius transplanted into distal stump of extensor pollicis longus.

Of course, this suture line will readily give way from the tension of such heavy muscular pull. Therefore, the muscle being repaired must be held in a relaxed position — flexion of elbow for the biceps brachii, extension of knee for quadriceps, equinus of foot with injuries of the Achilles tendon. Relaxation of the muscle might be enough in fresh injuries, but usually the belly of the muscle contracts and one finds constant tension necessary to hold the fragments in apposition. The best way to obtain relaxation at the site of injury is to apply traction to the muscle belly. This involves wire sutures running through the muscle, preferably just at the musculotendinous junction, then through a portion of tendon and, finally, attachment to some firm object beyond the site of rupture so that the muscle belly and the attachment of tendon beyond the rupture site may be approximated. Thus, the suture line can be placed and will hold without tension.

A clever method of attaching this heavy wire suture to bolts placed through appropriate bone, such as in the os calcis or the patella, has been devised and used by Dr. McLaughlin and is well illustrated in his article. [6] However, this necessitates incision for removal and some small difficulty in removing the screw from the bony area plus the irritating prominence at the site where these metallic ends lie free under the skin. The simple Bunnell pullout wire cannot be readily used, since the force of the heavy muscles under consideration here would cause necrosis of the skin at the site where the wire is tied and rests on the button. Therefore, at the Hospital for Special Surgery, both for the Achilles tendon and the quadriceps rupture we have on several occasions placed the wire traction suture with pullout wire, then run it through the skin distally out through the cast that is applied postoperatively (fig. 1).

Of course, during the operative procedure, once this suture is placed and tendon rupture is approximated, the traction must be maintained until closure is completed and the cast applied. The plaster must be applied around these wire sutures; after cast has set, the sutures are tied over plaster. Thus, traction is maintained on muscle belly using plaster cast against the extremity

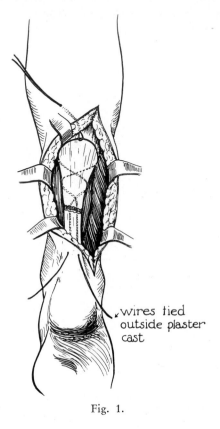

wires tied outside plaster cast

Fig. 1.

as a counter force. With a well fitting plaster cast, the force is distributed well over the entire skin surface and one need not be afraid of pressure sores. Also, with the area well immobilized, the wire coming through the skin does not seem to chafe back and forth, and although there is direct communication from external surface to deep tissues, no infection has yet been encountered in the few cases done. The Bunnell pullout wire has been used frequently enough to be quite familiar to all and to show that infection is not a problem with this method. If there is approximation of rupture site without tension, traction wire is not needed, but certainly there should be no hesitation about applying traction wire to obtain sufficient approximation.

The third principle, to prevent adhesions between site of repair and surrounding tissues, is important. Adherence of skin to tendons will prevent complete excursion in many cases, and thus limit function. One important facet of the problem is to give consideration to the skin incision. Placing the incision well to one side or the other of the damaged area and raising a flap by going through fascial or muscular planes will do much to prevent troublesome scar formation. Care to preserve what tendon sheath or fascial sheaths remain and to suture these when closing will do much to prevent adherent scars. Of course, proper débridement of non-viable tissue and careful approximation of clean, healthy tissue will do a great deal to produce a small, nonadherent scar resulting in good functioning.

Finally, after a period of three to six weeks, most fascial and tendinous tissue is healed well enough to begin careful usage. Therefore the cast is cut off. Skin sutures probably were removed through a window in the plaster at ten to fourteen days. The wire traction suture is taken out by use of pullout wire. If these are stuck, a rubber band under tension attached to the pullout wire for a period of 24 hours will usually suffice to loosen this up and permit easy removal. Then motion is begun. This is best performed under supervision of a physiotherapist; activity in a pool or a tank will reduce strain by removing gravity initially, as will employment of a splint for resting periods or to prevent long periods of usage. Such things as high heels to decrease stretching of muscle and tendon in calf will do much to prevent strain and possible rupture of suture line, but since use will loosen up muscles and the suture line will heal more firmly as usage increases, the patient should return to normal function as soon as possible. Of course, with larger tendons this return to normal will be slower. It may take up to one year with quadriceps and in some cases completely normal range of motion may never be reached; however, flexion of 90 degrees is sufficient for most purposes, particularly for older people, in whom this injury is most likely to occur.

Specific Injuries

Calf Muscle Group

Rupture of calf muscles or Achilles tendon may be of varying degrees. Rupture of plantaris tendon, although quite painful, does not need to be resutured. Use of an elevated heel, putting foot in equinus, and crutches during the acute phase will allow relaxation of muscles and tendons sufficient to relieve some of the pain, and after a period of three to six weeks all tenderness disappears and normal function resumes. However, total rupture of any other portion of this mechanism, musculotendinous junction, or Achilles tendon itself demands open operation and resuture. Incision is made on medial or lateral aspect of Achilles tendon and carried from os calcis to musculotendinous junction. Equinus of foot and flexion of knee may give sufficient relaxation to preclude use of traction suture, but if approximation is not easy or if tension exists across suture line, it will be necessary to employ pullout type of traction suture extending proximally up through tendon, transversely across musculotendinous junction and back down parallel to first portion of suture. The wire may run through the distal portion of tendon and out through the skin on either side of the calcaneus. This wire must be heavy. No. 28 or no. 26 stainless steel wire can be used. Traction is then applied to the muscle and must be maintained while interrupted silk mattress sutures are placed at rupture site. Subcutaneous tissue and skin are closed and plaster applied, the traction wires having been held out through the plaster and tied over a button and protected from injury.

The cast is maintained for four to six weeks, then removed. Function is resumed gradually with pool walking and splint for night use, gradually increasing weight-bearing and dorsiflexion of foot until normal function recurs.

In case of long-standing rupture where approximation of rupture site is impossible despite all measures, a strip of tendon cut from the tendo achillis itself can be used to bridge the gap, according to Bosworth's method. [2] The strip is removed beginning at the musculotendinous junction and brought distally, but left attached above the site of rupture. The free end is attached to a needle and used as a suture inserted transversely into proximal portion, then carried down and inserted transversely into distal tendon, back again transversely through distal portion, then into proximal end, and resutured on itself. Silk sutures are used to tack down the edge where tendon suture is inserted into Achilles tendon. Dr. Bosworth does not suggest use of wire traction suture into calf muscles, but it probably would be of value. The patient is kept in plaster for six weeks, then gradual resumption of normal activities is begun.

Knee Extensor Group

Injury to quadriceps tendon — and rarely, patellar tendon — will usually be associated with extensive tearing of the capsule of the knee. If the patellar tendon is torn, traction suture may be readily placed in the patella, but if quadriceps tendon is torn (and this is much more commonly the case) a traction suture will have to be used. The tendon itself is a broad fascial band rather than a round, thick chord, so that one cannot thread the suture up the tendon for any great distance; also, the lateral expansions of the quadriceps tendon — the attachments of vastus lateralis and vastus medialis — may be ruptured. If not ruptured, these attachments will slide laterally and posteriorly so that one must be careful to reapproximate all the tendons and also to be sure to pull them back anteriorly to a more normal position. The skin incisions in this case can be made along the medial border of quadriceps tendon, patella and patellar tendon, and extended down to the tibial tubercle and upwards as far as necessary.

In a fresh case of rupture of quadriceps tendon, mattress suture of braided silk or fascia lata suture and extension cast may be sufficient to keep rupture edge approximated, but if any retraction of muscle and tension across suture line occurs, a traction suture in the muscle will be necessary. It can run through patella, out the skin, and be tied over button outside the cast.

In any case of neglected injury, permanent contracture of muscle will take place and a gap in the mechanism will exist. Fascia lata is readily available in this instance and provides us with a large sheet of tissue. The fascia can be attached by multiple mattress sutures to the proximal side of rupture, then folded longitudinally on itself to narrow down the distal portion to fit into tendinous area at the patella. Mattress sutures can be used here, or else the folded end can be incised for a short distance and these strips inserted in stab wounds made in the portion of tendon attached to patella and sutured to themselves (fig. 2).

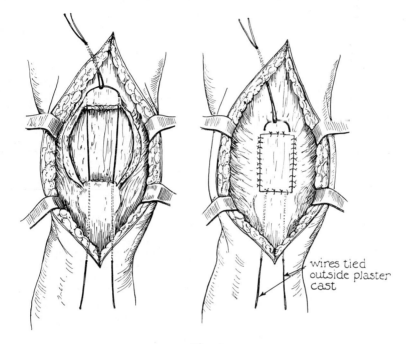

wires tied
outside plaster
cast

Fig. 2.

A cast from thigh to toes with leg in extension is advised. The skin sutures can be removed through a window at two weeks, and the cast removed at four weeks. Slow, supervised motion can be started at this time, with posterior molded splint for use after sessions of supervised motion. After eight weeks, flexion to 90 degrees should be obtained. It is possible that flexion much beyond 90 degrees will never be obtained, but it is sufficient for most activity in these cases; such limitation is much better than an unstable, weak extensor mechanism.

Biceps Brachii

When biceps brachii is injured, one must determine the site. If the long head is ruptured (Gilchreest in his study states that over 50 per cent occur here), it usually occurs in the tendon just at or within bicipital groove. In this instance, one may reapproximate tendons by direct suture. If, however, the long head is avulsed from attachment or if much of the tendon is atrophic and useless, one may resuture this free end to the short head of the biceps and/or the coracoid process. In cases in which the muscle belly is ruptured, diagnosis can usually be made by the obvious hiatus with muscle mass on either side. Heavy silk mattress sutures will hold this together. If rupture occurs at insertion into radius, the long amount of dissection necessary and the threat of osteophytic growth occurring after reinsertion of the tendon into the bicipital tubercle of the radius by means of pullout wire cautions us to plan to reinsert the muscle into the ulna either directly or into the origin of brachialis muscle. This gives acceptable function and practically is the most acceptable method.

Extensor Pollicis Longus

Rupture of tendons has been reported for all the tendons in the hand under various circumstances where bony prominences rub against the tendons. However, the most common occurrence is for the extensor pollicis longus tendon to rupture after mal-union of a Colles' fracture. The long, oblique pathway of this tendon over the bony prominence and the wide excursion of the tendon are probably contributing factors to this injury. If end-to-end apposition cannot be obtained, and this is usually the case since retraction takes place and the injury results in a fraying out of the tendon over a moderately long area, the tendon can be replaced by a free graft such as palmaris longus, or more easily the extensor indicis proprius can be transferred. An incision is made on the radial side of the second metacarpal. The tendon of the extensor indicis proprius can be transected and the distal end sutured into extensor communis tendon, thus maintaining function adequately. Then the tendon of the extensor indicis proprius is rerouted into the path of the extensor pollicis longus and the tendon sutured into the distal stump of the extensor pollicis longus with Bunnell type wire pullout suture. Before rerouting the tendon, one must be sure to remove any offending bony spurs or spicules which were the cause of the original pathology. The proximal portion of the extensor pollicis longus is sutured into the muscle belly of the extensor indicis proprius to provide further strength. This work can be done through one large incision from the area of the second metacarpo-phalangeal joint, radial aspect, proximally to the wrist, transversely across wrist, then extending proximally up the forearm. However, two incisions can be used, one small one distally parallel to the second metacarpal distal end, and a second along the extensor pollicis longus, transversely across wrist, then again up the forearm extending proximally between ulma radius.

Supraspinatus Tendon

Diagnosis of "shoulder cuff tear" is difficult to make. Also, the decision of whether or not to operate on this demands acute perception and diagnostic ability. Finally, the repair of this injury demands thought and careful execution of principles laid down by McLaughlin and P. D. Wilson. If there is a tear of shoulder cuff, the patient lacks ability to sustain abduction, particularly against any force. Pain and tenderness are present in this area. In cases of complete rupture of shoulder cuff abduction cannot be initiated or maintained even if the arm is positioned passively. We advise the use of the McLaughlin repair, opening the shoulder joint by a sabre cut incision, then splitting the deltoid fibers to see the area of pathology. The cuff is repaired by freshening the edge of the tear, then suturing this wound side to side. No effort is made to bring retracted tendon and muscle back down to normal position — rather, merely to close the defect in the position where it remains. After suturing the wound side-to-side distally to a point where tension is just beginning, the exposed portion of cartilaginous surface is removed from the head of the humerus and the tendon attached to raw bone by running suture through bone and out through the lateral aspect. Gravity pendulum exercises are used to mobilize the shoulder. Active motion begins in the third to seventh week under supervision of surgeon or physiotherapist.

Extensor Digitorum Communis Tendon

In this instance the insertion of the extensor tendon to distal phalanx is avulsed, usually in the third or long finger, resulting in a dropping of the distal tip of finger — "mallet finger" or "baseball finger." In freshly injured cases, placing the finger in a splint or cast with distal interphalangeal joint hyperextended and proximal interphalangeal joint flexed, permits a few millimeters of slack to take place in distal extensor tendon. This permits the tendon to reattach to site of avulsion. In cases where the injury is old or where this treatment has not been successful, Bunnell suture with pullout wire can be used, either bringing wire out through the nail or else through the phalanx and out through the skin of the palmar side. In the past few years cases have been treated by drilling through phalanges with Kirschner wire to hold the finger with distal interphalangeal joint in hyperextension and proximal interphalangeal joint in flexion, the wire being inserted through tip of finger retrograde through distal phalanx longitudinally, part of middle phalanx, and into the anterior surface and transversely across proximal phalanx. We have not had any experience with this method, but feel that careful application of splint or cast should give the same result with less risk. Care should be taken to be sure that in cases so treated the results obtained are worth the risks involved.

Tendon injuries are often missed by examiners in the immediate post-traumatic period. Not until a later time when lack of muscular effect is quite evident, is the diagnosis made. Certainly, immediate anatomic repair is to be desired in all cases of acute trauma. In the immediate postinjury phase, anatomic repair is usually possible with ease. The longer an injury is left untreated, the greater the need for a secondary type of repair and the less likely a good, normally functioning result. Skillful attention to detail in the physical examination will prevent many subsequent difficult repairs, problems and poor results.

References

[1] CONWELL, H. E., and ALDREDGE, R. H.: Ruptures and tears of muscles and tendons. Am. J. Surg. *35*: 22—33, 1957.

[2] BOSWORTH, D. M.: Repair of defects in the tendon achillis. J. Bone & Joint Surg. *38 A*: 111—114, (Jan.) 1956.

[3] CHRISTOPHE, K.: Rupture of extensor pollicis longus tendon. J. Bone & Joint Surg. *35 A*: 1003—1005 (Oct.) 1953.

[4] DAVIS, W. M., and YASSINO, Z.: An etiological factor in tear of the distal tendon of the biceps brachii. J. Bone & Joint Surg. *38 A*: 1365—1368, (Dec.) 1956.

[5] GILCHREEST, E. L.: Ruptures and tears of muscles and tendons of lower extremities. J. A.M.A., *100*: 153—160, (Jan.) 1933.

[6] MCLAUGHLIN, H. L.: Repair of major tendon ruptures by buried removable suture. Am. J. Surg. vol. *74*: 758—764, 1944.

[7] MCMASTER: Tendon and muscle ruptures. J. Bone & Joint Surg. *15*: 705, 1932.

[8] WAUGH, R. L., HATHCOCK, J. A., and ELLIOT, J. L.: Rupture of muscles and tendon, Surgery *25*: 370—392, 1949

[9] SPEED, J. S., ed.: Campbell's Operative Orthopedics, ed. 3, Chap. XXI: 1593—1622, St. Louis, C. V. Mosby Co., 1956.

INDEX

A

Abdominal distention, in spinal cord injury, 335, 339
Abdominal injuries, 362—371
  abdominal wall, 364
  duodenum, 365
  evaluation of, 53
  gallbladder and bile ducts, 369
  intestines, 366—367
  liver, 368—369
  pancreas, 370
  rectum, 367
  spleen, 369—370
  stomach, 364—365
  symptoms of, 362
  thoracoabdominal wounds, 360, 364
Abrasions, facial, 280
Abscess, intracranial, 242
Acetabulum fractures, 539—558. *See also* Hip injuries
Achilles tendon rupture, 755
Acidosis
  in anesthesia, 39
  in trauma, 23
Acromioclavicular joint injuries, 407—408
ACTH, and wound healing process, 10
Adhesions, after tendon repair, 754
Adrenal hormones, and wound healing, 9
Aged patients. *See* Geriatrics
Airway patency, maintenance of, 29, 31—32, 38, 48, 52, 237, 289. *See also* Tracheotomy
Alkalosis, with trauma, 23
Amputations, 734—735
  of finger tuft, accidental, 536
  incidence of, after arterial wounds, 748
  in pathologic fracture, 190
Anastomosis, vascular, 748
Androgen therapy, in osteoporosis, 15
Anesthesia, 37—41
  acidosis in, 39
  agents for, 40
  crash induction of, 39
  in face and neck area trauma, 40
  in femoral fractures, 566, 589
  in fracture reduction in children, 216
  full stomach in, 38—39
  in hand surgery, 526
  in head trauma, 40
  in humerus fracture reduction, 413
  hypovolemic shock in, 39
  in mandible fracture reduction, 268—269
  narcotics, 37
  premedication, 38
  in thoracic trauma, 41
Ankle
  fractured, 133, 701—721, 728
    bimalleolar, 705
    comminuted, 720
    malleolar, 704
    slipping of, 710, 720
    stress films of, 713
    trimalleolar, 714
  injuries of, 701—721
    in adult, 703—721
    in children, 701—703
    second-degree, 705—721
  intramedullary nailing of, 156
  splinting of, 34
  sprained, 703—704
Ankylosis, in burns of hand, 84—85
Anoxia, with pulmonary edema, 353—354
Antibiotics, 41—45
  in abdominal injuries, 363
  in arterial wounds, 749
  in burns, 79—83
  drug sensitivity tests, 43
  in liver injuries, 368
  in mandible fractures, 257, 277
  in open fractures, 113
Anticoagulants, in arterial injuries, 749
Arm. *See also specific arm regions*
  biceps brachii injury, 757
  splinting of, 33
Arterial injuries, 746—751
  diagnosis of, 747
  grafts and prostheses for, 749—750
  treatment of, 747—749
Arthritis, traumatic
  after dislocation of hip, 543
  after fracture, 105
Asphyxia, traumatic, 358—359
Astragalus. *See* Ankle

pelvic fractures, 400—401
tibial shaft fracture, 670—671
of Russell traction, 565
Compound fractures. See Open fractures
Compression fractures of spine, 326, 341
mobilization after, 182
Compression injuries of nerves, 741
Concussion, syndrome after, 244
Contaminated wounds, healing of, 5—6
Contracture, after burns, 86—87
Contusions
of bladder, 378
facial, 280
of kidney, 372
ocular, 251
of urethra, 384
Convalescence, 21—22
Convulsions, after head injury, 243
Coracoclavicular ligament injury, 407
Cortical grafts, 163
Cotton-Loder pronation position, 468
Coxa vara deformity, after femoral extra-
capsular fracture, 562, 587, 592
Cranial injuries. See Head injuries
Cranioplasty, 244
Crepitus, in mandible fracture, 256
Cross-leg flaps, 682—694
Cruciate ligaments of knee, injured, 624
Crush injury
of hand, 509, 536
of pelvis, 396—400
Crutchfield tongs, in cervical spine injury,
307, 339
Cuboid fracture, in foot, 727
Cuneiform fracture, in foot, 727
Cystogram, in bladder injury, 380
Cystostomy, in bladder and urethral in-
juries, 379, 383

D

Darrach ulnar excision, after Colles fracture,
486
Débridement, 674
antibiotics with, 44
in burns, 72
chemical or enzymatic, 77—79
in fractures, open, 113—114, 121
in hand wounds, 526
in mass casualties, 61
in multiple injuries, 54
wound healing after, 5
Debris impact, in atomic disasters, 62
Decompressive surgery
in dorsolumbar fractures, 330, 331
in spinal cord injury, 339—340
Delayed union. See Union of fractures

Deltoid ligament rupture, 711
Depressed fracture of skull, 238—239
Dermatomes, use of, 682
Diaphragm, ruptured, 357—358
Diet, in mandible fractures, 275—277
Dietary requirements, in wound healing, 9
Digital conditions. See Foot; Hand
Diplopia, in facial fractures, 293
Disaster plans, need for, 46, 59
Dislocations. See also Fracture dislocations
of carpal lunate, 498—500
of cervical spine, 306—319, 341
of elbow joint, 438—440
of eyeball, 292
of foot, 722—733
of glenohumeral joint, 408—409
of hip, 539—558
of interphalangeal joints of hand, 518
intrapelvic, of hip, 551
of pelvis, 393—396
of shoulder girdle, 405—411
of sternoclavicular joint, 406
subtalar, 728
of tarsus, 722—733
of wrist, 495—505
Dorsolumbar conditions. See Spine
Drainage
in bladder injuries, 379
in gallbladder injuries, 369
in liver injuries, 368
of peritoneal cavity, 367
in urethral injuries, 383
Drop foot, 565, 739
Dunlop's traction, in humerus fracture, 421
Duodenal injuries, 365

E

Ear, loss of tissue from, 288
Ecchymosis
of eye, 251
of mandible, 255
Edema, pulmonary, anoxia with, 353—354
Elbow injuries, 416—445
capitellum of humerus, fractured, 128,
427—428. See also Humerus
comminuted fractures, 423—425
dislocations of joint, 438—440
fracture, 128
in childhood, 214, 223—226
fracture-dislocation, 441
intercondylar fractures, 423—425
lateral condyle fractures, 128, 426
lower humeral epiphysis displacement, anterior, 422—423
manipulation in, passive, 185

medial epicondyle fractures, 128, 427
Monteggia fracture, 442—445, 456
myositis ossificans, 105, 214, 417—418
olecranon fractures, 127, 435—438
radial head fractures, in adults, 123, 431
    —434. See also Radius
radial neck fracture, in children, 428—431
stiffness after humerus fractures, 414
supracondylar fractures, 418—422
ulnar head fracture, 442. See also Ulna
Volkmann's ischemic paralysis, 214, 416
    —417
Electrical burns, treatment of, 69, 77
Electrolyte balance in trauma, 20
Emergency care
    in burns, 72—74
    in facial injuries, 278
    in femoral fractures, 588
    first aid, 31—36. See also First aid
    in fractures, open, 111—113
    in hand injuries, 522
    in mass casualties, 65
    in maxilla fractures, 294
    in multiple injuries, 47—53
    tracheotomy, 301—305. See also Trache-
        otomy
    transportation, 35—36. See also Trans-
        portation of injured
Endotracheal tube. See Airway patency,
    maintenance of
Enzymatic débridement, 77—79
Epiphyseal displacements, in childhood frac-
    tures, 206
Epithelium
    scar tissue in, 86
    wound healing in, 7
Erythromycin, 44. See also Antibiotics
Estrogen therapy, in osteoporosis, 15
Excision
    of carpal lunate, 499
    of deep burns, 76—77
    of femoral head, 547
    of pathologic fracture, 189
    ulnar, after Colles fracture, 486
Exercise. See Mobilization and exercise
Extremities, wounds of, 673—698
Eye injuries, 245—251
    burns, 245—246
    contusions, 251
    diplopia in facial fractures, 293
    dislocation of eyeball, 292
    foreign bodies, 246—247
    lacerations, 247—251
    loss of eyelid, 286
    pupillary responses in head injuries, 236

F
Facial injuries, 278—300
    abrasions, 280
    anesthesia in, 40
    contusions, 280
    diplopia in, 293
    ear, 288
    eyes, 245—251, 286, 292
    fractures, 288—299
    lacerations, 281—288
        with avulsion flap, 284—286
        with fractures, 288
        with loss of soft tissue, 286—288
        into oral cavity, 288
    malar bone fractures, 292—293
    mandible fractures, 252—277, 297—299.
        See also Mandible fracture
    maxilla fractures, 293—296
    nose, 286, 289—291
    soft tissue wounds, 278—288
    zygomatic arch fracture, 291—292
Felons, 535
Femur injuries, 596—616
    in adults, 602—613
    in aged, 613
    anatomy of femur, 584—586
    bayonet displacement, 227, 599
    birth fracture, 217
    in childhood, 227—228, 598—602
    coxa vara deformity after, 587, 592
    evaluation of, 51
    first aid in, 596—598
    of head. See also Hip injuries
        avascular necrosis after hip dislocation,
            543
        central dislocation of, 551—552
        fracture, with hip dislocation, 547—
            549
        prosthetic replacement of head, 544,
            547, 552, 579, 594
    intramedullary nailing of fractures, 144
        —147, 184, 606
    lower third injuries, 609, 626
        epiphyseal separation, 628
    of medial and lateral condyle, 627. See
        also Knee
    of neck, 559—583
        abduction type, 559—561
        adduction type, 562
        complications of, 582
        extracapsular, 584—595
        intracapsular, 130, 559—583
        MacMurray operation, 577
        nonunion of fracture, 573, 576
        postoperative care, 572—576

replacement prostheses, 579
technic of operation, 566—572
time of operation, 565—566
valgus fracture, impacted, 559—561
varus fracture, displaced, 562
nonunion of fractures, 159, 166, 573, 576
open fractures, 598
pathologic fractures, 611—613
prostheses, 544, 547, 552, 579, 594
Russell traction in, 565, 600, 602
segmental fractures, 611
shaft fractures, 132
with hip dislocation, 552—558
middle of shaft, 606—608
splinting of, 34
trochanteric fractures, 584—595
anesthesia in, 589
classification of, 587—588
complications of, 591—594
incision for, 590
mortality in, 591
operation for, 589
postoperative care in, 591
reduction procedure, 590
treatment of, 588—589
upper third fractures, 608—609
Fibula fractures, 633
in children, 228—231
intramedullary nailing of, 156
mobilization after, 182
open fracture, bipedicled flap for, 679
at upper end, 633. See also Knee
Fibulocalcaneal ligament tears, 703
Fibulotibial ligament tears, 718
Fingers. See Hand
First aid treatment, 31—36
airway patency maintenance, 29, 31—32,
38, 48, 52, 237, 289. See also Tracheotomy
in femur fractures, 596—598
hemorrhage control, 32, 747
in open fractures, 110
in open wounds of chest wall, 32
shock prevention, 32—33
splinting of fractures, 33—35. See also
Casts, slings and splints
tension pneumothorax, 32
transportation of injured, 35—36. See
also Transportation of injured
Fishhook traction, in vervical spine injury,
309, 339
Fishtail deformity, in humerus fracture, 223,
421
Fistula
bronchopleural, anesthesia in, 41

carotid artery-cavernous sinus, 243
cerebrospinal fluid, 241
Fixation
external. See Casts; Traction
internal, 139—156, 180
in acromioclavicular joint injury, 407
in ankle fracture, 156
bands for, 140. See also Wires and
bands
in cervical spine injury, 306, 309, 316,
318, 339
in childhood fractures, 139, 210—213
in clavicle fractures, 407
in Colles fracture, 468—482
Crutchfield tongs, in cervical spine injury, 307, 339
in dorsolumbar fractures, 330
in elbow fracture, 421, 423
in femoral dislocation, 551
in femoral fractures, 142—147, 184,
602—606
in forearm fractures, 151—156, 453
in hand fractures, 507
in humerus fractures, 156, 413—414,
428
in joint injuries, 179
in mallet finger, 533
in maxilla fractures, 271, 274, 295—296
in metacarpal fractures, 515
nailing, intramedullary, 142—156. See
also Nail fixation
in olecranon fractures, 436—437
in open fractures, 177
os calcis traction, 637, 644, 717
in pathologic fractures, 190—200
in pelvic dislocation, 395
in phalangeal fracture-dislocations, 514
plates for, 141. See also Plate fixation
in pubic fracture, 396
in radius fractures, 450
screws for, 142. See also Screw fixation
in tibia fractures, 147—151, 637, 644
in ulna fractures, 450—452
wires for, 140. See also Wires and
bands
Flaps, skin. See Reconstruction of soft tissues
Fluid therapy
in burns, 73, 74—75
in shock, 28
Fluorescein test of burn damage, 71
Food
diet in mandible fractures, 275—277
requirements in wound healing, 9

Foot injuries, 722—733
  drop foot, 565, 739
  metatarsal fractures, 726—727
    intramedullary nailing of, 156
    mobilization after, 182
  midtarsal bones, 727
  nerve injuries, 739
  os calcis, 722—726
    mobilization after fracture, 182
  tarsus, 722—733
  toes, 726—727
Forearm fractures, 447—459
  in adults, 447—458
  both bones, 452—456
  in childhood, 221—223, 447
  Colles fracture, 460—494. See also Colles
    fracture
  intramedullary nailing of, 151—156, 171
  Monteggia fracture, 456
  nonunion of, 159, 449, 452, 456—458
  radius, 449—450. See also Radius
  single bone fractures, 449—452
  splinting of, 34
  ulnar shaft fracture, 450—452. See also
    Ulna
Foreign bodies
  in eye, 246—247
  in liver, 368
  in rectum, 367
Fracture(s)
  of acetabulum, 539—558. See also Hip
    injuries
  of ankle, 133, 701—721, 728. See also
    Ankle
  Bennett's, 517
  birth fractures, 217—218
  of carpal bones, 495—505
  of cervical spine, 306—319, 341. See also
    Spine
  in children, 203—231. See also Pediatric
    fractures
  of clavicle, 406—407. See also Clavicle
    injuries
  of coccyx, 389—390
  Colles, 460—494. See also Colles fracture
  comminuted
    of elbow, 423—425
    pelvic, 397
    of spine, 332
  complications of, 22, 105. See also Com-
    plications of injuries
  compression, vertebral, 326, 341
    mobilization after, 182
  consolidation of, 102

  of dorsal and lumbar spine, 321—332,
    341. See also Spine
  of facial bones, 288—299. See also Facial
    injuries
  of femur, 596—616. See also Femur in-
    juries
  of fibula, 633. See also Fibula fracture
  of foot, 722—733. See alo Foot injuries
  of forearm, 447—459. See also Forearm
    fractures
  greenstick
    in forearm, 221
    in leg bones, 228—231
  of hand, 506—520. See also Hand injuries
  healing of, course of, 101—104
  of humerus, 412—415. See also Humerus
    fractures
  of ilium, 388—389
  impacted, 182, 559
  of ischium, 392
  of knee, 626—634. See also Knee
  lumbar, 321—332, 341. See also Spine
  of malar bone, 292—293
  of malleolus, 704. See also Ankle
  of mandible, 252—277, 297—299. See
    also Mandible fractures
  of maxilla, 293—296
    internal fixation in, 271, 274, 295—296
  of metacarpal shafts, 515—516. See also
    Hand
  mobilization of joints after, 179—187
  Monteggia, 442—445, 456
  in multiple injuries, 53—57
  of nasal bones, 289—291
  nonunion of, 104, 158—178. See also
    Nonunion of fractures
  occult, 100
  of olecranon, 127, 435—438. See also
    Elbow
  open, 109—119. See also Open fractures
  operative treatment of, 115—118, 120—
    157, 171. See also Operative treatment
    of injuries
  of os calcis, 722—726
    mobilization after, 182
  pathologic, 188—202. See also Pathologic
    fractures
  of pelvis, 388—401. See also Pelvis
  of phalanges, 509—511. See also Hand
  pseudofractures in osteomalacia, 18—19
  of pubis, 391—393
  of radius, 449—450. See also Radius
    fractures
  rehabilitation after, 186—187

of ribs, 359—360
  anesthesia in, 41
  mobilization after, 182
of sacrum, 389—390. *See also* Spine
of scaphoid
  in foot, 727
  in hand, 498
of scapula, 408
  mobilization after, 182
of shoulder girdle, 405—411
of skull, depressed, 217, 238—289. *See
  also* Head injuries
Smith's, 486—487
of spine, 321—332, 341. *See also* Spine
splinting of, 33—35. *See also* Casts, slings
  and splints
of tarsus, 722—733. *See also* Foot
of thumb, 516—520
of tibial shaft, 635—672. *See also* Tibia
of toes, 726—727. *See also* Foot injuries
of ulna shaft, 450—452. *See also* Ulna
union of, 102
unstable
  of ankle, 710, 720
  Colles, 466
  dorsolumbar, 330–331
  of hip, 547
  of tibial shaft, 637
weight-bearing after, 103
of wrist, 495—505
x-ray examination in, 95—108. *See also*
  X-ray examination
of zygomatic arch, 291—292
Fracture-dislocation
  of elbow, 441
  of hip, 544—547
  of interphalangeal joints of hand, 511—
   514, 518—520
  of shoulder, 410
Fusion
  cervical spine, 318
  os calcis, 726
  sacroiliac, 395
  spinal, 318, 327, 332
  wrist, 500, 503

G

Gallbladder injuries, 369
Gas gangrene, 44
  serum, in open fractures, 113
Gastric injuries, 364—365
Genitalia injuries, 386—387
Genitourinary tract injuries, 372—387
Geriatrics
  femur fractures, 613

of neck, 565
  trochanteric, 584—595
osteoporosis, 14
risk related to trauma, 23
spine fractures, pathologic, 324
Glenohumeral joint injuries, 408—410
Grafts
  bone
   calcellous, 163—165
    in forearm fractures, 455
    and intramedullary nailing, 165—171
   cortical, 163
   inlay, 161
   intramedullary nailing with, 165—171
   in nonunion, 161—171
   onlay
    in forearm fractures, 456
    massive, 163
   in open fractures, 177
   sliding graft, 161
  skin, 673—698. *See also* Reconstruction of
   soft tissues, 673—698
  vascular, 749
Granulation
  contractile effect of, 86—87
  wound closure by, 6
Greenstick fractures in children
  in forearm, 221
  in leg bones, 228—231
Guide wires, in femoral fractures, 570, 590
Gunning splint, in mandible fractures, 299

H

Hand injuries, 521—537
  amputations of finger tuft, 536
  anesthesia in surgery of, 526
  Bennett's fracture, 517
  boutonnière deformity, 514, 534
  burns, 84—85
  closed wounds, 536—537
  crush injury with fracture, 509, 536
  débridement in, 526
  diagnosis of, 526
  emergency treatment of, 522
  felons, 535
  fracture, 506—520
  fracture-dislocations of interphalangeal
   joints, 511—514
  hematoma, subungual, 537
  immobilization period in fractures, 508
  incisions, palmar, 523
  infections, 535
  mallet finger, 514, 533—534, 759
  metacarpal fracture, 515—516

intramedullary nailing in, 156
mobilization after, 182
nail injuries, 509
nerve injuries, 736
nonunion of fractures, 159, 166
lacerations, 530
open injury, 508, 521
palmar spaces, 522
paronychia, 535
phalanges fractures, 509—511
mobilization after, 182
oblique, 511
transverse, 509
radiography in, 526
splint for, 507, 509, 527, 533
synovial sheaths, 522
tendon injuries, 528—533
lacerations, 528, 530
ruptures, 531—533, 758
thenar spaces, 522
thumb fracture, 516—520
tourniquet, use of, 525
Hanson-Street nail, 144
Head cap
in mandible fractures, 259
in maxilla fractures, 295
Head injuries, 235—244
abscess, 242
anesthesia in, 40
birth fracture, 217
carotid artery-cavernous sinus fistula, 243
cerebrospinal fluid leak, 241
convulions after, 243
cranioplasty in, 244
depressed fractures, 238—239
evaluation of, 51
hematoma
chronic subdural, 241—242
intracerebral, 240—241
hemorrhage
acute subdural, 240
extradural, 239—240
hygroma, subdural, 242
motor responses in, 236
osteomyelitis, 242
penetrating wounds of brain, 239
postconcussion syndrome, 244
pupillary responses in, 236
spinal puncture in, 237
x-ray examination in, 236—237
Healing of wounds, 3—10, 674—676. See also Wound healing
Heart, tamponade, 361
Heat injuries. See Burns

Hematoma
dangers of, 676
intracerebral, 240—241
in metatarsal fractures, 727
subdural, chronic, 241—242
subungual, 537
Hematuria
in bladder injuries, 379
in pelvic fractures, 392
Hemorrhage
accident room care of, 48
in arterial injuries, 747
control of, 32, 747
in crushed pelvis, 398
extradural, 239—240
in facial injuries, 288
in kidney injuries, 373
in liver injuries, 368
in mandible fractures, 254
retroperitoneal, in pelvic injury, 393, 400
shock with, 26—30
in splenic injury, 369
subdural, acute, 240
Hemostasis, importance of, 676
Hemothorax, 354—355
Herniation of vertebral disk, 332, 333, 340
Hip injuries, 539—558
dislocation
central, of femoral head, 551—552
with femoral head fracture, 547—549
with femoral shaft fracture, 552—558
intrapelvic, 551
posterior, 539—544
evaluation of, 51
fracture dislocations, 544—547
Pauwell's classification of fractures, 564
splinting of, 34
Histamine wheal test of vascular sufficiency, 689, 692
Hooks, at zygomatic arch, in cervical spine injuries, 309, 339
Humerus fractures, 412—415
anatomic head, 133
birth fracture, 217
capitellum, 128, 427—428
elbow region. See Elbow
epiphyseal displacement, lower anterior, 422—423
fishtail deformity, 223, 421
glenohumeral joint injuries, 408—410
greater tuberosity fracture, with displacement, 128
hanging cast for, 159, 165, 181, 413
intramedullary nailing of, 156
lateral condyle, 128, 426

medial epicondyle, 128, 427
nonunion of, 159
prosthetic humeral head, 410
shoulder region. *See* Shoulder
splinting of, 33, 181
supracondylar, 418—422
Hygroma, subdural, 242
Hyperextension injury of cervical spine, 313, 317
Hyperparathyroidism, 17—18
pathologic fracture with, 613
Hypothermia treatment of shock, 29
Hypovolemic shock, 26—30
in anesthesia, 39
Hypoxia, cerebral, after trauma, 37

I

Ileum, injuries of, 366
Ilium
fractures of, 388—389
sacroiliac dislocation, 393—396
Immobilization, prolonged, effects of, 181—182. *See also* Casts; Traction
Impacted fracture, 182, 559
Incision
in femoral fracture repair, 569, 590
healing of, 3—10
palmar, 523
relaxing, 115, 167, 171
Infections
antibiotics in, 41—45
in arterial wounds, 749
in bone grafts, 166, 171
in forearm fractures, 458
in fractures, 105
in hand, 535
and healing process, 5
joint stiffness from, 180—181
in mandible fractures, 277
prevention of, 676
role in shock, 29
Injury. *See* Wound healing
Intestinal injuries, 366—367
Ischial fractures, 392

J

Jaws. *See* Mandible; Maxilla
Jejunum, injuries of, 366
Jewett nail, in femur fractures, 576, 589, 608
Joints
early mobilization of, after fracture, 179—187
fractured, 118—119, 128
immobilization of, prolonged, 181—182
stiffness of, causes of, 179—182

K

Ken-Pugh nail, 576
Kidney injuries, 372—377
Kienböck disease, lunate fracture in, 500
Kingsley splint, in maxilla fractures, 295
Kirschner
pin, in mandible fractures, 266
wire. *See* Wires and bands
Knee
epiphyseal separations, 628
fractures, 626—634
femoral, 626, 627. *See also* Femur
fibula, 633. *See also* Fibula fractures
intercondylar, 626
lateral condyles, 627
medial condyles, 627
patellar, 124—125, 629
supracondylar, 626
tibial, 630, 632. *See also* Tibia
ligament injury, patellar, 624
locking of joint, 619
meniscus injuries, 617—625
splinting of, 34
tendon injuries, 756—757
Küntscher nail, in femur fractures, 144, 555, 595, 608, 614

L

Lacerations
of face, 281—288. *See also* Facial injuries
of hand nerves, 530
of hand tendons, 528
of kidney, 373
ocular, 247—251
subcutaneous, 676
of urethra, 384
Laminectomy, in cord injuries, 342
Leadbetter maneuver, in femoral neck fracture, 569
Leg injuries. *See also specific leg regions*
calf muscle, 755—756
evaluation of, 51
splinting of, 34
Ligament
coracoclavicular, ruptured, 407
deltoid, rupture of, 711
fibulocalcaneal, tears of, 703
knee joint, injured, 617—625
tibiofibular, tears of, 718
Liver injuries, 368—369
Locking of knee joint, 619
Lorenzo screw and plate, 577, 589
Lottes nails, 144, 647, 651, 664
Lumbar conditions. *See* Spine
Lunate, carpal

dislocations of, 498—500
  fractures of, 500
Lungs
  edema, anoxia with, 353—354
  perforated, anesthesia in, 41

M

MacMurray operation, in femoral neck
  fracture, 577
McMurray sign in knee injuries, 619
Malar bone fractures, 292—293
Malleolus fractures, 704. *See also* Ankle
Mallet finger, 514, 533—534, 759
Malunion. *See* Nonunion of fracture
Manchot chart of skin blood supply, 676
Mandible fractures, 252—297, 297—299
  abnormal jaw movement in, 255
  arch bars in, 264
  bite block, plastic, 266—267
  bleeding from ear in, 256
  bone plating in, 269
  closed reduction of, 267
  complications in, treatment of, 277
  crepitus in, 256
  diagnosis of, 254
  diet in, 275—277
  endentulous anterior fragment, 269—271
    with displacement, 267—269
    with no displacement, 266—267
  emergency care of, 253—254
  evaluation of patient, 254
  fixation, intermaxillary, 264, 271
    length of time of, 274
  hyperesthesia of lip in, 256
  Kirschner pins for, 266
  looseness of teeth in, 256
  at neck of condyle, 272—274
  occlusion of teeth, changes in, 254
  open reduction of, 267—269
  oral hygiene in, 275
  pain and tenderness in, 255
  of ramus, 272
  splints for, 264—266, 299
  swelling and ecchymosis in, 255
  teeth in all fragments, 261—266
  treatment of, 257—277
  wiring for
    circumferential, 269—271
    interdental, 261—264
      clove hitch twist, 262
      loops, 261
      multiple loop, 262
    interosseous, 267—269
  x-ray examination in, 256—257
Marjolin's ulcer, 87—88

Mass casualties, 59—66
  in atomic disasters, 61—66
  sorting of patients in, 65
Massage and passive motion after fractures,
  185
  in childhood, 216
Massie nail, 576
Maxilla fractures, 293—296
  internal fixation in, 271, 274, 295—296
Median nerve injury, 737
  in Colles fracture, 491
Medullary nails, in fixation of fractures,
  142—156. *See also* Nail fixation
Meniscus medialis injuries, 617—625
Mesothelium, wound healing in, 7
Metabolic response to trauma, 20—25
  complications, 22
  convalescence, 21—22
  homeostatic mechanisms in, 20—21, 22
  risk related to trauma, 23—25
Metabolism of bone, 12—19
Metacarpal fractures, 515—516. *See also*
  Hand
Metastatic carcinoma, pathologic fractures
  with, 188—202, 331. *See also* Carcinoma
Metatarsal fractures, 726—727. *See also*
  Foot injuries
Migration of cross-leg flap, 689—692
Milk-alkali syndrome, 17
Milkman's syndrome, 18
Minerva plaster jacket, in cervical spine injuries, 309
Mobilization and exercise after injuries,
  179—187
  exercise and mobility, 182—183
  femoral fractures, 572, 591
  hip dislocation, 543
  humerus fractures, 414
  massage and passive motion, 185
    in childhood, 216
  os calcis fracture, 725
  rehabilitation, 186—187
  shoulder dislocations, 408, 410
  spinal fractures, 332
  stiffness, causes of, 179—182
Monteggia fracture, 442—445, 456
Moore
  femoral head replacement, 579
  nails, in femoral neck fracture, 563, 573
Morphine. *See* Narcotics
Mortality, in femoral extracapsular fractures, 591
Multiple injuries, 46—58
  accident room care in, 47—53
  fractures in, 53—57

Muscle
  cntractions, spinal fracture from, 323
    —324
  injuries
    biceps brachii, 757
    calf muscle group, 755—756
  ruptured, 752—759
  wound healing in, 7
Mustarde flap, 694—696
Myelograms, in spinal cord injury, 337—338
Myositis ossificans
  in elbow injuries, 417—418
    in childhood, 214
  after fracture, 105
  after hip dislocation, 543, 558

N

Nail, of finger. *See* Hand
Nail, or pin fixation, 142—156, 180
  in ankle fractures, 156
  and bone graft, cancellous, 165—171
  in clavicle fractures, 407
  collapsible nail, 576
  in Colles fracture, 473, 481
  in femur fractures, 606
    of neck, 563, 564, 570
    of shaft, 142—147, 184
    trochanteric, 589
  in forearm fractures, 151—156, 171, 455
  in hand fractures, 507
  Hanson-Street nail, 144
  in humerus fractures, 156, 413—414
  Jewett nail, 576, 589, 608
  Ken-Pugh nail, 576
  Kirschner pin in mandible fracture, 266
  Küntscher nail, 144, 555, 595, 608, 614
  Lottes nails, 144, 647, 651, 664
  Massie nail, 576
  Moore nail, 563, 573
  in pathologic fracture, 194—197
  in radius fracture, 450
  Rush nail, 144
    in ankle fracture, 708
    in femur fractures, 609
    in forearm fractures, 453
    in humerus fractures, 413—414
    in tibial shaft fractures, 664
  Smith-Petersen nail, 563, 564, 570
  Steinmann pins
    in acromioclavicular joint injury, 407
    in femur fractures, 602
    insertion of, 180
    in pelvic dislocation, 395

  in tibia fractures, 147—151, 664—666
  in ulna fractures, 452
Nalline, in opiate overdosage, 38
Narcotics, use of, 33, 37—38, 49, 112, 236, 238, 279
  in burns, 73
Nasal injuries, 286, 289—291
Navicular fractures, carpal, 133, 501—505
Neck, anesthesia in trauma of 40. *See also* Spine, cervical
Necrosis
  after cross-leg flaps, 685
  of femoral head, 543, 564, 574
Neomycin, 44. *See also* Antibiotics
Nerves
  axillary nerve paralysis, in shoulder joint injury, 409
  brachial plexus injury, in shoulder joint injury, 409
  causalgia, 744
  closed injuries of, 739
  compression injuries of, 741
  of hand, lacerated, 530
  median nerve, 737
    palsy in Colles fracture, 491
  open injuries of, 741
  peripheral nerve injuries, 736—745
  peroneal nerve, 739
    in femoral neck fractures, 565
    in fibula fractures, 634
  postoperative care of injuries, 743—744
  radial nerve injury, 736
    in humerus fracture, 413
  regeneration of, 744
  sciatic injury, in hip dislocation, 544
  sympathetic, in spinal cord injury, 335
  tibial nerve injury, 739
  treatment of injuries, 739—743
    technic of repair, 741—743
  ulnar nerve injury, 737
    after humerus fractures, 128, 226
  wound healing in nerve tissue, 7
Nonunion of fractures, 104, 158—178
  bone grafting in, 161—171
  in childhood, 203, 431
  of femur, 573, 576, 602
  of forearm, 452, 456—458
  of mandible, 277
  open fractures, 177
  operative treatment in, 131—132
  prevention of, 171—177
  of radius, 449
    in children, 431
  of shafts of long bones, 159
  of tibia, 668

of wrist, 501—503
Norepinephrine, in shock, 29
Nose injuries, 286, 289—291
Novobiocin, 44. *See also* Antibiotics
Nutrition
   in mandible fractures, 275—277
   and wound healing, 9

O

Occlusion of teeth, changes in, in mandible
   fractures, 254
Ocular injuries, 245—251. *See also* Eye injuries
Olecranon fractures, 127, 435—438. *See
also* Elbow
Open fractures, 109—119
   antibiotics in, 113
   in childhood, 218
   closure of wound, 115—118
   débridement in, 113—114, 121
   dressings for, 112
   drugs for, 112
   emergency room care in, 111—113
   of femur, 598
   first aid care in, 110
   gas gangrene serum in, 113
   of hand, 508, 521
   of joints, 118—119
   operating room procedure in, 113—118,
   121
   splinting of, 110—111
   tetanus antitoxin and toxoid in, 112—
   113
   tourniquets, use of, 111
   x-rax examination, 112
Open reduction of fractures, 138. *See also*
   Operative treatment of injuries
Open wounds
   of chest, 360
      control of, 48
      first aid treatment of, 32
   of nerves, 741
Operative treatment of injuries, 115—118,
   120—157, 171
   in ankle fractures, 133
   in carpal navicular fractures, 133, 499
   decompressive surgery
      in dorsolumbar fractures, 330, 331
      in spinal cord injury, 339—340
   in deltoid ligament tears, 712
   excision. *See* Excision
   in femoral dislocation, 551
   in femoral fracture, 130, 132, 569, 590
   in fractures, 137—138
      technic of, 137—138

in humerus fracture, 128, 133
incisions. *See* Incisions
indications for, 121—132
internal fixation methods, 139—156. *See
   also* Fixation, internal
in joint injuries, 128, 179
in metatarsal fractures, 727
as method of choice, 132—133
nerve repair technic, 741—743
in nonunion of fractures, 131—132
in olecranon fracture, 127
in open fractures, 113—118, 121
in os calcis fracture, 725
in patella fracture, 124—125
plastic surgery. *See* Reconstruction of soft
   tissue
in radial head or neck fracture, 123
tendon repair, 528, 756
in tibia fractures, 133
tissue interposition in adults, 130
Ophthalmic injuries, 245—251. *See also* Eye
   injuries
Opiates, use of. *See* Narcotics
Oral cavity, lacerations into, 288
Os calcis fracture, 722—726
   mobilization after, 182
Os calcis traction
   in ankle fracture, trimalleolar, 717
   in tibial shaft fracture, 637, 644
Osgood-Schlatter's disease, differential diagnosis of, 633
Osteoarthritis
   after dislocation of hip, 543
   after fractures, 105
Osteomalacia, 18—19
Osteomyelitis of skull, 242
Osteoporosis, 13—17
   treatment of, 14—17

P

Pain
   in abdominal injuries, 362
   backache, acute, 345—350
   in burns, 71
   in mandible fracture, 255
   in open fractures, 112
   in pathologic fractures, 188
   post-traumatic, 33, 37
   in spinal cord injuries, 334
Palliative agents, in tumors, 201
Palmar spaces, 522. *See also* Hand
Palmer reduction of os calcid fracture, 725,
   726
Palsy
   axillary nerve, in shoulder joint injury,
   409

median nerve, in Colles fracture, 491
peroneal nerve, after femoral neck frac-
    tures, 565
radial nerve, in humerus fractures, 413
ulnar nerve, after humerus fracture, 128,
    226
Pancreas injuries, 370
Paralysis, Volkmann's ischemic
    after elbow injuries, 416—417
    in children, 214
    after femur fractures, 227
Paraplegia in spinal cord injuries, 330, 333
    —344
    care of patients, 342—343
Parathyroid conditions. See Hyperpara-
    thyroidism
    pathologic fracture with, 613
Parham band, use of, 140, 656
Patella
    fracture of, 124—125, 629. See also Knee
    ligament injuries, 624
    tendon injury, 756
Pathologic fractures, 188—202
    amputation in, 190
    excision of, 189
    of femur, 595, 611—613
    fixation, internal, 190—200
    immobilization, external, 190
    source of, 188
    of spine, 324, 331
    symptoms of, 188
Pauwell's classification of hip fractures, 564
Pediatric fractures, 203—231
    anesthesia in reduction of, 216
    of ankle, 701—703
    bayonet position in femur fractures, 227
    birth fractures, 217—218
    Bryant's traction in femur fractures, 227
    of clavicle, 406
    of elbow, 214, 223—226
    epiphyseal displacements, 206
    of femur, 227—228, 598—602
    of fibula, 228—231
    fish-tail appearance of elbow fractures,
        223, 421
    fixation, internal, 139, 210—213
    of forearm, 221—223, 447
    greenstick fractures
        in forearm, 221
        in leg bones, 228—231
    growth potential of bones, 203
    of humerus
        lateral condyle, 128, 426
        medial epicondyle, 128, 427
        supracondylar, 422

massage and passive motion in, 216
nonunion of, 203
open fractures, 218
of radius, 123, 428—431
removal of splints and casts, 216
risk related to trauma, 23
Russell traction in femur fractures, 228
of tibia, 228—231
of wrist, 221—223
Pelvis
    crushed, 396—400
    dislocations of, 393—396
    evaluation of injuries, 53
    fractures of, 388—401
        cephalopelvic disproportion after, 401
        of coccyx, 389—390
        complications of, 400—401
        diagnosis of, 400
        of ilium, 388—389
        mobilization after, 182
        muscle avulsion in, 388
        of pubis, 391—393
        of sacrum, 389—390
        seat belt syndrome, 401
    intrapelvic dislocation of hip, 551
Penicillin, 44. See also Antibiotics
Penis, injuries of, 387
Perforation
    of bladder, 379
    of gallbladder, 369
    gastrointestinal, 364, 365, 366, 367
Periosteum, reflection of, in operative
    fracture treatment, 137
Peripheral nerve injuries, 736—745
Peritoneum
    drainage of cavity, 367
    wound healing in, 7
Peroneal nerve injury, 739
    in femoral neck fractures, 565
    in fibula fractures, 634
Phalanges. See Foot; Hand
Physiotherapy after fractures, 185
    in spinal fractures, 332
Pin traction. See Nail fixation
Plantaris tendon rupture, 755
Plaster casts. See Casts
Plastic surgery of extremities, 673—698.
    See also Reconstruction of soft tissue
Plate fixation, 141
    in dorsolumbar fractures, 330
    in femur fractures, 576, 609
    in forearm fractures, 452, 453
    in humerus fractures, 414
    in joint injuries, 179
    Lorenzo plate, 577, 589

in mandible fractures, 269
in Monteggia fracture, 444
in pathologic fracture, 194
Thornton plate, in femoral neck fractures, 576
in tibial shaft fractures, 663
Pneumothorax, tension, 355—357
anesthesia in, 41
first aid treatment of, 32
Polymixin E, in burns, 80
Pressure breathing, in thoracic trauma, 41
Pressure dressing, in hemorrhage, 32, 747
Pronation position, after Colles fracture, 468
Prostate injuries, 382—386
Prosthesis
for femoral head, 544, 547, 552, 579, 594
for humeral head, 410
vascular, 749
Protein
dietary requirements in osteoporosis, 14—15
and wound healing process, 9
Proteus vulgaris, 43
Pseudofractures, in osteomalacia, 18—19
Pseudomonas pyocyaneus, 43
in burns, 80
Pubis fractures, 391—393
Pugh nail, 576
Pulmonary
edema, anoxia with, 353—354
perforation, anesthesia in, 41
Pupillary responses in head injuries, 236
Pyelogram, in kidney injury, 373—374
Pyruvic acid starch paste, in burns, 78—79

Q
Quadriceps tendon injury, 756

R
Radial nerve injury, 736
in humerus fractures, 413
Radiant energy exposure, eye burns from, 246
Radiation injuries effects of, 8, 62, 88
Radiography. See X-ray examination
Radius fractures, 449—450. See also Forearm
carpal fractures with, 497
in childhood, 221
Colles fracture, 460—494. See also Colles fracture
of head or neck, 123. See also Elbow
in adults, 431—434
in children, 428—431
nonunion of, 431

intramedullary nailing of, 156, 171
Monteggia fracture, 442, 456
nonunion of, 159, 431, 449
Smith fracture, 487
ulnar fracture with, 452—456
Reconstruction of soft tissues, 673—698
avulsion flaps of soft tissue, 676
bipedicled flap, 679
broad-based flap, 682
in burns, 69, 76—77, 82—83
cross-leg flap, 682—694
migration of, 689—692
severance of, 692—694
technic of, 686—694
débridement in, 674
hemostasis in, 676
infection, prevention of, 676
lacerations, subcutaneous, 676
Mustarde flap, 694—696
open fracture of tibia and fibula, 678—680
tubed pedicle, 680
Rectum, injuries of, 367, 400
Reflexes, in spinal cord injury, 335
Regeneration of nerves, 744
Rehabilitation after fractures, 186—187
Relaxing incisions, 115, 167, 171
Renal injuries, 372—377
Respiration
in chest injuries, 353
in spinal cord injuries, 335
Respiratory function in shock, 29
Rib fractures, 359—360
anesthesia in, 41
mobilization after, 182
Rickets, 18—19
Rod fixation. See Nail fixation
Roentgenography. See X-ray examination
Roger-Anderson transfixion splinting, 473, 481
Rupture
of bladder, 378
of coracoclavicular ligament, 407
of deltoid ligament, 711
of diaphragm, 357—358
of duodenum, 365
of extensor pollicis longus, 531—533
of kidney, 373
of liver, 368
of meniscus medialis, 617
of small intestine, 365
of spleen, 369
of stomach, 365
of tendons and muscles, 752—759
of urethra, 382

Rush nail, 144. *See also under* Nail fixation

Russell traction, in femur fractures, 228, 565, 589, 600, 602

S

Sacroiliac dislocation, 393—396
Sacrum fractures, 389—390. *See also* Spine
Sayre head sling, in cervical spine injury, 306
Scaphoid fracture
    of foot, 727
    of hand, 498
Scapula injuries, 408
    mobilization after, 182
Scar epithelium, 86
    joint stiffness from, 180
    after tendon repair, 755
Sciatic nerve injury, in hip dislocation, 544
Screw fixation, 142
    Collison screw
        in ankle fracture, 707
        in femoral shaft injury, 590
    in elbow fracture, 423
    in femoral fractures, 589, 590
    in hip fracture dislocations, 544
    in humerus fractures, 414
    in joint injuries, 179
    Lorenzo screw and plate, 577, 589
    metacarpal, 515
    in olecranon fractures, 437
    in pathologic fractures, 190
    in tibial shaft fractures, 652
Scrotum, injuries of, 386
Seat belts, use of, and pelvic fractures, 401
Shanz collar, in cervical spine injuries, 310
Shock
    in facial injuries, 279, 288
    hypovolemic, 26—30
        in anesthesia, 39
    in liver injuries, 368
    prevention of, 32—33, 48
    traumatic, 26—30
Shoulder
    cuff tear, 758
    fracture dislocations of, 410
    girdle injuries, 405—411
    stiffness after humerus fractures, 414
Silver fork deformity, 460
Skeletal traction. *See* Fixation, internal
Skin
    grafts and flaps. *See* Reconstruction of soft tissue
    wound healing in, 7, 86

Skull. *See* Head injuries
Slings. *See* Casts, slings and splints
Slipping of ankle fracture, 710, 720
Smith fracture, 486—487
Smith-Petersen
    nail, in femoral fracture, 563, 564, 570, 589
    sacroiliac fusion, 395
Soft tissue
    reconstruction of, 673—698. *See also* Reconstruction of soft tissue
    wounds of face, 278—288
Spinal cord injuries, 333—344
    cauda equina lesions, 339
    cervical, 341
    herniated disk with, 340
    laminectomy in, 342
    lumbar, 341
    lumbar puncture in, 337
    myelogram in, 337—338
    prognosis of, 343
    reflexes in, 335
    respiration in, 335
    root compression in, 336
    sympathetic nerve involvement, 335
    symptoms of, 334—337
    syndrome of acute anterior cord injury, 340
    thoracic, 341
    treatment of, 338—343
    x-rax examination in, 337
Spinal puncture
    in head injuries, 237
    in spinal cord injury, 337
Spine
    cervical
        anesthesia in trauma of, 40
        fractures and dislocations of, 306—319, 341
        hyperextension injury, 313, 317
    coccyx, fractured, 389—390
    compression fractures, 326
        mobilization after, 182
    dorsolumbar injuries, 321—332, 341
        diagnosis of, 324—326
        evaluation of, 52
        fractures, 321—332
            treatment of, 326—330
            unstable, 330—331
        herniation of disk, 332, 333, 340
        pain, acute, 345—350
    herniation of disks, 332, 333, 340
    lumbosacral pain, 345—350
    muscular contractions causing fractures, 323—324

sacrum
  fractured, 389—390
  pain in, 345
  thoracic spine fractures, 341
  transportation with fractures of, 34
  wedge injury, 327—330
Spleen injuries, 369—370
Splinting of fractures, 33—35. *See also* Casts, slings and splints
Sprain, of ankle, 703—704
Staphylococcus infections, 42
  in burns, 79
  drug resistant, 45, 72
Steinmann pins. *See under* Nail fixation
Sternoclavicular joint injuries, 406
Stiffness of joints, causes of, 179—182
Stomach
  emptying of, before anesthesia, 38—39
  injuries of, 364—365
Straddle injuries, 384—385
Streptococcal infections, 42
  in burns, 80
Streptomycin, 44. *See also* Antibiotics
Stress films, in ankle fractures, 713
Strontium therapy, in osteoporosis, 16
Sudeck's atrophy, after fracture, 105
Surgery. *See* Operative treatment of injuries
Sutures, wire
  in hip fracture dislocations, 545
  in muscle repair, 753
  in olecranon fractures, 437
Sympathetic nerve involvement, in spinal cord injury, 335
Synovial
  effusion, in knee injuries, 618
  sheaths of hand, 522
Synovitis, after extensor tendon rupture in hand, 532

T

Talus. *See* Ankle
Tamponade, cardiac, 361
Tarsus injuries, 722—733. *See also* Foot
Tears
  of fibulocalcaneal ligaments, 703
  of meniscus medialis, 617
  of tibiofibular ligaments, 718
Teeth
  changes in occlusion of, in mandible fractures, 254
  looseness of, in mandible fractures, 256
  wiring, interdental, 261—264
Tendon injuries
  in hands, 528—533
  repair of

Bosworth, 756
Bunnell, 528
  ruptures, 752—759
  wound healing, 7
Tension pneumothorax, 355—357
  anesthesia in, 41
  first aid treatment of, 32
Tension of tissues, in healing wound, 675
Testosterone, in osteporosis, 15
Tetanus, 44
  antitoxin and toxoid, in open fractures, 112—113
Tetracycline, 44. *See also* Antibiotics
Thenar spaces, 522
Thermal injury. *See* Burns
Thigh. *See* Femur
Thomas
  collar, in cervical spine injuries, 310
  splint for lower extremitis, 34. *See also under* Casts, slings and splints
Thompson femoral head replacement, 579, 594
  splint for lower extremities, 34. *See also* Spine
Thorax. *See* Chest injuries
Thornton plate, in femoral neck fractures, 576
Thrombosis, after arterial injuries, 748
Thumb fractures, 516—520
  Benett's fracture, 517
Tibia fractures
  bumper fracture, 133
  in children, 228—231
  of condyle, 630
  intramedullary nailing of, 147—151, 664—666
  at lower end. *See* Ankle
  nonunion of, 159, 668
  open fracture, bipedicled flap for, 679
  of posterior lip, 133
  of shaft, 635—672
    butterfly fragments, 643
    comminuted, 648
    complications of, 670—671
    healing times compared, 666, 669
    immediate care of, 635—657
    internal fixation of, 641, 652
    intramedullary nails in, 147—151, 664—666
    long leg cast, 640
    nonunion of, 159, 668
    oblique-spiral, 644
    open reduction of, 640
    Parham bands in, 656
    plates in, 663

screws in, 652—655
segmental fragments, 643
traction in, 637—640
transfixion wires in, 656—663
transverse, 647
of spine, 632
of tuberosity, 632
Tibial nerve, 739
Tibiofibular ligament tears, 718
Tinel's sign, in nerve injuries, 743
Tissue tension, in healing wound, 675
Toes, fractured, 726—727. See also Foot
Tongs, in cervical spine injuries, 307, 339
Tourniquet, use of, 32, 48—49, 111, 137,
    525
Tracheobronchial aspiration, in anesthesia, 38
Tracheotomy, 29, 41, 48, 301—305
    in facial injuries, 289
    in head injuries, 238
    in mandible fractures, 253
    procedure for, 52
    in rib fractures, 359
Traction methods. See also Casts, slings and
    splints
    Bell traction table, 566
    Böhler frame, 547, 637—640
    Bryant traction, 227, 599
    Buck's traction, 589
    Dunlop traction, in humerus fracture, 421
    muscle and skin
        fishhook, in cervical spine injury, 309,
            339
        in muscle rupture, 753
    Russell traction, 228, 565, 589, 600, 602
    skeletal traction. See Fixation, internal
Transportation of injured, 35—36
    in femur fractures, 559, 562, 565, 589,
        596
    in spinal cord injuries, 338
    in spine fractures, 324
Trauma. See Wound healing
Triage system in disasters, 59—60
Trochanteric fractures of femur, 584—595
Tumors. See Carcinoma

U

Ulceration
    after burns, 86—87
    Marjolin's ulcer, 87—88
Ulna. See also Forearm
    Darrach excision of, after Colles fracture,
        486
    fractures
        in childhood, 221
        intramedullary nailing of, 156, 171

Monteggia fracture, 442, 456
    nonunion of, 159
    radius fracture with, 452—456
    of shaft, 450—452
    of upper end, 442. See also Elbow
Ulnar nerve injury, 737
    after humerus fracture, 128, 226
Ultraviolet exposure, eye burns from, 246
Union of fractures, 102
    delayed
        in femur fractures, 602
        in tibial fractures, 668
    nonunion, 104, 158—178. See also Non-
        union of fractures
Universal splint for hand, 507, 509, 527
Ureteral injuries, 377—378
Urethral injuries, 382—386
    straddle injuries, 384—385
Urinary tract injuries, 372—387
Urine retention, in spinal cord injuries, 335,
    339

V

Vascular
    grafts, 749
    injuries, 746—751
    sufficiency, histamine wheal test of, 689,
        692
Vein grafts, 749
Vertebral conditions. See Spine
Vitamin D therapy
    in osteomalacia, 19
    in osteoporosis, 16
Volkmann's ischemic paralysis
    in elbow injuries, 416—417
        in children, 214
    in femur fractures, 227

W

Watson-Jones
    apparatus in tibial shaft fractures, 644
    reduction of spinal fractures, 329
Wedge injury, vertebral, 327—330
Weight-bearing, after fractures, 103
Whitman abduction method, in femoral neck
    fractures, 564
Winke tongs, in cervical spine injury, 307
Wire sutures. See Sutures
Wires and bands in fixation of fractures,
    140, 180
    in acromioclavicular joint injury, 407
    in cervical spine injury, 307, 339
    in elbow fracture, 423
    in femur fractures, 602
    in forearm fractures, 453

guide wires in femoral fractures, 570, 590
in hip joint reduction, 555
in humerus fracture, 422, 426, 427, 428
insertion of Kirschner wire, 180
interdental, 261—264
in mallet finger, 533
in mandible fracture
  circumferential, 269—271
  interosseous, 267—269
in maxillar fractures, 295—296
in metacarpal fractures, 515
in Monteggia fracture, 444, 456
Parham band, 140, 656
in phalangeal fracture-dislocation, 514
in pubic fracture, 396
in radial fracture in children, 429
in tibial fractures, 656
Wound closure, 4—7
in abdominal injuries, 367
in fractures, 138
  open fractures, 115—118
Wound healing, 3—10, 674—676
in bone, 7
in cartilage, 7
clean wounds, 4
contaminated wounds, 5—6
in epithelium, 7
in fractures, 101—104
local factors in, 8
in mesothelium, 7
metabolic response to injury, 20—25
in muscle, 7
in nerve tissue, 7
shock, traumatic, 26—30
systemic factors in, 8—10
in tendons, 7
Wrinkle lines of face, 283
Wrist fractures and dislocations, 495—505
in childhood, 221—223

Colles fracture, 460—494. See also Colles fracture
examination of, 496—498
lunate dislocations, 498—500
lunate fractures, 500
mobilization after, 182
navicular fractures, 501—505
nonunion of, 501—503

X

X-ray examination
in abdominal injuries, 362
in accident room, 49
in ankle fractures, 713
complications of, 105
in dorsolumbar fractures, 324—325
errors in diagnosis, 97—100
in femoral fracture, 568, 573, 589
fish-tail appearance of elbow fractures, 223, 421
in fractures, 95—108
in hand injury, 526
in head injury, 236—237
healing, signs of, 101—104
in hip dislocations, 543
in malunion of fractures, 104
in mandible fractures, 256—257
in occult fracture, 100
in open fractures, 112
in operating room, 138
protection of patient in, 105
in spinal cord injury, 337
weight-bearing decisions, 103
in wrist fractures, 496

Z

Zygomatic arch fracture, 291—292